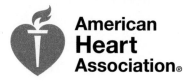

American
Heart
Association®

# 2010 American Heart Association Guidelines for Cardiopulmonary Resuscitation and Emergency Cardiovascular Care

Supplement to *Circulation* • Volume 122 • Issue 18 • Supplement 3 • November 2, 2010

ISBN 978-0-61669-043-4
Printed in the United States of America

First American Heart Association Printing November 2010
5 4 3 2 1

# Supplement to
# Circulation
JOURNAL OF THE AMERICAN HEART ASSOCIATION

Volume 122 ■ Number 18 ■ Supplement 3
November 2, 2010

**Editorial Board** . . . . . . . . . . . . . . . . . . . . . . . . . . . . . . . . . . . . . . . . . . . . . . . . . . . . . . . . . . . . . . . . . . . . . . . . . . . . . . . . . . . . . . . . . . . . . . . . **S639**

## 2010 American Heart Association Guidelines for Cardiopulmonary Resuscitation and Emergency Cardiovascular Care Science

**Part 1: Executive Summary**
*John M. Field, Co-Chair; Mary Fran Hazinski, Co-Chair; Michael R. Sayre; Leon Chameides;*
*Stephen M. Schexnayder; Robin Hemphill; Ricardo A. Samson; John Kattwinkel; Robert A. Berg;*
*Farhan Bhanji; Diana M. Cave; Edward C. Jauch; Peter J. Kudenchuk; Robert W. Neumar;*
*Mary Ann Peberdy; Jeffrey M. Perlman; Elizabeth Sinz; Andrew H. Travers; Marc D. Berg; John E. Billi;*
*Brian Eigel; Robert W. Hickey; Monica E. Kleinman; Mark S. Link; Laurie J. Morrison; Robert E. O'Connor;*
*Michael Shuster; Clifton W. Callaway; Brett Cucchiara; Jeffrey D. Ferguson; Thomas D. Rea;*
*Terry L. Vanden Hoek* . . . . . . . . . . . . . . . . . . . . . . . . . . . . . . . . . . . . . . . . . . . . . . . . . . . . . . . . . . . . . . **S640**

**Part 2: Evidence Evaluation and Management of Potential or Perceived Conflicts of Interest**
*Michael R. Sayre, Co-Chair; Robert E. O'Connor, Co-Chair; Dianne L. Atkins; John E. Billi;*
*Clifton W. Callaway; Michael Shuster; Brian Eigel; William H. Montgomery; Robert W. Hickey;*
*Ian Jacobs; Vinay M. Nadkarni; Peter T. Morley; Tanya I. Semenko; Mary Fran Hazinski* . . . . . . . . . . . . . . . . **S657**

**Part 3: Ethics**
*Laurie J. Morrison, Chair; Gerald Kierzek; Douglas S. Diekema; Michael R. Sayre;*
*Scott M. Silvers; Ahamed H. Idris; Mary E. Mancini* . . . . . . . . . . . . . . . . . . . . . . . . . . . . . . . . . . . . . **S665**

**Part 4: CPR Overview**
*Andrew H. Travers, Co-Chair; Thomas D. Rea, Co-Chair; Bentley J. Bobrow;*
*Dana P. Edelson; Robert A. Berg; Michael R. Sayre; Marc D. Berg; Leon Chameides;*
*Robert E. O'Connor; Robert A. Swor* . . . . . . . . . . . . . . . . . . . . . . . . . . . . . . . . . . . . . . . . . . . **S676**

**Part 5: Adult Basic Life Support**
*Robert A. Berg, Chair; Robin Hemphill; Benjamin S. Abella; Tom P. Aufderheide; Diana M. Cave;*
*Mary Fran Hazinski; E. Brooke Lerner; Thomas D. Rea; Michael R. Sayre; Robert A. Swor* . . . . . . . . . . . . . . **S685**

**Part 6: Electrical Therapies: Automated External Defibrillators, Defibrillation, Cardioversion, and Pacing**
*Mark S. Link, Chair; Dianne L. Atkins; Rod S. Passman; Henry R. Halperin; Ricardo A. Samson;*
*Roger D. White; Michael T. Cudnik; Marc D. Berg; Peter J. Kudenchuk; Richard E. Kerber* . . . . . . . . . . . . . . **S706**

**Part 7: CPR Techniques and Devices**
*Diana M. Cave, Chair; Raul J. Gazmuri; Charles W. Otto; Vinay M. Nadkarni; Adam Cheng;*
*Steven C. Brooks; Mohamud Daya; Robert M. Sutton; Richard Branson; Mary Fran Hazinski* . . . . . . . . . . . . . . **S720**

**Part 8: Adult Advanced Cardiovascular Life Support**
*Robert W. Neumar, Chair; Charles W. Otto; Mark S. Link; Steven L. Kronick;*
*Michael Shuster; Clifton W. Callaway; Peter J. Kudenchuk; Joseph P. Ornato; Bryan McNally;*
*Scott M. Silvers; Rod S. Passman; Roger D. White; Erik P. Hess; Wanchun Tang;*
*Daniel Davis; Elizabeth Sinz; Laurie J. Morrison* . . . . . . . . . . . . . . . . . . . . . . . . . . . . . . . . . . . . . . **S729**

**Part 9: Post–Cardiac Arrest Care**
*Mary Ann Peberdy, Co-Chair; Clifton W. Callaway, Co-Chair; Robert W. Neumar; Romergryko G. Geocadin;*
*Janice L. Zimmerman; Michael Donnino; Andrea Gabrielli; Scott M. Silvers; Arno L. Zaritsky;*
*Raina Merchant; Terry L. Vanden Hoek; Steven L. Kronick* . . . . . . . . . . . . . . . . . . . . . . . . . . . . . . . . . **S768**

CIRCULATION (ISSN 0009-7322) is published weekly except combined the first two weeks in January and the last two weeks in December by Lippincott Williams & Wilkins at 16522 Hunters Green Parkway, Hagerstown, MD 21740. Business offices are located at 530 Walnut Street, Philadelphia, PA 19106-3621. Production offices are located at 351 West Camden Street, Baltimore, MD 21201-2436. Individuals may subscribe for their personal use at the following rates: $216 for members of an American Heart Association scientific council and $386 for nonmembers; international: $371 for members of an American Heart Association scientific council and $649 for nonmembers. Periodicals postage paid at Hagerstown, MD, and additional mailing offices. POSTMASTER: Send address changes to CIRCULATION, American Heart Association, Lippincott Williams & Wilkins, 16522 Hunters Green Parkway, Hagerstown, MD 21740.

**Part 10: Acute Coronary Syndromes**
*Robert E. O'Connor, Chair; William Brady; Steven C. Brooks; Deborah Diercks; Jonathan Egan;*
*Chris Ghaemmaghami; Venu Menon; Brian J. O'Neil; Andrew H. Travers; Demetris Yannopoulos* .......... **S787**

**Part 11: Adult Stroke**
*Edward C. Jauch, Co-Chair; Brett Cucchiara, Co-Chair; Opeolu Adeoye; William Meurer;*
*Jane Brice; Yvonne (Yu-Feng) Chan; Nina Gentile; Mary Fran Hazinski* ............................. **S818**

**Part 12: Cardiac Arrest in Special Situations**
*Terry L. Vanden Hoek, Chair; Laurie J. Morrison; Michael Shuster; Michael Donnino;*
*Elizabeth Sinz; Eric J. Lavonas; Farida M. Jeejeebhoy; Andrea Gabrielli* ............................. **S829**

**Part 13: Pediatric Basic Life Support**
*Marc D. Berg, Chair; Stephen M. Schexnayder; Leon Chameides; Mark Terry; Aaron Donoghue;*
*Robert W. Hickey; Robert A. Berg; Robert M. Sutton; Mary Fran Hazinski* ........................... **S862**

**Part 14: Pediatric Advanced Life Support**
*Monica E. Kleinman, Chair; Leon Chameides; Stephen M. Schexnayder; Ricardo A. Samson;*
*Mary Fran Hazinski; Dianne L. Atkins; Marc D. Berg; Allan R. de Caen; Ericka L. Fink; Eugene B. Freid;*
*Robert W. Hickey; Bradley S. Marino; Vinay M. Nadkarni; Lester T. Proctor; Faiqa A. Qureshi;*
*Kennith Sartorelli; Alexis Topjian; Elise W. van der Jagt; Arno L. Zaritsky* ......................... **S876**

**Part 15: Neonatal Resuscitation**
*John Kattwinkel, Co-Chair; Jeffrey M. Perlman, Co-Chair; Khalid Aziz; Christopher Colby; Karen Fairchild;*
*John Gallagher; Mary Fran Hazinski; Louis P. Halamek; Praveen Kumar; George Little;*
*Jane E. McGowan; Barbara Nightengale; Mildred M. Ramirez; Steven Ringer; Wendy M. Simon;*
*Gary M. Weiner; Myra Wyckoff; Jeanette Zaichkin* .................................................. **S909**

**Part 16: Education, Implementation, and Teams**
*Farhan Bhanji, Chair; Mary E. Mancini; Elizabeth Sinz; David L. Rodgers; Mary Ann McNeil;*
*Theresa A. Hoadley; Reylon A. Meeks; Melinda Fiedor Hamilton; Peter A. Meaney;*
*Elizabeth A. Hunt; Vinay M. Nadkarni; Mary Fran Hazinski* ........................................ **S920**

# 2010 American Heart Association and American Red Cross Guidelines for First Aid

**Part 17: First Aid**
*David Markenson, Co-Chair; Jeffrey D. Ferguson, Co-Chair; Leon Chameides; Pascal Cassan;*
*Kin-Lai Chung; Jonathan Epstein; Louis Gonzales; Rita Ann Herrington; Jeffrey L. Pellegrino; Norda Ratcliff;*
*Adam Singer* ......................................................................................... **S934**

This supplement is also available online at: http://circ.ahajournals.org/content/vol122/18_suppl_3/. All articles are open access.

If the AHA Guidelines for CPR and ECC Science are to be cited, we suggest using the Executive Summary. The citation is:
Field JM, Hazinski MF, Sayre MR, Chameides L, Schexnayder SM, Hemphill R, Samson RA, Kattwinkel J, Berg RA, Bhanji F, Cave DM, Jauch EC, Kudenchuk PJ, Neumar RW, Peberdy MA, Perlman JM, Sinz E, Travers AH, Berg MD, Billi JE, Eigel B, Hickey RW, Kleinman ME, Link MS, Morrison LJ, O'Connor RE, Shuster M, Callaway CW, Cucchiara B, Ferguson JD, Rea TD, Vanden Hoek TL. Part 1: executive summary: 2010 American Heart Association Guidelines for Cardiopulmonary Resuscitation and Emergency Cardiovascular Care. *Circulation.* 2010;122(suppl 3): S640–S656.

Otherwise, each article should be cited individually. The complete citation of each article is included in the footnotes section on the first page of its respective article.

If the AHA/American Red Cross Guidelines for First Aid are to be cited, the following citation should be used:
Markenson D, Ferguson JD, Chameides L, Cassan P, Chung K-L, Epstein J, Gonzales L, Herrington RA, Pellegrino JL, Ratcliff N, Singer A. Part 17: first aid: 2010 American Heart Association and American Red Cross Guidelines for First Aid. *Circulation.* 2010;122(suppl 3):S934–S946.

Supplement to
# Circulation

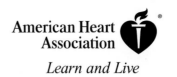

American Heart
Association

*Learn and Live*

# 2010 American Heart Association Guidelines for Cardiopulmonary Resuscitation and Emergency Cardiovascular Care Science

## Senior Science Editors
Mary Fran Hazinski*
John M. Field*

**Associate Science Editors**
Leon Chameides
Robin Hemphill
Peter J. Kudenchuk
Ricardo A. Samson
Stephen M. Schexnayder
Elizabeth Sinz

**Special Contributors**
Brenda Schoolfield
Janet Butler
Heba Costandy
Cathryn Evans
Pierce Goetz
Sallie Young,
    Pharmacotherapy Editor

**Acknowledgments**
Jeannette Allison
David Barnes
Jennifer Denton
Lana M. Gent
Colleen C. Halverson
Jody Hundley
Alicia Pederson
Kara Robinson
Tanya Semenko
Nina Tran
Paige Walker

# 2010 American Heart Association and American Red Cross Guidelines for First Aid

## AHA/American Red Cross First Aid Science Advisory Board
David Markenson (Co-Chair)
Jeffrey D. Ferguson (Co-Chair)

*Co-lead senior science editors for Part 1. Ms Hazinski also served as senior science editor for Parts 2, 3, 4, 5, 7, 13, 14, 15, 16, 17, and for the basic life support and/or pediatric portions of Parts 6 and 11. Dr Field also served as senior science editor for Parts 6, 8, 9, 10, 11, and 12.

# Part 1: Executive Summary
## 2010 American Heart Association Guidelines for Cardiopulmonary Resuscitation and Emergency Cardiovascular Care

John M. Field, Co-Chair*; Mary Fran Hazinski, Co-Chair*; Michael R. Sayre; Leon Chameides;
Stephen M. Schexnayder; Robin Hemphill; Ricardo A. Samson; John Kattwinkel; Robert A. Berg;
Farhan Bhanji; Diana M. Cave; Edward C. Jauch; Peter J. Kudenchuk; Robert W. Neumar;
Mary Ann Peberdy; Jeffrey M. Perlman; Elizabeth Sinz; Andrew H. Travers; Marc D. Berg;
John E. Billi; Brian Eigel; Robert W. Hickey; Monica E. Kleinman; Mark S. Link; Laurie J. Morrison;
Robert E. O'Connor; Michael Shuster; Clifton W. Callaway; Brett Cucchiara; Jeffrey D. Ferguson;
Thomas D. Rea; Terry L. Vanden Hoek

The publication of the *2010 American Heart Association Guidelines for Cardiopulmonary Resuscitation and Emergency Cardiovascular Care* marks the 50th anniversary of modern CPR. In 1960 Kouwenhoven, Knickerbocker, and Jude documented 14 patients who survived cardiac arrest with the application of closed chest cardiac massage.[1] That same year, at the meeting of the Maryland Medical Society in Ocean City, MD, the combination of chest compressions and rescue breathing was introduced.[2] Two years later, in 1962, direct-current, monophasic waveform defibrillation was described.[3] In 1966 the American Heart Association (AHA) developed the first cardiopulmonary resuscitation (CPR) guidelines, which have been followed by periodic updates.[4] During the past 50 years the fundamentals of early recognition and activation, early CPR, early defibrillation, and early access to emergency medical care have saved hundreds of thousands of lives around the world. These lives demonstrate the importance of resuscitation research and clinical translation and are cause to celebrate this 50th anniversary of CPR.

Challenges remain if we are to fulfill the potential offered by the pioneer resuscitation scientists. We know that there is a striking disparity in survival outcomes from cardiac arrest across systems of care, with some systems reporting 5-fold higher survival rates than others.[5–9] Although technology, such as that incorporated in automated external defibrillators (AEDs), has contributed to increased survival from cardiac arrest, no initial intervention can be delivered to the victim of cardiac arrest unless bystanders are ready, willing, and able to act. Moreover, to be successful, the actions of bystanders and other care providers must occur within a system that coordinates and integrates each facet of care into a comprehensive whole, focusing on survival to discharge from the hospital.

This executive summary highlights the major changes and most provocative recommendations in the *2010 AHA Guidelines for CPR and Emergency Cardiovascular Care (ECC)*.

The scientists and healthcare providers participating in a comprehensive evidence evaluation process analyzed the sequence and priorities of the steps of CPR in light of current scientific advances to identify factors with the greatest potential impact on survival. On the basis of the strength of the available evidence, they developed recommendations to support the interventions that showed the most promise. There was unanimous support for continued emphasis on high-quality CPR, with compressions of adequate rate and depth, allowing complete chest recoil, minimizing interruptions in chest compressions and avoiding excessive ventilation. High-quality CPR is the cornerstone of a system of care that can optimize outcomes beyond return of spontaneous circulation (ROSC). Return to a prior quality of life and functional state of health is the ultimate goal of a resuscitation system of care.

The *2010 AHA Guidelines for CPR and ECC* are based on the most current and comprehensive review of resuscitation literature ever published, the *2010 ILCOR International Consensus on CPR and ECC Science With Treatment Recommendations*.[10] The 2010 evidence evaluation process included 356 resuscitation experts from 29 countries who reviewed, analyzed, evaluated, debated, and discussed research and hypotheses through in-person meetings, teleconferences, and online sessions ("webinars") during the 36-month period before the 2010 Consensus Conference. The experts produced 411 scientific evidence reviews on 277 topics in resuscitation and emergency cardiovascular care. The process included structured evidence evaluation, analysis, and cataloging of the literature. It also included rigor-

The American Heart Association requests that this document be cited as follows: Field JM, Hazinski MF, Sayre MR, Chameides L, Schexnayder SM, Hemphill R, Samson RA, Kattwinkel J, Berg RA, Bhanji F, Cave DM, Jauch EC, Kudenchuk PJ, Neumar RW, Peberdy MA, Perlman JM, Sinz E, Travers AH, Berg MD, Billi JE, Eigel B, Hickey RW, Kleinman ME, Link MS, Morrison LJ, O'Connor RE, Shuster M, Callaway CW, Cucchiara B, Ferguson JD, Rea TD, Vanden Hoek TL. Part 1: executive summary: 2010 American Heart Association Guidelines for Cardiopulmonary Resuscitation and Emergency Cardiovascular Care. *Circulation*. 2010;122(suppl 3):S640–S656.
*Co-chairs and equal first co-authors.
(*Circulation.* 2010;122[suppl 3]:S640–S656.)

*Circulation* is available at http://circ.ahajournals.org          DOI: 10.1161/CIRCULATIONAHA.110.970889

ous disclosure and management of potential conflicts of interest, which are detailed in Part 2: "Evidence Evaluation and Management of Potential and Perceived Conflicts of Interest."

The recommendations in the 2010 Guidelines confirm the safety and effectiveness of many approaches, acknowledge ineffectiveness of others, and introduce new treatments based on intensive evidence evaluation and consensus of experts. These new recommendations do not imply that care using past guidelines is either unsafe or ineffective. In addition, it is important to note that they will not apply to all rescuers and all victims in all situations. The leader of a resuscitation attempt may need to adapt application of these recommendations to unique circumstances.

## New Developments in Resuscitation Science Since 2005

A universal compression-ventilation ratio of 30:2 performed by lone rescuers for victims of all ages was one of the most controversial topics discussed during the 2005 International Consensus Conference, and it was a major change in the *2005 AHA Guidelines for CPR and ECC.*[11] In 2005 rates of survival to hospital discharge from witnessed out-of-hospital sudden cardiac arrest due to ventricular fibrillation (VF) were low, averaging ≤6% worldwide with little improvement in the years immediately preceding the 2005 conference.[5] Two studies published just before the 2005 International Consensus Conference documented poor quality of CPR performed in both out-of-hospital and in-hospital resuscitations.[12,13] The changes in the compression-ventilation ratio and in the defibrillation sequence (from 3 stacked shocks to 1 shock followed by immediate CPR) were recommended to minimize interruptions in chest compressions.[11–13]

There have been many developments in resuscitation science since 2005, and these are highlighted below.

### Emergency Medical Services Systems and CPR Quality

Emergency medical services (EMS) systems and healthcare providers should identify and strengthen "weak links" in the Chain of Survival. There is evidence of considerable regional variation in the reported incidence and outcome from cardiac arrest within the United States.[5,14] This evidence supports the importance of accurately identifying each instance of treated cardiac arrest and measuring outcomes and suggests additional opportunities for improving survival rates in many communities. Recent studies have demonstrated improved outcome from out-of-hospital cardiac arrest, particularly from shockable rhythms, and have reaffirmed the importance of a stronger emphasis on compressions of adequate rate and depth, allowing complete chest recoil after each compression, minimizing interruptions in compressions and avoiding excessive ventilation.[15–22]

Implementation of new resuscitation guidelines has been shown to improve outcomes.[18,20–22] A means of expediting guidelines implementation (a process that may take from 18 months to 4 years[23–26]) is needed. Impediments to implementation include delays in instruction (eg, time needed to produce new training materials and update instructors and providers), technology upgrades (eg, reprogramming AEDs), and decision making (eg, coordination with allied agencies

and government regulators, medical direction, and participation in research).

### Documenting the Effects of CPR Performance by Lay Rescuers

During the past 5 years there has been an effort to simplify CPR recommendations and emphasize the fundamental importance of high-quality CPR. Large observational studies from investigators in member countries of the Resuscitation Council of Asia (the newest member of ILCOR)[27,28–30] and other studies[31,32] have provided important information about the positive impact of bystander CPR on survival after out-of-hospital cardiac arrest. For most adults with out-of-hospital cardiac arrest, bystander CPR with chest compression only (Hands-Only CPR) appears to achieve outcomes similar to those of conventional CPR (compressions with rescue breathing).[28–32] However, for children, conventional CPR is superior.[27]

### CPR Quality

Minimizing the interval between stopping chest compressions and delivering a shock (ie, minimizing the preshock pause) improves the chances of shock success[33,34] and patient survival.[33–35] Data downloaded from CPR-sensing and feedback-enabled defibrillators provide valuable information to resuscitation teams, which can improve CPR quality.[36] These data are driving major changes in the training of in-hospital resuscitation teams and out-of-hospital healthcare providers.

### In-Hospital CPR Registries

The National Registry of CardioPulmonary Resuscitation (NRCPR)[37] and other large databases are providing new information about the epidemiology and outcomes of in-hospital resuscitation in adults and children.[8,38–44] Although observational in nature, registries provide valuable descriptive information to better characterize cardiac arrest and resuscitation outcomes as well as identify areas for further research.

### Deemphasis on Devices and Advanced Cardiovascular Life Support Drugs During Cardiac Arrest

At the time of the 2010 International Consensus Conference there were still insufficient data to demonstrate that any drugs or mechanical CPR devices improve long-term outcome after cardiac arrest.[45] Clearly further studies, adequately powered to detect clinically important outcome differences with these interventions, are needed.

### Importance of Post–Cardiac Arrest Care

Organized post–cardiac arrest care with an emphasis on multidisciplinary programs that focus on optimizing hemodynamic, neurologic, and metabolic function (including therapeutic hypothermia) may improve survival to hospital discharge among victims who achieve ROSC following cardiac arrest either in- or out-of-hospital.[46–48] Although it is not yet possible to determine the individual effect of many of these therapies, when bundled as an integrated system of care, their deployment may well improve outcomes.

Therapeutic hypothermia is one intervention that has been shown to improve outcome for comatose adult victims of witnessed out-of-hospital cardiac arrest when the presenting rhythm was VF.[49,50] Since 2005, two nonrandomized studies with concurrent controls as well as other studies using historic controls have indicated the possible benefit of hypothermia following in- and out-of-hospital cardiac arrest from all other initial rhythms in adults.[46,51–56] Hypothermia has also been shown to be effective in improving intact neurologic survival in neonates with hypoxic-ischemic encephalopathy,[57–61] and the results of a prospective multicenter pediatric study of therapeutic hypothermia after cardiac arrest are eagerly awaited.

Many studies have attempted to identify comatose post–cardiac arrest patients who have no prospect for meaningful neurologic recovery, and decision rules for prognostication of poor outcome have been proposed.[62] Therapeutic hypothermia changes the specificity of prognostication decision rules that were previously established from studies of post–cardiac arrest patients not treated with hypothermia. Recent reports have documented occasional good outcomes in post–cardiac arrest patients who were treated with therapeutic hypothermia, despite neurologic exam or neuroelectrophysiologic studies that predicted poor outcome.[63,64]

### Education and Implementation

The quality of rescuer education and frequency of retraining are critical factors in improving the effectiveness of resuscitation.[65–83] Ideally retraining should not be limited to 2-year intervals. More frequent renewal of skills is needed, with a commitment to maintenance of certification similar to that embraced by many healthcare-credentialing organizations.

Resuscitation interventions are often performed simultaneously, and rescuers must be able to work collaboratively to minimize interruptions in chest compressions. Teamwork and leadership skills continue to be important, particularly for advanced cardiovascular life support (ACLS) and pediatric advanced life support (PALS) providers.[36,84–89]

Community and hospital-based resuscitation programs should systematically monitor cardiac arrests, the level of resuscitation care provided, and outcome. The cycle of measurement, interpretation, feedback, and continuous quality improvement provides fundamental information necessary to optimize resuscitation care and should help to narrow the knowledge and clinical gaps between ideal and actual resuscitation performance.

## Highlights of the 2010 Guidelines

### The Change From "A-B-C" to "C-A-B"

The newest development in the *2010 AHA Guidelines for CPR and ECC* is a change in the basic life support (BLS) sequence of steps from "A-B-C" (Airway, Breathing, Chest compressions) to "C-A-B" (Chest compressions, Airway, Breathing) for adults and pediatric patients (children and infants, excluding newly borns). Although the experts agreed that it is important to reduce time to first chest compressions, they were aware that a change in something as established as the A-B-C sequence would require re-education of everyone who has ever learned CPR. The *2010 AHA Guidelines for CPR and ECC* recommend this change for the following reasons:

- The vast majority of cardiac arrests occur in adults, and the highest survival rates from cardiac arrest are reported among patients of all ages with witnessed arrest and a rhythm of VF or pulseless ventricular tachycardia (VT). In these patients the critical initial elements of CPR are chest compressions and early defibrillation.[90]

- In the A-B-C sequence chest compressions are often delayed while the responder opens the airway to give mouth-to-mouth breaths or retrieves a barrier device or other ventilation equipment. By changing the sequence to C-A-B, chest compressions will be initiated sooner and ventilation only minimally delayed until completion of the first cycle of chest compressions (30 compressions should be accomplished in approximately 18 seconds).

- Fewer than 50% of persons in cardiac arrest receive bystander CPR. There are probably many reasons for this, but one impediment may be the A-B-C sequence, which starts with the procedures that rescuers find most difficult: opening the airway and delivering rescue breaths. Starting with chest compressions might ensure that more victims receive CPR and that rescuers who are unable or unwilling to provide ventilations will at least perform chest compressions.

- It is reasonable for healthcare providers to tailor the sequence of rescue actions to the most likely cause of arrest. For example, if a lone healthcare provider sees a victim suddenly collapse, the provider may assume that the victim has suffered a sudden VF cardiac arrest; once the provider has verified that the victim is unresponsive and not breathing or is only gasping, the provider should immediately activate the emergency response system, get and use an AED, and give CPR. But for a presumed victim of drowning or other likely asphyxial arrest the priority would be to provide about 5 cycles (about 2 minutes) of conventional CPR (including rescue breathing) before activating the emergency response system. Also, in newly born infants, arrest is more likely to be of a respiratory etiology, and resuscitation should be attempted with the A-B-C sequence unless there is a known cardiac etiology.

### Ethical Issues

The ethical issues surrounding resuscitation are complex and vary across settings (in- or out-of-hospital), providers (basic or advanced), and whether to start or how to terminate CPR. Recent work suggests that acknowledgment of a verbal do-not-attempt-resuscitation order (DNAR) in addition to the current standard—a written, signed, and dated DNAR document—may decrease the number of futile resuscitation attempts.[91,92] This is an important first step in expanding the clinical decision rule pertaining to when to start resuscitation in out-of-hospital cardiac arrest. However, there is insufficient evidence to support this approach without further validation.

When only BLS-trained EMS personnel are available, termination of resuscitative efforts should be guided by a validated termination of resuscitation rule that reduces the transport rate of attempted resuscitations without compromising the care of potentially viable patients.[93] Advanced life support (ALS) EMS providers may use the same termination of resuscitation rule[94–99] or a derived nonvalidated rule specific to ALS providers that when applied will decrease the number of futile transports to the emergency department (ED).[95,97–100]

Certain characteristics of a neonatal in-hospital cardiac arrest are associated with death, and these may be helpful in guiding physicians in the decision to start and stop a neonatal resuscitation attempt.[101–104] There is more variability in terminating resuscitation rates across systems and physicians when clinical decision rules are not followed, suggesting that these validated and generalized rules may promote uniformity in access to resuscitation attempts and full protocol care.[105]

Offering select family members the opportunity to be present during the resuscitation and designating staff within the team to respond to their questions and offer comfort may enhance the emotional support provided to the family during cardiac arrest and after termination of a resuscitation attempt.

Identifying patients during the post–cardiac arrest period who do not have the potential for meaningful neurologic recovery is a major clinical challenge that requires further research. Caution is advised when considering limiting care or withdrawing life-sustaining therapy. Characteristics or test results that are predictive of poor outcome in post–cardiac arrest patients not treated with therapeutic hypothermia may not be as predictive of poor outcome after administration of therapeutic hypothermia. Because of the growing need for transplant tissue and organs, all provider teams who treat postarrest patients should also plan and implement a system of tissue and organ donation that is timely, effective, and supportive of family members for the subset of patients in whom brain death is confirmed or for organ donation after cardiac arrest.

Resuscitation research is challenging. It must be scientifically rigorous while confronting ethical, regulatory, and public relations concerns that arise from the need to conduct such research with exception to informed consent. Regulatory requirements, community notification, and consultation requirements often impose expensive and time-consuming demands that may not only delay important research but also render it cost-prohibitive, with little significant evidence that these measures effectively address the concerns about research.[106–109]

## Basic Life Support

BLS is the foundation for saving lives following cardiac arrest. Fundamental aspects of adult BLS include immediate **recognition** of sudden cardiac arrest and **activation** of the emergency response system, early performance of **high-quality CPR**, and rapid **defibrillation** when appropriate. The *2010 AHA Guidelines for CPR and ECC* contain several important changes but also have areas of continued emphasis based on evidence presented in prior years.

### Key Changes in the 2010 AHA Guidelines for CPR and ECC

- The BLS algorithm has been simplified, and "Look, Listen and Feel" has been removed from the algorithm. Performance of these steps is inconsistent and time consuming. For this reason the *2010 AHA Guidelines for CPR and ECC* stress immediate activation of the emergency response system and starting chest compressions for any unresponsive adult victim with no breathing or no normal breathing (ie, only gasps).

- Encourage **Hands-Only (compression only) CPR** for the untrained lay rescuer. Hands-Only CPR is easier to perform by those with no training and can be more readily guided by dispatchers over the telephone.

- Initiate chest compressions before giving rescue breaths (**C-A-B rather than A-B-C**). Chest compressions can be started immediately, whereas positioning the head, attaining a seal for mouth-to-mouth rescue breathing, or obtaining or assembling a bag-mask device for rescue breathing all take time. Beginning CPR with 30 compressions rather than 2 ventilations leads to a shorter delay to first compression.

- There is an increased focus on methods to ensure that high-quality CPR is performed. Adequate chest compressions require that compressions be provided at the appropriate depth and rate, allowing complete recoil of the chest after each compression and an emphasis on minimizing any pauses in compressions and avoiding excessive ventilation. Training should focus on ensuring that chest compressions are performed correctly. The recommended depth of compression for adult victims has increased from a depth of 1½ to 2 inches to a depth of at least 2 inches.

- Many tasks performed by healthcare providers during resuscitation attempts, such as chest compressions, airway management, rescue breathing, rhythm detection, shock delivery, and drug administration (if appropriate), can be performed concurrently by an integrated team of highly trained rescuers in appropriate settings. Some resuscitations start with a lone rescuer who calls for help, resulting in the arrival of additional team members. Healthcare provider training should focus on building the team as each member arrives or quickly delegating roles if multiple rescuers are present. As additional personnel arrive, responsibilities for tasks that would ordinarily be performed sequentially by fewer rescuers may now be delegated to a team of providers who should perform them simultaneously.

### Key Points of Continued Emphasis for the 2010 AHA Guidelines for CPR and ECC

- Early recognition of sudden cardiac arrest in adults is based on assessing responsiveness and the absence of normal breathing. Victims of cardiac arrest may initially have gasping respirations or even appear to be having a seizure. These atypical presentations may confuse a rescuer, causing a delay in calling for help or beginning CPR. Training should focus on alerting potential rescuers to the unusual presentations of sudden cardiac arrest.

- Minimize interruptions in effective chest compressions until ROSC or termination of resuscitative efforts. Any unnecessary interruptions in chest compressions (including longer than necessary pauses for rescue breathing) decreases CPR effectiveness.

- Minimize the importance of pulse checks by healthcare providers. Detection of a pulse can be difficult, and even highly trained healthcare providers often incorrectly assess the presence or absence of a pulse when blood pressure is abnormally low or absent. Healthcare providers should take no more than 10 seconds to determine if a pulse is present. Chest compressions delivered to patients subsequently found not to be in cardiac arrest rarely lead to significant injury.[110] The lay rescuer should activate the emergency response system if he or she finds an unresponsive adult. The lay rescuer should not attempt to check for a pulse and should assume that cardiac arrest is present if an adult suddenly collapses, is unresponsive, and is not breathing or not breathing normally (ie, only gasping).

## CPR Techniques and Devices

Alternatives to conventional manual CPR have been developed in an effort to enhance perfusion during resuscitation from cardiac arrest and to improve survival. Compared with conventional CPR, these techniques and devices typically require more personnel, training, and equipment, or apply to a specific setting. Some alternative CPR techniques and devices may improve hemodynamics or short-term survival when used by well-trained providers in selected patients.

Several devices have been the focus of recent clinical trials. Use of the impedance threshold device (ITD) improved ROSC and short-term survival when used in adults with out-of-hospital cardiac arrest, but there was no significant improvement in either survival to hospital discharge or neurologically-intact survival to discharge.[111] One multicenter, prospective, randomized controlled trial[112,112a] comparing load-distributing band CPR (Autopulse) with manual CPR for out-of-hospital cardiac arrest demonstrated no improvement in 4-hour survival and worse neurologic outcome when the device was used. More research is needed to determine if site-specific factors[113] or experience with deployment of the device[114] influence effectiveness of the load-distributing band CPR device. Case series employing mechanical piston devices have reported variable degrees of success.[115–119]

To prevent delays and maximize efficiency, initial training, ongoing monitoring, and retraining programs should be offered on a frequent basis to providers using CPR devices. To date, no adjunct has consistently been shown to be superior to standard conventional (manual) CPR for out-of-hospital BLS, and no device other than a defibrillator has consistently improved long-term survival from out-of-hospital cardiac arrest.

## Electrical Therapies

The *2010 AHA Guidelines for CPR and ECC* have been updated to reflect new data on the use of pacing in bradycardia, and on cardioversion and defibrillation for tachycardic rhythm disturbances. Integration of AEDs into a system of care is critical in the Chain of Survival in public places outside of hospitals. To give the victim the best chance of survival, 3 actions must occur within the first moments of a cardiac arrest[120]: activation of the EMS system,[121] provision of CPR, and operation of a defibrillator.[122]

One area of continued interest is whether delivering a longer period of CPR before defibrillation improves outcomes in cardiac arrest. In early studies, survival was improved when 1.5 to 3 minutes of CPR preceded defibrillation for patients with cardiac arrest of >4 to 5 minutes duration prior to EMS arrival.[123,124] However, in 2 more recent randomized controlled trials, CPR performed before defibrillation did not improve outcome.[125,126] If ≥2 rescuers are present CPR should be performed while a defibrillator is being obtained and readied for use.

The 1-shock protocol for VF has not been changed. Evidence has accumulated that even short interruptions in CPR are harmful. Thus, rescuers should minimize the interval between stopping compressions and delivering shocks and should resume CPR immediately after shock delivery.

Over the last decade biphasic waveforms have been shown to be more effective than monophasic waveforms in cardioversion and defibrillation.[127–135] However, there are no clinical data comparing one specific biphasic waveform with another. Whether escalating or fixed subsequent doses of energy are superior has not been tested with different waveforms. However, if higher energy levels are available in the device at hand, they may be considered if initial shocks are unsuccessful in terminating the arrhythmia.

In the last 5 to 10 years a number of randomized trials have compared biphasic with monophasic cardioversion in atrial fibrillation. The efficacy of shock energies for cardioversion of atrial fibrillation is waveform-specific and can vary from 120 to 200 J depending on the defibrillator manufacturer. Thus, the recommended initial biphasic energy dose for cardioversion of atrial fibrillation is 120 to 200 J using the manufacturer's recommended setting.[136–140] If the initial shock fails, providers should increase the dose in a stepwise fashion. Cardioversion of adult atrial flutter and other supraventricular tachycardias generally requires less energy; an initial energy of 50 J to 100 J is often sufficient.[140] If the initial shock fails, providers should increase the dose in a stepwise fashion.[141] Adult cardioversion of atrial fibrillation with monophasic waveforms should begin at 200 J and increase in a stepwise fashion if not successful.

Transcutaneous pacing has also been the focus of several recent trials. Pacing is not generally recommended for patients in asystolic cardiac arrest. Three randomized controlled trials[142–144] indicate no improvement in rate of admission to hospital or survival to hospital discharge when paramedics or physicians attempted pacing in patients with cardiac arrest due to asystole in the prehospital or hospital (ED) setting. However, it is reasonable for healthcare providers to be prepared to initiate pacing in patients with bradyarrhythmias in the event the heart rate does not respond to atropine or other chronotropic (rate-accelerating) drugs.[145,146]

## Advanced Cardiovascular Life Support

ACLS affects multiple links in the Chain of Survival, including interventions to prevent cardiac arrest, treat cardiac arrest, and improve outcomes of patients who achieve ROSC after cardiac arrest. The *2010 AHA Guidelines for CPR and ECC* continue to emphasize that the foundation of successful ACLS is good BLS, beginning with prompt high-quality CPR with minimal interruptions, and for VF/pulseless VT, attempted defibrillation within minutes of collapse. The new fifth link in the Chain of Survival and Part 9: "Post–Cardiac Arrest Care" (expanded from a subsection of the ACLS part of the *2005 AHA Guidelines for CPR and ECC*) emphasize the importance of comprehensive multidisciplinary care that begins with recognition of cardiac arrest and continues after ROSC through hospital discharge and beyond. Key ACLS assessments and interventions provide an essential bridge between BLS and long-term survival with good neurologic function.

In terms of airway management the *2010 AHA Guidelines for CPR and ECC* have a major new Class I recommendation for adults: use of quantitative waveform capnography for confirmation and monitoring of endotracheal tube placement. In addition, the use of supraglottic advanced airways continues to be supported as an alternative to endotracheal intubation for airway management during CPR. Finally, the routine use of cricoid pressure during airway management of patients in cardiac arrest is no longer recommended.

There are several important changes in the *2010 AHA Guidelines for CPR and ECC* regarding management of symptomatic arrhythmias. On the basis of new evidence of safety and potential efficacy, adenosine can now be considered for the diagnosis and treatment of stable undifferentiated wide-complex tachycardia when the rhythm is regular and the QRS waveform is monomorphic. For symptomatic or unstable bradycardia, intravenous (IV) infusion of chronotropic agents is now recommended as an equally effective alternative to external pacing when atropine is ineffective.

For 2010 a new circular AHA ACLS Cardiac Arrest Algorithm has been introduced as an alternative to the traditional box-and-line format. Both algorithms represent restructured and simplified formats that focus on interventions that have the greatest impact on outcome. To that end, emphasis has been placed on delivery of high-quality CPR with minimal interruptions and defibrillation of VF/pulseless VT. Vascular access, drug delivery, and advanced airway placement, while still recommended, should not cause significant interruptions in chest compression or delay shocks. In addition, atropine is no longer recommended for routine use in the management of pulseless electrical activity (PEA)/asystole.

Real-time monitoring and optimization of CPR quality using either mechanical parameters (eg, monitoring of chest compression rate and depth, adequacy of chest wall relaxation, length and duration of pauses in compression and number and depth of ventilations delivered) or, when feasible, physiologic parameters (partial pressure of end-tidal $CO_2$ [$\text{Petco}_2$], arterial pressure during the relaxation phase of chest compressions, or central venous oxygen saturation [$\text{Scvo}_2$]) are encouraged. When quantitative waveform capnography is used for adults, guidelines now include recommendations for monitoring CPR quality and detecting ROSC based on $\text{Petco}_2$ values.

Finally the *2010 AHA Guidelines for CPR and ECC* continue to recognize that ACLS does not end when a patient achieves ROSC. Guidelines for post–cardiac arrest management have been significantly expanded (see Part 9) and now include a new Early Post–Cardiac Arrest Treatment Algorithm.

## Post–Cardiac Arrest Care

The *2010 AHA Guidelines for CPR and ECC* recognize the increased importance of systematic care and advancements in the multispecialty management of patients following ROSC and admission to the hospital that can affect neurologically intact survival. Part 9: "Post–Cardiac Arrest Care" recognizes the importance of bundled goal-oriented management and interventions to achieve optimal outcome in victims of cardiac arrest who are admitted to a hospital following ROSC. We recommend that a comprehensive, structured, integrated, multidisciplinary system of care should be implemented in a consistent manner for the treatment of post–cardiac arrest patients.

Initial and later key objectives of post–cardiac arrest care include

- Optimizing cardiopulmonary function and vital organ perfusion after ROSC
- Transportation to an appropriate hospital or critical-care unit with a comprehensive post–cardiac arrest treatment system of care
- Identification and intervention for acute coronary syndromes (ACS)
- Temperature control to optimize neurologic recovery
- Anticipation, treatment, and prevention of multiple organ dysfunction

The primary goal of a bundled treatment strategy for the patient after cardiac arrest includes a consistently applied comprehensive therapeutic plan delivered in a multidisciplinary environment leading to the return of normal or near-normal functional status. Patients with suspected ACS should be triaged to a facility with reperfusion capabilities and a multidisciplinary team prepared to monitor patients for multi-organ dysfunction and initiate appropriate post–cardiac arrest therapy, including hypothermia. Prognostic assessment in the setting of hypothermia is changing, and experts qualified in neurologic assessment in this patient population and integration of prognostic tools are essential for patients, caregivers, and families and are reviewed in detail in Part 9. As a guide to therapy, a new algorithm and a table of integrated goal therapy care were developed.

## Stabilization of the Patient With ACS

The *2010 AHA Guidelines for CPR and ECC* recommendations for the evaluation and management of ACS have been updated to define the scope of training for healthcare providers who treat patients with suspected or definite ACS within the first hours after onset of symptoms. Within this context several important strategies and components of care are defined and emphasized by these guidelines and include systems of care for patients with ST-elevation myocardial infarction (STEMI), prehospital 12-lead electrocardiograms (ECGs), triage to hospitals capable of performing percutaneous coronary intervention (PCI), and comprehensive care for patients following cardiac arrest with confirmed STEMI or suspected ACS.

A well-organized approach to STEMI care requires integration of community, EMS, physician, and hospital resources in a bundled STEMI system of care. An important and key component of STEMI systems of care is the performance of prehospital 12-lead ECGs with transmission or interpretation by EMS providers and advance notification of the receiving facility. Use of prehospital 12-lead ECGs has been recommended by the *AHA Guidelines for CPR and ECC* since 2000 and has been documented to reduce time to reperfusion with fibrinolytic therapy.[147–153] More recently, prehospital 12-lead ECGs have also been shown to reduce the time to primary percutaneous coronary intervention (PCI) and can facilitate triage to specific hospitals when PCI is the chosen strategy.[154–161] When EMS or ED physicians activate the cardiac care team, including the cardiac catheterization laboratory, significant reductions in reperfusion times are observed.

The ACS guidelines also make new recommendations for triage of patients to PCI centers after cardiac arrest. The performance of PCI has been associated with favorable outcomes in adult patients resuscitated from cardiac arrest, and it is reasonable to include cardiac catheterization in standardized post–cardiac arrest protocols as part of an overall strategy to improve neurologically intact survival in this patient group. In patients with out-of-hospital cardiac arrest due to VF, emergent angiography with prompt revascularization of the infarct-related artery is recommended. The ECG may be insensitive or misleading following cardiac arrest, and coronary angiography after ROSC in subjects with arrest of presumed ischemic cardiac etiology may be reasonable, even in the absence of a clearly defined STEMI. Clinical findings of coma in patients before PCI are common following out-of-hospital cardiac arrest and should not be a contraindication to consideration of immediate angiography and PCI.

### Adult Stroke

Part 11 emphasizes the early management of acute ischemic stroke in adult patients. It summarizes out-of-hospital care through the first hours of therapy. Approximately 795 000 people suffer a new or repeat stroke each year, and stroke remains the third leading cause of death in the United States. By integrating public education, 911 dispatch, prehospital detection and triage, hospital stroke system development, and stroke unit management, significant improvements in stroke care have been made. Important components of the stroke system of care are summarized in Part 11.

As with STEMI patients, prearrival hospital notification by the transporting EMS unit has been found to significantly increase the percentage of patients with acute stroke who receive fibrinolytic therapy. The *2010 AHA Guidelines for CPR and ECC* recommend that every hospital with an ED have a written plan that is communicated to EMS systems describing how patients with acute stroke are to be managed in that institution. Triage of patients with acute stroke directly to designated stroke centers is a new Class I recommendation, which has been added to the Stroke Algorithm. Another new Class I recommendation is admission of the stroke patient to a dedicated stroke unit managed by a multidisciplinary team experienced in stroke care.

Since publication of the *2005 AHA Guidelines for CPR and ECC*, additional data have emerged extending the time window for administration of IV rtPA to select patients with acute ischemic stroke. These guidelines now recommend IV rtPA for patients who meet the eligibility criteria for the National Institute of Neurological Disorders and Stroke (NINDS) or the Third European Cooperative Acute Stroke Study (ECASS-3) if rtPA is administered by physicians in the setting of a clearly defined protocol with a knowledgeable

team and institutional commitment. However, it is important to emphasize the continued time-dependent reperfusion window and that earlier treatment is better and is associated with improved outcome. Patients ineligible for standard IV fibrinolytic therapy may be considered for intra-arterial fibrinolytic therapy or mechanical revascularization at selected centers with specialized capabilities.

Finally these guidelines recommend admission to a stroke unit within 3 hours of presentation to the ED. Recent studies establish that stroke unit care is superior to care in general medical wards, and positive effects of stroke unit care can persist for years. The benefits from treatment in a stroke unit are comparable to the beneficial effects achieved with IV rtPA.

Overall stroke care has progressed dramatically since it was first incorporated into the ECC mission. Improvements in education, prehospital management, hospital system development, and acute treatments have lead to significant improvements in patient outcomes.

### Special Situations

Cardiac arrest in special situations may require special treatments or procedures beyond those provided during standard BLS or ACLS. Because of difficulty in conducting randomized clinical trials in these areas or their infrequent occurrence, these unique situations call for an experienced provider to go "beyond basics," using clinical consensus and extrapolation from typical circumstances. The topics covered in the *2005 AHA Guidelines for CPR and ECC* have been reviewed, updated, and expanded to 15 specific cardiac arrest situations. These guidelines emphasize the "above and beyond" knowledge required as well as the anticipatory clinical acumen to provide timely care and unique interventions.

Topics include significant periarrest features that may be important to prevent cardiac arrest or that require special post–cardiac arrest care and intervention beyond the usual care defined in these guidelines. Topics with these potentially unique features include asthma, anaphylaxis, pregnancy, morbid obesity, pulmonary embolism, electrolyte imbalance, ingestion of toxic substances, trauma, accidental hypothermia, avalanche, drowning, electric shock/lightning strikes, and special procedural situations affecting the heart, including PCI, cardiac tamponade, and cardiac surgery.

### Pediatric Basic Life Support

The majority of pediatric cardiac arrests are asphyxial, with only approximately 5% to 15% attributable to VF.[8,9,27,162,163] Animal studies[164–166] have shown that resuscitation from asphyxial arrest is best accomplished by a combination of ventilations and chest compressions. This has recently been confirmed in a large community pediatric study,[27] which not only showed that the best resuscitation results from asphyxial arrest were from a combination of ventilations and chest compressions but also that the small number of children with asphyxial arrest who received compression-only CPR had no better results than those who received no bystander CPR.

Although animal studies and pediatric series support the importance of ventilation for asphyxial arrest, data in adults suggest that chest compressions are critical for resuscitation from VF arrest, with ventilations being less important. Therefore we continue to support a combination of ventilations and chest compressions for pediatric resuscitation but emphasize that sudden witnessed cardiac arrest in the adolescent, such as might occur during an athletic event, should be treated as a VF arrest, with emphasis on chest compressions and early defibrillation. Compression-only CPR is encouraged for bystanders who are not trained in giving ventilations or are hesitant to do so.

Despite the importance of providing a combination of ventilations and chest compressions for resuscitation of victims from asphyxial arrest (including most children) as described above, a switch to a C-A-B (Chest compressions, Airway, Breathing) sequence was recommended for ease of teaching. Theoretically this should delay ventilation by a maximum of about 18 seconds (less time if 2 recuers are present).

There is again great emphasis on "push hard, push fast," allowing the chest to completely recoil after each compression, minimizing interruptions in chest compressions, and avoiding excessive ventilation. To achieve effective chest compressions, rescuers are advised to compress at least one third the anterior-posterior dimension of the chest. This corresponds to approximately 1½ inches (4 cm) in most infants and 2 inches (5 cm) in most children.

## Pediatric Advanced Life Support

The following are the most important changes and reinforcements to recommendations in the *2005 AHA Guidelines for CPR and ECC*:

- There is additional evidence that many healthcare providers cannot quickly and reliably determine the presence or absence of a pulse in infants or children.[167] The pulse assessment is therefore again deemphasized for healthcare providers. For a child who is unresponsive and not breathing normally, if a pulse cannot be detected within 10 seconds, healthcare providers should begin CPR.
- More data support the safety and effectiveness of cuffed endotracheal tubes in infants and young children, and the formula for selecting the appropriately sized cuffed tube has been updated.
- The safety and value of using cricoid pressure during emergency intubation has been questioned. It is therefore recommended that the application of cricoid pressure should be modified or discontinued if it impedes ventilation or the speed or ease of intubation.
- Monitoring capnography/capnometry is again recommended to confirm proper endotracheal tube (and other advanced airway) position and may be useful during CPR to assess and optimize quality of chest compressions.
- The optimal energy dose required for defibrillation (using either a monophasic or biphasic waveform) in infants and children is unknown. When shocks are indicated for VF or pulseless VT in infants and children, an initial energy dose of 2 to 4 J/kg of either waveform is reasonable; doses higher than 4 J/kg, especially if delivered with a biphasic defibrillator, may also be safe and effective.
- On the basis of increasing evidence of potential harm from high oxygen exposure after cardiac arrest, once spontaneous circulation is restored, inspired oxygen should be titrated to limit the risk of hyperoxemia.

- New sections have been added on resuscitation of infants and children with a single ventricle, after a variety of palliative procedures, and with pulmonary hypertension.
- There is recognition that for some young victims of sudden death, no cause of death is found on routine autopsy but these victims are found to have a genetic ion channel defect (channelopathy) that predisposes them to a fatal arrhythmia. It is therefore recommended that young victims of a sudden, unexpected cardiac arrest should have an unrestricted, complete autopsy when possible with appropriate preservation and genetic analysis of tissue. Detailed testing may reveal an inherited channelopathy that may also be present in surviving family members.

## Neonatal Resuscitation

The etiology of neonatal arrests is nearly always asphyxia. Therefore, the A-B-C sequence has been retained for resuscitation of neonates unless there is a known cardiac etiology.

### Assessment, Supplementary Oxygen, and Peripartum Suctioning

When assessing an infant's cardiorespiratory transition and need for resuscitation, the best indicators were found to be increasing heart rate, effective respirations, and good tone. Pulse oximetry, with the probe attached to the right upper extremity, should be used to assess any need for supplementary oxygen. Studies demonstrate that healthy babies born at term start with an oxygen saturation of <60% and will take >10 minutes to reach a saturation of >90%. Hyperoxia can be toxic, particularly to the preterm infant. For babies born at term, it is best to begin resuscitation with room air rather than 100% oxygen. Any supplementary oxygen administered should be regulated by blending oxygen and air, using oximetry to guide titration of the blend delivered.

The role of peripartum suctioning has been deemphasized. There is no evidence to support airway suctioning in active babies, even in the presence of meconium. The available evidence does not support or refute the routine endotracheal suctioning of non-vigorous infants born through meconium-stained amniotic fluid.

### Chest Compressions

The recommended compression-ventilation ratio remains 3:1 because ventilation is critical to reversal of newborn asphyxial arrest and higher ratios may decrease minute ventilation. If the arrest is known to be of cardiac etiology, a higher ratio (15:2) should be considered. If epinephrine is indicated, a dose of 0.01 to 0.03 mg/kg should be administered IV as soon as possible. When using the endotracheal route it is likely that a larger dose (0.05 mg/kg to 0.1 mg/kg) will be required.

### Postresuscitation Care (Post-Cardiac Arrest Care)

Therapeutic hypothermia is recommended for babies born near term with evolving moderate to severe hypoxic-ischemic encephalopathy. Cooling should be initiated and conducted under clearly defined protocols with treatment in neonatal intensive care facilities and the capabilities for multidisciplinary care.

## Ethics

The duration of resuscitation for newborns with prolonged cardiac arrest was reviewed. In a newly born baby with no detectable heart rate that remains undetectable for 10 minutes, it is appropriate to consider stopping resuscitation. When gestation, birth weight, or congenital anomalies are associated with almost certain early death and an unacceptably high morbidity is likely among the rare survivors, resuscitation is not indicated.

The role of simulation in education was assessed. The task force concluded that although it is reasonable to use simulation in resuscitation education, the most effective methodologies remain to be defined. Briefings and debriefings during learning improve acquisition of content knowledge, technical skills, or behavioral skills required for effective, safe resuscitation.

## Education

"Education, Implementation, and Teams" is a new section in the *2010 AHA Guidelines for CPR and ECC*. Major recommendations and points of emphasis in this new section include the following:

- Bystander CPR dramatically improves survival from cardiac arrest, yet far less than half of arrest victims receive this potentially lifesaving therapy.
- Methods to improve bystander willingness to perform CPR include formal training in CPR techniques, including compression-only (Hands-Only) CPR for those who may be unwilling or unable to perform conventional CPR; educating providers on the low risk of acquiring an infection by performing CPR; and specific training directed at helping providers overcome fear or panic when faced with an actual cardiac arrest victim.
- EMS should provide dispatcher instructions over the telephone to help bystanders recognize victims of cardiac arrest, including victims who may still be gasping, and to encourage bystanders to provide CPR if arrest is likely. Dispatchers may also instruct untrained bystanders in the performance of compression-only (Hands-Only) CPR.
- BLS skills can be learned equally well with "practice while watching" (video-based) training as through longer, traditional instructor-led courses.
- To reduce the time to defibrillation for cardiac arrest victims, AED use should not be limited only to persons with formal training in their use. However, AED training does improve performance in simulation and continues to be recommended.
- Training in teamwork and leadership skills should continue to be included in ALS courses.
- Manikins with realistic features such as the capability to replicate chest expansion and breath sounds, generate a pulse and blood pressure, and speak may be useful for integrating the knowledge, skills, and behaviors required in ALS training. However, there is insufficient evidence to recommend their routine use in ALS courses.
- Written tests should not be used exclusively to assess the competence of a participant in an advanced life support (ACLS or PALS) course (ie, there needs to be a performance assessment as well).

- Formal assessment should continue to be included in resuscitation courses, both as a method of evaluating the success of the student in achieving the learning objectives and of evaluating the effectiveness of the course.
- The current 2-year certification period for basic and advanced life support courses should include periodic assessment of rescuer knowledge and skills with reinforcement provided as needed. The optimal timing and method for this assessment and reinforcement are not known and warrant further investigation.
- CPR prompt and feedback devices may be useful for training rescuers and may be useful as part of an overall strategy to improve the quality of CPR for actual cardiac arrests.
- Debriefing is a learner-focused, nonthreatening technique to assist individual rescuers or teams to reflect on and improve performance. Debriefing should be included in advanced life support courses to facilitate learning and can be used to review performance in the clinical setting to improve subsequent performance.
- Systems-based approaches to improving resuscitation performance, such as regional systems of care and rapid response systems, may be useful to reduce the variability of survival for cardiac arrest.

## First Aid

Once again, a review of the literature on many topics relevant to first aid found that little investigation is being carried out in this field, and many recommendations have had to be extrapolated from research published in related fields. The following are new recommendations or reinforcements of previous recommendations.

- Evidence suggests that, without training, laypersons and some healthcare professionals may be unable to recognize the signs and symptoms of anaphylaxis. Therefore, initial or subsequent administration of epinephrine for anaphylaxis by either of these groups may be problematic. This issue takes on added importance in view of legislation permitting the practice in some jurisdictions.
- Except in diving decompression injuries, there is no evidence of any benefit of administration of oxygen by first aid providers.
- The administration of aspirin by a first aid provider to a victim experiencing chest discomfort is problematic. The literature is clear on the benefit of early administration of aspirin to victims experiencing a coronary ischemic event except when there is a contraindication, such as true aspirin allergy or a bleeding disorder. Less clear, however, is whether first aid providers can recognize the signs and symptoms of an acute coronary syndrome or contraindications to aspirin and whether administration of aspirin by first aid providers delays definitive therapy in an advanced medical facility.
- No evidence of benefit was found for placing an unresponsive victim who is breathing in a "recovery" position. Studies performed with volunteers appear to show that if a victim is turned because of emesis or copious secretions, the HAINES (High Arm IN Endangered Spine) position is an example of a recovery position that may have some theoretic advantages.

- Since 2005 considerable new data have emerged on the use of tourniquets to control bleeding. This experience comes primarily from the battlefields of Iraq and Afghanistan. There is no question that tourniquets do control bleeding, but if left on too long, they can cause gangrene distal to the application and systemic complications, including shock and death. Protocols for the proper use of tourniquets to control bleeding exist, but there is no experience with civilian use or how to teach the proper application of tourniquets to first aid providers. Studies have shown that not all tourniquets are the same, and some manufactured tourniquets perform better than others and better than tourniquets that are improvised.

- Because of its importance, the issue of spinal stabilization was once again reviewed. Unfortunately very little new data are available, and it is still not clear whether secondary spinal cord injury is a real problem and whether the methods recommended for spinal stabilization or movement restriction are effective.

- The literature regarding first aid for snake bites was once again reviewed. In the 2005 review evidence was found for a beneficial effect from pressure immobilization for neurotoxic snake bites, but it now appears that there is a benefit even for non-neurotoxic snake bites. The challenge is that the range of pressure needed under the immobilization bandage appears to be critical and may be difficult to teach or estimate in the field.

- A new section on jellyfish stings has been added and new recommendations for treatment have been made.

- The literature on the first aid treatment of frostbite was reviewed. There continues to be evidence of potential harm in thawing of a frozen body part if there is any chance of refreezing. The literature is mixed on the benefit of nonsteroidal anti-inflammatory agents as a first aid treatment for frostbite. Chemical warmers should not be used because they may generate temperatures capable of causing tissue injury.

- Oral fluid replacement has been found to be as effective as IV fluid in exercise- or heat-induced dehydration. The best oral fluid appears to be a carbohydrate-electrolyte mixture.

## Conflict of Interest Management

Throughout the 2010 evidence evaluation process the AHA and the International Liaison Committee on Resuscitation (ILCOR) followed rigorous conflict of interest (COI) policies to ensure that the potential for commercial bias was minimized. The COI process was based on the successful policies and actions used in developing the *2005 International Consensus on CPR and ECC Science With Treatment Recommendations*.[168,169] In 2007 ILCOR modified the COI management policies to be used for the 2010 evidence evaluation process, further enhancing and building on the process used in 2005. Modifications ensured that commercial relationships were identified as early as possible to avoid potential conflicts by reassigning the role to a participant who had no conflicts *before* work began. The revisions also took into account changes in AHA policies, approved by the AHA Science Advisory and Coordinating Committee in 2009, regarding requirements for scientific statement and guideline writing group chairs and members.

The COI policies and actions for the 2010 evidence evaluation process[170] described in full in Part 2 of this publication applied to the entire 5-year consensus development process—before, during, and after the actual 2010 International Consensus Conference. The policies applied to all aspects of the evidence evaluation process, including selection of leaders and members of ILCOR task forces and writing groups, selection of topics for worksheets, selection of worksheet authors, presentation and discussion of worksheets, development of final Consensus on Science statements, and, for the AHA, creation of the *2010 AHA Guidelines for CPR and ECC* that follow in this publication. The policies applied to all volunteers and staff involved in the process, including all leaders and members of ILCOR committees (Conference Planning Committee, Editorial Board, and Task Forces for resuscitation areas), all evidence evaluation worksheet authors, and all 2010 International Consensus Conference participants.

As in 2005, during the entire 2010 International Consensus Conference every participant used his or her assigned number when speaking as a presenter, panelist, moderator, or commentator from the floor. For the duration of each speaker's comments, a slide was displayed with the speaker's name, institution, and any commercial relationships the speaker had disclosed so that the audience could assess the impact these relationships might have on the speaker's input. All participants were encouraged to raise any concerns with the moderators or identified COI leads for the conference. Depending on the nature of the relationship and their role in the guidelines process, participants were restricted from some activities (ie, leading, voting, deciding, writing) that directly or indirectly related to that commercial interest. Although the focus of the evidence evaluation process was evaluation of the scientific data and translation of that evidence into treatment recommendations and guidelines, attention to potential conflicts of interest was omnipresent throughout the process, helping ensure evidence-based guidelines free of commercial influence.

## Summary

As we mark the 50th anniversary of modern-era CPR, we must acknowledge that, despite measurable progress aimed at its prevention, cardiac arrest—both in and out of the hospital—continues to be a major public health challenge. Over these 50 years, scientific knowledge about arrest pathophysiology and resuscitation mechanisms has increased substantially. In our ongoing commitment to ensure optimal community-based care for all victims of cardiac arrest, we must continue to effectively translate the science of resuscitation into clinical care and improved resuscitation outcomes.

## Acknowledgments

The writing group gratefully acknowledges the extraordinary dedication and contributions of the AHA ECC staff, especially Kara Robinson, as well as David Barnes, Jennifer Denton, Lana Gent, Colleen Halverson, Jody Hundley, Alicia Pederson, Tanya Semenko, and Nina Tran. In addition, the writing group acknowledges additional outstanding contributions, especially from Brenda Schoolfield, and also from Jeanette Allison, Janet Butler, Heba Costandy, Cathryn Evans, Pierce Goetz, and Sallie Young.

# Disclosures

## Guidelines Part 1: Executive Summary: Writing Group Disclosures

| Writing Group Member | Employment | Research Grant | Other Research Support | Speakers' Bureau/Honoraria | Ownership Interest | Consultant/Advisory Board | Other |
|---|---|---|---|---|---|---|---|
| John M. Field | Penn State University COM & Heart and Vascular Institute–Professor of Medicine and Surgery. AHA ECC Senior Science Editor | None | None | None | None | None | None |
| Mary Fran Hazinski | Vanderbilt University School of Nursing—Professor; AHA ECC Product Development-Senior Science Editor †Significant AHA compensation to write, edit and review documents such as the 2010 AHA Guidelines for CPR and ECC. | None | None | None | None | None | None |
| Michael R. Sayre | The Ohio State University-Associate Professor | None | None | None | None | None | None |
| Leon Chameides | Emeritus Director Pediatric Cardiology, Connecticut Children's Hospital; Clinical Professor, University of Connecticut | None | None | None | None | None | None |
| Stephen M. Schexnayder | University of Arkansas for Medical Sciences–Professor/Division Chief; AHA Compensated Consultant as Associate Senior Science Editor | *Pharmacokinetics of proton pump inhibitors in critically ill children | None | *Contemporary Forums (nursing conferences) | None | None | *Various medical legal cases involving pediatric critical care & emergency medicine |
| Robin Hemphill | Emory University, Dept. of Emergency Medicine–Associate Professor †Paid AHA writer | None | None | None | None | None | None |
| Ricardo A. Samson | The University of Arizona, providing clinical care, teaching, and research associated with an academic pediatric cardiology practice. Professor of Pediatrics | None | None | None | None | †Consultant-American Heart Association-Associate Science Editor Salary support received to devote 30% time to AHA for the development of ECC materials | None |
| John Kattwinkel | University of Virginia—Professor of Pediatrics | None | None | None | None | None | None |
| Robert A. Berg | U of Pennsylvania-Professor | Co-I, Laerdal Foundation, Sarver Heart Center (U of Arizona) Cardiac Arrest and CPR Program Support Grant, 2007–2009 | None | None | None. | None | None |
| Farhan Bhanji | Montreal Children's Hospital, McGill University; Assistant Professor of Pediatrics | None | None | None | None | None | None |
| Diana M. Cave | Legacy Health System, Emergency Services, RN | None | None | None | None | None | None |
| Edward C. Jauch | Medical University of South Carolina; Emergency medicine physician, Stroke team physician, Professor | †NIH (EC) IMS-3 U01 NS052220 (not related) NIH study, all money to University *NIH (Co-I) ALIAS II Study U01 NS054630 NIH study, all money to University | None | None | None | None | *Member, DSMB Field Administration of Stroke Therapy–Magnesium Trial (U01NS044364) No money involved |
| Peter J. Kudenchuk | University of Washington–Professor of Medicine | †NHLBI Resuscitation Outcomes Consortium (Principal Investigator); funding comes to institution | None | *Network for Continuing Medical Education, Academy for Healthcare Education, Sanofi-Aventis, Pri-Med, Horiizon CME, with honoraria | *Sanofi-Aventis, Novartis | None | †Medical-legal Consultation |
| Robert W. Neumar | University of Pennsylvania–Associate Professor of Emergency Medicine | †Funding Source: NIH/NINDS Grant Number: R21 NS054654 Funding Period 06/01/07 to 06/31/2010 Role on Project: Principal Investigator Title: Optimizing Therapeutic Hypothermia After Cardiac Arrest Description: The goal of this project is to evaluate how the onset and duration of therapeutic hypothermia after cardiac arrest impacts survival and neuroprotection | None | None | None | None | None |

*(Continued)*

## Guidelines Part 1: Executive Summary: Writing Group Disclosures, *Continued*

| Writing Group Member | Employment | Research Grant | Other Research Support | Speakers' Bureau/Honoraria | Ownership Interest | Consultant/Advisory Board | Other |
|---|---|---|---|---|---|---|---|
| Mary Ann Peberdy | Virginia Commonwealth University-Professor of Internal Medicine and Emergency Medicine | None | None | None | None | None | None |
| Jeffrey M. Perlman | Weill Cornell Medical College-Professor of Pediatrics | *NIH Grant –Co-PI-Antimicrobial Dosing in the NIH | None | None | None | None | None |
| Elizabeth Sinz | Penn State Hershey Medical Center– Professor of Anesthesiology and Neurosurgery *Associate Science Editor for AHA | None | None | None | None | None | None |
| Andrew H. Travers | Emergency Health Services NS-Provincial Medical Director | None | None | None | None | None | None |
| Marc D. Berg | University of Arizona/University Physician's Healthcare (UPH)– Asso. Prof. Clinical Pediatrics Attending Intensivist, Pediatric Critical Care Medicine | None | None | None | None | None | None |
| John E. Billi | University of Michigan Medical School -Professor | None | None | None | None | None | None |
| Brian Eigel | American Heart Association–Director of Science, ECC Programs | None | None | None | None | None | None |
| Robert W. Hickey | University of Pittsburgh–MD | †NIH sponsored research on the effect of cyclopentenone prostaglandins upon post-ischemic brain | None | None | None | None | *Occasional expert witness in medical malpractice cases (1–2 times/yr) |
| Monica E. Kleinman | Children's Hospital Anesthesia Foundation: Not-for-profit foundation– Senior Associate in Critical Care Medicine | None | None | None | None | None | None |
| Mark S. Link | Tufts Medical Center Academic Medical Institution-Attending Physician | None | None | None | None | None | None |
| Laurie J. Morrison | St. Michael Hospital, clinician | None | None | None | None | None | None |
| Robert E. O'Connor | University of Virginia Health System–Professor and Chair of Emergency Medicine | None | None | None | None | None | None |
| Michael Shuster | Self-employed; Emergency Physician | None | None | None | None | None | None |
| Clifton W. Callaway | University of Pittsburgh School of Medicine; Associate Professor UPMC Health System; Physician | †NHLBI-Resuscitation Outcomes Consortium | *Loan of cooling equipment from Medivance, Inc., a manufacturer of hypothermia devices | None | †Coinventor on patents related to timing of defibrillation. Patents licensed to Medtronic ERS, by the University of Pittsburgh. *Own stock in Apple Computer, Inc. | None | None |
| Brett Cucchiara | University of Pennsylvania Assistant Professor of Neurology | †NIH RO1-migraine imaging research | None | *Multiple CME talks at different institutions | None | None | *Occasionally serves as expert witness for medicolegal cases |
| Jeffrey D. Ferguson | Brody School of Medicine at East Carolina University– Assistant Professor | None | None | None | None | None | *Currently involved as expert witness on two pending cases. Fees to date total less than $10,000 over previous 12 months |
| Thomas D. Rea | University of Washington-Associate Professor | †Medtronic Foundation to develop community approaches to improve resuscitation. Monies to the institution. †Laerdal Foundation to evaluate optimal approaches for bystander CPR. Monies to the institution. *Philips Medical Inc PhysioControl Inc | †Philips Medical and PhysioControl provided equipment to support research. Equipment went to the institution. | None | None | None | None |

(Continued)

**Guidelines Part 1: Executive Summary: Writing Group Disclosures,** *Continued*

| Writing Group Member | Employment | Research Grant | Other Research Support | Speakers' Bureau/Honoraria | Ownership Interest | Consultant/Advisory Board | Other |
|---|---|---|---|---|---|---|---|
| Terry L. Vanden Hoek | The University of Chicago; Associate Professor | *Principal Investigator Department of Defense, Office of Naval Research "Proteomic Development of Molecular Vital Signs: Mapping a Mitochondrial Injury Severity Score to Triage and Guide Resuscitation of Hemorrhagic Shock" 9/6/04–4/31/10 $885,639 (current year) Research grant awarded to the University of Chicago | None | None | None | None | None |

This table represents the relationships of writing group members that may be perceived as actual or reasonably perceived conflicts of interest as reported on the Disclosure Questionnaire, which all members of the writing group are required to complete and submit. A relationship is considered to be "significant" if (a) the person receives $10 000 or more during any 12-month period, or 5% or more of the person's gross income; or (b) the person owns 5% or more of the voting stock or share of the entity, or owns $10 000 or more of the fair market value of the entity. A relationship is considered to be "modest" if it is less than "significant" under the preceding definition.

*Modest.
†Significant.

# References

1. Kouwenhoven WB, Jude JR, Knickerbocker GG. Closed-chest cardiac massage. *JAMA*. 1960;173:1064–1067.
2. Eisenberg M. *Resuscitate! How Your Community Can Improve Survival from Sudden Cardiac Arrest*. Seattle, WA: University of Washington Press; 2009.
3. Lown B, Neuman J, Amarasingham R, Berkovits BV. Comparison of alternating current with direct electroshock across the closed chest. *Am J Cardiol*. 1962;10:223–233.
4. Cardiopulmonary resuscitation: statement by the Ad Hoc Committee on Cardiopulmonary Resuscitation, of the Division of Medical Sciences, National Academy of Sciences, National Research Council. *JAMA*. 1966;198:372–379.
5. Nichol G, Thomas E, Callaway CW, Hedges J, Powell JL, Aufderheide TP, Rea T, Lowe R, Brown T, Dreyer J, Davis D, Idris A, Stiell I. Regional variation in out-of-hospital cardiac arrest incidence and outcome. *JAMA*. 2008;300:1423–1431.
6. Mogayzel C, Quan L, Graves JR, Tiedeman D, Fahrenbruch C, Herndon P. Out-of-hospital ventricular fibrillation in children and adolescents: causes and outcomes. *Ann Emerg Med*. 1995;25:484–491.
7. Donoghue AJ, Nadkarni V, Berg RA, Osmond MH, Wells G, Nesbitt L, Stiell IG. Out-of-hospital pediatric cardiac arrest: an epidemiologic review and assessment of current knowledge. *Ann Emerg Med*. 2005; 46:512–522.
8. Samson RA, Nadkarni VM, Meaney PA, Carey SM, Berg MD, Berg RA. Outcomes of in-hospital ventricular fibrillation in children. *N Engl J Med*. 2006;354:2328–2339.
9. Atkins DL, Everson-Stewart S, Sears GK, Daya M, Osmond MH, Warden CR, Berg RA. Epidemiology and outcomes from out-of-hospital cardiac arrest in children: the Resuscitation Outcomes Consortium Epistry-Cardiac Arrest. *Circulation*. 2009;119:1484–1491.
10. Hazinski MF, Nolan JP, Billi JE, Böttiger BW, Bossaert L, de Caen AR, Deakin CD, Drajer S, Eigel B, Hickey RW, Jacobs I, Kleinman ME, Kloeck W, Koster RW, Lim SH, Mancini ME, Montgomery WH, Morley PT, Morrison LJ, Nadkarni VM, O'Connor RE, Okada K, Perlman JM, Sayre MR, Shuster M, Soar J, Sunde K, Travers AH, Wyllie J, Zideman D. Part 1: executive summary: 2010 International Consensus on Cardiopulmonary Resuscitation and Emergency Cardiovascular Care Science With Treatment Recommendations. *Circulation*. 2010;122(suppl 2):S250–S275.
11. American Heart Association Guidelines for Cardiopulmonary Resuscitation and Emergency Cardiovascular Care. *Circulation*. 2005; 112(Suppl):IV1–203.
12. Wik L, Kramer-Johansen J, Myklebust H, Sorebo H, Svensson L, Fellows B, Steen PA. Quality of cardiopulmonary resuscitation during out-of-hospital cardiac arrest. *JAMA*. 2005;293:299–304.
13. Abella BS, Alvarado JP, Myklebust H, Edelson DP, Barry A, O'Hearn N, Vanden Hoek TL, Becker LB. Quality of cardiopulmonary resuscitation during in-hospital cardiac arrest. *JAMA*. 2005;293:305–310.
14. Callaway CW, Schmicker R, Kampmeyer M, Powell J, Rea TD, Daya MR, Aufderheide TP, Davis DP, Rittenberger JC, Idris AH, Nichol G. Receiving hospital characteristics associated with survival after out-of-hospital cardiac arrest. *Resuscitation*. 2010;81:524–529.
15. Hollenberg J, Herlitz J, Lindqvist J, Riva G, Bohm K, Rosenqvist M, Svensson L. Improved survival after out-of-hospital cardiac arrest is associated with an increase in proportion of emergency crew–witnessed cases and bystander cardiopulmonary resuscitation. *Circulation*. 2008; 118:389–396.
16. Lund-Kordahl I, Olasveengen TM, Lorem T, Samdal M, Wik L, Sunde K. Improving outcome after out-of-hospital cardiac arrest by strengthening weak links of the local Chain of Survival: quality of advanced life support and post-resuscitation care. *Resuscitation*. 2010; 81:422–426.
17. Iwami T, Nichol G, Hiraide A, Hayashi Y, Nishiuchi T, Kajino K, Morita H, Yukioka H, Ikeuchi H, Sugimoto H, Nonogi H, Kawamura T. Continuous improvements in "chain of survival" increased survival after out-of-hospital cardiac arrests: a large-scale population-based study. *Circulation*. 2009;119:728–734.
18. Rea TD, Helbock M, Perry S, Garcia M, Cloyd D, Becker L, Eisenberg M. Increasing use of cardiopulmonary resuscitation during out-of-hospital ventricular fibrillation arrest: survival implications of guideline changes. *Circulation*. 2006;114:2760–2765.
19. Bobrow BJ, Clark LL, Ewy GA, Chikani V, Sanders AB, Berg RA, Richman PB, Kern KB. Minimally interrupted cardiac resuscitation by emergency medical services for out-of-hospital cardiac arrest. *JAMA*. 2008;299:1158–1165.
20. Sayre MR, Cantrell SA, White LJ, Hiestand BC, Keseg DP, Koser S. Impact of the 2005 American Heart Association cardiopulmonary resuscitation and emergency cardiovascular care guidelines on out-of-hospital cardiac arrest survival. *Prehosp Emerg Care*. 2009;13:469–477.
21. Steinmetz J, Barnung S, Nielsen SL, Risom M, Rasmussen LS. Improved survival after an out-of-hospital cardiac arrest using new guidelines. *Acta Anaesthesiol Scand*. 2008;52:908–913.
22. Hinchey PR, Myers JB, Lewis R, De Maio VJ, Reyer E, Licatese D, Zalkin J, Snyder G. Improved out-of-hospital cardiac arrest survival after the sequential implementation of 2005 AHA guidelines for compressions, ventilations, and induced hypothermia: the Wake County Experience. *Ann Emerg Med*. 2010; Mar 30. Epub.
23. Berdowski J, Schmohl A, Tijssen JG, Koster RW. Time needed for a regional emergency medical system to implement resuscitation guidelines 2005–the Netherlands experience. *Resuscitation*. 2009;80: 1336–1341.
24. Bigham BL, Koprowicz K, Aufderheide TP, Davis DP, Donn S, Powell J, Suffoletto B, Nafziger S, Stouffer J, Idris A, Morrison LJ. Delayed prehospital implementation of the 2005 American Heart Association guidelines for cardiopulmonary resuscitation and emergency cardiac care. *Prehosp Emerg Care*. 2010;14:355–360.
25. Bigham B, Aufderheide T, Davis D, Powell J, Donn S, Suffoletto B, Nafziger S, Stouffer J, Morrison LJ, the ROC Investigators. Knowledge translation in emergency medical services: a qualitative survey of barriers to guideline implementation. *Resuscitation*. 2010; Apr 14. Epub.
26. Binks AC, Murphy RE, Prout RE, Bhayani S, Griffiths CA, Mitchell T, Padkin A, Nolan JP. Therapeutic hypothermia after cardiac arrest—

implementation in UK intensive care units. *Anaesthesia.* 2010;65:260–265.

27. Kitamura T, Iwami T, Kawamura T, Nagao K, Tanaka H, Nadkarni VM, Berg RA, Hiraide A. Conventional and chest-compression-only cardiopulmonary resuscitation by bystanders for children who have out-of-hospital cardiac arrests: a prospective, nationwide, population-based cohort study. *Lancet.* 2010;375:1347–1354.

28. Iwami T, Kawamura T, Hiraide A, Berg RA, Hayashi Y, Nishiuchi T, Kajino K, Yonemoto N, Yukioka H, Sugimoto H, Kakuchi H, Sase K, Yokoyama H, Nonogi H. Effectiveness of bystander-initiated cardiac-only resuscitation for patients with out-of-hospital cardiac arrest. *Circulation.* 2007;116:2900–2907.

29. SOS-KANTO Study Group. Cardiopulmonary resuscitation by bystanders with chest compression only (SOS-KANTO): an observational study. *Lancet.* 2007;369(9565):920–926.

30. Ong ME, Ng FS, Anushia P, Tham LP, Leong BS, Ong VY, Tiah L, Lim SH, Anantharaman V. Comparison of chest compression only and standard cardiopulmonary resuscitation for out-of-hospital cardiac arrest in Singapore. *Resuscitation.* 2008;78:119–126.

31. Bohm K, Rosenqvist M, Herlitz J, Hollenberg J, Svensson L. Survival is similar after standard treatment and chest compression only in out-of-hospital bystander cardiopulmonary resuscitation. *Circulation.* 2007;116:2908–2912.

32. Olasveengen TM, Wik L, Steen PA. Standard basic life support vs continuous chest compressions only in out-of-hospital cardiac arrest. *Acta Anaesthesiol Scand.* 2008;52:914–919.

33. Edelson DP, Abella BS, Kramer-Johansen J, Wik L, Myklebust H, Barry AM, Merchant RM, Hoek TL, Steen PA, Becker LB. Effects of compression depth and pre-shock pauses predict defibrillation failure during cardiac arrest. *Resuscitation.* 2006;71:137–145.

34. Eftestol T, Sunde K, Steen PA. Effects of interrupting precordial compressions on the calculated probability of defibrillation success during out-of-hospital cardiac arrest. *Circulation.* 2002;105:2270–2273.

35. Christenson J, Andrusiek D, Everson-Stewart S, Kudenchuk P, Hostler D, Powell J, Callaway CW, Bishop D, Vaillancourt C, Davis D, Aufderheide TP, Idris A, Stouffer JA, Stiell I, Berg R. Chest compression fraction determines survival in patients with out-of-hospital ventricular fibrillation. *Circulation.* 2009;120:1241–1247.

36. Edelson DP, Litzinger B, Arora V, Walsh D, Kim S, Lauderdale DS, Vanden Hoek TL, Becker LB, Abella BS. Improving in-hospital cardiac arrest process and outcomes with performance debriefing. *Arch Intern Med.* 2008;168:1063–1069.

37. National Registry of CPR (NRCPR). http://www.nrcpr.org/. Accessed May 5, 2010.

38. Meaney PA, Nadkarni VM, Kern KB, Indik JH, Halperin HR, Berg RA. Rhythms and outcomes of adult in-hospital cardiac arrest. *Crit Care Med.* 2010;38:101–108.

39. Topjian AA, Localio AR, Berg RA, Alessandrini EA, Meaney PA, Pepe PE, Larkin GL, Peberdy MA, Becker LB, Nadkarni VM. Women of child-bearing age have better inhospital cardiac arrest survival outcomes than do equal-aged men. *Crit Care Med.* 2010;38:1254–1260.

40. Chan PS, Nichol G, Krumholz HM, Spertus JA, Jones PG, Peterson ED, Rathore SS, Nallamothu BK. Racial differences in survival after in-hospital cardiac arrest. *JAMA.* 2009;302:1195–1201.

41. Kayser RG, Ornato JP, Peberdy MA. Cardiac arrest in the Emergency Department: a report from the National Registry of Cardiopulmonary Resuscitation. *Resuscitation.* 2008;78:151–160.

42. Peberdy MA, Ornato JP, Larkin GL, Braithwaite RS, Kashner TM, Carey SM, Meaney PA, Cen L, Nadkarni VM, Praestgaard AH, Berg RA. Survival from in-hospital cardiac arrest during nights and weekends. *JAMA.* 2008;299:785–792.

43. Nadkarni VM, Larkin GL, Peberdy MA, Carey SM, Kaye W, Mancini ME, Nichol G, Lane-Truitt T, Potts J, Ornato JP, Berg RA. First documented rhythm and clinical outcome from in-hospital cardiac arrest among children and adults. *JAMA.* 2006;295:50–57.

44. Peberdy MA, Kaye W, Ornato JP, Larkin GL, Nadkarni V, Mancini ME, Berg RA, Nichol G, Lane-Trultt T. Cardiopulmonary resuscitation of adults in the hospital: a report of 14720 cardiac arrests from the National Registry of Cardiopulmonary Resuscitation. *Resuscitation.* 2003;58:297–308.

45. Olasveengen TM, Sunde K, Brunborg C, Thowsen J, Steen PA, Wik L. Intravenous drug administration during out-of-hospital cardiac arrest: a randomized trial. *JAMA.* 2009;302:2222–2229.

46. Sunde K, Pytte M, Jacobsen D, Mangschau A, Jensen LP, Smedsrud C, Draegni T, Steen PA. Implementation of a standardised treatment protocol for post resuscitation care after out-of-hospital cardiac arrest. *Resuscitation.* 2007;73:29–39.

47. Rittenberger JC, Guyette FX, Tisherman SA, DeVita MA, Alvarez RJ, Callaway CW. Outcomes of a hospital-wide plan to improve care of comatose survivors of cardiac arrest. *Resuscitation.* 2008;79:198–204.

48. Gaieski DF, Band RA, Abella BS, Neumar RW, Fuchs BD, Kolansky DM, Merchant RM, Carr BG, Becker LB, Maguire C, Klair A, Hylton J, Goyal M. Early goal-directed hemodynamic optimization combined with therapeutic hypothermia in comatose survivors of out-of-hospital cardiac arrest. *Resuscitation.* 2009;80:418–424.

49. Mild therapeutic hypothermia to improve the neurologic outcome after cardiac arrest. *N Engl J Med.* 2002;346:549–556.

50. Bernard SA, Gray TW, Buist MD, Jones BM, Silvester W, Gutteridge G, Smith K. Treatment of comatose survivors of out-of-hospital cardiac arrest with induced hypothermia. *N Engl J Med.* 2002;346:557–563.

51. Arrich J. Clinical application of mild therapeutic hypothermia after cardiac arrest. *Crit Care Med.* 2007;35:1041–1047.

52. Holzer M, Mullner M, Sterz F, Robak O, Kliegel A, Losert H, Sodeck G, Uray T, Zeiner A, Laggner AN. Efficacy and safety of endovascular cooling after cardiac arrest: cohort study and Bayesian approach. *Stroke.* 2006;37:1792–1797.

53. Oddo M, Schaller MD, Feihl F, Ribordy V, Liaudet L. From evidence to clinical practice: effective implementation of therapeutic hypothermia to improve patient outcome after cardiac arrest. *Crit Care Med.* 2006;34:1865–1873.

54. Busch M, Soreide E, Lossius HM, Lexow K, Dickstein K. Rapid implementation of therapeutic hypothermia in comatose out-of-hospital cardiac arrest survivors. *Acta Anaesthesiol Scand.* 2006;50:1277–1283.

55. Storm C, Steffen I, Schefold JC, Krueger A, Oppert M, Jorres A, Hasper D. Mild therapeutic hypothermia shortens intensive care unit stay of survivors after out-of-hospital cardiac arrest compared to historical controls. *Crit Care.* 2008;12:R78.

56. Don CW, Longstreth WT Jr, Maynard C, Olsufka M, Nichol G, Ray T, Kupchik N, Deem S, Copass MK, Cobb LA, Kim F. Active surface cooling protocol to induce mild therapeutic hypothermia after out-of-hospital cardiac arrest: a retrospective before-and-after comparison in a single hospital. *Crit Care Med.* 2009;37:3062–3069.

57. Gluckman PD, Wyatt JS, Azzopardi D, Ballard R, Edwards AD, Ferriero DM, Polin RA, Robertson CM, Thoresen M, Whitelaw A, Gunn AJ. Selective head cooling with mild systemic hypothermia after neonatal encephalopathy: multicentre randomised trial. *Lancet.* 2005;365(9460):663–670.

58. Shankaran S, Laptook AR, Ehrenkranz RA, Tyson JE, McDonald SA, Donovan EF, Fanaroff AA, Poole WK, Wright LL, Higgins RD, Finer NN, Carlo WA, Duara S, Oh W, Cotten CM, Stevenson DK, Stoll BJ, Lemons JA, Guillet R, Jobe AH. Whole-body hypothermia for neonates with hypoxic-ischemic encephalopathy. *N Engl J Med.* 2005;353:1574–1584.

59. Azzopardi DV, Strohm B, Edwards AD, Dyet L, Halliday HL, Juszczak E, Kapellou O, Levene M, Marlow N, Porter E, Thoresen M, Whitelaw A, Brocklehurst P. Moderate hypothermia to treat perinatal asphyxial encephalopathy. *N Engl J Med.* 2009;361:1349–1358.

60. Eicher DJ, Wagner CL, Katikaneni LP, Hulsey TC, Bass WT, Kaufman DA, Horgan MJ, Languani S, Bhatia JJ, Givelichian LM, Sankaran K, Yager JY. Moderate hypothermia in neonatal encephalopathy: safety outcomes. *Pediatr Neurol.* 2005;32:18–24.

61. Gluckman PD, Wyatt JS, Azzopardi D, Ballard R, Edwards AD, Ferriero DM, Polin RA, Robertson CM, Thoresen M, Whitelaw A, Gunn AJ. Selective head cooling with mild systemic hypothermia after neonatal encephalopathy: multicentre randomised trial. *Lancet.* 2005;365:663–670.

62. Wijdicks EF, Hijdra A, Young GB, Bassetti CL, Wiebe S. Practice parameter: prediction of outcome in comatose survivors after cardiopulmonary resuscitation (an evidence-based review): report of the Quality Standards Subcommittee of the American Academy of Neurology. *Neurology.* 2006;67:203–210.

63. Rossetti AO, Oddo M, Logroscino G, Kaplan PW. Prognostication after cardiac arrest and hypothermia: a prospective study. *Ann Neurol.* 2010;67:301–307.

64. Leithner C, Ploner CJ, Hasper D, Storm C. Does hypothermia influence the predictive value of bilateral absent N20 after cardiac arrest? *Neurology.* 2010;74:965–969.

65. Smith KK, Gilcreast D, Pierce K. Evaluation of staff's retention of ACLS and BLS skills. *Resuscitation.* 2008;78:59–65.

66. Woollard M, Whitfeild R, Smith A, Colquhoun M, Newcombe RG, Vetteer N, Chamberlain D. Skill acquisition and retention in automated external defibrillator (AED) use and CPR by lay responders: a prospective study. *Resuscitation.* 2004;60:17–28.

67. Spooner BB, Fallaha JF, Kocierz L, Smith CM, Smith SC, Perkins GD. An evaluation of objective feedback in basic life support (BLS) training. *Resuscitation.* 2007;73:417–424.

68. Einspruch EL, Lynch B, Aufderheide TP, Nichol G, Becker L. Retention of CPR skills learned in a traditional AHA Heartsaver course versus 30-min video self-training: a controlled randomized study. *Resuscitation.* 2007;74: 476–486.

69. Roppolo LP, Pepe PE, Campbell L, Ohman K, Kulkarni H, Miller R, Idris A, Bean L, Bettes TN, Idris AH. Prospective, randomized trial of the effectiveness and retention of 30-min layperson training for cardiopulmonary resuscitation and automated external defibrillators: the American Airlines Study. *Resuscitation.* 2007;74:276–285.

70. Berden HJ, Willems FF, Hendrick JM, Pijls NH, Knape JT. How frequently should basic cardiopulmonary resuscitation training be repeated to maintain adequate skills? *BMJ.* 1993;306(6892):1576–1577.

71. Woollard M, Whitfield R, Newcombe RG, Colquhoun M, Vetter N, Chamberlain D. Optimal refresher training intervals for AED and CPR skills: a randomised controlled trial. *Resuscitation.* 2006;71:237–247.

72. Duran R, Aladag N, Vatansever U, Kucukugurluoglu Y, Sut N, Acunas B. Proficiency and knowledge gained and retained by pediatric residents after neonatal resuscitation course. *Pediatr Int.* 2008;50:644–647.

73. Anthonypillai F. Retention of advanced cardiopulmonary resuscitation knowledge by intensive care trained nurses. *Intensive Crit Care Nurs.* 1992;8:180–184.

74. Boonmak P, Boonmak S, Srichaipanha S, Poomsawat S. Knowledge and skill after brief ACLS training. *J Med Assoc Thai.* 2004;87:1311–1314.

75. Kaye W, Wynne G, Marteau T, Dubin HG, Rallis SF, Simons RS, Evans TR. An advanced resuscitation training course for preregistration house officers. *J R Coll Physicians Lond.* 1990;24:51–54.

76. Skidmore MB, Urquhart H. Retention of skills in neonatal resuscitation. *Paediatr Child Health.* 2001;6:31–35.

77. Semeraro F, Signore L, Cerchiari EL. Retention of CPR performance in anaesthetists. *Resuscitation.* 2006;68:101–108.

78. Trevisanuto D, Ferrarese P, Cavicchioli P, Fasson A, Zanardo V, Zacchello F. Knowledge gained by pediatric residents after neonatal resuscitation program courses. *Paediatr Anaesth.* 2005;15:944–947.

79. Young R, King L. An evaluation of knowledge and skill retention following an in-house advanced life support course. *Nurs Crit Care.* 2000;5:7–14.

80. Duran R, Sen F, N A, Vatansever U, Acunaş B. Knowledge gained and retained by neonatal nurses following neonatal resuscitation program course. *Turk Pediatr Ars.* 2007;42:153–155.

81. Grant EC, Marczinski CA, Menon K. Using pediatric advanced life support in pediatric residency training: does the curriculum need resuscitation? *Pediatr Crit Care Med.* 2007;8:433–439.

82. O'Steen DS, Kee CC, Minick MP. The retention of advanced cardiac life support knowledge among registered nurses. *J Nurs Staff Dev.* 1996;12: 66–72.

83. Hammond F, Saba M, Simes T, Cross R. Advanced life support: retention of registered nurses' knowledge 18 months after initial training. *Aust Crit Care.* 2000;13:99–104.

84. Hunziker S, Buhlmann C, Tschan F, Balestra G, Legeret C, Schumacher C, Semmer NK, Hunziker P, Marsch S. Brief leadership instructions improve cardiopulmonary resuscitation in a high-fidelity simulation: a randomized controlled trial. *Crit Care Med.* 2010;38:1086–1091.

85. Thomas EJ, Taggart B, Crandell S, Lasky RE, Williams AL, Love LJ, Sexton JB, Tyson JE, Helmreich RL. Teaching teamwork during the Neonatal Resuscitation Program: a randomized trial. *J Perinatol.* 2007; 27:409–414.

86. Gilfoyle E, Gottesman R, Razack S. Development of a leadership skills workshop in paediatric advanced resuscitation. *Med Teach.* 2007;29: e276–e283.

87. DeVita MA, Schaefer J, Lutz J, Wang H, Dongilli T. Improving medical emergency team (MET) performance using a novel curriculum and a computerized human patient simulator. *Qual Saf Health Care.* 2005;14: 326–331.

88. Makinen M, Aune S, Niemi-Murola L, Herlitz J, Varpula T, Nurmi J, Axelsson AB, Thoren AB, Castren M. Assessment of CPR-D skills of nurses in Goteborg, Sweden and Espoo, Finland: teaching leadership makes a difference. *Resuscitation.* 2007;72:264–269.

89. Morey JC, Simon R, Jay GD, Wears RL, Salisbury M, Dukes KA, Berns SD. Error reduction and performance improvement in the emergency department through formal teamwork training: evaluation results of the MedTeams project. *Health Serv Res.* 2002;37:1553–1581.

90. Rea TD, Cook AJ, Stiell IG, Powell J, Bigham B, Callaway CW, Chugh S, Aufderheide TP, Morrison L, Terndrup TE, Beaudoin T, Wittwer L, Davis D, Idris A, Nichol G. Predicting survival after out-of-hospital cardiac arrest: role of the Utstein data elements. *Ann Emerg Med.* 2010;55:249–257.

91. Feder S, Matheny RL, Loveless RS, Jr, Rea TD. Withholding resuscitation: a new approach to prehospital end-of-life decisions. *Ann Intern Med.* 2006;144:634–640.

92. Kellermann A, Lynn J. Withholding resuscitation in prehospital care. *Ann Intern Med.* 2006;144:692–693.

93. Morrison LJ, Visentin LM, Kiss A, Theriault R, Eby D, Vermeulen M, Sherbino J, Verbeek PR. Validation of a rule for termination of resuscitation in out-of-hospital cardiac arrest. *N Engl J Med.* 2006;355: 478–487.

94. Richman PB, Vadeboncoeur TF, Chikani V, Clark L, Bobrow BJ. Independent evaluation of an out-of-hospital termination of resuscitation (TOR) clinical decision rule. *Acad Emerg Med.* 2008;15:517–521.

95. Morrison LJ, Verbeek PR, Zhan C, Kiss A, Allan KS. Validation of a universal prehospital termination of resuscitation clinical prediction rule for advanced and basic life support providers. *Resuscitation.* 2009;80: 324–328.

96. Ong ME, Jaffey J, Stiell I, Nesbitt L. Comparison of termination-of-resuscitation guidelines for basic life support: defibrillator providers in out-of-hospital cardiac arrest. *Ann Emerg Med.* 2006;47:337–343.

97. Sasson C, Hegg AJ, Macy M, Park A, Kellermann A, McNally B. Prehospital termination of resuscitation in cases of refractory out-of-hospital cardiac arrest. *JAMA.* 2008;300:1432–1438.

98. Ruygrok ML, Byyny RL, Haukoos JS. Validation of 3 termination of resuscitation criteria for good neurologic survival after out-of-hospital cardiac arrest. *Ann Emerg Med.* 2009;54:239–247.

99. Skrifvars MB, Vayrynen T, Kuisma M, Castren M, Parr MJ, Silfverstople J, Svensson L, Jonsson L, Herlitz J. Comparison of Helsinki and European Resuscitation Council "do not attempt to resuscitate" guidelines, and a termination of resuscitation clinical prediction rule for out-of-hospital cardiac arrest patients found in asystole or pulseless electrical activity. *Resuscitation.* 2010;81:679–684.

100. Morrison LJ, Verbeek PR, Vermeulen MJ, Kiss A, Allan KS, Nesbitt L, Stiell I. Derivation and evaluation of a termination of resuscitation clinical prediction rule for advanced life support providers. *Resuscitation.* 2007;74:266–275.

101. De Leeuw R, Cuttini M, Nadai M, Berbik I, Hansen G, Kucinskas A, Lenoir S, Levin A, Persson J, Rebagliato M, Reid M, Schroell M, de Vonderweid U. Treatment choices for extremely preterm infants: an international perspective. *J Pediatr.* 2000;137:608–616.

102. Jain L, Ferre C, Vidyasagar D, Nath S, Sheftel D. Cardiopulmonary resuscitation of apparently stillborn infants: survival and long-term outcome. *J Pediatr.* 1991;118:778–782.

103. Casalaz DM, Marlow N, Speidel BD. Outcome of resuscitation following unexpected apparent stillbirth. *Arch Dis Child Fetal Neonatal Ed.* 1998;78:F112–F115.

104. Laptook AR, Shankaran S, Ambalavanan N, Carlo WA, McDonald SA, Higgins RD, Das A. Outcome of term infants using apgar scores at 10 minutes following hypoxic-ischemic encephalopathy. *Pediatrics.* 2009; 124:1619–1626.

105. Eckstein M, Stratton SJ, Chan LS. Termination of resuscitative efforts for out-of-hospital cardiac arrests. *Acad Emerg Med.* 2005;12:65–70.

106. Weisfeldt ML, Sugarman J, Bandeen-Roche K. Toward definitive trials and improved outcomes of cardiac arrest. *Circulation.* 2010;121: 1586–1588.

107. Sugarman J. Examining the provisions for research without consent in the emergency setting. *Hastings Cent Rep.* 2007;37:12–13.

108. Tisherman SA, Powell JL, Schmidt TA, Aufderheide TP, Kudenchuk PJ, Spence J, Climer D, Kelly D, Marcantonio A, Brown T, Sopko G, Kerber R, Sugarman J, Hoyt D. Regulatory challenges for the resuscitation outcomes consortium. *Circulation.* 2008;118:1585–1592.

109. Dickert NW, Sugarman J. Getting the ethics right regarding research in the emergency setting: lessons from the PolyHeme study. *Kennedy Inst Ethics J.* 2007;17:153–169.

110. White L, Rogers J, Bloomingdale M, Fahrenbruch C, Culley L, Subido C, Eisenberg M, Rea T. Dispatcher-assisted cardiopulmonary resusci-

tation: risks for patients not in cardiac arrest. *Circulation*. 2010;121: 91–97.

111. Cabrini L, Beccaria P, Landoni G, Biondi-Zoccai GG, Sheiban I, Cristofolini M, Fochi O, Maj G, Zangrillo A. Impact of impedance threshold devices on cardiopulmonary resuscitation: a systematic review and meta-analysis of randomized controlled studies. *Crit Care Med*. 2008; 36:1625–1632.

112. Hallstrom A, Rea TD, Sayre MR, Christenson J, Anton AR, Mosesso VN, Jr, Van Ottingham L, Olsufka M, Pennington S, White LJ, Yahn S, Husar J, Morris MF, Cobb LA. Manual chest compression vs use of an automated chest compression device during resuscitation following out-of-hospital cardiac arrest: a randomized trial. *JAMA*. 2006;295: 2620–2628.

112a. Hallstrom A, Rea TD, Sayre MR, Christenson J, Cobb LA, Mosesso VN Jr, Anton AR. The ASPIRE trial investigators respond to inhomogenity and temporal effects assertion. *Am J Emerg Med*. August 16, 2010. doi:10.1016/j.ajem.2010.07.001. Available at: http://www.ajemjournal.com/article/S0735-6757(10)00307-4/fulltext.

113. Paradis N, Young G, Lemeshow S, Brewer J, Halperin H. Inhomogeneity and temporal effects in AutoPulse Assisted Prehospital International Resuscitation—an exception from consent trial terminated early. *Am J Emerg Med*. 2010;28:391–398.

114. Tomte O, Sunde K, Lorem T, Auestad B, Souders C, Jensen J, Wik L. Advanced life support performance with manual and mechanical chest compressions in a randomized, multicentre manikin study. *Resuscitation*. 2009;80:1152–1157.

115. Axelsson C, Nestin J, Svensson L, Axelsson AB, Herlitz J. Clinical consequences of the introduction of mechanical chest compression in the EMS system for treatment of out-of-hospital cardiac arrest-a pilot study. *Resuscitation*. 2006;71:47–55.

116. Larsen AI, Hjornevik AS, Ellingsen CL, Nilsen DW. Cardiac arrest with continuous mechanical chest compression during percutaneous coronary intervention. A report on the use of the LUCAS device. *Resuscitation*. 2007;75:454–459.

117. Deakin CD, O'Neill JF, Tabor T. Does compression-only cardiopulmonary resuscitation generate adequate passive ventilation during cardiac arrest? *Resuscitation*. 2007;75:53–59.

118. Bonnemeier H, Olivecrona G, Simonis G, Gotberg M, Weitz G, Iblher P, Gerling I, Schunkert H. Automated continuous chest compression for in-hospital cardiopulmonary resuscitation of patients with pulseless electrical activity: a report of five cases. *Int J Cardiol*. 2009;136: e39–e50.

119. Wagner H, Terkelsen CJ, Friberg H, Harnek J, Kern K, Lassen JF, Olivecrona GK. Cardiac arrest in the catheterisation laboratory: a 5-year experience of using mechanical chest compressions to facilitate PCI during prolonged resuscitation efforts. *Resuscitation*. 2010;81:383–387.

120. Larsen MP, Eisenberg MS, Cummins RO, Hallstrom AP. Predicting survival from out-of-hospital cardiac arrest: a graphic model. *Ann Emerg Med*. 1993;22:1652–1658.

121. Valenzuela TD, Roe DJ, Cretin S, Spaite DW, Larsen MP. Estimating effectiveness of cardiac arrest interventions: a logistic regression survival model. *Circulation*. 1997;96:3308–3313.

122. Swor RA, Jackson RE, Cynar M, Sadler E, Basse E, Boji B, Rivera-Rivera EJ, Maher A, Grubb W, Jacobson R, et al. Bystander CPR, ventricular fibrillation, and survival in witnessed, unmonitored out-of-hospital cardiac arrest. *Ann Emerg Med*. 1995;25:780–784.

123. Cobb LA, Fahrenbruch CE, Walsh TR, Copass MK, Olsufka M, Breskin M, Hallstrom AP. Influence of cardiopulmonary resuscitation prior to defibrillation in patients with out-of-hospital ventricular fibrillation. *JAMA*. 1999;281:1182–1188.

124. Wik L, Hansen TB, Fylling F, Steen T, Vaagenes P, Auestad BH, Steen PA. Delaying defibrillation to give basic cardiopulmonary resuscitation to patients with out-of-hospital ventricular fibrillation: a randomized trial. *JAMA*. 2003;289:1389–1395.

125. Baker PW, Conway J, Cotton C, Ashby DT, Smyth J, Woodman RJ, Grantham H. Defibrillation or cardiopulmonary resuscitation first for patients with out-of-hospital cardiac arrests found by paramedics to be in ventricular fibrillation? A randomised control trial. *Resuscitation*. 2008; 79:424–431.

126. Jacobs IG, Finn JC, Oxer HF, Jelinek GA. CPR before defibrillation in out-of-hospital cardiac arrest: a randomized trial. *Emerg Med Australas*. 2005;17:39–45.

127. Morrison LJ, Dorian P, Long J, Vermeulen M, Schwartz B, Sawadsky B, Frank J, Cameron B, Burgess R, Shield J, Bagley P, Mausz V, Brewer JE, Lerman BB. Out-of-hospital cardiac arrest rectilinear biphasic to

128. Schneider T, Martens PR, Paschen H, Kuisma M, Wolcke B, Gliner BE, Russell JK, Weaver WD, Bossaert L, Chamberlain D. Multicenter, randomized, controlled trial of 150-J biphasic shocks compared with 200- to 360-J monophasic shocks in the resuscitation of out-of-hospital cardiac arrest victims. Optimized Response to Cardiac Arrest (ORCA) Investigators. *Circulation*. 2000;102:1780–1787.

129. van Alem AP, Chapman FW, Lank P, Hart AA, Koster RW. A prospective, randomised and blinded comparison of first shock success of monophasic and biphasic waveforms in out-of-hospital cardiac arrest. *Resuscitation*. 2003;58:17–24.

130. Carpenter J, Rea TD, Murray JA, Kudenchuk PJ, Eisenberg MS. Defibrillation waveform and post-shock rhythm in out-of-hospital ventricular fibrillation cardiac arrest. *Resuscitation*. 2003;59:189–196.

131. Freeman K, Hendey GW, Shalit M, Stroh G. Biphasic defibrillation does not improve outcomes compared to monophasic defibrillation in out-of-hospital cardiac arrest. *Prehosp Emerg Care*. 2008;12:152–156.

132. Gliner BE, White RD. Electrocardiographic evaluation of defibrillation shocks delivered to out-of-hospital sudden cardiac arrest patients. *Resuscitation*. 1999;41:133–144.

133. White RD, Hankins DG, Bugliosi TF. Seven years' experience with early defibrillation by police and paramedics in an emergency medical services system. *Resuscitation*. 1998;39:145–151.

134. Cummins RO, Eisenberg MS, Bergner L, Hallstrom A, Hearne T, Murray JA. Automatic external defibrillation: evaluations of its role in the home and in emergency medical services. *Ann Emerg Med*. 1984;13(pt 2):798–801.

135. White RD, Vukov LF, Bugliosi TF. Early defibrillation by police: initial experience with measurement of critical time intervals and patient outcome. *Ann Emerg Med*. 1994;23:1009–1013.

136. Mittal S, Ayati S, Stein KM, Schwartzman D, Cavlovich D, Tchou PJ, Markowitz SM, Slotwiner DJ, Scheiner MA, Lerman BB. Transthoracic cardioversion of atrial fibrillation: comparison of rectilinear biphasic versus damped sine wave monophasic shocks. *Circulation*. 2000;101: 1282–1287.

137. Page RL, Kerber RE, Russell JK, Trouton T, Waktare J, Gallik D, Olgin JE, Ricard P, Dalzell GW, Reddy R, Lazzara R, Lee K, Carlson M, Halperin B, Bardy GH. Biphasic versus monophasic shock waveform for conversion of atrial fibrillation: the results of an international randomized, double-blind multicenter trial. *J Am Coll Cardiol*. 2002;39: 1956–1963.

138. Scholten M, Szili-Torok T, Klootwijk P, Jordaens L. Comparison of monophasic and biphasic shocks for transthoracic cardioversion of atrial fibrillation. *Heart*. 2003;89:1032–1034.

139. Glover BM, Walsh SJ, McCann CJ, Moore MJ, Manoharan G, Dalzell GW, McAllister A, McClements B, McEneaney DJ, Trouton TG, Mathew TP, Adgey AA. Biphasic energy selection for transthoracic cardioversion of atrial fibrillation. The BEST AF Trial. *Heart*. 2008;94: 884–887.

140. Reisinger J, Gstrein C, Winter T, Zeindlhofer E, Hollinger K, Mori M, Schiller A, Winter A, Geiger H, Siostrzonek P. Optimization of initial energy for cardioversion of atrial tachyarrhythmias with biphasic shocks. *Am J Emerg Med*. 2010;28:159–165.

141. Kerber RE, Martins JB, Kienzle MG, Constantin L, Olshansky B, Hopson R, Charbonnier F. Energy, current, and success in defibrillation and cardioversion: clinical studies using an automated impedance-based method of energy adjustment. *Circulation*. 1988;77:1038–1046.

142. Hedges JR, Syverud SA, Dalsey WC, Feero S, Easter R, Shultz B. Prehospital trial of emergency transcutaneous cardiac pacing. *Circulation*. 1987;76:1337–1343.

143. Barthell E, Troiano P, Olson D, Stueven HA, Hendley G. Prehospital external cardiac pacing: a prospective, controlled clinical trial. *Ann Emerg Med*. 1988;17:1221–1226.

144. Cummins RO, Graves JR, Larsen MP, Hallstrom AP, Hearne TR, Ciliberti J, Nicola RM, Horan S. Out-of-hospital transcutaneous pacing by emergency medical technicians in patients with asystolic cardiac arrest. *N Engl J Med*. 1993;328:1377–1382.

145. Smith I, Monk TG, White PF. Comparison of transesophageal atrial pacing with anticholinergic drugs for the treatment of intraoperative bradycardia. *Anesth Analg*. 1994;78:245–252.

146. Morrison LJ, Long J, Vermeulen M, Schwartz B, Sawadsky B, Frank J, Cameron B, Burgess R, Shield J, Bagley P, Mausz V, Brewer JE, Dorian P. A randomized controlled feasibility trial comparing safety and effec-

tiveness of prehospital pacing versus conventional treatment: 'PrePACE.' *Resuscitation.* 2008;76:341–349.

147. Karagounis L, Ipsen SK, Jessop MR, Gilmore KM, Valenti DA, Clawson JJ, Teichman S, Anderson JL. Impact of field-transmitted electrocardiography on time to in-hospital thrombolytic therapy in acute myocardial infarction. *Am J Cardiol.* 1990;66:786–791.

148. Kereiakes DJ, Gibler WB, Martin LH, Pieper KS, Anderson LC. Relative importance of emergency medical system transport and the prehospital electrocardiogram on reducing hospital time delay to therapy for acute myocardial infarction: a preliminary report from the Cincinnati Heart Project. *Am Heart J.* 1992;123(4 Pt 1):835–840.

149. Banerjee S, Rhoden WE. Fast-tracking of myocardial infarction by paramedics. *J R Coll Physicians Lond.* 1998;32:36–38.

150. Melville MR, Gray D, Hinchley M. The potential impact of prehospital electrocardiography and telemetry on time to thrombolysis in a United Kingdom center. *Ann Noninvasive Electrocardiol.* 1998;3:327–332.

151. Millar-Craig MW, Joy AV, Adamowicz M, Furber R, Thomas B. Reduction in treatment delay by paramedic ECG diagnosis of myocardial infarction with direct CCU admission. *Heart.* 1997;78:456–461.

152. Brainard AH, Raynovich W, Tandberg D, Bedrick EJ. The prehospital 12-lead electrocardiogram's effect on time to initiation of reperfusion therapy: a systematic review and meta-analysis of existing literature. *Am J Emerg Med.* 2005;23:351–356.

153. Morrison LJ, Brooks S, Sawadsky B, McDonald A, Verbeek PR. Prehospital 12-lead electrocardiography impact on acute myocardial infarction treatment times and mortality: a systematic review. *Acad Emerg Med.* 2006;13:84–89.

154. Adams GL, Campbell PT, Adams JM, Strauss DG, Wall K, Patterson J, Shuping KB, Maynard C, Young D, Corey C, Thompson A, Lee BA, Wagner GS. Effectiveness of prehospital wireless transmission of electrocardiograms to a cardiologist via hand-held device for patients with acute myocardial infarction (from the Timely Intervention in Myocardial Emergency, NorthEast Experience [TIME-NE]). *Am J Cardiol.* 2006;98:1160–1164.

155. Afolabi BA, Novaro GM, Pinski SL, Fromkin KR, Bush HS. Use of the prehospital ECG improves door-to-balloon times in ST segment elevation myocardial infarction irrespective of time of day or day of week. *Emerg Med J.* 2007;24:588–591.

156. Terkelsen CJ, Lassen JF, Norgaard BL, Gerdes JC, Poulsen SH, Bendix K, Ankersen JP, Gotzsche LB, Romer FK, Nielsen TT, Andersen HR. Reduction of treatment delay in patients with ST-elevation myocardial infarction: impact of pre-hospital diagnosis and direct referral to primary percutaneous coronary intervention. *Eur Heart J.* 2005;26:770–777.

157. Wall T, Albright J, Livingston B, Isley L, Young D, Nanny M, Jacobowitz S, Maynard C, Mayer N, Pierce K, Rathbone C, Stuckey T, Savona M, Leibrandt P, Brodie B, Wagner G. Prehospital ECG transmission speeds reperfusion for patients with acute myocardial infarction. *N C Med J.* 2000;61:104–108.

158. Dhruva VN, Abdelhadi SI, Anis A, Gluckman W, Hom D, Dougan W, Kaluski E, Haider B, Klapholz M. ST-Segment Analysis Using Wireless Technology in Acute Myocardial Infarction (STAT-MI) trial. *J Am Coll Cardiol.* 2007;50:509–513.

159. Sekulic M, Hassunizadeh B, McGraw S, David S. Feasibility of early emergency room notification to improve door-to-balloon times for patients with acute ST segment elevation myocardial infarction. *Catheter Cardiovasc Interv.* 2005;66:316–319.

160. Swor R, Hegerberg S, McHugh-McNally A, Goldstein M, McEachin CC. Prehospital 12-lead ECG: efficacy or effectiveness? *Prehosp Emerg Care.* 2006;10:374–377.

161. Campbell PT, Patterson J, Cromer D, Wall K, Adams GL, Albano A, Corey C, Fox P, Gardner J, Hawthorne B, Lipton J, Sejersten M, Thompson A, Wilfong S, Maynard C, Wagner G. Prehospital triage of acute myocardial infarction: wireless transmission of electrocardiograms to the on-call cardiologist via a handheld computer. *J Electrocardiol.* 2005;38:300–309.

162. Lopez-Herce J, Garcia C, Dominguez P, Carrillo A, Rodriguez-Nunez A, Calvo C, Delgado MA. Characteristics and outcome of cardiorespiratory arrest in children. *Resuscitation.* 2004;63:311–320.

163. Rodriguez-Nunez A, Lopez-Herce J, Garcia C, Dominguez P, Carrillo A, Bellon JM. Pediatric defibrillation after cardiac arrest: initial response and outcome. *Crit Care.* 2006;10:R113.

164. Berg RA, Hilwig RW, Kern KB, Babar I, Ewy GA. Simulated mouth-to-mouth ventilation and chest compressions (bystander cardiopulmonary resuscitation) improves outcome in a swine model of prehospital pediatric asphyxial cardiac arrest. *Crit Care Med.* 1999;27:1893–1899.

165. Berg RA, Hilwig RW, Kern KB, Ewy GA. "Bystander" chest compressions and assisted ventilation independently improve outcome from piglet asphyxial pulseless "cardiac arrest." *Circulation.* 2000;101:1743–1748.

166. Iglesias JM, Lopez-Herce J, Urbano J, Solana MJ, Mencia S, Del Castillo J. Chest compressions versus ventilation plus chest compressions in a pediatric asphyxial cardiac arrest animal model. *Intensive Care Med.* 2010;36:712–716.

167. Tibballs J, Weeranatna C. The influence of time on the accuracy of healthcare personnel to diagnose paediatric cardiac arrest by pulse palpation. *Resuscitation.* 2010;81:671–675.

168. Billi JE, Zideman DA, Eigel B, Nolan JP, Montgomery WH, Nadkarni VM; from the International Liaison Committee on Resuscitation and the American Heart Association. Conflict of interest management before, during, and after the 2005 International Consensus Conference on Cardiopulmonary Resuscitation and Emergency Cardiovascular Care Science With Treatment Recommendations. *Circulation.* 2005;112(22suppl):III 131–132.

169. Billi JE, Eigel B, Montgomery WH, Nadkarni VM, Hazinski MF. Management of conflict of interest issues in the activities of the American Heart Association Emergency Cardiovascular Care Committee, 2000–2005. *Circulation.* 2005;112(24 Suppl):IV204–205.

170. Billi JE, Shuster M, Bossaert L, de Caen AR, Deakin CD, Eigel B, Hazinski MF, Hickey RW, Jacobs I, Kleinman ME, Koster RW, Mancini ME, Montgomery WH, Morley PT, Morrison LJ, Munoz H, Nadkarni VM, Nolan JP, O'Connor RE, Perlman JM, Richmond S, Sayre MR, Soar J, Wyllie J, Zideman D; for the International Liaison Committee on Resuscitation and the American Heart Association. Part 4: conflict of interest management before, during, and after the 2010 International Consensus on Cardiopulmonary Resuscitation and Emergency Cardiovascular Care Science With Treatment Recommendations. *Circulation.* 2010;122(suppl 2):S291–S297.

KEY WORDS: cardiac arrest ■ cardiopulmonary resuscitation ■ emergency ■ resuscitation

# Part 2: Evidence Evaluation and Management of Potential or Perceived Conflicts of Interest

## 2010 American Heart Association Guidelines for Cardiopulmonary Resuscitation and Emergency Cardiovascular Care

Michael R. Sayre, Co-Chair*; Robert E. O'Connor, Co-Chair*; Dianne L. Atkins; John E. Billi; Clifton W. Callaway; Michael Shuster; Brian Eigel; William H. Montgomery; Robert W. Hickey; Ian Jacobs; Vinay M. Nadkarni; Peter T. Morley; Tanya I. Semenko; Mary Fran Hazinski

Evidence-based medicine integrates the best available evidence and clinical expertise to deliver the finest possible patient care.[1] The victim of cardiac arrest requires immediate action, and potential rescuers must be ready to respond. Evidence must be compiled, analyzed, and discussed; clear recommendations must be established prior to the patient encounter. The *2010 American Heart Association (AHA) Guidelines for Cardiopulmonary Resuscitation (CPR) and Emergency Cardiovascular Care (ECC) (2010 AHA Guidelines for CPR and ECC)* are based on a transparent, expert review of scientific evidence, informed by the clinical expertise of the writing teams. These guidelines are designed to provide rescuers and clinicians with a strategy for action that can save lives from cardiac arrest. Clinicians should always apply these evidence-based guidelines in combination with clinical judgment.

The International Liaison Committee on Resuscitation (ILCOR), an international consortium of many of the world's resuscitation councils, was formed in 1992, in part to collect, discuss, and debate scientific data on resuscitation. The majority of ILCOR's work focuses on reviewing published, peer-reviewed evidence on resuscitation to produce science-based consensus summaries.[2] As one of ILCOR's member councils, the AHA transforms international scientific consensus statements into periodic revisions of the *AHA Guidelines for CPR and ECC.*

During production of the 1992 *AHA Guidelines for CPR and ECC,* an evidence evaluation process was developed to guide topic experts in conducting a thorough evidence review, distilling the evidence, and producing treatment recommendations. This evidence evaluation process was revised in 2000, when an international set of CPR and ECC guidelines was developed. The evidence evaluation process was refined for the creation of the *2005 International Consensus on Cardiopulmonary Resuscitation and Emergency Cardiovascular Care Science With Treatment Recommendations*

*(ILCOR 2005 CPR Consensus).*[3] For the *2010 AHA Guidelines for CPR and ECC,* the process was further refined, and a comprehensive description of the 2010 process has been published.[4] The purpose of this chapter is to briefly describe this evidence evaluation process and its translation to the *2010 AHA Guidelines for CPR and ECC.*

## Evidence Evaluation Process

To begin the 2010 review process, ILCOR representatives established six task forces: basic life support; advanced life support; acute coronary syndromes; pediatric life support; neonatal life support; and a task force for education, implementation, and teams. The AHA established two additional task forces that were not part of the ILCOR process, one for stroke and one for first aid. Two co-chairs were recruited for each task force to oversee the processes of evidence evaluation and consensus development. For most task forces, one co-chair was recruited from the AHA and the other from the international resuscitation councils. Within the advanced life support (ALS) task force, five domain subgroups were created: electrical therapy, CPR and airway devices, drugs, special situations, and post–cardiac arrest care. The ALS co-chairs designated leaders for these domains to direct completion of the evidence reviews. Three worksheet experts (Atkins, Callaway, and Jacobs) and one evidence evaluation expert (Morley) were recruited to oversee the evidence evaluation worksheets, review the search strategies, ensure correct assignment of levels of evidence (LOE), and verify completeness. The lead evidence evaluation expert, trained in the Cochrane methodology and experienced in the CPR and ECC evidence evaluation process, and the three similarly trained worksheet experts shepherded individual evidence evaluation worksheet authors through the established ILCOR process.

The process included the appointment of two co-chairs (Billi and Shuster) to review conflict of interest (COI)

---

The American Heart Association requests that this document be cited as follows: Sayre MR, O'Connor RE, Atkins DL, Billi JE, Callaway CW, Shuster M, Eigel B, Montgomery WH, Hickey RW, Jacobs I, Nadkarni VM, Morley PT, Semenko TI, Hazinski MF. Part 2: evidence evaluation and management of potential or perceived conflicts of interest: 2010 American Heart Association Guidelines for Cardiopulmonary Resuscitation and Emergency Cardiovascular Care. *Circulation.* 2010;122(suppl 3):S657–S664.

*Co-chairs and equal first co-authors.

**(*Circulation***. 2010;122[suppl 3]:S657–S664.)

*Circulation* is available at http://circ.ahajournals.org

DOI: 10.1161/CIRCULATIONAHA.110.966861

**Table 1. Population, Intervention, Control, Outcome (PICO) Question Examples**

| Type of Question | Example Question in PICO Format |
|---|---|
| Outcome | In adult patients in cardiac arrest (asystole, pulseless electrical activity, pulseless VT and VF) (prehospital or in-hospital) (P), does the use of vasopressors (epinephrine, norepinephrine, others) or combination of vasopressors (I) compared with not using drugs (or a standard drug regimen) (C), improve outcomes (e.g. ROSC, survival) (O)? |
| Diagnosis | In adult and pediatric patients with presumed cardiac arrest (prehospital or in-hospital) (P), are there any factors (eg, on clinical exam) (I), as opposed to standard care (C), that increase the likelihood of diagnosing cardiac arrest (as opposed to nonarrest conditions, eg, post-seizure, hypoglycemia, intoxication) (O)? |
| Prognosis | In adult cardiac arrest (prehospital or in-hospital) (P), does the use of end-tidal $CO_2$ (eg, absolute $CO_2$ values or changes in waveform) (I), compared with not using end-tidal $CO_2$ (C), accurately predict outcomes (e.g. ROSC, survival) (O)? |

disclosures and to manage COI issues. All task force members and co-chairs completed rigorous COI disclosures, and potential conflicts were managed as noted below.

To begin the process, the evidence evaluation expert updated the 2005 evidence review worksheet for use in the 2010 process. The template was designed to facilitate the structured evidence reviews for the production of the final consensus on science and treatment recommendation documents. Successful completion of the evidence evaluation worksheet was required to ensure consistent application of the process by many different worksheet authors from around the world.

## Use of PICO Format
Shortly after the *2005 AHA Guidelines for CPR and ECC* were published, the task forces generated a comprehensive list of questions for evidence evaluation. Questions were selected based on controversy, new information, and previously identified knowledge gaps.[5] The clinical questions posed during the 2005 guidelines process and the knowledge gaps identified during the 2005 Consensus on Science process provided the initial basis for this list, which was supplemented during in-person meetings and conference calls among the task forces. Questions were then refined to fit the Population Intervention Comparator Outcome (PICO) format (see Table 1 for examples).[6]

The task forces selected and invited topic experts from around the world to serve as evidence evaluation worksheet authors. Specialty organizations were also solicited to suggest potential worksheet authors. The qualifications of each worksheet author were reviewed by the task force, and potential conflicts of interest were disclosed and evaluated by the task force co-chairs and COI co-chairs. Worksheet authors could not have any significant COI issues pertaining to their assigned worksheet. If a COI was identified, the topic was assigned to a different worksheet author. Generally two authors were invited to complete independent reviews of each

PICO question. A total of 356 worksheet authors from 29 countries completed 411 evidence reviews on 277 topics.

After generating formal search strategies directly from the PICO questions, the worksheet authors searched, at a minimum, four databases: the Cochrane Library (The Cochrane Collaboration, Oxford, England), PubMed (National Library of Medicine, Washington, DC), Embase (Elsevier B.V., Amsterdam, Netherlands), and an internal database of articles constructed from previous ILCOR and ILCOR council CPR guidelines development cycles. Worksheet authors were asked to review the references cited in key articles to identify other relevant articles, and authors were encouraged to review any articles that cited the key studies found. Worksheet authors then submitted their search strategies, criteria for inclusion and exclusion of articles, and initial search results for review by the task force co-chairs, worksheet experts, and an evidence evaluation expert before initiating their literature review. If necessary, the search strategy was modified and repeated based on feedback from the reviewers. The complete search strategy was documented in the evidence evaluation worksheet; this process provided transparency and enabled the worksheet authors to use the same strategy to update the literature search just prior to the 2010 Consensus Conference. Articles could be included in the evidence review only if the full manuscript was published or accepted for publication in a peer-reviewed journal. Abstracts and unpublished data were excluded.

## Classification of Evidence
After a search strategy was approved, worksheet authors identified and reviewed each relevant study. Each relevant study was assigned both a numeric level of evidence (LOE) and a quality of evidence. The numeric LOE classification system was updated from the system used for the 2005 process based on a review of available classification schemes (see Table 2). The levels of evidence were reduced from seven categories in 2005 to five in 2010 (see Table 3). The LOEs were subdivided into three major categories, depending on the type of question being asked: intervention, diagnosis, or prognosis. The quality of evidence categories were reduced from five categories in 2005 to three (good, fair, poor) in 2010.

Several characteristics within each LOE were defined to guide the worksheet authors. Examples included methods of randomization, blinding, similarity of groups, and equal treatment of all groups. Complete instructions for both LOE and quality of evidence were provided to the worksheet authors.[7] Worksheet authors also created a short summary of each article including the LOE, quality of evidence, direction of outcome effect for the question asked (supporting, neutral, or opposing), and outcome measured. Worksheet authors also noted industry support for the study and wrote a one- or two-sentence synopsis.

## Worksheet Author Summary
The worksheet authors summarized the evidence in a form similar to that typically used in published systematic reviews, using the evidence evaluation worksheet "grid" to position relevant studies in three dimensions: LOE, Quality, and

**Table 2.**    **ILCOR Levels of Evidence**

| Studies of Interventions | Studies of Prognostic Tests | Studies of Diagnostic Tests | Level of AHA Recommendation |
|---|---|---|---|
| LOE 1: Randomized controlled trials (RCTs) or meta-analyses of RCTs | LOE P1: Inception (prospective) cohort studies (or meta-analyses of inception cohort studies), or validation of Clinical Decision Rule (CDR) | LOE D1: Validating cohort studies (or meta-analyses of validating cohort studies), or validation of Clinical Decision Rule (CDR) | Level A |
| LOE 2: Studies using concurrent controls without true randomization (e.g. "pseudo"-randomized) | LOE P2: Follow-up of untreated control groups in RCTs (or meta-analyses of follow-up studies), or derivation of CDR, or validated on split-sample only | LOE D2: Exploratory cohort study (or meta-analyses of follow-up studies), or derivation of CDR, or a CDR validated on a split-sample only | Level B |
| LOE 3: Studies using retrospective controls | LOE P3: Retrospective cohort studies | LOE D3: Diagnostic case control study | Level B |
| LOE 4: Studies without a control group (eg, case series) | LOE P4: Case series | LOE D4: Study of diagnostic yield (no reference standard) | Level C |
| LOE 5: Studies not directly related to the specific patient/population (eg, different patient/population, animal models, mechanical models etc.) | LOE P5: Studies not directly related to the specific patient/population (eg, different patient/population, animal models, mechanical models etc.) | LOE D5: Studies not directly related to the specific patient/population (eg, different patient/population, animal models, mechanical models etc.) | Level C |
| Expert Opinion | Expert Opinion | Expert Opinion | Level C |

Direction of Effect. In the later section of the worksheet template, authors summarized the evidence, noting merits and shortcomings of the published literature. Finally the worksheet authors proposed draft Consensus on Science statements and draft Treatment Recommendations.

## Evidence Evaluation Expert and Task Force Reviews

Several iterative reviews were completed for each worksheet. As noted above, the search strategies were first reviewed by the task force co-chairs and worksheet experts to confirm accuracy and completeness. Once the search strategy was approved, the worksheet authors independently performed the evidence evaluation. The evidence evaluation was again reviewed by the task force co-chairs and the worksheet experts, and the authors were asked to offer revisions when necessary. The evidence evaluation expert approved each final worksheet. For evidence reviews completed earlier than August 2009, the literature search was repeated just prior to the February 2010 ILCOR International Consensus on CPR and ECC Science With Treatment Recommendations Conference so that any new publications could be identified and then incorporated into the final worksheet.

From 2007 to 2010, the worksheet authors summarized their evidence evaluation for the task force using a standardized presentation format, either during one of six international

face-to-face meetings or during Web conferences using Microsoft Live Meeting collaboration software. Task force co-chairs occasionally asked worksheet authors who reviewed the same question to work together after their initial review, either to reconcile different interpretations of the scientific evidence or to consider studies identified by only one author. During those meetings and Web conferences, the task forces debated and discussed the evidence presented by the worksheet authors and developed final Task Force Consensus on Science and Treatment Recommendations statements. Starting in May 2009, worksheets approved by the task forces were posted on the Internet for external review and comments from the broader resuscitation community.[7] Authors of comments disclosed conflicts of interest, if any, and the task forces and worksheet authors carefully considered those comments.

## 2010 International Consensus on Science Conference

Reviews culminated in the 2010 Consensus Conference held in Dallas, TX, in February 2010. A total of 313 international experts from 30 countries attended the conference to discuss and debate the evidence evaluation reviews presented by invited worksheet authors and experts. The program provided ample time for open discussion of each topic with the audience. Prior to the meeting, each participant completed an AHA Conflict of Interest (COI) Form. Whenever anyone spoke, whether that person was speaking as a scheduled presenter, panelist, or moderator or was asking questions or making comments from the floor, the speaker's COI disclosure was projected on a screen separate from the screen used to display presentation slides.

Immediately following the conference, ILCOR Consensus on Science writing groups compiled, discussed, reviewed and edited the draft Consensus on Science and Treatment Recommendations statements of the task forces to create the *2010 ILCOR International Consensus on CPR and ECC Science With Treatment Recommendations*, published simultaneously in *Circulation*[8] and *Resuscitation*.[9] If the writing groups

**Table 3.**    **Comparison of ILCOR Levels of Evidence for 2005 and 2010**

| Type of Evidence | 2005 Level | 2010 Level |
|---|---|---|
| Randomized clinical trials | 1 or 2 | 1 |
| Meta-analyses | 1 | 1 or 2 |
| Concurrent controls | 3 | 2 |
| Retrospective controls | 4 | 3 |
| Case series without controls | 5 | 4 |
| Animal/mechanical/model | 6 | 5 |
| Extrapolations from data collected for other purposes; theoretical analyses | 7 | 5 |

**Table 4.    AHA Levels of Evidence[10]**

| ESTIMATE OF CERTAINTY (PRECISION) OF TREATMENT EFFECT | | SIZE OF TREATMENT EFFECT → | | | |
|---|---|---|---|---|---|
| | | **CLASS I**<br>*Benefit >>> Risk*<br>**Procedure/Treatment SHOULD be performed/administered** | **CLASS IIa**<br>*Benefit >> Risk*<br>*Additional studies with focused objectives needed*<br>**IT IS REASONABLE to perform procedure/administer treatment** | **CLASS IIb**<br>*Benefit ≥ Risk*<br>*Additional studies with broad objectives needed; additional registry data would be helpful*<br>**Procedure/Treatment MAY BE CONSIDERED** | **CLASS III**<br>*Risk ≥ Benefit*<br>**Procedure/Treatment should NOT be performed/administered SINCE IT IS NOT HELPFUL AND MAY BE HARMFUL** |
| | **LEVEL A**<br>Multiple populations evaluated*<br>Data derived from multiple randomized clinical trials or meta-analyses | ■ Recommendation that procedure or treatment is useful/effective<br>■ Sufficient evidence from multiple randomized trials or meta-analyses | ■ Recommendation in favor of treatment or procedure being useful/effective<br>■ Some conflicting evidence from multiple randomized trials or meta-analyses | ■ Recommendation's usefulness/efficacy less well established<br>■ Greater conflicting evidence from multiple randomized trials or meta-analyses | ■ Recommendation that procedure or treatment is not useful/effective and may be harmful<br>■ Sufficient evidence from multiple randomized trials or meta-analyses |
| | **LEVEL B**<br>Limited populations evaluated*<br>Data derived from a single randomized trial or nonrandomized studies | ■ Recommendation that procedure or treatment is useful/effective<br>■ Evidence from single randomized trial or nonrandomized studies | ■ Recommendation in favor of treatment or procedure being useful/effective<br>■ Some conflicting evidence from single randomized trial or nonrandomized studies | ■ Recommendation's usefulness/efficacy less well established<br>■ Greater conflicting evidence from single randomized trial or nonrandomized studies | ■ Recommendation that procedure or treatment is not useful/effective and may be harmful<br>■ Evidence from single randomized trial or nonrandomized studies |
| | **LEVEL C**<br>Very limited populations evaluated*<br>Only consensus opinion of experts, case studies, or standard of care | ■ Recommendation that procedure or treatment is useful/effective<br>■ Only expert opinion, case studies, or standard of care | ■ Recommendation in favor of treatment or procedure being useful/effective<br>■ Only diverging expert opinion, case studies, or standard of care | ■ Recommendation's usefulness/efficacy less well established<br>■ Only diverging expert opinion, case studies, or standard of care | ■ Recommendation that procedure or treatment is not useful/effective and may be harmful<br>■ Only expert opinion, case studies, or standard of care |
| | Suggested phrases for writing recommendations† | should<br>is recommended<br>is indicated<br>is useful/effective/beneficial | is reasonable<br>can be useful/effective/beneficial<br>is probably recommended<br> or indicated | may/might be considered<br>may/might be reasonable<br>usefulness/effectiveness is<br>unknown/unclear/uncertain<br>or not well established | is not recommended<br>is not indicated<br>should not<br>is not useful/effective/beneficial<br>may be harmful |

*Data available from clinical trials or registries about the usefulness/efficacy in different subpopulations, such as gender, age, history of diabetes, history of prior myocardial infarction, history of heart failure, and prior aspirin use. A recommendation with Level of Evidence B or C does not imply that the recommendation is weak. Many important clinical questions addressed in the guidelines do not lend themselves to clinical trials. Even though randomized trials are not available, there may be a very clear clinical consensus that a particular test or therapy is useful or effective.

†In 2003, the ACCF/AHA Task Force on Practice Guidelines developed a list of suggested phrases to use when writing recommendations. All guideline recommendations have been written in full sentences that express a complete thought, such that a recommendation, even if separated and presented apart from the rest of the document (including headings above sets of recommendations), would still convey the full intent of the recommendation. It is hoped that this will increase readers' comprehension of the guidelines and will allow queries at the individual recommendation level.

agreed on common treatment recommendations, those recommendations were included with the Consensus on Science statements.

## Development of the AHA Guidelines

### AHA Writing Groups

In 2009 the chairs and writing group members for each chapter of the *2010 AHA Guidelines for CPR and ECC* were nominated and required to complete an AHA conflict of interest disclosure that was reviewed by AHA staff and the AHA officers. Writing group chairs and most of the writing group members were required to be free of relevant conflicts of interest.

After the 2010 Consensus Conference, seventeen AHA writing groups developed the *2010 AHA Guidelines for CPR and ECC* based on the ILCOR Consensus on Science state-

ments, citations, and treatment recommendations. In essence, the *2010 ILCOR International Consensus on CPR and ECC Science With Treatment Recommendations* summarizes what is known in each subject area. The ILCOR Treatment Recommendations present the evidence-supported treatment approach for each problem. The *2010 AHA Guidelines for CPR and ECC* expand on the details of how and when to provide treatment, and they address the training requirements for treatment providers. Other resuscitation councils around the world performed a similar process to develop their versions of the 2010 guidelines.

In developing these guidelines, the writing groups used a recommendation system consistent with that used by the American College of Cardiology Foundation/American Heart Association (ACCF/AHA) collaboration on evidence-based guidelines (see Table 4).[10] These classes represent the integration of the weight of scientific evidence with contextual factors such as expert assessment of the magnitude of benefit, usefulness, or efficacy; cost; educational and training challenges; and difficulties in implementation.

## AHA Classes of Recommendations and Levels of Evidence

Generally for Class I recommendations, high-level prospective studies support the action or therapy, and the benefit substantially outweighs the potential for harm. An exception is possible for actions or therapies with extraordinarily large treatment effects for which expert consensus alone may suffice.[11] Under ideal conditions all CPR and ECC recommendations should be based on large, prospective, randomized, controlled clinical trials that find substantial treatment effects on long-term survival and carry a Class I label. In reality, more questions exist than there are studies attempting to answer them; and when studies have been done, they are not typically large, randomized trials on human subjects. As a result, the writing groups were often confronted with the need to make recommendations based on results from human trials that reported only intermediate outcomes, nonrandomized or retrospective observational studies, animal models, or extrapolations from studies of human subjects who were not in cardiac arrest.

For Class IIa recommendations, the weight of available evidence supports the action or therapy, and the therapy is considered reasonable and generally useful. Recommendations were generally labeled Class IIb when the evidence documented only short-term benefits from the therapy or weakly positive or mixed results. Class IIb recommendations are identified by terms such as "can be considered" or "may be useful" or "usefulness/effectiveness is unknown or unclear or not well established."

Class III recommendations were reserved for interventions for which the available evidence suggests more harm than good, and experts agreed that the intervention should be avoided.

"Class Indeterminate" recommendations, which were used in 2005, are not included in the *2010 AHA Guidelines for CPR and ECC*. The elimination of the term "Class Indeterminate" is consistent with the ACCF–AHA Classes of Recommendation. When the AHA writing groups felt that the evidence was insufficient to offer a recommendation either for or against the use of a drug or intervention, no recommendation was given.

The Levels of Evidence used by the ACCF/AHA Task Force on Practice Guidelines employs an alphabetic system (LOE A, B, or C) to describe the body of evidence supporting a given recommendation, in comparison to the numeric system used for the ILCOR evidence evaluation. Generally a level-A body of evidence means there are 2 or more ILCOR LOE 1 studies in support of the recommendation: multiple populations have been evaluated, or data are derived from multiple randomized clinical trials or meta-analyses. A level-B body of evidence indicates that most studies supporting the recommendation are ILCOR LOE 2 or 3 studies: limited populations have been evaluated, or data are derived from a single randomized trial or nonrandomized trial. A level-C body of evidence means that very limited populations have been evaluated or that only the consensus opinions of experts, case studies, or standards of care support the recommendation.

## Management of Potential Conflicts of Interest

Rescuers rely on the AHA ECC Guidelines development process to distill the extensive and diverse scientific evidence into straightforward recommendations on how to manage critical emergencies. They trust that the *2010 AHA Guidelines for CPR and ECC* will be evidence based and free of commercial bias. For creation of the *2005 AHA Guidelines for CPR and ECC*, the AHA and ILCOR adopted extensive conflict of interest (COI) management principles.[12,13] For 2010 those principles were revised to incorporate what was learned from the 2005 COI process and to incorporate new COI guidelines developed by the AHA.[14]

The revised COI policy governed the entire development process for the *2010 ILCOR International Consensus on CPR and ECC Science With Treatment Recommendations* and *2010 AHA Guidelines for CPR and ECC*, including selection of ILCOR task force and writing group leaders and members, selection of questions for review, selection of worksheet authors, creation of worksheets, presentation and discussion of worksheets, distillation into the *2010 ILCOR International Consensus on CPR and ECC Science With Treatment Recommendations*, and development of the *2010 AHA Guidelines for CPR and ECC*. All participants completed the detailed AHA online COI disclosure form and updated it annually and when changes occurred. Relationships were considered inactive if they terminated over 12 months prior to the AHA activity, consistent with AHA policy. The policy requires all participants to disclose all commercial relationships, including consulting agreements; speakers' bureau memberships; membership in advisory boards; equity or stock ownership; patents or intellectual property; grant funding from industry or foundations; roles on industry-sponsored, data–safety monitoring boards;, and any other commercial relationship. Individuals with a commercial relationship were not selected to serve in roles for which they had a possible conflict.

Because of their greater potential to influence discussion and outcomes, those in leadership positions (task force or writing group leaders) were held to a higher standard, having no commercial relationships with the issues or industries under discussion and review by their group. Consistent with new AHA guidelines for manuscript authorship,[15] the writing group chairs had no relevant industry relationships, the majority of the members of each writing group had no significant commercial relationships, and no two individuals with relationships with the same industry entity were permitted to serve on the same writing group (ILCOR COI policy can be found at http://ecccanadaheart.com/presenter.jhtml?identifier=3033464). Participants with limited relationships (eg, industry-funded research) were permitted to comment during discussions, with full concurrent disclosure of their relationships, but they were required to recuse themselves from voting and writing about issues related to that relationship for the *2010 ILCOR International Consensus on CPR and ECC Science With Treatment Recommendations* and the *2010 AHA Guidelines for CPR and ECC*. Participants with more direct commercial relationships (eg, consultant, equity ownership) were precluded from participation in decisions, votes, or writing for any topic directly relating to the company's business (Please see *2010 ILCOR International Consensus on CPR and ECC Science With Treatment Recommendations* for details of the worksheet author selection process and the management of COI during the 2010 Consensus Conference.)[14]

The AHA is committed to the most transparent and influence-free evidence-based guidelines process possible. To help improve the process for the future, readers are encouraged to send their questions, suggestions, or comments to one of the authors who oversaw the COI effort (jbilli@umich.edu).

## Writing Group Voting Procedures

Writing group members voted on every recommendation contained in these guidelines, unless they had a conflict of interest related to the topic. In the case of a conflict, the writing group member abstained from the vote and that abstention was recorded.

## Integration of Science Into Practice Guidelines

The final *2010 AHA Guidelines for CPR and ECC* are not intended to repeat verbatim the International Consensus on Science because that document is available online[8,9] and

because it contains a more extensive review of the literature than is needed for a guidelines document. Instead these *2010 AHA Guidelines for CPR and ECC* are intended to reflect the interpretation of the Consensus on Science by the AHA writing groups and members of the ECC Committee and its subcommittees. Whenever possible, the *AHA Guidelines for CPR and ECC* are consistent with the *2010 ILCOR International Consensus on CPR and ECC Science With Treatment Recommendations* statements, and they reference the supporting science publications. However, the *2010 AHA Guidelines for CPR and ECC* also take into consideration local resources, training and education issues, available healthcare systems, and cost-effectiveness. That translation often must balance an acknowledgment of the limitations of systems with an effort to advocate for the care most likely to improve survival from cardiac arrest.

## Summary

In summary, the evidence review process has attempted to provide a systematic review of the scientific literature using *a priori* defined methods. The details and steps of the literature review are transparent and replicable. External opinions and community critique are highly valued, and the final products represent the combined labor of hundreds of participants.

## Disclosures
### Guidelines Part 2: Evidence Evaluation Process and Management of COI: Writing Group Disclosures

| Writing Group Member | Employment | Research Grant | Other Research Support | Speakers' Bureau/ Honoraria | Ownership Interest | Consultant/ Advisory Board | Other |
|---|---|---|---|---|---|---|---|
| Michael R. Sayre | The Ohio State University; Assoc. Professor | None | None | None | None | None | None |
| Robert E. O'Connor | University of Virginia Health System–Professor and Chair of Emergency Medicine | None | None | None | None | None | None |
| Dianne L. Atkins | University of Iowa: Medical School-Professor | None | None | None | None | None | None |
| John E. Billi | University of Michigan: Medical School-Professor | None | None | None | None | None | None |
| Clifton W. Callaway | University of Pittsburgh School of Medicine: Associate Professor; UPMC Health System—Physician †American Heart Association-Work Sheet Editor for 2010 Guidelines. My effort on this project is paid to University of Pittsburgh as a "contracted services agreement," and not paid directly to me | †Grants to University of Pittsburgh: NHLBI-Resuscitation Outcomes Consortium HRSA-Development and Dissemination of Program Tools for Uncontrolled Donation After Cardiac Death (UDCD) | None | None | None | None | None |
| Michael Shuster | Self-employed–emergency MD | None | None | None | None | None | None |
| Brian Eigel | American Heart Association–Director of Science, ECC Programs | None | None | None | None | None | None |
| William H. Montgomery | AHA consultant–C2010 Conference Coordinator; self employed anesthesiologist–private practice; | None | None | None | None | None | None |

*(Continued)*

## Guidelines Part 2: Evidence Evaluation Process and Management of COI: Writing Group Disclosures, *Continued*

| Writing Group Member | Employment | Research Grant | Other Research Support | Speakers' Bureau/ Honoraria | Ownership Interest | Consultant/ Advisory Board | Other |
|---|---|---|---|---|---|---|---|
| Robert W. Hickey | University of Pittsburgh–MD | †NIH sponsored research on the effect of cyclopentenone prostaglandins upon post-ischemic brain | None | None | None | None | None |
| Ian Jacobs | Univ of Western Australia; Emergency Med. Teaching and Research-Professor; AHA-Evidence Eval. Expert | a) National Health and Medical Research Council  b) The Department of Health-Western Australia  c) The National Heart Foundation of Australia  Funds to the Discipline of Emergency Medicine-University of Western Australia from the Ambulance Service-Western Australia and Laerdal (Australia) to maintain the Cardiac Arrest Registry for Western Australia. Our role is to independently maintain, analyze and report outcomes of cardiac arrest in Western Australia. I oversee the operation of the registry and reporting of outcomes. These funds are not used to provide any direct or indirect salary or other financial support | None | None | None | None | None |
| Vinay M. Nadkarni | University of Pennsylvania, Children's Hospital of Philadelphia-Attending Physician, Anesthesia, Critical Care and Pediatrics | None | None | None | None | None | None |
| Peter T. Morley | University of Melbourne-Director of Medical Education; Royal Melbourne Hospital; Hospital Intensivist  AHA Not for profit Evidence Evaluation Expert | None | None | None | None | None | None |
| Tanya I. Semenko | American Heart Association—Science Publications Manager | None | None | None | None | None | None |
| Mary Fran Hazinski | Vanderbilt University School of Nursing—Professor; American Heart Association–Senior Science Editor  †Significant AHA compensation for my editing responsibilities-writing and editing of the 2010 AHA Guidelines for CPR and ECC | None | None | None | None | None | None |

Table represents the relationships of writing group members that may be perceived as actual or reasonably perceived conflicts of interest as reported on the Disclosure Questionnaire, which all members of the writing group are required to complete and submit. A relationship is considered to be "significant" if (a) the person receives $10 000 or more during any 12-month period, or 5% or more of the person's gross income; or (b) the person owns 5% or more of the voting stock or share of the entity, or owns $10 000 or more of the fair market value of the entity. A relationship is considered to be "modest" if it is less than "significant" under the preceding definition.

*Modest.

†Significant.

# References

1. Sackett DL, Rosenberg WM, Gray JA, Haynes RB, Richardson WS. Evidence based medicine: what it is and what it isn't. *BMJ*. 1996;312: 71–72.

2. Cummins RO, Chamberlain D, Montgomery WH, Kloeck WGJ, Nadkarni VM. International collaboration in resuscitation medicine. *Circulation*. 2005; 112(suppl):III-126–III-127.

3. Zaritsky A, Morley PT. The evidence evaluation process for the 2005 International Consensus Conference on Cardiopulmonary Resuscitation and Emergency Cardiovascular Care Science With Treatment Recommendations. *Circulation*. 2005;112(suppl):III-128–III-130.

4. Morley PT, Atkins DL, Billi JE, Bossaert L, Callaway CW, de Caen AR, Deakin CD, Eigel B, Hazinski MF, Hickey RW, Jacobs I, Kleinman ME, Koster RW, Mancini ME, Montgomery WH, Morrison LJ, Nadkarni VM,

Nolan JP, O'Connor RE, Perlman JM, Sayre MR, Semenko TI, Shuster M, Soar J, Wyllie J, Zideman D. Part 3: evidence evaluation process: 2010 International Consensus on Cardiopulmonary Resuscitation and Emergency Cardiovascular Care Science With Treatment Recommendations. *Circulation.* 2010;122(suppl 2):S325–S337.

5. Gazmuri RJ, Nadkarni VM, Nolan JP, Arntz HR, Billi JE, Bossaert L, Deakin CD, Finn J, Hammill WW, Handley AJ, Hazinski MF, Hickey RW, Jacobs I, Jauch EC, Kloeck WG, Mattes MH, Montgomery WH, Morley P, Morrison LJ, Nichol G, O'Connor RE, Perlman J, Richmond S, Sayre M, Shuster M, Timerman S, Weil MH, Weisfeldt ML, Zaritsky A, Zideman DA. Scientific knowledge gaps and clinical research priorities for cardiopulmonary resuscitation and emergency cardiovascular care identified during the 2005 International Consensus Conference on ECC [corrected] and CPR science with treatment recommendations: a consensus statement from the International Liaison Committee on Resuscitation (American Heart Association, Australian Resuscitation Council, European Resuscitation Council, Heart and Stroke Foundation of Canada, InterAmerican Heart Foundation, Resuscitation Council of Southern Africa, and the New Zealand Resuscitation Council); the American Heart Association Emergency Cardiovascular Care Committee; the Stroke Council; and the Cardiovascular Nursing Council. *Circulation.* 2007;116:2501–2512.

6. Centre for Evidence Based Medicine. Asking focused questions. Available at: http://www.cebm.net/index.aspx?o=1036. Accessed April 30, 2010.

7. American Heart Association. International Liaison Committee on Resuscitation 2010 Consensus on ECC and CPR Science and Treatment Recommendations. Evidence evaluation worksheets. Available at: www.heart.org/ILCOR.

8. Hazinski MF, Nolan JP, Billi JE, Böttiger BW, Bossaert L, de Caen AR, Deakin CD, Drajer S, Eigel B, Hickey RW, Jacobs I, Kleinman ME, Kloeck W, Koster RW, Lim SH, Mancini ME, Montgomery WH, Morley PT, Morrison LJ, Nadkarni VM, O'Connor RE, Okada K, Perlman JM, Sayre MR, Shuster M, Soar J, Sunde K, Travers AH, Wyllie J, Zideman D. Part 1: executive summary: 2010 International Consensus on Cardiopulmonary Resuscitation and Emergency Cardiovascular Care Science With Treatment Recommendations. *Circulation.* 2010;122(suppl 2):S250–S275.

9. Nolan JP, Hazinski MF, Billi JE, Boettiger BW, Bossaert L, de Caen AR, Deakin CD, Drajer S, Eigel B, Hickey RW, Jacobs I, Kleinman ME, Kloeck W, Koster RW, Lim SH, Mancini ME, Montgomery WH, Morley PT, Morrison LJ, Nadkarni VM, O'Connor RE, Okada K, Perlman JM, Sayre MR, Shuster M, Soar J, Sunde K, Travers AH, Wyllie J, Zideman D. Part 1: executive summary: 2010 International Consensus on Cardio-pulmonary Resuscitation and Emergency Cardiovascular Care Science With Treatment Recommendations. *Circulation.* 2010;122(suppl 2):S250–S275.

10. Kushner FG, Hand M, Smith SC Jr, King SB III, Anderson JL, Antman EM, Bailey SR, Bates ER, Blankenship JC, Casey DE Jr, Green LA, Hochman JS, Jacobs AK, Krumholz HM, Morrison DA, Ornato JP, Pearle DL, Peterson ED, Sloan MA, Whitlow PL, Williams DO. 2009 Focused updates: ACC/AHA guidelines for the management of patients with ST-elevation myocardial infarction (updating the 2004 guideline and 2007 focused update) and ACC/AHA/SCAI guidelines on percutaneous coronary intervention (updating the 2005 guideline and 2007 focused update): a report of the American College of Cardiology Foundation/American Heart Association Task Force on Practice Guidelines [published correction appears in *Circulation.* 2010;121:e257; dosage error in article text]. *Circulation.* 2009;120:2271–2306.

11. Smith GC, Pell JP. Parachute use to prevent death and major trauma related to gravitational challenge: systematic review of randomised controlled trials. *BMJ.* 2003;327:1459–1461.

12. Billi JE, Zideman DA, Eigel B, Nolan JP, Montgomery WH, Nadkarni VM; International Liaison Committee on Resuscitation and the American Heart Association. Conflict of interest management before, during, and after the 2005 International Consensus Conference on Cardiopulmonary Resuscitation and Emergency Cardiovascular Care Science With Treatment Recommendations. *Circulation.* 2005;112(suppl):III-131–III-132.

13. 2005 American Heart Association Guidelines for Cardiopulmonary Resuscitation and Emergency Cardiovascular Care, part 1: introduction. *Circulation.* 2005;112(suppl):IV-1–IV-5.

14. Billi JE, Shuster M, Bossaert L, de Caen A, Deakin C, Eigel B, Hazinski MF, Hickey RW, Jacobs I, Kleinman ME, Koster RW, Mancini ME, Montgomery WH, Morley PT, Morrison LJ, Munoz H, Nadkarni VM, Nolan JP, O'Connor RE, Perlman JM, Richmond S, Sayre MR, Soar J, Wyllie J, Zideman D; for the International Liaison Committee on Resuscitation and the American Heart Association. Part 4: conflict of interest management before, during, and after the 2010 International Consensus Conference on Cardiopulmonary Resuscitation and Emergency Cardiovascular Care Science With Treatment Recommendations. *Circulation.* 2010;122(suppl 2):S291–S297.

15. ILCOR/AHA COI. Available at: http://www.americanheart.org/presenter.jhtml?identifier=3049576.

KEY WORDS: resuscitation

# Part 3: Ethics

## 2010 American Heart Association Guidelines for Cardiopulmonary Resuscitation and Emergency Cardiovascular Care

Laurie J. Morrison, Chair; Gerald Kierzek; Douglas S. Diekema; Michael R. Sayre;
Scott M. Silvers; Ahamed H. Idris; Mary E. Mancini

The goals of resuscitation are to preserve life, restore health, relieve suffering, limit disability, and respect the individual's decisions, rights, and privacy. Decisions about cardiopulmonary resuscitation (CPR) efforts are often made in seconds by rescuers who may not know the victim of cardiac arrest or whether an advance directive exists. As a result, administration of CPR may be contrary to the individual's desires or best interests.[1–3] However, practice is evolving as more emergency physicians reportedly honor legal advance directives in decisions about resuscitation.[4–7] This section provides guidelines for healthcare providers who are faced with the difficult decision to provide or withhold emergency cardiovascular care.

## Ethical Principles

Healthcare professionals should consider ethical, legal, and cultural factors[8,9] when caring for those in need of CPR. Although healthcare providers must play a role in resuscitation decision making, they should be guided by science, the individual patient or surrogate preferences, local policy, and legal requirements.

### Principle of Respect for Autonomy[10]

The principle of respect for autonomy is an important social value in medical ethics and law. The principle is based on society's respect for a competent individual's ability to make decisions about his or her own healthcare. Adults are presumed to have decision-making capability unless they are incapacitated or declared incompetent by a court of law. Truly informed decisions require that individuals receive and understand accurate information about their condition and prognosis, as well as the nature, risks, benefits, and alternatives of any proposed interventions. The individual must deliberate and choose among alternatives by linking the decision to his or her framework of values. Truly informed decisions require a strong healthcare provider–patient relationship/communication and a 3-step process: (1) the patient receives and understands accurate information about his or her condition, prognosis, the nature of any proposed interventions, alternatives, and risks and benefits; (2) the patient is asked to paraphrase the information to give the provider the opportunity to assess his or her understanding and

to correct any misimpressions; and (3) the patient deliberates and chooses among alternatives and justifies his or her decision.[11]

When decision-making capacity is temporarily impaired by factors such as active illness, treatment of these conditions may restore capacity. When the individual's preferences are unknown or uncertain, emergency conditions should be treated until further information is available.

### Advance Directives, Living Wills, and Patient Self-Determination

A recent study documented that more than a quarter of elderly patients require surrogate decision making at the end of life. Advance directives, living wills, and executing a durable power of attorney for health care ensure that when the patient is unable to make decisions, the preferences that the individual established in advance can guide care. These decisions are associated with less aggressive medical care near death, earlier hospice referrals for palliation, better quality of life, and caregiver's bereavement adjustment.[12]

A **healthcare advance directive** is a legal binding document that in the United States (US) is based on the Patient Self-Determination Act of 1990.[13] It communicates the thoughts, wishes, or preferences for healthcare decisions that might need to be made during periods of incapacity. The Patient Self-Determination Act mandated that healthcare institutions should facilitate the completion of advance directives if patients desire them.[13] Advance directives can be verbal or written and may be based on conversations, written directives, living wills, or durable power of attorney for health care. The legal validity of various forms of advance directives varies from jurisdiction to jurisdiction. Courts consider written advance directives to be more trustworthy than recollections of conversations.

A **living will** may be referred to as a "medical directive" or "declaration" or "directive to physicians," and it provides written direction to healthcare providers about the care that the individual approves should he or she become terminally ill and be unable to make decisions. A living will constitutes evidence of the individual's wishes, and in most areas it can be legally enforced.

A **durable power of attorney for health care** is a legal document that appoints an authorized person to make healthcare decisions (not limited to end-of-life decisions). Simply put, a

The American Heart Association requests that this document be cited as follows: Morrison LJ, Kierzek G, Diekema DS, Sayre MR, Silvers SM, Idris AH, Mancini ME. Part 3: ethics: 2010 American Heart Association Guidelines for Cardiopulmonary Resuscitation and Emergency Cardiovascular Care. *Circulation.* 2010;122(suppl 3):S665–S675.

**(*Circulation.* 2010;122[suppl 3]:S665–S675.)**

*Circulation* is available at http://circ.ahajournals.org        DOI: 10.1161/CIRCULATIONAHA.110.970905

living will affects the care received, and a durable power of attorney accounts for unforeseen circumstances. The latter decisions may be in conflict with the living will or advance directive; at the time of the unforeseen circumstances they are considered to be valid expressions of the patient's best interests.[14]

A **comprehensive healthcare advance directive** combines the living will and the durable power of attorney for health care into one legally binding document.

As a patient's medical condition and desire for types of medical treatment may change over time, all types of advance directives should be revisited regularly. Most importantly the presence of an advance directive, a living will, or a durable power of attorney for health care is closely associated with ensuring that personal preferences match the actual care received, as documented in a survey of surrogates for patients of at least 60 years of age who died between 2000 and 2006 and required surrogate decision making at some point in their care.[14]

A **Do Not Attempt Resuscitation (DNAR) order** is given by a licensed physician or alternative authority as per local regulation, and it must be signed and dated to be valid.[15,16] In many settings, "Allow Natural Death" (AND) is becoming a preferred term to replace DNAR, to emphasize that the order is to allow natural consequences of a disease or injury, and to emphasize ongoing end-of-life care.[17] The DNAR order should explicitly describe the resuscitation interventions to be performed in the event of a life-threatening emergency. In most cases, a DNAR order is preceded by a documented discussion with the patient, family, or surrogate decision maker addressing the patient's wishes about resuscitation interventions. In addition, some jurisdictions may require confirmation by a witness or a second treating physician.

### Surrogate Decision Makers

In the event of incapacity, an adult may require a surrogate decision maker to make medical decisions. In the event that the individual has a durable power of attorney for health care, the person appointed by that document is authorized to make medical decisions within the scope of authority granted by the document. If the individual has a court-appointed guardian with authority to make healthcare decisions, the guardian becomes the authorized surrogate.

If there is no court-appointed or other authority, a close relative or friend can become a surrogate decision maker. Most jurisdictions have laws that designate the legally authorized surrogate decision maker for an incompetent patient who has not identified a decision maker through a durable power of attorney for health care. Surrogate decision makers should base their decisions on the individual's previously expressed preferences, if known; otherwise, surrogates should make decisions based on their understanding of what constitutes the best interests of the individual.

### Pediatric Decision Making

As a general rule, minors are considered incompetent to provide legally binding consent about their health care. Parents or guardians are generally empowered to make healthcare decisions on their behalf, and in most situations, parents are given wide latitude in terms of the decisions they make on behalf of their children. Parental authority is not absolute, however, and when a parent or guardian's decision appears to place the child at significant risk of serious harm as compared to other options, medical providers may seek to involve state agencies (eg, child

protective services or a court determination) to allow treatment of the child over parental objections.[18]

A child should be involved in decision making at a level appropriate for the child's maturity. Children should be asked to consent to healthcare decisions when able within the legal definition of a consenting adult based on local policy and legislation. Children <14 years of age (in Canada) and <18 years of age (in the US) rarely possess the legal authority to consent to their health care except under specific legally defined situations (emancipated minors, mature minors, and for specific health conditions such as sexually transmitted diseases and pregnancy-related care). In situations where an older child will not consent, the dissent should be carefully considered by the treating provider.

### Principle of Futility

Patients or families may ask for care that is highly unlikely to improve health outcomes. Healthcare providers, however, are not obliged to provide such care when there is scientific and social consensus that the treatment is ineffective. If the purpose of a medical treatment cannot be achieved, the treatment can be considered futile.

An objective criterion for medical futility was defined in 1990 for interventions and drug therapy as imparting a <1% chance of survival.[19] Although this criterion may be controversial, it remains a basis for current futility research. An obvious example of an inappropriate or futile intervention is providing CPR for a patient who has suffered irreversible death. Without objective signs of irreversible death (eg, decapitation, rigor mortis, or decomposition) and in the absence of known advance directives declining resuscitative attempts, full resuscitation should be offered.

Conditions such as irreversible brain damage or brain death cannot be reliably assessed or predicted at the time of cardiac arrest. Withholding resuscitation and the discontinuation of life-sustaining treatment during or after resuscitation are ethically equivalent. In situations where the prognosis is uncertain, a trial of treatment may be initiated while further information is gathered to help determine the likelihood of survival, the patient's preferences, and the expected clinical course (Class IIb, LOE C).

## Witholding and Withdrawing CPR (Termination of Resuscitative Efforts) Related to Out-of Hospital Cardiac Arrest (OHCA)

### Criteria for Not Starting CPR in All OHCA

Basic life support (BLS) training urges all potential rescuers to immediately begin CPR without seeking consent, because any delay in care dramatically decreases the chances of survival. While the general rule is to provide emergency treatment to a victim of cardiac arrest, there are a few exceptions where withholding CPR might be appropriate, as follows:

- Situations where attempts to perform CPR would place the rescuer at risk of serious injury or mortal peril
- Obvious clinical signs of irreversible death (eg, rigor mortis, dependent lividity, decapitation, transection, or decomposition)
- A valid, signed, and dated advance directive indicating that resuscitation is not desired, or a valid, signed, and dated DNAR order

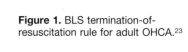

**Figure 1.** BLS termination-of-resuscitation rule for adult OHCA.[23]

## DNAR Orders in OHCA

Out-of-hospital DNAR protocols must be clearly written and easily implemented for all involved (all members of the healthcare team, patients, family members, and loved ones). DNAR documentation can take many forms (eg, written bedside orders, wallet identification cards, identification bracelets, or predefined paper documents approved by the local emergency medical services [EMS] authority). The ideal out-of-hospital DNAR documentation is portable and can be carried on the person.[16]

Delayed or token efforts such as so-called "slow-codes" (knowingly providing ineffective resuscitative efforts) are inappropriate. This practice compromises the ethical integrity of healthcare providers, uses deception to create a false impression, and may undermine the provider-patient relationship. The practice of "pseudo resuscitation" was self-reported by paramedics to occur in 27% of cardiac arrests in a community where a prehospital DNAR and termination-of-resuscitation protocols were not in place.[20]

Some EMS systems have extended the DNAR protocol to include verbal DNAR requests from family members as grounds to withhold therapy.[21,22] Paramedics withheld care to patients in cardiac arrest with a history of a terminal illness, who were under the care of a physician, and when at the time of the cardiac arrest the family requested that resuscitation not be attempted. The numbers of patients for whom resuscitation was withheld doubled after implementation (from 45 to 99 a year). This is an important first step in expanding the clinical decision rule pertaining to when to start resuscitation in OHCA, however there is insufficient evidence to support this approach without further validation.

## Advance Directives in OHCA

Advance directives do not have to include a DNAR order, and a DNAR order is valid without an advance directive. A significant number of cardiac arrest victims for whom EMS is summoned have a terminal illness, and many have written advance directives. Laws detailing the actions of a prehospital provider in response to an out-of-hospital DNAR order vary across jurisdictions. In general, EMS professionals should initiate CPR and advanced life support if there is reasonable doubt about the validity of a DNAR order, if there is concern that the victim may have had a change of mind, or if there is a question about whether the patient intended the advance directive to be applied under the actual conditions for which EMS has been called.

The DNAR order should be shown to EMS responders as soon as they arrive on the scene. If the EMS professional cannot obtain clear information about the victim's wishes, they should not hesitate to start resuscitation. Sometimes within a few minutes of starting resuscitation, relatives or other medical personnel will arrive and confirm that the victim had clearly expressed a wish that resuscitation not be attempted. CPR or other life-support measures may be discontinued by following local directives or protocols, which may include real-time consultation with medical direction.

## Terminating Resuscitative Efforts in OHCA

### Terminating Resuscitative Efforts in Neonatal or Pediatric OHCA

No predictors of neonatal or pediatric (infant or child) out-of-hospital resuscitation success or failure have been established. No validated clinical decision rules have been derived and evaluated. Further research in this area is needed.

In the absence of clinical decision rules for the neonatal or pediatric OHCA victim, the responsible prehospital provider should follow BLS pediatric and advanced cardiovascular life support protocols and consult with real-time medical direction or transport the victim to the most appropriate facility per local directives.

### Terminating Resuscitative Efforts in Adult OHCA

*Terminating Resuscitative Efforts in a BLS Out-of-Hospital System*

Rescuers who start BLS should continue resuscitation until one of the following occurs:

- Restoration of effective, spontaneous circulation
- Care is transferred to a team providing advanced life support
- The rescuer is unable to continue because of exhaustion, the presence of dangerous environmental hazards, or because continuation of the resuscitative efforts places others in jeopardy
- Reliable and valid criteria indicating irreversible death are met, criteria of obvious death are identified, or criteria for termination of resuscitation are met.

One set of reliable and valid criteria for termination of resuscitation is termed the "BLS termination of resuscitation rule" (see Figure 1).[23] All 3 of the following criteria must be present before moving to the ambulance for transport, to consider terminating BLS resuscitative attempts for adult victims of out-of-hospital cardiac arrest: (1) arrest was not witnessed by EMS provider or first responder; (2) no return of spontaneous

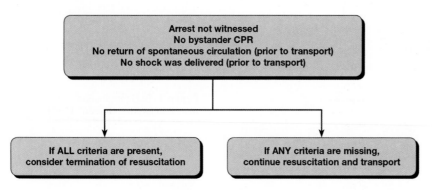

**Figure 2.** ALS termination-of-resuscitation rule for adult OHCA.[33]

circulation (ROSC) after 3 full rounds of CPR and automated external defibrillator (AED) analysis; and (3) no AED shocks were delivered.

The BLS termination of resuscitation rule can reduce the rate of hospital transport to 37% of cardiac arrests without compromising the care of potentially viable patients. This was prospectively validated in rural and urban EMS services[23] and externally validated in additional locations in the US, Canada, and Europe.[24–29] The rule should be applied before moving to the ambulance for transport.[30] This clinical prediction rule consistently generates the highest specificity and positive predictive values when compared to previous guidelines.[29] It is recommended that regional or local EMS authorities use the BLS termination rule to develop protocols for the termination of resuscitative efforts by BLS providers for adult victims of cardiac arrest in areas where advanced life support is not available or may be significantly delayed (Class I, LOE A). The reliability and validity of this rule is uncertain if modified (Class IIb, LOE A).

Implementation of the rule includes real-time contacting of medical control when the rule suggests termination. Before the protocol is implemented, EMS providers require training in sensitive communication with the family about the outcome of the resuscitative attempt.[31] This strategy will help to ensure comfort of the provider and appropriate support of the grieving family. Support for the prehospital protocol should be sought from collaborating external agencies (eg, destination hospital emergency departments [EDs], coroner, medical directors, and police) before implementation.

*Terminating Resuscitative Efforts in an ALS Out-of-Hospital System*
A different rule may be useful when the additional diagnostic and therapeutic capabilities of an advanced life support EMS response are available to the victim. The National Association of EMS Physicians (NAEMSP) suggested that resuscitative efforts could be terminated in patients who do not respond to at least 20 minutes of ALS care.[32] An ALS termination of resuscitation rule was derived from a diverse population of rural and urban EMS settings.[33] This rule recommends considering terminating resuscitation when ALL of the following criteria apply before moving to the ambulance for transport (see Figure 2): (1) arrest was not witnessed; (2) no bystander CPR was provided; (3) no ROSC after full ALS care in the field; and (4) no AED shocks were delivered.

This rule has been retrospectively externally validated for adult patients in several regions in the US, Canada, and Europe,[25,27–29] and it is reasonable to employ this rule in all ALS services (Class IIa, LOE B).

*Terminating Resuscitative Efforts in a Combined BLS and ALS Out-of-Hospital System*
In a tiered ALS- and BLS-provider system, the use of a universal rule can avoid confusion at the scene of a cardiac arrest without compromising diagnostic accuracy.[25,28,29] The BLS rule is reasonable to use in these services (Class IIa, LOE B).

*Termination of Resuscitative Efforts and Transport Implications*
Field termination reduces unnecessary transport to the hospital by 60% with the BLS rule and 40% with the ALS rule,[25] reducing associated road hazards[34,35] that put the provider, patient, and public at risk. In addition field termination reduces inadvertent paramedic exposure to potential biohazards and the higher cost of ED pronouncement.[36–38] More importantly the quality of CPR is compromised during transport, and survival is linked to optimizing scene care rather than rushing to hospital.[39–41]

## Withholding and Withdrawing CPR (Termination of Resuscitative Efforts) Related To In-Hospital Cardiac Arrest

### Criteria for Not Starting CPR in Newly Born Infant IHCA
There are prescribed recommendations to guide the initiation of resuscitative efforts in newly born infants. When gestational age, birth weight, or congenital anomalies are associated with almost certain early death and when unacceptably high morbidity is likely among the rare survivors, resuscitation is not indicated. Examples may include extreme prematurity (gestational age <23 weeks or birth weight <400 g), anencephaly, and some major chromosomal abnormalities such as trisomy 13 (Class IIb, LOE C).

In conditions associated with uncertain prognosis where survival is borderline, the morbidity rate is relatively high, and the anticipated burden to the child is high, parental desires concerning initiation of resuscitation should be supported (Class IIb, LOE C).

There should be a consistent and coordinated approach from the obstetric and neonatal teams in applying these guidelines and in communicating with the parents in developing an agreed-upon management plan when possible.

## Criteria for Not Starting CPR in Pediatric and Adult IHCA

Few criteria can accurately predict the futility of continued resuscitation. In light of this uncertainty, all pediatric and adult patients who suffer cardiac arrest in the hospital setting should have resuscitative attempts initiated unless the patient has a valid DNAR order or has objective signs of irreversible death (eg, dependent lividity).

## DNAR Orders in IHCA

Unlike other medical interventions, CPR is initiated without a physician's order, based on implied consent for emergency treatment. A licensed physician's order is necessary to withhold CPR in the hospital setting. Physicians should initiate a discussion about the use of CPR with all patients admitted for medical and surgical care or with their surrogates. Terminally ill patients may fear abandonment and pain more than death, so physicians should also reassure the patient and family that control of pain and other symptoms as well as other aspects of support will continue even if resuscitation is withheld.

The attending physician should write the DNAR order in accordance with local policy in the patient's chart, with a note explaining the rationale for the DNAR order, other specific limitations of care, and documenting discussions with the patient, surrogate, and family. Oral DNAR orders are not acceptable. The limitation-of-treatment order should provide explicit instructions for specific emergency interventions that may arise, including the use of vasopressor agents, mechanical ventilation, blood products, or antibiotics. The scope of a DNAR order should specify which interventions are to be withheld.

It is important to emphasize that all other care should be administered without delay and as appropriate for all patients. A DNAR order does not automatically preclude interventions such as administration of parenteral fluids, nutrition, oxygen, analgesia, sedation, antiarrhythmics, or vasopressors, unless these are included in the order. Some patients may choose to accept defibrillation and chest compressions but not intubation and mechanical ventilation. DNAR orders carry no implications about other forms of treatment, and other aspects of the treatment plan should be documented separately and communicated to members of the healthcare team. DNAR orders should be reviewed periodically as per local protocol, particularly if the patient's condition changes.[42] DNAR orders should also be reviewed before surgery by the anesthesiologist, attending surgeon, and patient or surrogate to determine their applicability in the operating suite and during the immediate postoperative recovery period.[43]

## Terminating Resuscitative Efforts in IHCA

### Terminating Cardiac Arrest Resuscitative Efforts in Neonatal IHCA

Noninitiation of resuscitation and discontinuation of life-sustaining treatment during or after resuscitation are ethically equivalent, and clinicians should not hesitate to withdraw support when functional survival is highly unlikely.[44] The following guidelines must be interpreted according to current regional outcomes.[45]

In a newly born infant with no detectable heart rate, it is appropriate to consider stopping resuscitation if the heart rate remains undetectable for 10 minutes (Class IIb, LOE C[46–48]).

The decision to continue resuscitative efforts beyond 10 minutes with no heart rate should take into consideration factors such as presumed etiology of arrest, gestational age, presence or absence of complications, and the parents' previous expressed feelings about the acceptable risk of morbidity.

In the absence of clinical decision rules to guide the termination of resuscitation in the neonatal patient, the responsible clinician should stop the resuscitative attempt if there is a high degree of certainty that the newborn will not respond to further advanced life support.

### Terminating Cardiac Arrest Resuscitative Efforts in Pediatric IHCA

No predictors of pediatric (infant or child) resuscitative success or failure have been established.[49–51] No validated clinical decision rules to guide the termination of resuscitative efforts in pediatric cardiac arrest have been reported, and the decision to stop resuscitation may vary considerably across physicians and institutions. Further research in this area is needed.

In the absence of clinical decision rules, the responsible clinician should stop the resuscitative attempt if there is a high degree of certainty that the patient will not respond to further pediatric advanced life support. Arrest characteristics to be considered by physicians making decisions may include duration of CPR, witnessed event, number of doses of epinephrine, etiology of arrest, first and subsequent rhythm, and age.[49,52–56] Prolonged efforts are typically made for infants and children with recurring or refractory VF or VT, those who demonstrate some ROSC, those with drug toxicity, or those experiencing an event causing primary hypothermia. Prolonged efforts are also indicated when a decision to employ extracorporeal CPR (ECPR) has been made (see Part 14: "Pediatric Advanced Life Support").

### Terminating Cardiac Arrest Resuscitative Efforts in Adult IHCA

In the hospital the decision to terminate resuscitative efforts rests with the treating physician and is based on consideration of many factors, including witnessed versus unwitnessed arrest, time to CPR, initial arrest rhythm, time to defibrillation, comorbid disease, prearrest state, and whether there is ROSC at some point during the resuscitative efforts. Clinical decision rules for in-hospital termination of resuscitation may be helpful in reducing variability in decision making[57]; however, the evidence for their reliability is limited, and rules should be prospectively validated before adoption.

## Providing Emotional Support to the Family

### Providing Emotional Support to the Family During Resuscitative Efforts in Cardiac Arrest

In the past, family members have often been excluded from being present during the attempted resuscitation of a child or other relative. Surveys suggest that healthcare providers hold a range of opinions about the presence of family members during resuscitative attempts.[58–69] One theoretical concern is the potential for family members to become disruptive, interfere with resuscitative procedures, or develop syncope, and another is the possibility of increased exposure to legal liability; however, these are not reported in the literature.

Several surveys suggested that most family members wish to be present during a resuscitative attempt.[62–66] Family members with no medical background have reported that being at a loved one's side and saying goodbye during the final moments of life was comforting.[62,63,67] Family members have also reported that it helped them to adjust to the death of their loved one,[68,70] and most indicated that they would do so again.[67] Several retrospective reports note positive reactions from family members,[58–60] many of whom said that they felt a sense of having helped their loved one and of easing their own grieving.[61] Most parents surveyed indicated that they wanted to be offered the option of being present during the resuscitative effort for their child.[60,71–79]

In the absence of data documenting harm and in light of data suggesting that it may be helpful, offering select family members the opportunity to be present during a resuscitation is reasonable and desirable (assuming that the patient, if an adult, has not raised a prior objection) (Class IIa, LOE C for adults and Class I, LOE B for pediatric patients). Parents and other family members seldom ask if they can be present unless they are encouraged to do so by healthcare providers. Resuscitation team members should be sensitive to the presence of family members during resuscitative efforts, assigning a team member to remain with the family to answer questions, clarify information, and otherwise offer comfort.[66]

### Providing Emotional Support to the Family After Termination of Resuscitative Efforts in Cardiac Arrest

Notifying family members of the death of a loved one is an important aspect of a resuscitation that should be performed compassionately, with care taken to consider the family's culture, religious beliefs and preconceptions surrounding death, and any guilt they may feel associated with the event or circumstances preceding the event.[80]

## Limitation of Care and Withdrawal of Life-Sustaining Therapies

Limitation of care or withdrawal of life-sustaining therapies is an emotionally complex decision for family and staff. Withholding and withdrawing life support are ethically similar. A decision to limit care or withdraw life support is justifiable if the patient is determined to be brain dead, if the physician and patient or surrogate agree that treatment goals cannot be met, or if the burden to the patient of continued treatment is believed to exceed any benefits.

Patients in the end stage of an incurable disease should receive care that ensures their autonomy, comfort, and dignity. Interventions that minimize suffering and pain, dyspnea, delirium, convulsions, and other terminal complications should always be provided. For such patients it is ethically acceptable to gradually increase the doses of narcotics and sedatives to relieve pain and other suffering, even to levels that might concomitantly shorten the patient's life. The care team should initiate plans for future care by collaborative discussions and the resolution of any conflicts with nurses, consultants, residents, fellows, the patient (when capable of participating), surrogate decision makers, and the family. Nursing and comfort care (eg, oral hygiene, skin care, patient positioning, and measures to relieve pain and suffering) must always be continued.

In the absence of evidence of an incurable disease in the end stage, decisions to withdraw or limit care in the post-arrest

patient are often challenging, given the difficulties of accurate prognostication, especially in the era of treatment advances such as therapeutic hypothermia.

### Prognostication in Neonatal and Pediatric Patients After Cardiac Arrest—Determining When to Withdraw Life-Sustaining Therapies

There is insufficient evidence about clinical neurologic signs, electrophysiologic studies, biomarkers, or imaging modalities to describe an approach to prognostication in the neonatal or pediatric patient after cardiac arrest. In the absence of prognostication guidelines, the decision to withdraw life-sustaining therapies rests with the treating physician and may vary considerably across physicians and institutions. Further research in this area is needed.

### Prognostication in Adult Patients After Cardiac Arrest—Determining When to Withdraw Life-Sustaining Therapies

There are no clinical neurologic signs, electrophysiologic studies, biomarkers, or imaging modalities that can reliably predict death or poor neurologic outcome (eg, Cerebral Performance Category of 3, 4, or 5) within the first 24 hours after cardiac arrest in patients treated with or without therapeutic hypothermia (see Part 9: "Post–Cardiac Arrest Care"). There is a tendency to withdraw care prematurely in the post-arrest patient, and this has contributed to a selection bias in the current literature on prognostic testing.

#### Prognostic Testing in the Adult Post-Arrest Patient Not Treated With Therapeutic Hypothermia

In adult post–cardiac arrest patients who are *not* treated with therapeutic hypothermia, it is recommended in comatose patients that pupillary light and corneal reflexes as well as vestibular-ocular reflexes and Glasgow Coma Scale (GCS) Motor Score be documented at 72 hours after sustained ROSC and thereafter at least daily (Class I, LOE B). When available, recording the unprocessed electroencephalography interpretation between 24 and 72 hours after sustained ROSC may be helpful to assist in the prediction of a poor outcome in the absence of sedatives, hypotension, accidental hypothermia, or hypoxemia; specifically the finding of generalized suppression to $<20\ \mu V$, burst suppression pattern with generalized epileptic activity, or diffuse periodic complexes on a flat background (Class IIb, LOE B[81]).

#### Prognostic Testing in the Adult Post-Arrest Patient Treated With Therapeutic Hypothermia

Based on limited available evidence, potentially reliable prognosticators of poor outcome in patients treated with therapeutic hypothermia after cardiac arrest include bilateral absence of N20 peak on median nerve somatosensory evoked potential $\geq 24$ hours after cardiac arrest[82,83] and the absence of both corneal and pupillary reflexes $\geq 3$ days after cardiac arrest. Limited available evidence also suggests that (1) GCS Motor Score of 2 or less at day 3 after sustained ROSC,[82] and (2) presence of status epilepticus[84–86] are potentially unreliable prognosticators of poor outcome in post–cardiac arrest patients treated with therapeutic hypothermia. Similarly, recovery of consciousness and cognitive functions is possible in a few post–cardiac arrest patients treated with therapeutic hypothermia despite bilateral absent or minimally present N20 responses of median nerve somatosensory-evoked potentials, suggesting that they may be unreliable as well.[87] Serum biomarkers such as neuron-specific enolase[88–90] are potentially valuable as adjunctive studies in prognostication of poor outcome in patients treated with hypothermia, but their reliability is limited by the relatively small number of patients studied and the lack of assay standardization.

In the adult post–cardiac arrest patient treated with therapeutic hypothermia, it is recommended that clinical neurologic signs, electrophysiologic studies, biomarkers, and imaging be done where available at 3 days after cardiac arrest. There is limited evidence to guide decisions to withdraw life-sustaining therapy currently and the clinician should document all available prognostic testing after 72 hours post–cardiac arrest for patients treated with therapeutic hypothermia (Class I, LOE C) and use clinical judgment based on this testing to make a decision to withdraw life-sustaining therapy when appropriate.

## Ethics of Organ and Tissue Donation

Most communities do not optimize the retrieval of organ and tissue donations; this has created protracted waiting time and greater suffering for patients awaiting organ transplantation. The Emergency Cardiovascular Care community of the American Heart Association supports efforts to optimize the ethical acquisition of organ and tissue donations. Studies suggest no difference in functional outcomes of organs transplanted from patients who are determined to be brain dead as a consequence of cardiac arrest when compared with donors who are brain dead from other causes.[91–94] Therefore it is reasonable to suggest that all communities should optimize retrieval of tissue and organ donations in brain dead post–cardiac arrest patients (in-hospital) and those pronounced dead in the out-of-hospital setting (Class IIa, LOE B).

Most important to this process is advance planning and infrastructure support to allow organ donation to occur in a manner sensitive to the needs of the donor's family and without undue burden on the staff. Medical directors of EMS agencies, emergency departments (EDs), and critical care units (CCUs) should develop protocols and implementation plans with the regional organ and tissue donation program to optimize donation following a cardiac arrest death (Class I, LOE C), including

- A process by which permission for organ and tissue donations will be obtained
- The establishment of clearly defined guidelines for organ and tissue procurement that will be available to all healthcare providers both in and out of the hospital
- Information to address the possible differences between applicable laws and societal values in procedures for organ procurement
- The emotional support to be offered to providers post event
- A system to acquire organ and tissue donations from individuals pronounced dead in the out-of-hospital setting. This discussion should include input from the coroner, EMS, police, and lay people representing the target community

## Ethics and Privacy Issues Related to Resuscitation Research

Conducting clinical research in patients with cardiopulmonary arrest is challenging. In general, research involving human subjects requires the consent of the subject or, in some cases, a legally authorized surrogate decision-maker.[95,96] This has proven to be a challenge for research involving patients in cardiac arrest because research interventions must frequently be implemented at a time when it is impossible to obtain consent.[97,98] After much public discussion and in recognition of the value of this type of human research, the United States government, through the Food and Drug Administration and the National Institutes of Health, adopted regulations that allow an exception for the need to obtain informed consent in certain limited circumstances.[99] These exceptions to informed consent for research enrollment apply only if the following conditions are met:

- The subject is unconscious or incapacitated and facing a life-threatening or permanently disabling situation for which the only known therapy is investigational, unproven, or unsatisfactory.
- The subject is incapable or unable to provide valid consent and the surrogate decision maker cannot be reached for permission before the time the investigational treatment must be started.
- The investigational therapy offers the prospect of direct benefit to the participant, and there is no accepted therapy that is clearly superior to the experimental therapy.
- The research protocol is approved by an institutional research board (IRB).

In addition these regulations require that input from community representatives be sought before IRB approval in order to gain a form of "community consultation" to proceed with the research.[96,100,101] Before its initiation, public disclosure of the research and its risks and benefits must be made to the community from which potential participants will come. Public disclosure of study results is also required. This process attempts to assess the opinions and thoughts of the community in which the research will take place and enables a two-way exchange that may, in fact, modify the implementation or research design in light of the community dialogue.

If a patient is enrolled in such a study, once the legal decision maker has been identified and informed of the research, the decision maker may choose to discontinue participation at any time after being fully informed of the consequences of doing so.

Healthcare providers involved in training and research must be careful to protect patient privacy and the confidentiality of patient data and to minimize the collection of personal health information. Provisions to protect the privacy of patients' health information and medical records are included in the US Health Insurance Portability and Accountability Act, commonly referred to as HIPAA. For details pertaining to the US regulations see http://www.hhs.gov/ocr/privacy/hipaa/administrative/privacyrule/index.html (accessed April 22, 2010).

## Ethics of Training on the Newly Dead

The use of newly dead patients for training raises important ethical and legal issues. Obtaining consent from family members shows respect for the newly dead patient and those who will survive the patient. It may not always be possible or practical to obtain such consent immediately after the death of a patient. One argument is that presuming consent in these situations serves a "greater good" that will benefit the living. An alternate viewpoint is that consent is unnecessary because the body is "non persona" and without autonomy or interests. These arguments, however, fail to adequately weigh the potential for harm to surviving family members who may oppose using a recently deceased loved one for the purpose of training or research. This view also ignores significant cultural differences in the acceptance or nonacceptance of the use of cadavers in medical education. The American College of Emergency Physicians practice guidelines summarizes the issues on their website, offering a more detailed discussion at http://www.acep.org/content.aspx?id=30104 (accessed April 18, 2010).[102]

Ultimately, the respect for the individual should prevail over the need for healthcare providers to practice lifesaving techniques. The technical advances of high-fidelity simulation and the use of cadaver labs where consent has been obtained in advance should reduce the need for use of recently deceased patients for educational purposes.

## Acknowledgements

Neonatal Task Force Chair Jeffrey M. Perlman for his contributions to the manuscript and Andrew H. Travers and Thomas D. Rea for their insightful review and editing.

## Disclosures

**Guidelines Part 3: Ethics: Writing Group Disclosures**

| Writing Group Member | Employment | Research Grant | Other Research Support | Speakers' Bureau/ Honoraria | Ownership Interest | Consultant/ Advisory Board | Other |
|---|---|---|---|---|---|---|---|
| Laurie J. Morrison | St Michael's Hospital–Clinician Scientist, Director Rescu Robert and Dorothy Pitts Chair in Acute Care & Emergency Medicine Keenan Research Centre Li Ka Shing Knowledge Institute St Michael's Hosp. Univ of Toronto | None | None | None | None | None | None |
| Gerald Kierzek | Assistance Publique Hopitaux de Paris & Univ of Paris, Emerg Dept & EMS & Forensic Med, Hotel-Dieu Cochin Hosp; MD | †Pitts Foundation/ StMichaels Hosp Toronto, 1 yr research Fellow Emerg Med CCM | None | None | None | *Steering Com (Study LMWH in traumatic injury) GSK | None |
| Douglas S. Diekema | Children's University Medical Group-Professor of Pediatrics | None | None | None | None | None | None |
| Michael R. Sayre | The Ohio State University; Assoc Prof | none | None | None | None | None | None |
| Scott M. Silvers | Mayo Clinic Chair Emergency Medicine | None | None | None | None | None | None |
| Ahamed H. Idris | UT Southwestern Medical Center at Dallas–Professor of Surgery | †NIH grant for the Resuscitation Outcomes Consortium Dallas-Fort Worth Site. I serve as the site PI. All payments to UT SWMC, at which I'm employed | *In kind support from Philips, Medtronics, and ZOLL consisting of defibrillators, software, and manikins used for training purposes | None | None | None | None |
| Mary E. Mancini | Univ of Texas at Arlington, Professor | None | None | None | None | None | None |

This table represents the relationships of writing group members that may be perceived as actual or reasonably perceived conflicts of interest as reported on the Disclosure Questionnaire, which all members of the writing group are required to complete and submit. A relationship is considered to be "significant" if (a) the person receives $10 000 or more during any 12-month period, or 5% or more of the person's gross income; or (b) the person owns 5% or more of the voting stock or share of the entity, or owns $10 000 or more of the fair market value of the entity. A relationship is considered to be "modest" if it is less than "significant" under the preceding definition.

*Modest.

†Significant.

# References

1. Guru V, Verbeek PR, Morrison LJ. Response of paramedics to terminally ill patients with cardiac arrest: an ethical dilemma. *CMAJ.* 1999;161:1251–1254.

2. Wiese CH, Bartels UE, Zausig YA, Pfirstinger J, Graf BM, Hanekop GG. Prehospital emergency treatment of palliative care patients with cardiac arrest: a retrolective investigation. *Support Care Cancer.* 2009.

3. Miller W, Levy P, Lamba S, Zalenski RJ, Compton S. Descriptive analysis of the in-hospital course of patients who initially survive out-of-hospital cardiac arrest but die in-hospital. *J Palliat Med.* 2010;13: 19–22.

4. ACEP Policy Statement: Code of Ethics for Emergency Physicians. *Am College of Emergency Physicians.* Available at: http://www.acep.org/practres.aspx?id=29144. Accessed 5 May, 2010.

5. Marco CA, Bessman ES, Schoenfeld CN, Kelen GD. Ethical issues of cardiopulmonary resuscitation: current practice among emergency physicians. *Acad Emerg Med.* 1997;4:898–904.

6. Marco CA, Bessman ES, Kelen GD. Ethical issues of cardiopulmonary resuscitation: comparison of emergency physician practices from 1995 to 2007. *Acad Emerg Med.* 2009;16:270–273.

7. ACEP statement: Code of Ethics for Emergency Physicians.

8. Schmid B, Allen RS, Haley PP, Decoster J. Family matters: dyadic agreement in end-of-life medical decision making. *Gerontologist.* 2010; 50:226–237.

9. Barnato AE, Anthony DL, Skinner J, Gallagher PM, Fisher ES. Racial and ethnic differences in preferences for end-of-life treatment. *J Gen Intern Med.* 2009;24:695–701.

10. Beauchamp T, Childress J. *Principles of Biomedical Ethics.* 6th ed: Oxford University Press; 2008.

11. Simon JR. Refusal of care: the physician-patient relationship and decisionmaking capacity. *Ann Emerg Med.* 2007;50:456–461.

12. Wright AA, Zhang B, Ray A, Mack JW, Trice E, Balboni T, Mitchell SL, Jackson VA, Block SD, Maciejewski PK, Prigerson HG. Associations between end-of-life discussions, patient mental health, medical care near death, and caregiver bereavement adjustment. *JAMA.* 2008; 300:1665–1673.

13. Omnibus Budget Reconciliation Act of 1990, Pub. Law No. 1990; 101–508.

14. Silveira MJ, Kim SY, Langa KM. Advance directives and outcomes of surrogate decision making before death. *N Engl J Med.* 2010;362: 1211–1218.

15. Cerminara KL, Bogin SM. A paper about a piece of paper. Regulatory action as the most effective way to promote use of physician orders for life-sustaining treatment. *J Leg Med.* 2008;29:479–503.

16. Payne JK, Thornlow DK. Clinical perspectives on portable do-not-resuscitate orders. *J Gerontol Nurs.* 2008;34:11–16.

17. Venneman SS, Narnor-Harris P, Perish M, Hamilton M. "Allow natural death" versus "do not resuscitate": three words that can change a life. *J Med Ethics.* 2008;34:2–6.

18. Diekema DS. Parental refusals of medical treatment: the harm principle as threshold for state intervention. *Theor Med Bioeth.* 2004;25:243–264.

19. Schneiderman LJ, Jecker NS, Jonsen AR. Medical futility: its meaning and ethical implications. *Ann Intern Med.* 1990;112:949–954.

20. Sherbino J, Guru V, Verbeek PR, Morrison LJ. Prehospital emergency medical services. *CJEM.* 2000;2:246–251.

21. Kellermann A, Lynn J. Withholding resuscitation in prehospital care. *Ann Intern Med.* 2006;144:692–693.

22. Feder S, Matheny RL, Loveless RS Jr, Rea TD. Withholding resuscitation: a new approach to prehospital end-of-life decisions. *Ann Intern Med.* 2006;144:634–640.

23. Morrison LJ, Visentin LM, Kiss A, Theriault R, Eby D, Vermeulen M, Sherbino J, Verbeek PR. Validation of a rule for termination of resuscitation in out-of-hospital cardiac arrest. *N Engl J Med.* 2006;355: 478–487.

24. Richman PB, Vadeboncoeur TF, Chikani V, Clark L, Bobrow BJ. Independent evaluation of an out-of-hospital termination of resuscitation (TOR) clinical decision rule. *Acad Emerg Med.* 2008;15:517–521.

25. Morrison LJ, Verbeek PR, Zhan C, Kiss A, Allan KS. Validation of a universal prehospital termination of resuscitation clinical prediction rule for advanced and basic life support providers. *Resuscitation.* 2009;80: 324–328.

26. Ong ME, Jaffey J, Stiell I, Nesbitt L. Comparison of termination-of-resuscitation guidelines for basic life support: defibrillator providers in out-of-hospital cardiac arrest. *Ann Emerg Med.* 2006;47:337–343.

27. Sasson C, Hegg AJ, Macy M, Park A, Kellermann A, McNally B. Prehospital termination of resuscitation in cases of refractory out-of-hospital cardiac arrest. *JAMA.* 2008;300:1432–1438.

28. Ruygrok ML, Byyny RL, Haukoos JS. Validation of 3 termination of resuscitation criteria for good neurologic survival after out-of-hospital cardiac arrest. *Ann Emerg Med.* 2009;54:239–247.

29. Skrifvars MB, Vayrynen T, Kuisma M, Castren M, Parr MJ, Silfverstople J, Svensson L, Jonsson L, Herlitz J. Comparison of Helsinki and European Resuscitation Council "do not attempt to resuscitate" guidelines, and a termination of resuscitation clinical prediction rule for out-of-hospital cardiac arrest patients found in asystole or pulseless electrical activity. *Resuscitation.* 2010.

30. Verbeek PR, Vermeulen MJ, Ali FH, Messenger DW, Summers J, Morrison LJ. Derivation of a termination-of-resuscitation guideline for emergency medical technicians using automated external defibrillators. *Acad Emerg Med.* 2002;9:671–678.

31. Morrison LJ, Visentin LM, Vermeulen M, Kiss A, Theriault R, Eby D, Sherbino J, Verbeek R. Inter-rater reliability and comfort in the application of a basic life support termination of resuscitation clinical prediction rule for out of hospital cardiac arrest. *Resuscitation.* 2007;74: 150–157.

32. Bailey ED, Wydro GC, Cone DC. Termination of resuscitation in the prehospital setting for adult patients suffering nontraumatic cardiac arrest. National Association of EMS Physicians Standards and Clinical Practice Committee. *Prehosp Emerg Care.* 2000;4: 190–195.

33. Morrison LJ, Verbeek PR, Vermeulen MJ, Kiss A, Allan KS, Nesbitt L, Stiell I. Derivation and evaluation of a termination of resuscitation clinical prediction rule for advanced life support providers. *Resuscitation.* 2007;74: 266–275.

34. Auerbach PS, Morris JA Jr, Phillips JB Jr, Redlinger SR, Vaughn WK. An analysis of ambulance accidents in Tennessee. *JAMA.* 1987;258: 1487–1490.

35. Kellermann AL, Hackman BB. Terminating unsuccessful advanced cardiac life support in the field. *Am J Emerg Med.* 1987;5:548–549.

36. Morrison LJ, Cheung MC, Redelmeier DA. Evaluating paramedic comfort with field pronouncement: development and validation of an outcome measure. *Acad Emerg Med.* 2003;10:633–637.

37. Gray WA, Capone RJ, Most AS. Unsuccessful emergency medical resuscitation: are continued efforts in the emergency department justified? *N Engl J Med.* 1991;325:1393–1398.

38. Suchard JR, Fenton FR, Powers RD. Medicare expenditures on unsuccessful out-of-hospital resuscitations. *J Emerg Med.* 1999;17:801–805.

39. Olasveengen TM, Wik L, Steen PA. Quality of cardiopulmonary resuscitation before and during transport in out-of-hospital cardiac arrest. *Resuscitation.* 2008;76:185–190.

40. Eisenberg MS, Mengert TJ. Cardiac resuscitation. *N Engl J Med.* 2001; 344:1304–1313.

41. Chung TN, Kim SW, Cho YS, Chung SP, Park I, Kim SH. Effect of vehicle speed on the quality of closed-chest compression during ambulance transport. *Resuscitation.* 2010.

42. Loertscher L, Reed DA, Bannon MP, Mueller PS. Cardiopulmonary resuscitation and do-not-resuscitate orders: a guide for clinicians. *Am J Med.* 2010;123:4–9.

43. Do Not Attempt Resuscitation (DNAR) Decisions in the Perioperative Period. London: The Association of Anaesthetists of Great Britain and Ireland; 2009.

44. Paris JJ. What standards apply to resuscitation at the borderline of gestational age? *J Perinatol.* 2005;25:683–684.

45. De Leeuw R, Cuttini M, Nadai M, Berbik I, Hansen G, Kucinskas A, Lenoir S, Levin A, Persson J, Rebagliato M, Reid M, Schroell M, de Vonderweid U. Treatment choices for extremely preterm infants: an international perspective. *J Pediatr.* 2000;137:608–616.

46. Jain L, Ferre C, Vidyasagar D, Nath S, Sheftel D. Cardiopulmonary resuscitation of apparently stillborn infants: survival and long-term outcome. *J Pediatr.* 1991;118:778–782.

47. Casalaz DM, Marlow N, Speidel BD. Outcome of resuscitation following unexpected apparent stillbirth. *Arch Dis Child Fetal Neonatal Ed.* 1998;78:F112–F115.

48. Laptook AR, Shankaran S, Ambalavanan N, Carlo WA, McDonald SA, Higgins RD, Das A. Outcome of term infants using Apgar scores at 10

minutes following hypoxic-ischemic encephalopathy. *Pediatrics*. 2009; 124:1619–1626.

49. Atkins DL, Everson-Stewart S, Sears GK, Daya M, Osmond MH, Warden CR, Berg RA. Epidemiology and outcomes from out-of-hospital cardiac arrest in children: the Resuscitation Outcomes Consortium Epistry-Cardiac Arrest. *Circulation*. 2009;119:1484–1491.

50. Perron AD, Sing RF, Branas CC, Huynh T. Predicting survival in pediatric trauma patients receiving cardiopulmonary resuscitation in the prehospital setting. *Prehosp Emerg Care*. 2001;5:6–9.

51. Donoghue AJ, Nadkarni V, Berg RA, Osmond MH, Wells G, Nesbitt L, Stiell IG. Out-of-hospital pediatric cardiac arrest: an epidemiologic review and assessment of current knowledge. *Ann Emerg Med*. 2005; 46:512–522.

52. Reis AG, Nadkarni V, Perondi MB, Grisi S, Berg RA. A prospective investigation into the epidemiology of in-hospital pediatric cardiopulmonary resuscitation using the international Utstein reporting style. *Pediatrics*. 2002;109:200–209.

53. Rodriguez-Nunez A, Lopez-Herce J, Garcia C, Carrillo A, Dominguez P, Calvo C, Delgado MA. Effectiveness and long-term outcome of cardiopulmonary resuscitation in paediatric intensive care units in Spain. *Resuscitation*. 2006;71:301–309.

54. Samson RA, Nadkarni VM, Meaney PA, Carey SM, Berg MD, Berg RA. Outcomes of in-hospital ventricular fibrillation in children. *N Engl J Med*. 2006;354:2328–2339.

55. Nadkarni VM, Larkin GL, Peberdy MA, Carey SM, Kaye W, Mancini ME, Nichol G, Lane-Truitt T, Potts J, Ornato JP, Berg RA. First documented rhythm and clinical outcome from in-hospital cardiac arrest among children and adults. *JAMA*. 2006;295:50–57.

56. Meaney PA, Nadkarni VM, Cook EF, Testa M, Helfaer M, Kaye W, Larkin GL, Berg RA. Higher survival rates among younger patients after pediatric intensive care unit cardiac arrests. *Pediatrics*. 2006;118: 2424–2433.

57. Eckstein M, Stratton SJ, Chan LS. Termination of resuscitative efforts for out-of-hospital cardiac arrests. *Acad Emerg Med*. 2005; 12:65–70.

58. Meyers TA, Eichhorn DJ, Guzzetta CE. Do families want to be present during CPR? A retrospective survey. *J Emerg Nurs*. 1998; 24:400–405.

59. Robinson SM, Mackenzie-Ross S, Campbell Hewson GL, Egleston CV, Prevost AT. Psychological effect of witnessed resuscitation on bereaved relatives. *Lancet*. 1998;352:614–617.

60. Boie ET, Moore GP, Brummett C, Nelson DR. Do parents want to be present during invasive procedures performed on their children in the emergency department? A survey of 400 parents. *Ann Emerg Med*. 1999;34:70–74.

61. Adams S, Whitlock M, Higgs R, Bloomfield P, Baskett PJ. Should relatives be allowed to watch resuscitation? *BMJ*. 1994;308:1687–1692.

62. Boyd R. Witnessed resuscitation by relatives. *Resuscitation*. 2000;43: 171–176.

63. Hampe SO. Needs of the grieving spouse in a hospital setting. *Nurs Res*. 1975;24:113–120.

64. Offord RJ. Should relatives of patients with cardiac arrest be invited to be present during cardiopulmonary resuscitation? *Intensive Crit Care Nurs*. 1998;14:288–293.

65. Shaner K, Eckle N. Implementing a program to support the option of family presence during resuscitation. *The Association for the Care of Children's Health (ACCH) Advocate*. 1997;3:3–7.

66. Eichhorn DJ, Meyers TA, Mitchell TG, Guzzetta CE. Opening the doors: family presence during resuscitation. *J Cardiovasc Nurs*. 1996; 10:59–70.

67. Doyle CJ, Post H, Burney RE, Maino J, Keefe M, Rhee KJ. Family participation during resuscitation: an option. *Ann Emerg Med*. 1987;16: 673–675.

68. Barratt F, Wallis DN. Relatives in the resuscitation room: their point of view. *J Accid Emerg Med*. 1998;15:109–111.

69. Compton S, Madgy A, Goldstein M, Sandhu J, Dunne R, Swor R. Emergency medical service providers' experience with family presence during cardiopulmonary resuscitation. *Resuscitation*. 2006;70:223–228.

70. Beckman AW, Sloan BK, Moore GP, Cordell WH, Brizendine EJ, Boie ET, Knoop KJ, Goldman MJ, Geninatti MR. Should parents be present during emergency department procedures on children, and who should make that decision? A survey of emergency physician and nurse attitudes. *Acad Emerg Med*. 2002;9:154–158.

71. Dudley NC, Hansen KW, Furnival RA, Donaldson AE, Van Wagenen KL, Scaife ER. The effect of family presence on the efficiency of pediatric trauma resuscitations. *Ann Emerg Med*. 2009;53:777–784. e773.

72. Tinsley C, Hill JB, Shah J, Zimmerman G, Wilson M, Freier K, Abd-Allah S, Tinsley C, Hill JB, Shah J, Zimmerman G, Wilson M, Freier K, Abd-Allah S. Experience of families during cardiopulmonary resuscitation in a pediatric intensive care unit. *Pediatrics*. 2008;122: e799–e804.

73. Mangurten J, Scott SH, Guzzetta CE, Clark AP, Vinson L, Sperry J, Hicks B, Voelmeck W. Effects of family presence during resuscitation and invasive procedures in a pediatric emergency department. *Journal of Emergency Nursing*. 2006;32:225–233.

74. McGahey-Oakland PR, Lieder HS, Young A, Jefferson LS, McGahey-Oakland PR, Lieder HS, Young A, Jefferson LS. Family experiences during resuscitation at a children's hospital emergency department. *Journal of Pediatric Health Care*. 2007;21:217–225.

75. Jones M, Qazi M, Young KD. Ethnic differences in parent preference to be present for painful medical procedures. *Pediatrics*. 2005;116: e191–e197.

76. Andrews R, Andrews R. Family presence during a failed major trauma resuscitation attempt of a 15-year-old boy: lessons learned.[see comment]. *Journal of Emergency Nursing*. 2004;30: 556–558.

77. Dill K, Gance-Cleveland B, Dill K, Gance-Cleveland B. With you until the end: family presence during failed resuscitation. *Journal for Specialists in Pediatric Nursing: JSPN*. 2005;10:204–207.

78. Gold KJ, Gorenflo DW, Schwenk TL, Bratton SL, Gold KJ, Gorenflo DW, Schwenk TL, Bratton SL. Physician experience with family presence during cardiopulmonary resuscitation in children. [see comment]. *Pediatric Crit Care Med*. 2006;7:428–433.

79. Duran CR, Oman KS, Abel JJ, Koziel VM, Szymanski D. Attitudes Toward and Beliefs About Family Presence: A Survey of Healthcare Providers, Patients' Families, and Patients. *Am Journal of Critical Care*. 2007;16:270–279.

80. Iserson KV. Notifying survivors about sudden, unexpected deaths. *West J Med*. 2000;173:261–265.

81. Wijdicks EF, Hijdra A, Young GB, Bassetti CL, Wiebe S. Practice parameter: prediction of outcome in comatose survivors after cardiopulmonary resuscitation (an evidence-based review): report of the Quality Standards Subcommittee of the Am Academy of Neurology. *Neurology*. 2006;67:203–210.

82. Al Thenayan E, Savard M, Sharpe M, Norton L, Young B. Predictors of poor neurologic outcome after induced mild hypothermia following cardiac arrest. *Neurology*. 2008;71:1535–1537.

83. Tiainen M, Kovala TT, Takkunen OS, Roine RO. Somatosensory and brainstem auditory evoked potentials in cardiac arrest patients treated with hypothermia. *Crit Care Med*. 2005;33:1736–1740.

84. Rossetti AO, Oddo M, Liaudet L, Kaplan PW. Predictors of awakening from postanoxic status epilepticus after therapeutic hypothermia. *Neurology*. 2009;72:744–749.

85. Rossetti AO, Logroscino G, Liaudet L, Ruffieux C, Ribordy V, Schaller MD, Despland PA, Oddo M. Status epilepticus: an independent outcome predictor after cerebral anoxia. *Neurology*. 2007; 69:255–260.

86. Rossetti AO, Oddo M, Logroscino G, Kaplan PW. Prognostication after cardiac arrest and hypothermia: a prospective study. *Ann Neurol*. 2010; 67:301–307.

87. Leithner C, Ploner CJ, Hasper D, Storm C. Does hypothermia influence the predictive value of bilateral absent N20 after cardiac arrest? *Neurology*. 2010;74:965–969.

88. Tiainen M, Roine RO, Pettila V, Takkunen O. Serum neuron-specific enolase and S-100B protein in cardiac arrest patients treated with hypothermia. *Stroke*. 2003;34:2881–2886.

89. Oksanen T, Tiainen M, Skrifvars MB, Varpula T, Kuitunen A, Castren M, Pettila V. Predictive power of serum NSE and OHCA score regarding 6-month neurologic outcome after out-of-hospital ventricular fibrillation and therapeutic hypothermia. *Resuscitation*. 2009;80: 165–170.

90. Rundgren M, Karlsson T, Nielsen N, Cronberg T, Johnsson P, Friberg H. Neuron specific enolase and S-100B as predictors of outcome after cardiac arrest and induced hypothermia. *Resuscitation*. 2009;80: 784–789.

91. Adrie C, Haouache H, Saleh M, Memain N, Laurent I, Thuong M, Darques L, Guerrini P, Monchi M. An underrecognized source of organ donors: patients with brain death after successfully resuscitated cardiac arrest. *Intensive Care Med*. 2008;34:132–137.

92. Ali AA, Lim E, Thanikachalam M, Sudarshan C, White P, Parameshwar J, Dhital K, Large SR. Cardiac arrest in the organ donor does not negatively influence recipient survival after heart transplantation. *Eur J Cardiothorac Surg*. 2007;31:929–933.

93. Matsumoto CS, Kaufman SS, Girlanda R, Little CM, Rekhtman Y, Raofi V, Laurin JM, Shetty K, Fennelly EM, Johnson LB, Fishbein TM. Utilization of donors who have suffered cardiopulmonary arrest and resuscitation in intestinal transplantation. *Transplantation*. 2008;86:941–946.

94. Mercatello A, Roy P, Ng-Sing K, Choux C, Baude C, Garnier JL, Colpart JJ, Finaz J, Petit P, Moskovtchenko JF, et al. Organ transplants from out-of-hospital cardiac arrest patients. *Transplant Proc*. 1988;20:749–750.

95. Weisfeldt ML, Sugarman J, Bandeen-Roche K. Toward definitive trials and improved outcomes of cardiac arrest. *Circulation*. 2010;121:1586–1588.

96. Dickert N, Sugarman J. Ethical goals of community consultation in research. *Am J Public Health*. 2005;95:1123–1127.

97. Tisherman SA, Powell JL, Schmidt TA, Aufderheide TP, Kudenchuk PJ, Spence J, Climer D, Kelly D, Marcantonio A, Brown T, Sopko G, Kerber R, Sugarman J, Hoyt D. Regulatory challenges for the resuscitation outcomes consortium. *Circulation*. 2008;118:1585–1592.

98. Dickert NW, Sugarman J. Getting the ethics right regarding research in the emergency setting: lessons from the PolyHeme study. *Kennedy Inst Ethics J*. 2007;17:153–169.

99. Protection of human subjects; informed consent–FDA. Final rule. *Fed Regist*. 1996;61:51498–51533.

100. Dickert NW, Sugarman J. Community consultation: not the problem—an important part of the solution. *Am J Bioeth*. 2006;6:26–28.

101. Shah AN, Sugarman J. Protecting research subjects under the waiver of informed consent for emergency research: experiences with efforts to inform the community. *Ann Emerg Med*. 2003;41:72–78.

102. Marco C. Teaching Procedures Using the Newly Dead. Am College of Emergency Physicians. Ethics Committee; 2003.

KEY WORDS: arrhythmia ■ automatic external defibrillator ■ cardioversion ■ ventricular fibrillation

# Part 4: CPR Overview
## 2010 American Heart Association Guidelines for Cardiopulmonary Resuscitation and Emergency Cardiovascular Care

Andrew H. Travers, Co-Chair*; Thomas D. Rea, Co-Chair*; Bentley J. Bobrow;
Dana P. Edelson; Robert A. Berg; Michael R. Sayre; Marc D. Berg;
Leon Chameides; Robert E. O'Connor; Robert A. Swor

Cardiopulmonary resuscitation (CPR) is a series of life-saving actions that improve the chance of survival following cardiac arrest.[1] Although the optimal approach to CPR may vary, depending on the rescuer, the victim, and the available resources, the fundamental challenge remains: how to achieve early and effective CPR. Given this challenge, recognition of arrest and prompt action by the rescuer continue to be priorities for the *2010 AHA Guidelines for CPR and ECC*. This chapter provides an overview of cardiac arrest epidemiology, the principles behind each link in the Chain of Survival, an overview of the core components of CPR (see Table 1), and the approaches of the *2010 AHA Guidelines for CPR and ECC* to improving the quality of CPR. The goal of this chapter is to integrate resuscitation science with real-world practice in order to improve the outcomes of CPR.

## Epidemiology

Despite important advances in prevention, cardiac arrest remains a substantial public health problem and a leading cause of death in many parts of the world.[2] Cardiac arrest occurs both in and out of the hospital. In the US and Canada, approximately 350 000 people/year (approximately half of them in-hospital) suffer a cardiac arrest and receive attempted resuscitation.[3–7] This estimate does not include the substantial number of victims who suffer an arrest without attempted resuscitation. While attempted resuscitation is not always appropriate, there are many lives and life-years lost because appropriate resuscitation is not attempted.

The estimated incidence of EMS-treated out-of-hospital cardiac arrest in the US and Canada is about 50 to 55/100 000 persons/year and approximately 25% of these present with pulseless ventricular arrhythmias.[3,8] The estimated incidence of in-hospital cardiac arrest is 3 to 6/1000 admissions[4–6] and similarly, approximately 25% of these present with pulseless ventricular arrhythmias.[7] Cardiac arrest victims who present with ventricular fibrillation (VF) or pulseless ventricular tachycardia (VT) have a substantially better outcome compared with those who present with asystole or pulseless electric activity.[1,7,9]

The vast majority of cardiac arrest victims are adults, but thousands of infants and children suffer either an in-hospital or out-of-hospital cardiac arrest each year in the US and Canada.[7,10]

Cardiac arrest continues to be an all-too-common cause of premature death, and small incremental improvements in survival can translate into thousands of lives saved every year.

## Key Principles in Resuscitation: Strengthening the Links in the Chain of Survival

Successful resuscitation following cardiac arrest requires an integrated set of coordinated actions represented by the links in the Chain of Survival (see Figure 1).

The links include the following:

- Immediate **recognition** of cardiac arrest and **activation** of the emergency response system
- Early **CPR** with an emphasis on chest compressions
- Rapid **defibrillation**
- Effective **advanced life support**
- Integrated **post–cardiac arrest care**

Emergency systems that can effectively implement these links can achieve witnessed VF cardiac arrest survival of almost 50%.[11–14] In most emergency systems, however, survival is lower, indicating that there is an opportunity for improvement by carefully examining the links and strengthening those that are weak.[3] The individual links are interdependent, and the success of each link is dependent on the effectiveness of those that precede it.

Rescuers have a wide variety of training, experience, and skills. The cardiac arrest victim's status and response to CPR maneuvers, as well as the settings in which the arrests occur, can also be heterogeneous. The challenge is how to encourage early, effective CPR for as many victims as possible, taking

The American Heart Association requests that this document be cited as follows: Travers AH, Rea TD, Bobrow BJ, Edelson DP, Berg RA, Sayre MR, Berg MD, Chameides L, O'Connor RE, Swor RA. Part 4: CPR overview: 2010 American Heart Association Guidelines for Cardiopulmonary Resuscitation and Emergency Cardiovascular Care. *Circulation.* 2010;122(suppl 3):S676–S684.

*Co-chairs and equal first co-authors.

(*Circulation.* 2010;122[suppl 3]:S676–S684.)

*Circulation* is available at http://circ.ahajournals.org

DOI: 10.1161/CIRCULATIONAHA.110.970913

**Table 1.    Summary of Key BLS Components for Adults, Children and Infants**

| Component | Recommendations | | |
|---|---|---|---|
| | Adults | Children | Infants |
| Recognition | Unresponsive (for all ages) | | |
| | No breathing, not breathing normally (eg, only gasping) | No breathing or only gasping | |
| | No pulse palpated within 10 seconds (HCP Only) | | |
| CPR Sequence | CAB | CAB | CAB |
| Compression Rate | At least 100/min | | |
| Compression Depth | At least 2 inches (5 cm) | At least 1/3 AP Depth About 2 inches (5 cm) | At least 1/3 AP Depth About $1\frac{1}{2}$ inches (4 cm) |
| Chest Wall Recoil | Allow Complete Recoil Between Compressions HCPs Rotate Compressors Every 2 minutes | | |
| Compression Interruptions | Minimize Interruptions in Chest Compressions Attempt to limit interruptions to less than 10 seconds | | |
| Airway | Head tilt-chin lift (HCP suspected trauma: jaw thrust) | | |
| Compression to Ventilation Ratio (until advanced airway placed) | 30:2 (1 or 2 rescuers) | 30:2 Single Rescuer 15:2 2 HCP Rescuers | 30:2 Single Rescuer 15:2 2 HCP Rescuers |
| Ventilations: When rescuer Untrained or Trained and Not Proficient | Compressions Only | | |
| Ventilations with advanced airway (HCP) | 1 breath every 6–8 seconds (8–10 breaths/min) Asynchronous with chest compressions About 1 second per breath Visible Chest Rise | | |
| Defibrillation | Attach and use AED as soon as available. Minimize interruptions in chest compressions before and after shock, resume CPR beginning with compressions immediately after each shock | | |

into account the wide range of rescuers, victims, and available resources.

Solutions must be based on rigorous research and careful interpretation whenever possible. As with past guidelines,[15] the process of evidence evaluation for the *2010 AHA Guidelines for CPR and ECC* was comprehensive, systematic, and transparent. The *2010 AHA Guidelines for CPR and ECC* rest on a foundation of previous guidelines, but they are supported by new evidence whenever possible.

The following sections provide an overview of the first three links in the Chain of Survival: immediate recognition of

an arrest and activation of the emergency response system, early CPR, and rapid defibrillation. The information is provided in a manner that recognizes the real-world heterogeneity of the rescuer, victim, and resources.

## Conceptual Framework for CPR: Interaction of Rescuer(s) and Victim

CPR traditionally has integrated chest compressions and rescue breathing with the goal of optimizing circulation and oxygenation. Rescuer and victim characteristics may influence the optimal application of the components of CPR.

### *Rescuer*
Everyone can be a lifesaving rescuer for a cardiac arrest victim. CPR skills and their application depend on the rescuer's training, experience, and confidence.

Chest compressions are the foundation of CPR (see Figure 2). *All rescuers, regardless of training, should provide chest compressions to all cardiac arrest victims.* Because of their importance, chest compressions should be the initial CPR action for all victims regardless of age. Rescuers who are able should add ventilations to chest compressions. Highly trained rescuers working together should coordinate their care and perform chest compressions as well as ventilations in a team-based approach.

### *Victim*
Most cardiac arrests in adults are sudden, resulting from a primary cardiac cause; circulation produced by chest compressions is therefore paramount.[16] In contrast, cardiac arrest in children is most often asphyxial, which requires both ventilations and chest compressions for optimal results.[17] Thus rescue breathing may be more important for children than for adults in cardiac arrest.[17]

## Early Action: Integrating the Critical Components of CPR

The Universal Adult Basic Life Support (BLS) Algorithm is a conceptual framework for all levels of rescuers in all settings. It emphasizes the key components that any rescuer can and should perform (see Figure 3).

When encountering a victim of sudden adult cardiac arrest, the lone rescuer must first **recognize** that the victim has experienced a cardiac arrest, based on unresponsiveness and lack of normal breathing. After recognition, the rescuer should immediately **activate** the emergency response system, get an AED/defibrillator, if available, and start **CPR** with chest compressions. If an AED is not close by, the rescuer should proceed directly to CPR. If other rescuers are present, the first rescuer should direct them to activate the emergency response system and get

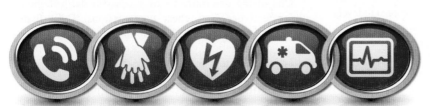

**Figure 1.** Chain of Survival. The links in this Chain are: Immediate recognition and activation, early CPR, rapid defibrillation, effective advanced life support and integrated post-cardiac arrest care.

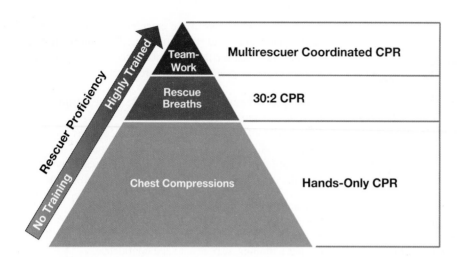

**Figure 2.** Building Blocks of CPR.

the AED/defibrillator; the first rescuer should start CPR immediately.

When the AED/defibrillator arrives, apply the pads, if possible, without interrupting chest compressions and turn the AED "on." The AED will analyze the rhythm and direct the rescuer either to provide a shock (ie, attempt **defibrillation**) or to continue CPR.

If an AED/defibrillator is not available, continue CPR without interruptions until more experienced rescuers assume care.

## Recognition and Activation of Emergency Response

Prompt emergency activation and initiation of CPR requires rapid recognition of cardiac arrest. A cardiac arrest victim is not responsive. Breathing is absent or is not normal.[18,19] Agonal gasps are common early after sudden cardiac arrest and can be confused with normal breathing.[20–23] Pulse detection alone is often unreliable, even when performed by trained rescuers, and it may require additional time.[24–27] Consequently, rescuers should start CPR immediately if the adult victim is unresponsive and not breathing or not breathing normally (ie, only gasping). The directive to "look, listen, and feel for breathing" to aid recognition is no longer recommended.

Emergency dispatchers can and should assist in the assessment and direction to start CPR.[18,28,29] A healthcare professional may incorporate additional information to aid arrest recognition.

## Chest Compressions

The prompt initiation of effective chest compressions is a fundamental aspect of cardiac arrest resuscitation. CPR improves the victim's chance of survival by providing heart and brain circulation. Rescuers should perform chest compressions for all victims in cardiac arrest, regardless of rescuer skill level, victim characteristics, or available resources.

Rescuers should focus on delivering high-quality CPR:

- providing chest compressions of adequate rate (at least 100/minute)
- providing chest compressions of adequate depth
  - adults: a compression depth of at least 2 inches (5 cm)

- infants and children: a depth of least one third the anterior-posterior (AP) diameter of the chest or about 1 ½ inches (4 cm) in infants and about 2 inches (5 cm) in children
- allowing complete chest recoil after each compression
- minimizing interruptions in compressions
- avoiding excessive ventilation

If multiple rescuers are available, they should rotate the task of compressions every 2 minutes.

## Airway and Ventilations

Opening the airway (with a head tilt–chin lift or jaw thrust) followed by rescue breaths can improve oxygenation and ventilation. However, these maneuvers can be technically challenging and require interruptions of chest compressions, particularly for a lone rescuer who has not been trained. Thus, the untrained rescuer will provide Hands-Only (compression-only) CPR (ie, compressions without ventilations), and the lone rescuer who is able should open the airway and give rescue breaths with chest compressions. Ventilations should be provided if the victim has a high likelihood of an asphyxial cause of the arrest (eg, infant, child, or drowning victim).

Once an advanced airway is in place, healthcare providers will deliver ventilations at a regular rate 1 breath every 6 to 8 seconds (8 to 10 breaths/minute) and chest compressions can be delivered without interruption.

## Defibrillation

The victim's chance of survival decreases with an increasing interval between the arrest and defibrillation.[30,31] Thus early defibrillation remains the cornerstone therapy for ventricular fibrillation and pulseless ventricular tachycardia. Community and hospital strategies should aggressively work to reduce the interval between arrest and defibrillation.[32]

One of the determinants of successful defibrillation is the effectiveness of chest compressions. Defibrillation outcome is improved if interruptions (for rhythm assessment, defibrillation, or advanced care) in chest compressions are kept to a minimum.[11,14,33–39]

## Translating Resuscitation Science Into Practice

In a community setting, the sole trained layperson responding to a cardiac arrest victim needs to perform an ordered

**Simplified Adult BLS**

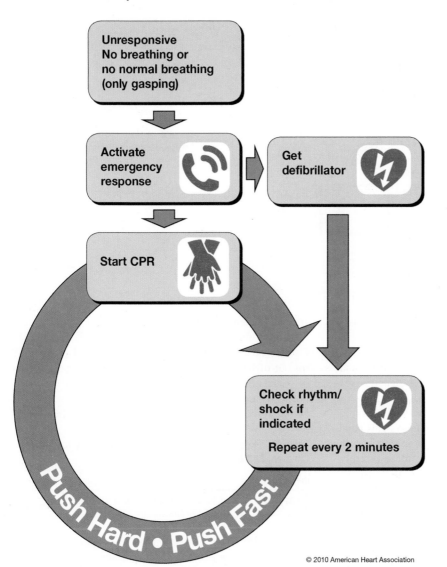

**Figure 3.** Simplified Adult BLS Algorithm.

sequence of CPR steps. Laypersons can learn these skills online and in courses.

In contrast, in a highly specialized environment, such as a critical care unit of a hospital, many of the individual components of CPR (compression-ventilation-defibrillation) may be managed simultaneously. This approach requires choreography among many highly-trained rescuers who work as an integrated team.

In the prehospital setting, the order of the CPR components performed by the healthcare provider may switch between a sequenced and choreographed model depending on the proficiency of the provider and the availability of resources.

## Quality Improvement in Resuscitation Systems, Process, and Outcomes

### A Systems Approach

Cardiac arrest is an important public health issue. Resuscitation involves a broad spectrum of individual stakeholders and groups. Individuals include victims, family members, rescuers, and healthcare providers. Key stakeholder groups include the public, emergency medical dispatchers, public safety organizations, EMS systems, hospitals, civic groups, and policy makers at the local, state, and federal levels.

Because the links in the Chain of Survival are interdependent, an effective resuscitation strategy requires these individuals and groups to work in an integrated fashion and function as a *system of care*.[40] Fundamental to a successful resuscitation system of care is the collective appreciation of the challenges and opportunities presented by the Chain of Survival. Thus individuals and groups must work together, sharing ideas and information, to evaluate and improve their resuscitation system. Leadership and accountability are important components of this team approach.

A conceptual appreciation of the system and its working components is only a starting point. Improving care requires assessment of performance. Only when performance is evaluated can participants in a system effectively

# Developing a culture of high quality resuscitation

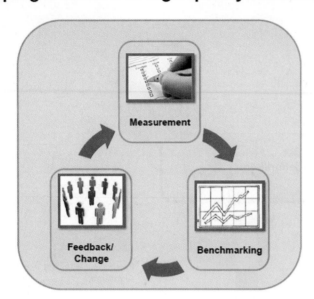

**Figure 4.** Quality Improvement Elements of a Resuscitation System.

intervene to improve care. This process of quality improvement consists of an iterative and continuous cycle of (1) systematic evaluation of resuscitation care and outcome, (2) benchmarking with stakeholder feedback, and (3) strategic efforts to address identified deficiencies (see Figure 4).

There is wide community and hospital variability in cardiac arrest survival.[3,8,13] High-performing systems have used this continuous quality improvement approach with great success,[41] as have systems that have more recently adopted this strategy.[42] These successes have occurred in a variety of systems, suggesting that all communities and hospitals can substantially improve care and outcomes. Since each system has different characteristics and challenges, there is no single prescriptive strategy for improvement. However, each system has an obligation to address the fundamental principles of quality improvement: measurement, benchmarking, and feedback and change.

## Measurement

Quality improvement relies on valid assessment of resuscitation performance and outcome. The Utstein Guidelines provide useful templates for measuring key aspects of resuscitation care and outcome.[43,44] Examples of core performance measures include the rate of bystander CPR, time to defibrillation, and survival to hospital discharge. Such measures are typically assessed based on review of dispatch, EMS, and hospital records, underscoring the importance of information sharing among all the links in the system of care. Additional measures can be incorporated to meet a system's individual quality improvement strategy. For example, individual CPR components can be measured through review of the electronic defibrillator recording and can provide a useful set of metrics for EMS and hospital providers.[45]

## Benchmarking and Feedback

These data should be systematically reviewed and compared internally to prior performance and externally to similar systems. Existing cardiac arrest registries can facilitate this benchmarking effort; examples include the Cardiac Arrest Registry to Enhance Survival (CARES)[46] for out-of-hospital cardiac arrest and the National Registry of CardioPulmonary Resuscitation (NRCPR)[47] for in-hospital cardiac arrest. The results of assessments should be regularly interpreted by all stakeholders and can iden-

**Table 2.   Key Challenges to Improve CPR Quality for Adults, Children, and Infants**

| CPR Component | Key Challenges to Improving Quality |
|---|---|
| Recognition | • Failure to recognize gasping as sign of cardiac arrest<br>• Unreliable pulse detection |
| Initiation of CPR | • Low bystander CPR response rates<br>• Incorrect dispatch instructions |
| Compression rate | • Slow compression rate |
| Compression depth | • Shallow compression depth |
| Chest wall recoil | • Rescuer leaning on the chest |
| Compression interruptions | • Excessive interruptions for<br>  – rhythm/pulse checks<br>  – ventilations<br>  – defibrillation<br>  – intubation<br>  – intravenous (IV) access<br>  – other |
| Ventilation | • Ineffective ventilations<br>• Prolonged interruptions in compressions to deliver breaths<br>• Excessive ventilation (especially with advanced airway) |
| Defibrillation | • Prolonged time to defibrillator availability<br>• Prolonged interruptions in chest compressions pre- and post-shocks |
| Team Performance | • Delayed rotation, leading to rescuer fatigue and decay in compression quality<br>• Poor communication among rescuers, leading to unnecessary interruptions in compressions |

tify key considerations for directed efforts of improvement (see Table 2).

### Change

The process of simply measuring and benchmarking care can positively influence outcome.[48] However, ongoing review and interpretation are necessary to identify areas for improvement. Local data may suggest the need to increase bystander CPR response rates, improve CPR performance, or shorten the time to defibrillation. Useful strategies might include programs targeting citizen awareness, education and training for citizens and professionals, and various technologic solutions. These programs need to be continually re-evaluated to ensure that potential areas for improvement are fully addressed.

## Important Lessons from CPR and Summary

The *2010 AHA Guidelines for CPR and ECC* mark the 50th anniversary of modern CPR. There is general agreement that the 1960 Meeting of the Maryland Medical Society in Ocean City, MD, formally introduced the combination of chest compressions and rescue breathing.[49] Two years later (1962) direct-current, monophasic waveform defibrillation was described.[50] In 1966, the American Heart Association developed the first CPR guidelines.[51] Over the past 50 years, these modern-era basic life support fundamentals of early recognition and activation, early CPR, and early defibrillation have saved hundreds of thousands of lives around the world. These lives stand as a testament to the importance of resuscitation research and clinical translation. They give us cause to celebrate this 50th anniversary of CPR.

And yet we still have a long road to travel if we are to fulfill the potential offered by the Chain of Survival. There is a striking disparity in survival across systems of care for cardiac arrest. Survival disparities that were present a generation ago appear to persist.[3,8,52] Although future discoveries will offer opportunities to improve survival, we currently possess the knowledge and tools—represented by the Chain of Survival—to address many of these care gaps.

The challenge is one of real-world translation across diverse systems. Since the *2005 AHA Guidelines for CPR and ECC*, many instructive and encouraging examples have been published, describing ways in which that translation can be accomplished. Each system, whether in the hospital or in the community, must assess its performance and implement a strategy for improving care in cases of cardiac arrest. That strategy should support the building blocks of resuscitation: the BLS links of immediate recognition and emergency activation, early CPR, and rapid defibrillation. If we accept this imperative to act, we can achieve the full potential offered by the Chain of Survival and, in turn, improve public health.

## Disclosures

**Guidelines Part 4: Overview of CPR Writing Group Disclosures**

| Writing Group Member | Employment | Research Grant | Other Research Support | Speakers' Bureau/Honoraria | Ownership Interest | Consultant/ Advisory Board | Other |
|---|---|---|---|---|---|---|---|
| Andrew H. Travers | Emergency Health Services Nova Scotia–Provincial Medical Director | None | None | None | None | None | None |
| Thomas D. Rea | University of Washington: Physician, Associate Professor of Medicine; Emergency Medical Services Division - Public Health Seattle & King County–Program Medical Director | *In the past, I have received modest grants from Philips Inc and PhysioControl to evaluate changes in resuscitation protocols. These investigations did not support evaluation of proprietary equipment. I am an investigator in the Resuscitation Outcomes Consortium so participate in studies evaluating dynamic CPR feedback available in a Philips defibrillator and the impedance threshold device which is developed and owned by a private company. These studies are funded primarily by the NIH and I receive no support from private industry related to these research activities. I participate in a trial of chest compression alone versus chest compression plus ventilation supported in part by the Laerdal Foundation. Collectively I receive < 5% of my salary from these research activities. | *We recently completed an AED training study for which Philips and PhysioControl provided equipment. I did not directly receive any equipment as part of the research activity. | None | None | None | *I participate as part of a DSMB in a trial sponsored by Philips Inc to evaluate quantitative VF waveform algorithm to guide care. I receive no financial support as part of the DSMB. |
| Bentley J. Bobrow | Arizona Department of Health Services–Medical Director, Bureau of EMS and Trauma System; Maricopa Medical Center-Clin. Associate. Professor, Emergency Medicine Department | †AHA. Ultra-Brief CPR Video Study, PI. *Medtronic Foundation. Arizona Statewide Resuscitation System of Care, 2010–2015, PI. | None | None | None | None | None |

*(Continued)*

## Guidelines Part 4: Overview of CPR Writing Group Disclosures, *Continued*

| Writing Group Member | Employment | Research Grant | Other Research Support | Speakers' Bureau/Honoraria | Ownership Interest | Consultant/ Advisory Board | Other |
|---|---|---|---|---|---|---|---|
| Dana P. Edelson | University of Chicago Assistant Professor | †CURRENT RESEARCH GRANTS Pending NHLBI Career Development Award Strategies to Predict and Prevent In-Hospital Cardiac Arrest (1K23HL097157–01) This study is to validate a clinical judgment based tool for predicting impending clinical deterioration of hospitalized floor patients and compare it to previously described physiology-based tools. Role: PI (funds delivered to university). 2009–present Philips Healthcare Research Grant Advancements in CPR and Emergency Care during Hemodynamic Crisis The purpose of this project is to measure capnography and pulse pressure, using a novel plethysmographic sensor, in critically ill patients and correlate quality of CPR with these measures during CA. Role: PI (funds delivered to university) 2008–present Philips Healthcare Research Grant Q-CPR Users & Development Research Alliance The purpose of this project is to establish a multi-center registry of in-hospital resuscitation quality data and a network for clinical trials of resuscitation. Role: PI (funds delivered to university) 2008–present NIH Clinical Research Loan Repayment Granted two years of student loan repayment aims to evaluate the effects of integrated team debriefing using actual performance data to improve CPR quality and patient survival following IHCA.Role: PI (funds delivered to loan servicing program) 2007–present AHA Scientist Development Grant Improving CPR Quality and Patient Outcomes Using a Novel Educational Program This project aims to evaluate the effects of integrated team debriefing using actual performance data to improve CPR quality & patient survival following IHCA. Role: PI (funds delivered to university) 2008–2009 NIH Agency for Healthcare Research and Quality Immersive Simulation Team Training–Impact on Rescue, Recovery and Safety Culture (5U18HS016664–02) The goal is to study the effects of simulation based training for Rapid Response Teams. Consultant (funds to univ.) | *Philips Healthcare, Andover, MA | *Philips Healthcare, Andover, MA | None | *Triage Wireless Inc, San Diego, CA | *Hanna Campbell & Powell LLP, Akron, OH-Hankton Vs Beeson |
| Robert A. Berg | University of Pennsylvania–Professor | | None | None | None | None | None |
| Michael R. Sayre | The Ohio State University–Associate Professor | None | None | None | None | None | None |
| Marc D. Berg | University of Arizona - Associate Professor of Clinical Pediatrics Attending Intensivist | None | None | *Travel expenses reimbursed (<$4000 USD) for participation in 13th Asian Australasian Congress of Anesthesiologists, Fukuoka, Japan, June 2010 | None | None | None |
| Leon Chameides | Emeritus–Director, Pediatric Cardiology, Connecticut Children's Hospital, Clinical Professor, University of Connecticut | None | None | None | None | None | None |
| Robert E. O'Connor | University of Virginia Health System–Professor and Chair of Emergency Medicine | None | None | None | None | None | None |
| Robert A. Swor | William Beaumont Hospital - Hospital Emergency Physician | None | None | None | None | None | None |

This table represents the relationships of writing group members that may be perceived as actual or reasonably perceived conflicts of interest as reported on the Disclosure Questionnaire, which all members of the writing group are required to complete and submit. A relationship is considered to be "significant" if (a) the person receives $ 00 or more during any 12-month period, or 5% or more of the person's gross income; or (b) the person owns 5% or more of the voting stock or share of the entity, or owns $10 000 or more of the fair market value of the entity. A relationship is considered to be "modest" if it is less than "significant" under the preceding definition.

*Modest.

†Significant.

# References

1. Sasson C, Rogers MA, Dahl J, Kellermann AL. Predictors of survival from out-of-hospital cardiac arrest: a systematic review and meta-analysis. *Circ Cardiovasc Qual Outcomes.* 2010;3:63–81.
2. Lloyd-Jones D, Adams RJ, Brown TM, Carnethon M, Dai S, De Simone G, Ferguson TB, Ford E, Furie K, Gillespie C, Go A, Greenlund K, Haase N, Hailpern S, Ho PM, Howard V, Kissela B, Kittner S, Lackland D, Lisabeth L, Marelli A, McDermott MM, Meigs J, Mozaffarian D, Mussolino M, Nichol G, Roger VL, Rosamond W, Sacco R, Sorlie P, Stafford R, Thom T, Wasserthiel-Smoller S, Wong ND, Wylie-Rosett J; American Heart Association Statistics Committee and Stroke Statistics Subcommittee. Heart disease and stroke statistics–2010 update: a report from the American Heart Association. *Circulation.* 2010;121:e46–e215.
3. Nichol G, Thomas E, Callaway CW, Hedges J, Powell JL, Aufderheide TP, Rea T, Lowe R, Brown T, Dreyer J, Davis D, Idris A, Stiell I. Regional variation in out-of-hospital cardiac arrest incidence and outcome. *JAMA.* 2008;300:1423–1431.
4. Hodgetts TJ, Kenward G, Vlackonikolis I, Payne S, Castle N, Crouch R, Ineson N, Shaikh L. Incidence, location and reasons for avoidable in-hospital cardiac arrest in a district general hospital. *Resuscitation.* 2002;54:115–123.
5. Jones-Crawford JL, Parish DC, Smith BE, Dane FC. Resuscitation in the hospital: circadian variation of cardiopulmonary arrest. *Am J Med.* 2007; 120:158–164.
6. Chan PS, Jain R, Nallmothu BK, Berg RA, Sasson C. Rapid response teams: a systematic review and meta-analysis. *Arch Intern Med.* 2010; 170:18–26.
7. Nadkarni VM, Larkin GL, Peberdy MA, Carey SM, Kaye W, Mancini ME, Nichol G, Lane-Truitt T, Potts J, Ornato JP, Berg RA. First documented rhythm and clinical outcome from in-hospital cardiac arrest among children and adults. *JAMA.* 2006;295:50–57.
8. Rea TD, Eisenberg MS, Sinibaldi G, White RD. Incidence of EMS-treated out-of-hospital cardiac arrest in the United States. *Resuscitation.* 2004;63:17–24.
9. Meaney PA, Nadkarni VM, Kern KB, Indik JH, Halperin HR, Berg RA. Rhythms and outcomes of adult in-hospital cardiac arrest. *Crit Care Med.* 2010;38:101–108.
10. Atkins DL, Everson-Stewart S, Sears GK, Daya M, Osmond MH, Warden CR, Berg RA. Epidemiology and outcomes from out-of-hospital cardiac arrest in children: the Resuscitation Outcomes Consortium Epistry-Cardiac Arrest. *Circulation.* 2009;119:1484–1491.
11. Rea TD, Helbock M, Perry S, Garcia M, Cloyd D, Becker L, Eisenberg M. Increasing use of cardiopulmonary resuscitation during out-of-hospital ventricular fibrillation arrest: survival implications of guideline changes. *Circulation.* 2006;114:2760–2765.
12. Agarwal DA, Hess EP, Atkinson EJ, White RD. Ventricular fibrillation in Rochester, Minnesota: experience over 18 years. *Resuscitation.* 2009;80: 1253–1258.
13. Chan PS, Nichol G, Krumholz HM, Spertus JA, Nallamothu BK. Hospital variation in time to defibrillation after in-hospital cardiac arrest. *Arch Intern Med.* 2009;169:1265–1273.
14. Hinchey PR, Myers JB, Lewis R, De Maio VJ, Reyer E, Licatese D, Zalkin J, Snyder G. Improved out-of-hospital cardiac arrest survival after the sequential implementation of 2005 AHA guidelines for compressions, ventilations, and induced hypothermia: the Wake County experience. *Ann Emerg Med.* 2010.[epub ahead of print].
15. 2005 American Heart Association Guidelines for Cardiopulmonary Resuscitation and Emergency Cardiovascular Care. Part 1: Introduction. *Circulation.* 2005;112(24 suppl):IV-1–5.
16. Rea TD, Cook AJ, Stiell IG, Powell J, Bigham B, Callaway CW, Chugh S, Aufderheide TP, Morrison L, Terndrup TE, Beaudoin T, Wittwer L, Davis D, Idris A, Nichol G. Predicting survival after out-of-hospital cardiac arrest: role of the Utstein data elements. *Ann Emerg Med.* 2010; 55:249–257.
17. Kitamura T, Iwami T, Kawamura T, Nagao K, Tanaka H, Nadkarni VM, Berg RA, Hiraide A. Conventional and chest-compression-only cardiopulmonary resuscitation by bystanders for children who have out-of-hospital cardiac arrests: a prospective, nationwide, population-based cohort study. *Lancet.* 2010;375:1347–1354.
18. Berdowski J, Beekhuis F, Zwinderman AH, Tijssen JG, Koster RW. Importance of the first link: description and recognition of an out-of-hospital cardiac arrest in an emergency call. *Circulation.* 2009;119: 2096–2102.
19. Clawson J, Olola C, Scott G, Heward A, Patterson B. Effect of a Medical Priority Dispatch System key question addition in the seizure/convulsion/

20. fitting protocol to improve recognition of ineffective (agonal) breathing. *Resuscitation.* 2008;79:257–264.
21. Bobrow BJ, Zuercher M, Ewy GA, Clark L, Chikani V, Donahue D, Sanders AB, Hilwig RW, Berg RA, Kern KB. Gasping during cardiac arrest in humans is frequent and associated with improved survival. *Circulation.* 2008;118:2550–2554.
22. Hauff SR, Rea TD, Culley LL, Kerry F, Becker L, Eisenberg MS. Factors impeding dispatcher-assisted telephone cardiopulmonary resuscitation. *Ann Emerg Med.* 2003;42:731–737.
23. Vaillancourt C, Verma A, Trickett J, Crete D, Beaudoin T, Nesbitt L, Wells GA, Stiell IG. Evaluating the effectiveness of dispatch-assisted cardiopulmonary resuscitation instructions. *Acad Emerg Med.* 2007;14: 877–883.
24. Bohm K, Rosenqvist M, Hollenberg J, Biber B, Engerstrom L, Svensson L. Dispatcher-assisted telephone-guided cardiopulmonary resuscitation: an underused lifesaving system. *Eur J Emerg Med.* 2007;14:256–259.
25. Eberle B, Dick WF, Schneider T, Wisser G, Doetsch S, Tzanova I. Checking the carotid pulse check: diagnostic accuracy of first responders in patients with and without a pulse. *Resuscitation.* 1996;33:107–116.
26. Tibballs J, Russell P. Reliability of pulse palpation by healthcare personnel to diagnose pediatric cardiac arrest. *Resuscitation.* 2009;80:61–64.
27. Chamberlain D, Smith A, Woollard M, Colquhoun M, Handley AJ, Leaves S, Kern KB. Trials of teaching methods in basic life support (3): comparison of simulated CPR performance after first training and at 6 months, with a note on the value of re-training. *Resuscitation.* 2002;53: 179–187.
28. Lapostolle F, Le Toumelin P, Agostinucci JM, Catineau J, Adnet F. Basic cardiac life support providers checking the carotid pulse: performance, degree of conviction, and influencing factors. *Acad Emerg Med.* 2004; 11:878–880.
29. Rea TD, Eisenberg MS, Culley LL, Becker L. Dispatcher-assisted cardiopulmonary resuscitation and survival in cardiac arrest. *Circulation.* 2001;104:2513–2516.
30. Roppolo LP, Westfall A, Pepe PE, Nobel LL, Cowan J, Kay JJ, Idris AH. Dispatcher assessments for agonal breathing improve detection of cardiac arrest. *Resuscitation.* 2009;80:769–772.
31. Chan PS, Krumholz HM, Nichol G, Nallamothu BK. Delayed time to defibrillation after in-hospital cardiac arrest. *N Engl J Med.* 2008; 358:9–17.
32. Valenzuela TD, Roe DJ, Nichol G, Clark LL, Spaite DW, Hardman RG. Outcomes of rapid defibrillation by security officers after cardiac arrest in casinos. *N Engl J Med.* 2000;343:1206–1209.
33. The Public Access Defibrillation Trial Investigators. Public-access defibrillation and survival after out-of-hospital cardiac arrest. *N Engl J Med.* 2004;351:637–646.
34. Christenson J, Andrusiek D, Everson-Stewart S, Kudenchuk P, Hostler D, Powell J, Callaway CW, Bishop D, Vaillancourt C, Davis D, Aufderheide TP, Idris A, Stouffer JA, Stiell I, Berg R. Chest compression fraction determines survival in patients with out-of-hospital ventricular fibrillation. *Circulation.* 2009;120:1241–1247.
35. Garza AG, Gratton MC, Salomone JA, Lindholm D, McElroy J, Archer R. Improved patient survival using a modified resuscitation protocol for out-of-hospital cardiac arrest. *Circulation.* 2009;119:2597–2605.
36. Bobrow BJ, Clark LL, Ewy GA, Chikani V, Sanders AB, Berg RA, Richman PB, Kern KB. Minimally interrupted cardiac resuscitation by emergency medical services for out-of-hospital cardiac arrest. *JAMA.* 2008;299:1158–1165.
37. Kellum MJ, Kennedy KW, Barney R, Keilhauer FA, Bellino M, Zuercher M, Ewy GA. Cardiocerebral resuscitation improves neurologically intact survival of patients with out-of-hospital cardiac arrest. *Ann Emerg Med.* 2008;52:244–252.
38. Sayre MR, Cantrell SA, White LJ, Hiestand BC, Keseg DP, Koser S. Impact of the 2005 American Heart Association cardiopulmonary resuscitation and emergency cardiovascular care guidelines on out-of-hospital cardiac arrest survival. *Prehosp Emerg Care.* 2009;13:469–477.
39. Steinmetz J, Barnung S, Nielsen SL, Risom M, Rasmussen LS. Improved survival after an out-of-hospital cardiac arrest using new guidelines. *Acta Anaesthesiol Scand.* 2008;52:908–913.
40. Aufderheide TP, Yannopoulos D, Lick CJ, Myers B, Romig LA, Stothert JC, Barnard J, Vartanian L, Pilgrim AJ, Benditt DG. Implementing the 2005 American Heart Association guidelines improves outcomes after out-of-hospital cardiac arrest. *Heart Rhythm.* 2010.[epub ahead of print].
41. Rea TD, Page RL. Community approaches to improve resuscitation after out-of-hospital sudden cardiac arrest. *Circulation.* 2010;121:1134–1140.

41. Cobb LA, Fahrenbruch CE, Walsh TR, Copass MK, Olsufka M, Breskin M, Hallstrom AP. Influence of cardiopulmonary resuscitation prior to defibrillation in patients with out-of-hospital ventricular fibrillation. *JAMA*. 1999;281:1182–1188.

42. Bobrow BJ, Vadeboncoeur TF, Clark L, Chikani V. Establishing Arizona's statewide cardiac arrest reporting and educational network. *Prehosp Emerg Care*. 2008;12:381–387.

43. Jacobs I, Nadkarni V, Bahr J, Berg RA, Billi JE, Bossaert L, Cassan P, Coovadia A, D'Este K, Finn J, Halperin H, Handley A, Herlitz J, Hickey R, Idris A, Kloeck W, Larkin GL, Mancini ME, Mason P, Mears G, Monsieurs K, Montgomery W, Morley P, Nichol G, Nolan J, Okada K, Perlman J, Shuster M, Steen PA, Sterz F, Tibballs J, Timerman S, Truitt T, Zideman D. Cardiac arrest and cardiopulmonary resuscitation outcome reports: update and simplification of the Utstein templates for resuscitation registries: a statement for healthcare professionals from a task force of the International Liaison Committee on Resuscitation (American Heart Association, European Resuscitation Council, Australian Resuscitation Council, New Zealand Resuscitation Council, Heart and Stroke Foundation of Canada, InterAmerican Heart Foundation, Resuscitation Councils of Southern Africa). *Circulation*. 2004;110:3385–3397.

44. Peberdy MA, Cretikos M, Abella BS, DeVita M, Goldhill D, Kloeck W, Kronick SL, Morrison LJ, Nadkarni VM, Nichol G, Nolan JP, Parr M, Tibballs J, van der Jagt EW, Young L. Recommended guidelines for monitoring, reporting, and conducting research on medical emergency team, outreach, and rapid response systems: an Utstein-style scientific statement: a scientific statement from the International Liaison Committee on Resuscitation (American Heart Association, Australian Resuscitation Council, European Resuscitation Council, Heart and Stroke Foundation of Canada, InterAmerican Heart Foundation, Resuscitation Council of Southern Africa, and the New Zealand Resuscitation Council); the American Heart Association Emergency Cardiovascular Care Committee; the Council on Cardiopulmonary, Perioperative, and Critical Care; and the Interdisciplinary Working Group on Quality of Care and Outcomes Research. *Circulation*. 2007;116:2481–2500.

45. Kramer-Johansen J, Edelson DP, Losert H, Kohler K, Abella BS. Uniform reporting of measured quality of cardiopulmonary resuscitation (CPR). *Resuscitation*. 2007;74:406–417.

46. Cardiac Arrest Registry to Enhance Survival (CARES): an out of hospital CPR registry. Available at: https://mycares.net. Accessed 5 May 2010.

47. National Registry of CPR (NRCPR). Available at: http://www.nrcpr.org/. Accessed 5 May 2010.

48. Kohli E, Ptak J, Smith R, Taylor E, Talbot EA, Kirkland KB. Variability in the Hawthorne effect with regard to hand hygiene performance in high- and low-performing inpatient care units. *Infect Control Hosp Epidemiol*. 2009;30:222–225.

49. Eisenberg M. *Resuscitate! How Your Community Can Improve Survival from Sudden Cardiac Arrest*. Seattle: University of Washington Press; 2009.

50. Lown B, Neuman J, Amarasingham R, Berkovits BV. Comparison of alternating current with direct electroshock across the closed chest. *Am J Cardiol*. 1962;10:223–233.

51. Cardiopulmonary resuscitation. *JAMA*. 1966;198:372–379.

52. Eisenberg MS, Horwood BT, Cummins RO, Reynolds-Haertle R, Hearne TR. Cardiac arrest and resuscitation: a tale of 29 cities. *Ann Emerg Med*. 1990;19:179–186.

KEY WORDS: cardiac arrest ■ defibrillation ■ emergency department

# Part 5: Adult Basic Life Support
## 2010 American Heart Association Guidelines for Cardiopulmonary Resuscitation and Emergency Cardiovascular Care

Robert A. Berg, Chair; Robin Hemphill; Benjamin S. Abella; Tom P. Aufderheide; Diana M. Cave;
Mary Fran Hazinski; E. Brooke Lerner; Thomas D. Rea; Michael R. Sayre; Robert A. Swor

Basic life support (BLS) is the foundation for saving lives following cardiac arrest. Fundamental aspects of BLS include immediate **recognition** of sudden cardiac arrest (SCA) and **activation** of the emergency response system, early **cardiopulmonary resuscitation** (*CPR*), and rapid **defibrillation** with an automated external defibrillator (*AED*). Initial recognition and response to heart attack and stroke are also considered part of BLS. This section presents the 2010 adult BLS guidelines for lay rescuers and healthcare providers. Key changes and continued points of emphasis from the 2005 BLS Guidelines include the following:

- Immediate recognition of SCA based on assessing unresponsiveness and absence of normal breathing (ie, the victim is not breathing or only gasping)
- "Look, Listen, and Feel" removed from the BLS algorithm
- Encouraging Hands-Only (chest compression only) CPR (ie, continuous chest compression over the middle of the chest) for the untrained lay-rescuer
- Sequence change to chest compressions before rescue breaths (CAB rather than ABC)
- Health care providers continue effective chest compressions/CPR until return of spontaneous circulation (ROSC) or termination of resuscitative efforts
- Increased focus on methods to ensure that high-quality CPR (compressions of adequate rate and depth, allowing full chest recoil between compressions, minimizing interruptions in chest compressions and avoiding excessive ventilation) is performed
- Continued de-emphasis on pulse check for health care providers
- A simplified adult BLS algorithm is introduced with the revised traditional algorithm
- Recommendation of a simultaneous, choreographed approach for chest compressions, airway management, rescue breathing, rhythm detection, and shocks (if appropriate) by an integrated team of highly-trained rescuers in appropriate settings

Despite important advances in prevention, SCA continues to be a leading cause of death in many parts of the world.[1]

SCA has many etiologies (ie, cardiac or noncardiac causes), circumstances (eg, witnessed or unwitnessed), and settings (eg, out-of-hospital or in-hospital). This heterogeneity suggests that a single approach to resuscitation is not practical, but a core set of actions provides a universal strategy for achieving successful resuscitation. These actions are termed the links in the "Chain of Survival." For adults they include

- Immediate recognition of cardiac arrest and activation of the emergency response system
- Early CPR that emphasizes chest compressions
- Rapid defibrillation if indicated
- Effective advanced life support
- Integrated post–cardiac arrest care

When these links are implemented in an effective way, survival rates can approach 50% following witnessed out-of-hospital ventricular fibrillation (VF) arrest.[2] Unfortunately survival rates in many out-of-hospital and in-hospital settings fall far short of this figure. For example, survival rates following cardiac arrest due to VF vary from approximately 5% to 50% in both out-of-hospital and in-hospital settings.[3,4] This variation in outcome underscores the opportunity for improvement in many settings.

Recognition of cardiac arrest is not always straightforward, especially for laypersons. Any confusion on the part of a rescuer can result in a delay or failure to activate the emergency response system or to start CPR. Precious time is lost if bystanders are too confused to act. Therefore, these adult BLS Guidelines focus on recognition of cardiac arrest with an appropriate set of rescuer actions. Once the lay bystander recognizes that the victim is unresponsive, that bystander must immediately activate (or send someone to activate) the emergency response system. Once the healthcare provider recognizes that the victim is unresponsive with no breathing or no normal breathing (ie, only gasping) the healthcare provider will activate the emergency response system. After activation, rescuers should immediately begin CPR.

Early CPR can improve the likelihood of survival, and yet CPR is often not provided until the arrival of professional emergency responders.[5] Chest compressions are an especially critical component of CPR because perfusion during CPR

The American Heart Association requests that this document be cited as follows: Berg RA, Hemphill R, Abella BS, Aufderheide TP, Cave DM, Hazinski MF, Lerner EB, Rea TD, Sayre MR, Swor RA. Part 5: Adult basic life support: 2010 American Heart Association Guidelines for Cardiopulmonary Resuscitation and Emergency Cardiovascular Care. *Circulation*. 2010;122(suppl 3):S685–S705.

(*Circulation*. 2010;122[suppl 3]:S685–S705.)

*Circulation* is available at http://circ.ahajournals.org          DOI: 10.1161/CIRCULATIONAHA.110.970939

depends on these compressions. Therefore, chest compressions should be the highest priority and the initial action when starting CPR in the adult victim of sudden cardiac arrest. The phrase "push hard and push fast" emphasizes some of these critical components of chest compression. High-quality CPR is important not only at the onset but throughout the course of resuscitation. Defibrillation and advanced care should be interfaced in a way that minimizes any interruption in CPR.[6]

Rapid defibrillation is a powerful predictor of successful resuscitation following VF SCA.[7,8] Efforts to reduce the interval from collapse to defibrillation can potentially improve survival in both out-of-hospital and in-hospital settings.[8,9] Depending on the setting and circumstances, earlier defibrillation may be achieved by a variety of strategies that include rescuers who are laypersons, nontraditional first responders, police, emergency medical services (EMS) professionals, and hospital professionals.[9–12] One of these strategies is the use of an AED. The AED correctly assesses heart rhythm, enabling a rescuer who is not trained in heart rhythm interpretation to accurately provide a potentially lifesaving shock to a victim of SCA.[13]

Immediate **recognition and activation**, early **CPR**, and rapid **defibrillation** (when appropriate) are the first three BLS links in the adult Chain of Survival. BLS care in the out-of-hospital setting is often provided by laypersons who may be involved in a resuscitation attempt only once in their lives. Thus, creating an effective strategy to translate BLS skills to real-world circumstances presents a challenge. This section updates the adult BLS guidelines with the goal of incorporating new scientific information while acknowledging the challenges of real-world application. Everyone, regardless of training or experience, can potentially be a lifesaving rescuer.

The rest of this chapter is organized in sections that address the emergency response system, adult BLS sequence, adult BLS skills, use of an AED, special resuscitation situations, and the quality of BLS. The "Adult BLS Sequence" section provides an overview and an abridged version of the BLS sequence. The "Adult BLS Skills" section provides greater detail regarding individual CPR skills and more information about Hands-Only (compression-only) CPR. The "Special Resuscitation Situations" section addresses acute coronary syndromes, stroke, hypothermia, and foreign body airway obstruction. Because of increasing interest in monitoring and ensuring the quality of CPR, the last section focuses on the quality of BLS.

## Activating the Emergency Response System

Emergency medical dispatch is an integral component of the EMS response.[14] Bystanders (lay responders) should immediately call their local emergency number to initiate a response anytime they find an unresponsive victim. Because dispatcher CPR instructions substantially increase the likelihood of bystander CPR performance and improve survival from cardiac arrest, all dispatchers should be appropriately trained to provide telephone CPR instructions (Class I, LOE B).[15–21]

When dispatchers ask bystanders to determine if breathing is present, bystanders often misinterpret agonal gasps or abnormal breathing as normal breathing. This erroneous information can result in failure by 911 dispatchers to instruct bystanders to initiate CPR for a victim of cardiac arrest.[19,22–26] To help bystanders recognize cardiac arrest, dispatchers should inquire about a victim's absence of consciousness and quality of breathing (normal versus not normal). Dispatchers should be specifically educated in recognition of abnormal breathing in order to improve recognition of gasping and cardiac arrest (Class I, LOE B). Notably, dispatchers should be aware that brief generalized seizures may be the first manifestation of cardiac arrest.[26,27] Dispatchers should recommend CPR for unresponsive victims who are not breathing normally because most are in cardiac arrest and the frequency of serious injury from chest compressions in the nonarrest group is very low (Class I, LOE B).[28] In summary, in addition to activating professional emergency responders, the dispatcher should ask straightforward questions about whether the patient is conscious and breathing normally in order to identify patients with possible cardiac arrest. The dispatcher should also provide CPR instructions to help bystanders initiate CPR when cardiac arrest is suspected.

Because it is easier for rescuers receiving telephone CPR instructions to perform Hands-Only (compression-only) CPR than conventional CPR (compressions plus rescue breathing), dispatchers should instruct untrained lay rescuers to provide Hands-Only CPR for adults with SCA (Class I, LOE B).[29] While Hands-Only CPR instructions have broad applicability, instances remain when rescue breaths are critically important. Dispatchers should include rescue breathing in their telephone CPR instructions to bystanders treating adult and pediatric victims with a high likelihood of an asphyxial cause of arrest (eg, drowning).[30]

The EMS system quality improvement process, including review of the quality of dispatcher CPR instructions provided to specific callers, is considered an important component of a high-quality lifesaving program (Class IIa, LOE B).[31–33]

## Adult BLS Sequence

The steps of BLS consist of a series of sequential assessments and actions, which are illustrated in the new simplified BLS algorithm (Figure 1). The intent of the algorithm is to present the steps of BLS in a logical and concise manner that is easy for all types of rescuers to learn, remember and perform. These actions have traditionally been presented as a sequence of distinct steps to help a single rescuer prioritize actions. However, many workplaces and most EMS and in-hospital resuscitations involve teams of providers who should perform several actions simultaneously (eg, one rescuer activates the emergency response system while another begins chest compressions, and a third either provides ventilations or retrieves the bag-mask for rescue breathing, and a fourth retrieves and sets up a defibrillator).

## Immediate Recognition and Activation of the Emergency Response System

If a lone rescuer finds an unresponsive adult (ie, no movement or response to stimulation) or witnesses an adult who suddenly collapses, after ensuring that the scene is safe, the rescuer should check for a response by tapping the victim on the shoulder and shouting at the victim. The trained or

**Simplified Adult BLS**

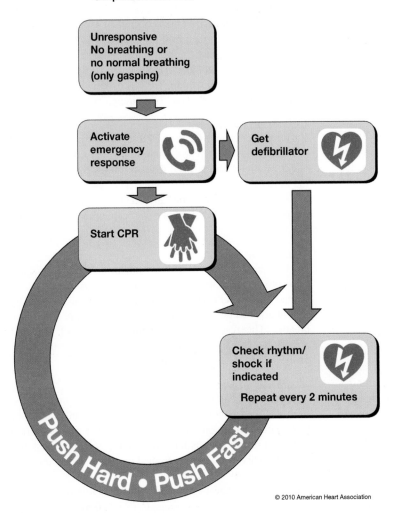

**Figure 1.** Simplified adult BLS algorithm.

untrained bystander should—at a minimum—activate the community emergency response system (eg, call 911, or if in an institution with an emergency response system, call that facility's emergency response number). If the victim also has absent or abnormal breathing (ie, only gasping), the rescuer should assume the victim is in cardiac arrest (Class I, LOE C).[19,24,34] The lay rescuer should phone the emergency response system once the rescuer finds that the victim is unresponsive—the dispatcher should be able to guide the lay rescuer through the check for breathing and the steps of CPR, if needed. The healthcare provider can check for response and look for no breathing or no normal breathing (ie, only gasping) almost simultaneously before activating the emergency response system. After activation of the emergency response system, all rescuers should immediately begin CPR (see steps below) for adult victims who are unresponsive with no breathing or no normal breathing (only gasping).

When phoning 911 for help, the rescuer should be prepared to answer the dispatcher's questions about the location of the incident, the events of the incident, the number and condition of the victim(s), and the type of aid provided. If rescuers never learned or have forgotten how to do CPR, they should also be prepared to follow the dispatcher's instructions. Finally the rescuer making the phone call should hang up only when instructed to do so by the dispatcher.

## Pulse Check

Studies have shown that both lay rescuers and healthcare providers have difficulty detecting a pulse.[35–44] Healthcare providers also may take too long to check for a pulse.[38,41]

- The lay rescuer should not check for a pulse and should assume that cardiac arrest is present if an adult suddenly collapses or an unresponsive victim is not breathing normally.
- The healthcare provider should take no more than 10 seconds to check for a pulse and, if the rescuer does not definitely feel a pulse within that time period, the rescuer should start chest compressions (Class IIa, LOE C).[45,46]

## Early CPR

### Chest Compressions

Chest compressions consist of forceful rhythmic applications of pressure over the lower half of the sternum. These compressions create blood flow by increasing intrathoracic pressure and directly compressing the heart. This generates blood flow and oxygen delivery to the myocardium and brain.

- Effective chest compressions are essential for providing blood flow during CPR. For this reason all patients in cardiac arrest should receive chest compressions (Class I, LOE B).[47–51]

- To provide effective chest compressions, push hard and push fast. It is reasonable for laypersons and healthcare providers to compress the adult chest at a rate of at least 100 compressions per minute (Class IIa, LOE B) with a compression depth of at least 2 inches/5 cm (Class IIa, LOE B). Rescuers should allow complete recoil of the chest after each compression, to allow the heart to fill completely before the next compression (Class IIa, LOE B).
- Rescuers should attempt to minimize the frequency and duration of interruptions in compressions to maximize the number of compressions delivered per minute (Class IIa, LOE B). A compression-ventilation ratio of 30:2 is recommended (Class IIa, LOE B).

### Rescue Breaths

A change in the *2010 AHA Guidelines for CPR and ECC* is to recommend the initiation of compressions before ventilations. While no published human or animal evidence demonstrates that starting CPR with 30 compressions rather than 2 ventilations leads to improved outcomes, it is clear that blood flow depends on chest compressions. Therefore, delays in, and interruptions of, chest compressions should be minimized throughout the entire resuscitation. Moreover, chest compressions can be started almost immediately, while positioning the head, achieving a seal for mouth-to-mouth rescue breathing, and getting a bag-mask apparatus for rescue breathing all take time. Beginning CPR with 30 compressions rather than 2 ventilations leads to a shorter delay to first compression (Class IIb, LOE C).[52–54]

Once chest compressions have been started, a trained rescuer should deliver rescue breaths by mouth-to-mouth or bag-mask to provide oxygenation and ventilation, as follows:

- Deliver each rescue breath over 1 second (Class IIa, LOE C).
- Give a sufficient tidal volume to produce *visible chest rise* (Class IIa, LOE C).[55]
- Use a compression to ventilation ratio of 30 chest compressions to 2 ventilations.

## Early Defibrillation With an AED

After activating the emergency response system the lone rescuer should next retrieve an AED (if nearby and easily accessible) and then return to the victim to attach and use the AED. The rescuer should then provide high-quality CPR. When 2 or more rescuers are present, one rescuer should begin chest compressions while a second rescuer activates the emergency response system and gets the AED (or a manual defibrillator in most hospitals) (Class IIa, LOE C). The AED should be used as rapidly as possible and both rescuers should provide CPR with chest compressions and ventilations.

### Defibrillation Sequence

- Turn the AED on.
- Follow the AED prompts.
- Resume chest compressions immediately after the shock (minimize interruptions).

## Rescuer Specific CPR Strategies: Putting It All Together

This section summarizes the sequence of CPR interventions that should be performed by 3 prototypical rescuers after they activate the emergency response system. The specific steps that rescuers should take (Hands-Only CPR, conventional CPR with rescue breathing, CPR and AED use) are determined by the rescuer's level of training.

### Untrained Lay Rescuer

If a bystander is not trained in CPR, then the bystander should provide Hands-Only (chest compression only) CPR, with an emphasis on "push hard and fast," or follow the directions of the emergency medical dispatcher. The rescuer should continue Hands-Only CPR until an AED arrives and is ready for use or healthcare providers take over care of the victim (Class IIa, LOE B).

### Trained Lay Rescuer

All lay rescuers should, at a minimum, provide chest compressions for victims of cardiac arrest. In addition, if the trained lay rescuer is able to perform rescue breaths, he or she should add rescue breaths in a ratio of 30 compressions to 2 breaths. The rescuer should continue CPR until an AED arrives and is ready for use or EMS providers take over care of the victim (Class I, LOE B).

### Healthcare Provider

Optimally all healthcare providers should be trained in BLS. In this trained population it is reasonable for both EMS and in-hospital professional rescuers to provide chest compressions and rescue breaths for cardiac arrest victims (Class IIa, LOE B). This should be performed in cycles of 30 compressions to 2 ventilations until an advanced airway is placed; then continuous chest compressions with ventilations at a rate of 1 breath every 6 to 8 seconds (8 to 10 ventilations per minute) should be performed. Care should be taken to minimize interruptions in chest compressions when placing, or ventilating with, an advanced airway. In addition, excessive ventilation should be avoided.

It is reasonable for healthcare providers to tailor the sequence of rescue actions to the most likely cause of arrest. For example, if a lone healthcare provider sees an adolescent suddenly collapse, the provider may assume that the victim has suffered a sudden cardiac arrest and call for help (phone 911 or the emergency response number), get an AED (if nearby), and return to the victim to attach and use the AED and then provide CPR. If a lone healthcare provider aids an adult drowning victim or a victim of foreign body airway obstruction who becomes unconscious, the healthcare provider may give about 5 cycles (approximately 2 minutes) of CPR before activating the emergency response system (Class IIa, LOE C).

## Adult BLS Skills

The sequence of BLS skills for the healthcare provider is depicted in the BLS Healthcare Provider Algorithm (see Figure 2).

## Recognition of Arrest (Box 1)

The necessary first step in the treatment of cardiac arrest is immediate recognition. Bystanders may witness the sudden

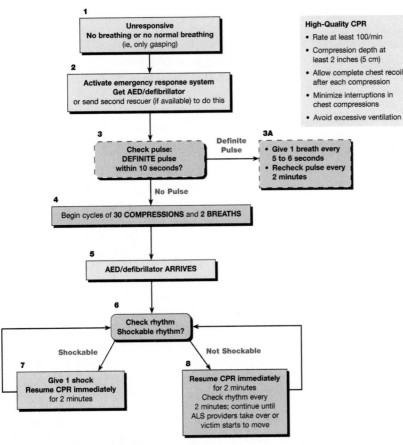

**Adult BLS Healthcare Providers**

**High-Quality CPR**
- Rate at least 100/min
- Compression depth at least 2 inches (5 cm)
- Allow complete chest recoil after each compression
- Minimize interruptions in chest compressions
- Avoid excessive ventilation

**1** Unresponsive
No breathing or no normal breathing
(ie, only gasping)

**2** Activate emergency response system
Get AED/defibrillator
or send second rescuer (if available) to do this

**3** Check pulse:
DEFINITE pulse
within 10 seconds? — Definite Pulse → **3A**
- Give 1 breath every 5 to 6 seconds
- Recheck pulse every 2 minutes

No Pulse

**4** Begin cycles of 30 COMPRESSIONS and 2 BREATHS

**5** AED/defibrillator ARRIVES

**6** Check rhythm
Shockable rhythm?

Shockable — **7** Give 1 shock
Resume CPR immediately for 2 minutes

Not Shockable — **8** Resume CPR immediately for 2 minutes
Check rhythm every 2 minutes; continue until ALS providers take over or victim starts to move

*Note:* The boxes bordered with dashed lines are performed by healthcare providers and not by lay rescuers

© 2010 American Heart Association

**Figure 2.** BLS healthcare provider algorithm.

collapse of a victim or find someone who appears lifeless. At that time several steps should be initiated. Before approaching a victim, the rescuer must ensure that the scene is safe and then check for response. To do this, tap the victim on the shoulder and shout, "Are you all right?" If the victim is responsive he or she will answer, move, or moan. If the victim remains unresponsive, the **lay rescuer** should activate the emergency response system. The **health care provider** should also check for no breathing or no normal breathing (ie, only gasping) while checking for responsiveness; if the healthcare provider finds the victim is unresponsive with no breathing or no normal breathing (ie, only gasping), the rescuer should assume the victim is in cardiac arrest and immediately activate the emergency response system (Class I, LOE C[19,24,34]).

These *2010 AHA Guidelines for CPR and ECC* deemphasize checking for breathing. Professional as well as lay rescuers may be unable to accurately determine the presence or absence of adequate or normal breathing in unresponsive victims[35,56] because the airway is not open[57] or because the victim has occasional gasps, which can occur in the first minutes after SCA and may be confused with adequate breathing. Occasional gasps do not necessarily result in adequate ventilation. The rescuer should treat the victim who has occasional gasps as if he or she is not breathing (Class I, LOE C). CPR training, both formal classroom training and "just in time" training such as that given through a dispatch

center, should emphasize how to recognize occasional gasps and should instruct rescuers to provide CPR even when the unresponsive victim demonstrates occasional gasps (Class I, LOE B).

These *2010 AHA Guidelines for CPR and ECC* also deemphasize the pulse check as a mechanism to identify cardiac arrest. Studies have shown that both laypersons and healthcare providers have difficulty detecting a pulse.[35–44] For this reason pulse check was deleted from training for lay rescuers several years ago, and is deemphasized in training for healthcare providers. The lay rescuer should assume that cardiac arrest is present and should begin CPR if an adult suddenly collapses or an unresponsive victim is not breathing or not breathing normally (ie, only gasping).

Healthcare providers may take too long to check for a pulse[38,41] and have difficulty determining if a pulse is present or absent.[38,41,45] There is no evidence, however, that checking for breathing, coughing, or movement is superior for detection of circulation.[58] Because delays in chest compressions should be minimized, the healthcare provider should take no more than 10 seconds to check for a pulse; and if the rescuer does not definitely feel a pulse within that time period the rescuer should start chest compressions (Class IIa, LOE C[45,46]).

## Technique: Chest Compressions (Box 4)
To maximize the effectiveness of chest compressions, place the victim on a firm surface when possible, in a supine

position with the rescuer kneeling beside the victim's chest (eg, out-of-hospital) or standing beside the bed (eg, in-hospital).[59] Because hospital beds are typically not firm and some of the force intended to compress the chest results in mattress displacement rather than chest compression, we have traditionally recommended the use of a backboard despite insufficient evidence for or against the use of backboards during CPR.[60–63] If a backboard is used, care should be taken to avoid delays in initiation of CPR, to minimize interruptions in CPR, and to avoid line/tube displacement.[61] Air-filled mattresses should be deflated when performing CPR.[64,65]

The rescuer should place the heel of one hand on the center (middle) of the victim's chest (which is the lower half of the sternum) and the heel of the other hand on top of the first so that the hands are overlapped and parallel (Class IIa, LOE B[66–69]).

Correct performance of chest compressions requires several essential skills. The adult sternum should be depressed at least 2 inches (5 cm) (Class IIa, LOE B[70–73]), with chest compression and chest recoil/relaxation times approximately equal (Class IIb, LOE C[74,75]). Allow the chest to completely recoil after each compression (Class IIa, LOE B[76–80]). In human studies of CPR in out-of-hospital[81] and in-hospital settings,[78–80] incomplete chest wall recoil was common, particularly when rescuers were fatigued.[78,81] Incomplete recoil during BLS CPR is associated with higher intrathoracic pressures and significantly decreased hemodynamics, including decreased coronary perfusion, cardiac index, myocardial blood flow, and cerebral perfusion.[76,82] Importantly, the incidence of incomplete chest wall recoil can be reduced during CPR by using electronic recording devices that provide real-time feedback.[80] Manikin studies suggest that lifting the heel of the hand slightly, but completely, off the chest can improve chest recoil.[77,81]

The total number of chest compressions delivered to the victim is a function of the chest compression rate and the proportion of time that chest compressions are delivered without interruption. The compression rate refers to the speed of compressions, not the actual number of compressions delivered per minute. The actual number of chest compressions delivered per minute is determined by the rate of chest compressions and the number and duration of interruptions to open the airway, deliver rescue breaths, and allow AED analysis.[83,84] The number of chest compressions delivered per minute is an important determinant of return of spontaneous circulation (ROSC) and neurologically intact survival.[6,85] One study of in-hospital cardiac arrest patients[85] showed that delivery of >80 compressions/min was associated with ROSC. Extrapolation of data from an out-of-hospital observational study[6] showed improved survival to hospital discharge when at least 68 to 89 chest compressions per minute were delivered; the study also demonstrated that improved survival occurred with chest compression rates as high as 120/min. It is therefore reasonable for lay rescuers and healthcare providers to perform chest compressions for adults at a rate of at least 100 compressions per minute (Class IIa, LOE B).

The term "duty cycle" refers to the time spent compressing the chest as a proportion of the time between the start of 1 cycle of compression and the start of the next. Coronary blood flow is determined partly by the duty cycle (reduced coronary perfusion is associated with a duty cycle of >50%) and partly by how fully the chest is relaxed at the end of each compression.[86] Although duty cycles ranging between 20% and 50% can result in adequate coronary and cerebral perfusion,[87–90] a duty cycle of 50% is recommended because it is easy to achieve with practice (Class IIb, LOE C[75]).

In 2005 3 human observational studies[91–93] showed that interruptions of chest compressions were common, averaging 24% to 57%[85,91–93] of the total arrest time.

The preponderance of *efficacy* data[94,95] suggests that limiting the frequency and duration of interruptions in chest compressions may improve clinically meaningful outcomes in cardiac arrest patients. Data are now accumulating regarding the *effectiveness* of these interventions in "the real world."[2,96–102] Therefore, despite some data to the contrary,[103] it is reasonable for rescuers to minimize interruption of chest compressions for checking the pulse, analyzing rhythm, or performing other activities throughout the entire resuscitation, particularly in the period immediately before and after a shock is delivered (Class IIa, LOE B[94–98]).

Additional evidence of the importance of minimizing interruptions in chest compressions comes from nonrandomized studies suggesting that survival from out-of-hospital cardiac arrest may be improved by the initial EMS provider delivery of continuous chest compressions without initial assisted ventilations,[97,98] or by EMS providers using a higher compression-to-ventilation ratio (50:2).[96] Notably, in each of these studies, the airway was opened, oxygen insufflations were provided, and assisted ventilation was recommended at some point during the EMS resuscitation. Other EMS systems have noted significant improvement in survival from out-of-hospital arrest with use of compressions-plus-ventilations with emphases on improved quality of compressions and minimization of hands-off time.[2,99] At this time there is insufficient evidence to support the removal of ventilations from CPR provided by EMS professionals.

Rescuer fatigue may lead to inadequate compression rates or depth.[104–106] Significant fatigue and shallow compressions are common after 1 minute of CPR, although rescuers may not recognize that fatigue is present for ≥5 minutes.[105] When 2 or more rescuers are available it is reasonable to switch chest compressors approximately every 2 minutes (or after about 5 cycles of compressions and ventilations at a ratio of 30:2) to prevent decreases in the quality of compressions (Class IIa, LOE B). Consider switching compressors during any intervention associated with appropriate interruptions in chest compressions (eg, when an AED is delivering a shock). Every effort should be made to accomplish this switch in <5 seconds. If the 2 rescuers are positioned on either side of the patient, 1 rescuer will be ready and waiting to relieve the "working compressor" every 2 minutes.

Interruptions of chest compressions to palpate for a spontaneous pulse or to otherwise check for return of spontaneous circulation (ROSC) can compromise vital organ perfusion.[2,94–99] Accordingly lay rescuers should not interrupt chest compressions to palpate pulses or check for ROSC (Class IIa, LOE C). In addition lay rescuers should continue

CPR until an AED arrives, the victim wakes up, or EMS personnel take over CPR (Class IIa, LOE B).

Healthcare providers should interrupt chest compressions as infrequently as possible and try to limit interruptions to no longer than 10 seconds, except for specific interventions such as insertion of an advanced airway or use of a defibrillator (Class IIa, LOE C). Because of difficulties with pulse assessments, interruptions in chest compressions for a pulse check should be minimized during the resuscitation, even to determine if ROSC has occurred.

Because of the difficulty in providing effective chest compressions while moving the patient during CPR, the resuscitation should generally be conducted where the patient is found (Class IIa, LOE C). This may not be possible if the environment is dangerous.

### Compression-Ventilation Ratio (Box 4)
A compression-ventilation ratio of 30:2 is reasonable in adults, but further validation of this guideline is needed (Class IIb, LOE B[83,107–111]). This 30:2 ratio in adults is based on a consensus among experts and on published case series.[2,99–102] Further studies are needed to define the best method for coordinating chest compressions and ventilations during CPR and to define the best compression-ventilation ratio in terms of survival and neurologic outcome in patients with or without an advanced airway in place.

Once an advanced airway is in place, 2 rescuers no longer need to pause chest compressions for ventilations. Instead, the compressing rescuer should give continuous chest compressions at a rate of at least 100 per minute without pauses for ventilation (Class IIa, LOE B). The rescuer delivering ventilation can provide a breath every 6 to 8 seconds (which yields 8 to 10 breaths per minute).

### Hands-Only CPR
Only about 20% to 30% of adults with out-of-hospital cardiac arrests receive any bystander CPR.[29,48–51,112,113] Hands-Only (compression-only) bystander CPR substantially improves survival following adult out-of-hospital cardiac arrests compared with no bystander CPR.[29,48–51] Observational studies of adults with cardiac arrest treated by lay rescuers showed similar survival rates among victims receiving Hands-Only CPR versus conventional CPR with rescue breaths.[29,48–51] Of note, some healthcare providers[114–116] and laypersons[116,117] indicate that reluctance to perform mouth-to-mouth ventilation for victims of cardiac arrest is a theoretical and potential barrier to performing bystander CPR. When actual bystanders were interviewed, however, such reluctance was not expressed; panic was cited as the major obstacle to laypersons performance of bystander CPR.[118] The simpler Hands-Only technique may help overcome panic and hesitation to act.

How can bystander CPR be effective without rescue breathing? Initially during SCA with VF, rescue breaths are not as important as chest compressions because the oxygen level in the blood remains adequate for the first several minutes after cardiac arrest. In addition, many cardiac arrest victims exhibit gasping or agonal gasps, and gas exchange allows for some oxygenation and carbon dioxide ($CO_2$) elimination.[110,111,119] If the airway is open, passive chest recoil during the relaxation phase of chest compressions can also provide some air exchange.[19,110,111,119–122] However, at some time during prolonged CPR, supplementary oxygen with assisted ventilation is necessary. The precise interval for which the performance of Hands-Only CPR is acceptable is not known at this time.[110,111,119,123–126]

Laypersons should be encouraged to provide chest compressions (either Hands-Only or conventional CPR, including rescue breaths) for anyone with a presumed cardiac arrest (Class I, LOE B). No prospective study of adult cardiac arrest has demonstrated that layperson conventional CPR provides better outcomes than Hands-Only CPR when provided before EMS arrival. A recent large study of out-of-hospital pediatric cardiac arrests showed that survival was better when conventional CPR (including rescue breaths) as opposed to Hands-Only CPR was provided for children in cardiac arrest due to noncardiac causes.[30] Because rescue breathing is an important component for successful resuscitation from pediatric arrests (other than sudden, witnessed collapse of adolescents), from asphyxial cardiac arrests in both adults and children (eg, drowning, drug overdose) and from prolonged cardiac arrests, conventional CPR with rescue breathing is recommended for all trained rescuers (both in hospital and out of hospital) for those specific situations (Class IIa, LOE C[109,123,127–129]).

## Managing the Airway
As previously stated, a significant change in these Guidelines is to recommend the initiation of chest compressions before ventilations (CAB rather than ABC). This change reflects the growing evidence of the importance of chest compressions and the reality that setting up airway equipment takes time. The ABC mindset may reinforce the idea that compressions should wait until ventilations have begun. This mindset can occur even when more than 1 rescuer is present because "airway and breathing before ventilations" is so ingrained in many rescuers. This new emphasis on CAB helps clarify that airway maneuvers should be performed quickly and efficiently so that interruptions in chest compressions are minimized and chest compressions should take priority in the resuscitation of an adult.

### Open the Airway: Lay Rescuer
The trained lay rescuer who feels confident that he or she can perform both compressions and ventilations should open the airway using a head tilt–chin lift maneuver (Class IIa, LOE B). For the rescuer providing Hands-Only CPR, there is insufficient evidence to recommend the use of any specific passive airway (such as hyperextending the neck to allow passive ventilation).

### Open the Airway: Healthcare Provider
A healthcare provider should use the head tilt–chin lift maneuver to open the airway of a victim with no evidence of head or neck trauma. Although the head tilt–chin lift technique was developed using unconscious, paralyzed adult volunteers and has not been studied in victims with cardiac arrest, clinical[130] and radiographic evidence[131,132] and a case series[133] have shown it to be effective (Class IIa, LOE B).

Between 0.12 and 3.7% of victims with blunt trauma have a spinal injury,[134–136] and the risk of spinal injury is increased if the victim has a craniofacial injury,[137,138] a Glasgow Coma

Scale score of <8,[139,140] or both.[138,139] For victims with suspected spinal injury, rescuers should initially use manual spinal motion restriction (eg, placing 1 hand on either side of the patient's head to hold it still) rather than immobilization devices (Class IIb, LOE C[141,142]). Spinal immobilization devices may interfere with maintaining a patent airway,[143,144] but ultimately the use of such a device may be necessary to maintain spinal alignment during transport.

If healthcare providers suspect a cervical spine injury, they should open the airway using a jaw thrust without head extension (Class IIb, LOE C[133]). Because maintaining a patent airway and providing adequate ventilation are priorities in CPR (Class I, LOE C), use the head tilt–chin lift maneuver if the jaw thrust does not adequately open the airway.

### Rescue Breathing (Box 3A, 4)

The *2010 AHA Guidelines for CPR and ECC* make many of the same recommendations regarding rescue breathing as in 2005:

- Deliver each rescue breath over 1 second (Class IIa, LOE C).
- Give a sufficient tidal volume to produce *visible chest rise* (Class IIa, LOE C).[55]
- Use a compression to ventilation ratio of 30 chest compressions to 2 ventilations.
- When an advanced airway (ie, endotracheal tube, Combitube, or laryngeal mask airway [LMA]) is in place during 2-person CPR, give 1 breath every 6 to 8 seconds without attempting to synchronize breaths between compressions (this will result in delivery of 8 to 10 breaths/minute). There should be no pause in chest compressions for delivery of ventilations (Class IIb, LOE C).

Studies in anesthetized adults (with normal perfusion) suggest that a tidal volume of 8 to 10 mL/kg maintains normal oxygenation and elimination of $CO_2$. During CPR, cardiac output is ≈25% to 33% of normal, so oxygen uptake from the lungs and $CO_2$ delivery to the lungs are also reduced. As a result, a low minute ventilation (lower than normal tidal volume and respiratory rate) can maintain effective oxygenation and ventilation.[55,110,111,119] For that reason during adult CPR tidal volumes of approximately 500 to 600 mL (6 to 7 mL/kg) should suffice (Class IIa, LOE B).[145–147] This is consistent with a tidal volume that produces visible chest rise.

Patients with airway obstruction or poor lung compliance may require high pressures to be properly ventilated (to make the chest visibly rise). A pressure-relief valve on a resuscitation bag-mask may prevent the delivery of a sufficient tidal volume in these patients.[148] Ensure that the bag-mask device allows you to bypass the pressure-relief valve and use high pressures, if necessary, to achieve visible chest expansion.[149]

Excessive ventilation is unnecessary and can cause gastric inflation and its resultant complications, such as regurgitation and aspiration (Class III, LOE B[150–152]). More important, excessive ventilation can be harmful because it increases intrathoracic pressure, decreases venous return to the heart, and diminishes cardiac output and survival.[152] In summary, rescuers should avoid excessive ventilation (too many breaths or too large a volume) during CPR (Class III, LOE B).

During CPR the primary purpose of assisted ventilation is to maintain adequate oxygenation; the secondary purpose is to eliminate $CO_2$. However, the optimal inspired oxygen concentration, tidal volume and respiratory rate to achieve those purposes are not known. As noted above, during the first minutes of sudden VF cardiac arrest, rescue breaths are not as important as chest compressions[29,108,153] because the oxygen content in the noncirculating arterial blood remains unchanged until CPR is started; the blood oxygen content then continues to be adequate during the first several minutes of CPR. In addition, attempts to open the airway and give rescue breaths (or to access and set up airway equipment) may delay the initiation of chest compressions.[154] These issues support the CAB approach of the *2010 AHA Guidelines for CPR and ECC* (ie, starting with **C**hest Compressions prior to **A**irway and **B**reathing).

For victims of prolonged cardiac arrest both ventilations and compressions are important because over time oxygen in the blood is consumed and oxygen in the lungs is depleted (although the precise time course is unknown). Ventilations and compressions are also important for victims of asphyxial arrest, such as children and drowning victims, because they are hypoxemic at the time of cardiac arrest.[30,109]

### Mouth-to-Mouth Rescue Breathing

Mouth-to-mouth rescue breathing provides oxygen and ventilation to the victim.[155] To provide mouth-to-mouth rescue breaths, open the victim's airway, pinch the victim's nose, and create an airtight mouth-to-mouth seal. Give 1 breath over 1 second, take a "regular" (not a deep) breath, and give a second rescue breath over 1 second (Class IIb, LOE C). Taking a regular rather than a deep breath prevents the rescuer from getting dizzy or lightheaded and prevents overinflation of the victim's lungs. The most common cause of ventilation difficulty is an improperly opened airway,[57] so if the victim's chest does not rise with the first rescue breath, reposition the head by performing the head tilt–chin lift again and then give the second rescue breath.

If an adult victim with spontaneous circulation (ie, strong and easily palpable pulses) requires support of ventilation, the healthcare provider should give rescue breaths at a rate of about 1 breath every 5 to 6 seconds, or about 10 to 12 breaths per minute (Class IIb, LOE C). Each breath should be given over 1 second regardless of whether an advanced airway is in place. Each breath should cause visible chest rise.

### Mouth-to–Barrier Device Breathing

Some healthcare providers[114–116] and lay rescuers state that they may hesitate to give mouth-to-mouth rescue breathing and prefer to use a barrier device. The risk of disease transmission through mouth to mouth ventilation is very low, and it is reasonable to initiate rescue breathing with or without a barrier device. When using a barrier device the rescuer should not delay chest compressions while setting up the device.

### Mouth-to-Nose and Mouth-to-Stoma Ventilation

Mouth-to-nose ventilation is recommended if ventilation through the victim's mouth is impossible (eg, the mouth is seriously injured), the mouth cannot be opened, the victim is in water, or a mouth-to-mouth seal is difficult to achieve

(Class IIa, LOE C). A case series suggests that mouth-to-nose ventilation in adults is feasible, safe, and effective.[156]

Give mouth-to-stoma rescue breaths to a victim with a tracheal stoma who requires rescue breathing. A reasonable alternative is to create a tight seal over the stoma with a round, pediatric face mask (Class IIb, LOE C). There is no published evidence on the safety, effectiveness, or feasibility of mouth-to-stoma ventilation. One study of patients with laryngectomies showed that a pediatric face mask created a better peristomal seal than a standard ventilation mask.[157]

### Ventilation With Bag and Mask
Rescuers can provide bag-mask ventilation with room air or oxygen. A bag-mask device provides positive-pressure ventilation without an advanced airway; therefore a bag-mask device may produce gastric inflation and its complications.

#### The Bag-Mask Device
A bag-mask device should have the following[158]: a nonjam inlet valve; either no pressure relief valve or a pressure relief valve that can be bypassed; standard 15-mm/22-mm fittings; an oxygen reservoir to allow delivery of high oxygen concentrations; a nonrebreathing outlet valve that cannot be obstructed by foreign material and will not jam with an oxygen flow of 30 L/min; and the capability to function satisfactorily under common environmental conditions and extremes of temperature.

Masks should be made of transparent material to allow detection of regurgitation. They should be capable of creating a tight seal on the face, covering both mouth and nose. Masks should be fitted with an oxygen (insufflation) inlet and have a standard 15-mm/22-mm connector.[159] They should be available in one adult and several pediatric sizes.

#### Bag-Mask Ventilation
Bag-mask ventilation is a challenging skill that requires considerable practice for competency.[160,161] Bag-mask ventilation is not the recommended method of ventilation for a lone rescuer during CPR. It is most effective when provided by 2 trained and experienced rescuers. One rescuer opens the airway and seals the mask to the face while the other squeezes the bag. Both rescuers watch for visible chest rise.[160,162]

The rescuer should use an adult (1 to 2 L) bag to deliver approximately 600 mL tidal volume[163–165] for adult victims. This amount is usually sufficient to produce visible chest rise and maintain oxygenation and normocarbia in apneic patients (Class IIa, LOE C[145–147]). If the airway is open and a good, tight seal is established between face and mask, this volume can be delivered by squeezing a 1-L adult bag about two thirds of its volume or a 2-L adult bag about one third of its volume. As long as the patient does not have an advanced airway in place, the rescuers should deliver cycles of 30 compressions and 2 breaths during CPR. The rescuer delivers ventilations during pauses in compressions and delivers each breath over 1 second (Class IIa, LOE C). The healthcare provider should use supplementary oxygen ($O_2$ concentration >40%, at a minimum flow rate of 10 to 12 L/min) when available.

### Ventilation With a Supraglottic Airway
Supraglottic airway devices such as the LMA, the esophageal-tracheal combitube and the King airway device, are currently within the scope of BLS practice in a number of regions (with specific authorization from medical control). Ventilation with a bag through these devices provides an acceptable alternative to bag-mask ventilation for well-trained healthcare providers who have sufficient experience to use the devices for airway management during cardiac arrest (Class IIa, LOE B[166–171]). It is not clear that these devices are any more or less complicated to use than a bag and mask; training is needed for safe and effective use of both the bag-mask device and each of the advanced airways. These devices are discussed in greater detail in Part 8.1 of these Guidelines.

### Ventilation With an Advanced Airway
When the victim has an advanced airway in place during CPR, rescuers no longer deliver cycles of 30 compressions and 2 breaths (ie, they no longer interrupt compressions to deliver 2 breaths). Instead, continuous chest compressions are performed at a rate of at least 100 per minute without pauses for ventilation, and ventilations are delivered at the rate of 1 breath about every 6 to 8 seconds (which will deliver approximately 8 to 10 breaths per minute).

### Passive Oxygen Versus Positive-Pressure Oxygen During CPR
Although many studies describe outcomes after compression-only CPR, these studies infrequently address additional techniques to improve ventilation or oxygenation. Two comparative studies[97,172] and 2 post hoc analysis studies[98,173] of passive ventilation airway techniques during cardiac arrest used the same protocol. The protocol included insertion of an oral airway and administration of oxygen with a nonrebreather mask, with interposed ventilations versus passive insufflation of oxygen during minimally interrupted chest compressions. These studies did not demonstrate a significant overall improvement in outcome measures. However, subgroup analysis showed better survival with passive oxygen insufflation among patients with witnessed VF cardiac arrest. For layperson Hands-Only CPR, evidence is insufficient to support recommending the use of any specific passive airway or ventilation technique.

### Cricoid Pressure
Cricoid pressure is a technique of applying pressure to the victim's cricoid cartilage to push the trachea posteriorly and compress the esophagus against the cervical vertebrae. Cricoid pressure can prevent gastric inflation and reduce the risk of regurgitation and aspiration during bag-mask ventilation, but it may also impede ventilation. Seven randomized, controlled studies demonstrated that cricoid pressure can delay or prevent the placement of an advanced airway and that aspiration can occur despite application of pressure.[174–180] Additional manikin studies[181–194] found training in the maneuver to be difficult for both expert and nonexpert rescuers. Neither expert nor nonexpert rescuers demonstrated mastery of the technique, and the applied pressure was frequently inconsistent and outside of effective limits. Cricoid pressure might be used in a few special circumstances (eg, to aid in viewing the vocal cords during tracheal intubation). However, the routine use of cricoid pressure in adult cardiac arrest is not recommended (Class III, LOE B).

## AED Defibrillation (Box 5, 6)

All BLS providers should be trained to provide defibrillation because VF is a common and treatable initial rhythm in adults with witnessed cardiac arrest.[195] For victims with VF, survival rates are highest when immediate bystander CPR is provided and defibrillation occurs within 3 to 5 minutes of collapse.[4,5,10,11,196,197] Rapid defibrillation is the treatment of choice for VF of short duration, such as for victims of witnessed out-of-hospital cardiac arrest or for hospitalized patients whose heart rhythm is monitored (Class I, LOE A).

In swine, microvascular blood flow is markedly reduced within 30 seconds of the onset of VF; chest compressions restore some of the diminished microvascular blood flow within 1 minute.[198] Performing chest compressions while another rescuer retrieves and charges a defibrillator improves the probability of survival.[6] After about 3 to 5 minutes of untreated VF, some animal models suggest that a period of chest compressions before defibrillation may be beneficial.[199] In 2 randomized controlled trials in adults with out-of-hospital VF/pulseless ventricular tachycardia (VT), a period of 1 ½ to 3 minutes of CPR by EMS before defibrillation did not improve ROSC or survival rates regardless of EMS response interval.[200,201] A third randomized controlled trial[202] and a cohort clinical trial with historic controls[203] also found no overall differences in outcomes. However, in two of these studies subgroups of patients with the EMS response interval intervals longer than 4 to 5 minutes showed increased survival to hospital discharge with a period of CPR prior to defibrillation.[202, 203]

There is insufficient evidence to recommend for or against delaying defibrillation to provide a period of CPR for patients in VF/pulseless VT out-of-hospital cardiac arrest. In settings with lay rescuer AED programs (AED onsite and available) and for in-hospital environments, or if the EMS rescuer witnesses the collapse, the rescuer should use the defibrillator as soon as it is available (Class IIa, LOE C). When more than one rescuer is available, one rescuer should provide chest compressions while another activates the emergency response system and retrieves the defibrillator. Defibrillation is discussed in further detail in Part 6: "Electrical Therapies."

## Recovery Position

The recovery position is used for unresponsive adult victims who clearly have normal breathing and effective circulation. This position is designed to maintain a patent airway and reduce the risk of airway obstruction and aspiration. The victim is placed on his or her side with the lower arm in front of the body.

There are several variations of the recovery position, each with its own advantages. No single position is perfect for all victims.[204,205] The position should be stable, near a true lateral position, with the head dependent and with no pressure on the chest to impair breathing (Class IIa, LOE C). Studies in normal volunteers[206] show that extending the lower arm above the head and rolling the head onto the arm, while bending both legs, may be feasible for victims with known or suspected spinal injury.[207]

## Special Resuscitation Situations

### Acute Coronary Syndromes

In the United States coronary heart disease was responsible for 1 of every 6 hospital admissions in 2005 and 1 in every 6 deaths in 2006.[208] The American Heart Association estimates that in 2010, 785 000 Americans will have a new coronary attack and 470 000 will have a recurrent attack.[208] Approximately 70% of deaths from acute myocardial infarction (AMI) occur outside of the hospital, most within the first 4 hours after the onset of symptoms.[208,209]

Early recognition, diagnosis, and treatment of AMI can improve outcome by limiting damage to the heart,[210] but treatment is most effective if provided within a few hours of the onset of symptoms.[211] Patients at risk for acute coronary syndromes (ACS) and their families should be taught to recognize the symptoms of ACS and to immediately activate the EMS system when symptoms appear, rather than delaying care by contacting family, calling a physician, or driving themselves to the hospital.

The classic symptoms associated with ACS are chest discomfort, discomfort in other areas of the upper body, shortness of breath, sweating, nausea, and lightheadedness. The symptoms of AMI characteristically last more than 15 minutes. Atypical symptoms of ACS may be more common in the elderly, women, and diabetic patients, but any patient may present with atypical signs and symptoms.[212–214] Signs and symptoms cannot be used to confirm or exclude the diagnosis of ACS because reported sensitivity ranges from 35% to 92% and specificity ranges from 28% of 91%. Numerous studies do not support the use of any clinical signs and symptoms independent of electrocardiograph (ECG) tracings, cardiac biomarkers, or other diagnostic tests to rule in or rule out ACS in prehospital or emergency department (ED) settings.[215–228]

To improve ACS outcome, all dispatchers and EMS providers must be trained to recognize ACS symptoms, even if atypical. It is reasonable for dispatchers to advise patients with potential cardiac symptoms to chew an aspirin (160 to 325 mg), providing the patient has no history of aspirin allergy and no signs of active or recent gastrointestinal bleeding (Class IIa, LOE C).[229–233]

EMS providers should obtain a 12-lead ECG, determine onset of ACS symptoms, and provide prearrival notification to the destination hospital.[229,234] Clinical trials have shown improved outcomes in ST-segment elevation myocardial infarction (STEMI) patients transported by EMS directly to a percutaneous coronary intervention (PCI)–capable hospital.[235–237] If the patient has a STEMI on ECG and if PCI is the chosen method of reperfusion, it is reasonable to transport the patient directly to a PCI facility, bypassing closer emergency departments as necessary, in systems where time intervals between first medical contact and balloon times are less than 90 minutes, and transport times are relatively short (ie, less than 30 minutes), or based on regional EMS protocols (Class IIa, LOE B).

Common practice has been for basic EMT's to administer oxygen during the initial assessment of patients with suspected ACS. However, there is insufficient evidence to 'support or refute oxygen use in uncomplicated ACS. If the patient is dyspneic, hypoxemic, has obvious signs of heart failure, or an oxyhemoglobin saturation <94%, providers should administer oxygen and titrate therapy to provide the lowest administered oxygen concentration that will maintain the oxyhemoglobin saturation ≥94% (Class I, LOE C).[238] If the patient has not taken aspirin and has no history of aspirin allergy and no evidence of recent gastrointestinal bleeding, EMS providers should give the patient nonenteric aspirin (160 to 325 mg) to chew (Class I, LOE C).[229,234,239,240]

EMS providers can administer nitroglycerin for patients with chest discomfort and suspected ACS. Although it is reasonable to consider the early administration of nitroglycerin in select hemodynamically stable patients, insufficient evidence exists to support or refute the routine administration of nitroglycerin in the ED or prehospital setting in patients with a suspected ACS (Class IIb, LOE B).[241-243] Nitrates in all forms are contraindicated in patients with initial systolic blood pressure <90 mm Hg or ≥30 mm Hg below baseline and in patients with right ventricular infarction (see Part 10). Caution is advised in patients with known inferior wall STEMI, and a right-sided ECG should be performed to evaluate right ventricular infarction. Administer nitrates with extreme caution, if at all, to patients with inferior STEMI and suspected RV involvement because these patients require adequate RV preload. Nitrates are contraindicated when patients have taken a phosphodiesterase-5 (PDE-5) inhibitor within 24 hours (48 hours for tadalafil).

For patients diagnosed with STEMI in the prehospital setting, EMS providers should administer appropriate analgesics, such as intravenous morphine, for persistent chest pain (Class IIa, LOE C). EMS providers may consider administering intravenous morphine for undifferentiated chest pain unresponsive to nitroglycerin (Class IIb, LOE C). However, morphine should be used with caution in unstable angina (UA)/NSTEMI due to an association with increased mortality in a large registry.

Additional information about the assessment and treatment of the patient with ACS and STEMI is included in Part 10: "Acute Coronary Syndromes."

## Stroke

Almost 800 000 people suffer stroke each year in the United States, and stroke is a leading cause of severe, long-term disability and death.[245] Fibrinolytic therapy administered within the first hours of the onset of symptoms limits neurological injury and improves outcome in selected patients with acute ischemic stroke.[246-249] The window of opportunity is extremely limited, however. Effective therapy requires early detection of the signs of stroke, prompt activation of the EMS system and dispatch of EMS personnel; appropriate triage to a stroke center; prearrival notification; rapid triage, evaluation, and management in the ED; and rapid delivery of fibrinolytic therapy to eligible patients. For additional information about these steps, see the AHA/American Stroke Association (ASA) Guidelines for the management of acute ischemic stroke and Part 11: "Adult Stroke."[250,251]

Patients at high risk for stroke, their family members, and BLS providers should learn to recognize the signs and symptoms

of stroke and to call EMS as soon as any signs of stroke are present (Class I, LOE C). The signs and symptoms of stroke are sudden numbness or weakness of the face, arm, or leg, especially on one side of the body; sudden confusion, trouble speaking or understanding; sudden trouble seeing in one or both eyes; sudden trouble walking, dizziness, loss of balance or coordination; and sudden severe headache with no known cause.[252,253] Community and professional education is essential to improve stroke recognition and early EMS activation.[254-256]

EMS dispatchers should be trained to suspect stroke and rapidly dispatch emergency responders. EMS personnel should be able to perform an out-of-hospital stroke assessment (Class I, LOE B[257-259]), establish the time of symptom onset when possible, provide cardiopulmonary support, and notify the receiving hospital that a patient with possible stroke is being transported.[260-262] EMS systems should have protocols that address triaging the patient when possible directly to a stroke center (Class I, LOE B[261,263,264]). It may be important for a family member to accompany the patient during transport to verify the time of symptom onset and provide consent for interventional therapy.

Patients with acute stroke are at risk for respiratory compromise, and the combination of poor perfusion and hypoxemia will exacerbate and extend ischemic brain injury leading to worse outcomes.[265] Both out-of-hospital and in-hospital medical personnel should administer supplementary oxygen to hypoxemic (ie, oxygen saturation <94%) stroke patients (Class 1, LOE C) or those with unknown oxygen saturation. There are no data to support initiation of hypertension intervention in the prehospital environment. Unless the patient is hypotensive (systolic blood pressure <90 mm Hg), prehospital intervention for blood pressure is not recommended (Class III, LOE C). Additional information about the assessment of stroke using stroke scales and the management of stroke is included in Part 11: "Adult Stroke."

## Drowning

Drowning is a preventable cause of death for more than 3500 Americans annually.[266] Over the last 25 years, the incidence of fatal drowning has declined significantly from 3.8 deaths per 100 000 population in 1970 to 1.2 in 2006.[266] The duration and severity of hypoxia sustained as a result of drowning is the single most important determinant of outcome.[267,268] Rescuers should provide CPR, particularly rescue breathing, as soon as an unresponsive submersion victim is removed from the water (Class I, LOE C). When rescuing a drowning victim of any age, it is reasonable for the lone healthcare provider to give 5 cycles (about 2 minutes) of CPR before leaving the victim to activate the EMS system.

Mouth-to-mouth ventilation in the water may be helpful when administered by a trained rescuer (Class IIb, LOE C[269]). Chest compressions are difficult to perform in water; they may not be effective and they could potentially cause harm to both the rescuer and the victim. There is no evidence that water acts as an obstructive foreign body. Maneuvers to relieve foreign-body airway obstruction (FBAO) are not recommended for drowning victims because such maneuvers are not necessary and they can cause injury, vomiting, aspiration, and delay of CPR.[270]

Rescuers should remove drowning victims from the water by the fastest means available and should begin resuscitation as quickly as possible. Spinal cord injury is rare among fatal drowning victims.[271] Victims with obvious clinical signs of injury, alcohol intoxication, or a history of diving into shallow water are at a higher risk of spinal cord injury, and health care providers may consider stabilization and possible immobilization of the cervical and thoracic spine for these victims.[272]

## Hypothermia

In an unresponsive victim with hypothermia, assessments of breathing and pulse are particularly difficult because heart rate and breathing may be very slow, depending on the degree of hypothermia.

If the victim is unresponsive with no normal breathing, lay rescuers should begin chest compressions immediately (see Part 12: "Cardiac Arrest in Special Situations"). If the adult victim is unresponsive with no breathing or no normal breathing (ie, only gasping), healthcare providers can check for a pulse, but should start CPR if a pulse is not definitely felt within 10 seconds. Do not wait to check the victim's temperature and do not wait until the victim is rewarmed to start CPR. To prevent further heat loss, remove wet clothes from the victim; insulate or shield the victim from wind, heat, or cold; and if possible, ventilate the victim with warm, humidified oxygen.

Avoid rough movement, and transport the victim to a hospital as soon as possible. If VF is detected, emergency personnel should deliver shocks using the same protocols used for the normothermic cardiac arrest victim (see Part 12: "Cardiac Arrest in Special Situations").

For the hypothermic patient in cardiac arrest, continue resuscitative efforts until the patient is evaluated by advanced care providers. In the out-of-hospital setting, passive warming can be used until active warming is available.

## Foreign-Body Airway Obstruction (Choking)

FBAO is an uncommon, but preventable, cause of death.[273] Most reported cases of FBAO occur in adults while they are eating.[274] Most reported episodes of choking in infants and children occur during eating or play when parents or child-care providers are present. The choking event is therefore commonly witnessed, and the rescuer usually intervenes while the victim is still responsive. Treatment is usually successful, and survival rates can exceed 95%.[275]

### Recognition of Foreign-Body Airway Obstruction

Because recognition of FBAO is the key to successful outcome, it is important to distinguish this emergency from fainting, heart attack, seizure, or other conditions that may cause sudden respiratory distress, cyanosis, or loss of consciousness.

Foreign bodies may cause either mild or severe airway obstruction. The rescuer should intervene if the choking victim shows signs of severe airway obstruction. These include signs of poor air exchange and increased breathing difficulty, such as a silent cough, cyanosis, or inability to speak or breathe. The victim may clutch the neck, demonstrating the universal choking sign. Quickly ask, "Are you choking?" If the victim indicates "yes" by nodding his head without speaking, this will verify that the victim has severe airway obstruction.

### Relief of Foreign-Body Airway Obstruction

When FBAO produces signs of severe airway obstruction, rescuers must act quickly to relieve the obstruction. If mild obstruction is present and the victim is coughing forcefully, do not interfere with the patient's spontaneous coughing and breathing efforts. Attempt to relieve the obstruction only if signs of severe obstruction develop: the cough becomes silent, respiratory difficulty increases and is accompanied by stridor, or the victim becomes unresponsive. Activate the EMS system quickly if the patient is having difficulty breathing. If more than one rescuer is present, one rescuer should phone 911 while the other rescuer attends to the choking victim.

The clinical data about effectiveness of maneuvers to relieve FBAO are largely retrospective and anecdotal. For responsive adults and children >1 year of age with severe FBAO, case reports show the feasibility and effectiveness of back blows or "slaps,"[276–278] abdominal thrusts,[275–277,279,280] and chest thrusts.[276,281] In 1 case series of 513 choking episodes for which EMS was summoned,[275] approximately 50% of the episodes of airway obstruction were relieved prior to arrival of EMS. EMS intervention with abdominal thrusts successfully relieved the obstruction in more than 85% of the remaining cases. The few patients with persistent obstruction usually responded to suction or the use of Magill forceps. Less than 4% died.[275]

Although chest thrusts, back slaps, and abdominal thrusts are feasible and effective for relieving severe FBAO in conscious (responsive) adults and children ≥1 year of age, for simplicity in training it is recommended that abdominal thrusts be applied in rapid sequence until the obstruction is relieved (Class IIb, LOE B). If abdominal thrusts are not effective, the rescuer may consider chest thrusts (Class IIb, LOE B). It is important to note that abdominal thrusts are not recommended for infants <1 year of age because thrusts may cause injuries.

Chest thrusts should be used for obese patients if the rescuer is unable to encircle the victim's abdomen. If the choking victim is in the late stages of pregnancy, the rescuer should use chest thrusts instead of abdominal thrusts.

If the adult victim with FBAO becomes unresponsive, the rescuer should carefully support the patient to the ground, immediately activate (or send someone to activate) EMS, and then begin CPR. The healthcare provider should carefully lower the victim to the ground, send someone to activate the emergency response system and begin CPR (without a pulse check). After 2 minutes, if someone has not already done so, the healthcare provider should activate the emeregency response system. A randomized trial of maneuvers to open the airway in cadavers[282] and 2 prospective studies in anesthetized volunteers[281,283] showed that higher sustained airway pressures can be generated using the chest thrust rather than the abdominal thrust. Each time the airway is opened during CPR, the rescuer should look for an object in the victim's mouth and if found, remove it. Simply looking into the mouth should not significantly increase the time needed to attempt the ventilations and proceed to the 30 chest compressions.

No studies have evaluated the routine use of the finger sweep to clear an airway in the absence of visible airway obstruction. The recommendation to use the finger sweep in past guidelines was based on anecdotal reports that suggested that it was helpful for relieving an airway obstruction.[276,277,284] However, case reports have also documented harm to the victim[236,285,286] or rescuer.

## The Quality of BLS

The quality of unprompted CPR in both in-hospital and out-of–hospital cardiac arrest events is often poor, and methods should be developed to improve the quality of CPR delivered to victims of cardiac arrest.[73,91–93,287] Several studies have demonstrated improvement in chest compression rate, depth, chest recoil, ventilation rate, and indicators of blood flow such as end-tidal $CO_2$ ($PETCO_2$) when real-time feedback or prompt devices are used to guide CPR performance.[72,73,80,288–293] However, there are no studies to date that demonstrate a significant improvement in patient survival related to the use of CPR feedback devices during actual cardiac arrest events. Other CPR feedback devices with accelerometers may overestimate compression depth when compressions are performed on a soft surface such as a mattress because the depth of sternal movement may be partly due to movement of the mattress rather than anterior-posterior (AP) compression of the chest.[62,294] Nevertheless, real-time CPR prompting and feedback technology such as visual and auditory prompting devices can improve the quality of CPR (Class IIa, LOE B).

## Summary

The critical lifesaving steps of BLS are

- Immediate **Recognition** and **Activation** of the emergency response system
- Early **CPR** and
- Rapid **Defibrillation** for VF

When an adult suddenly collapses, whoever is nearby should activate the emergency system and begin chest compressions (regardless of training). Trained lay rescuers who are able and healthcare providers should provide compressions and ventilations. Contrary to the belief of too many in this situation, *CPR is not harmful. Inaction is harmful and CPR can be lifesaving.* However, the quality of CPR is critical. Chest compressions should be delivered by pushing hard and fast in the center of the chest (ie, chest compressions should be of adequate rate and depth). Rescuers should allow complete chest recoil after each compression and minimize interruptions in chest compressions. They should also avoid excessive ventilation. If and when available, an AED should be applied and used without delaying chest compressions. With prompt and effective provision of these actions, lives are saved every day.

## Disclosures

**Guidelines Part 5: Adult Basic Life Support: Writing Group Disclosures**

**Guidelines Part 5: Adult Basic Life Support: Writing Group Disclosures,** *Continued*

| Writing Group Member | Employment | Research Grant | Other Research Support | Speakers' Bureau/Honoraria | Ownership Interest | Consultant/Advisory Board | Other |
|---|---|---|---|---|---|---|---|
| E. Brooke Lerner | Medical College of Wisconsin– Associate Professor | None | †Title: Circulation Improving Resuscitation Care Trial Source: Zoll Medical Corporation Role: Consultant Principal Investigator: Lars Wik, M.D. Dates: 12/2006–8/2010 Total Funding to MCW: $345,000 (funding is received by my employer to support my time on this trial. My institution receives support for 20% of my time and the remaining funds are used for other members of our staff and supplies. My role is to advise them on human subject protection issues and to assist with data management and report generation for the trial) | None | *Stockholder in Medtronic, Pfizer, and General Electric | None | None |
| Thomas D. Rea | University of Washington: Physician–Associate Professor of Medicine; Emergency Medical Services Division of Public Health-Seattle & King County–Program Medical Director | *In the past, I have received unrestricted (modest) grant support from Philips Inc and PhysioControl. The topics were related to improving resuscitation generally (changing resuscitation protocols) and not specific to proprietary information or equipment. I am currently an investigator in the ROC. As part of this, I am directly involved in the Feedback Trial to evaluate dynamic fdbk available on the Philips MRX. The ROC is also evaluating the impedance threshold device. These studies are supported by the NIH primarily and I receive no support from Philips or the company that makes the impedance threshold device. I am participating in a trial of chest compression only vs chest compression plus ventilation for dispatch-assisted CPR-supported in part by Laerdal Foundation. I receive less than 5% salary support | *We conducted an AED training study that recently completed where Philips and PhysioControl contributed equipment for the research. I did not receive any of this equipment | None | None | None | *I serve on a DSMB for a trial sponsored by Philips to evaluate quantitative VF waveform algorithm to guide care. I receive no support for this effort in order to minimize (eliminate) any conflict |
| Michael R. Sayre | The Ohio State University-Associate Professor | None | None | None | None | None | None |
| Robert A. Swor | Beaumont Hospital–Director EMS Programs | None | None | None | None | None | None |

This table represents the relationships of writing group members that may be perceived as actual or reasonably perceived conflicts of interest as reported on the Disclosure Questionnaire, which all members of the writing group are required to complete and submit. A relationship is considered to be "significant" if (a) the person receives $10 000 or more during any 12-month period, or 5% or more of the person's gross income; or (b) the person owns 5% or more of the voting stock or share of the entity, or owns $10 000 or more of the fair market value of the entity. A relationship is considered to be "modest" if it is less than "significant" under the preceding definition.

*Modest.

†Significant.

# References

1. Lloyd-Jones D, Adams RJ, Brown TM, Carnethon M, Dai S, De Simone G, Ferguson TB, Ford E, Furie K, Gillespie C, Go A, Greenlund K, Haase N, Hailpern S, Ho PM, Howard V, Kissela B, Kittner S, Lackland D, Lisabeth L, Marelli A, McDermott MM, Meigs J, Mozaffarian D, Mussolino M, Nichol G, Roger VL, Rosamond W, Sacco R, Sorlie P, Stafford R, Thom T, Wasserthiel-Smoller S, Wong ND, Wylie-Rosett J. Executive summary: heart disease and stroke statistics–2010 update: a report from the American Heart Association. *Circulation.* 2010;121: 948–954.

2. Rea TD, Helbock M, Perry S, Garcia M, Cloyd D, Becker L, Eisenberg M. Increasing use of cardiopulmonary resuscitation during out-of-hospital ventricular fibrillation arrest: survival implications of guideline changes. *Circulation.* 2006;114:2760–2765.

3. Nichol G, Thomas E, Callaway CW, Hedges J, Powell JL, Aufderheide TP, Rea T, Lowe R, Brown T, Dreyer J, Davis D, Idris A, Stiell I. Regional variation in out-of-hospital cardiac arrest incidence and outcome. *JAMA.* 2008;300:1423–1431.

4. Chan PS, Nichol G, Krumholz HM, Spertus JA, Nallamothu BK. Hospital variation in time to defibrillation after in-hospital cardiac arrest. *Arch Intern Med.* 2009;169:1265–1273.

5. Sasson C, Rogers MA, Dahl J, Kellermann AL. Predictors of survival from out-of-hospital cardiac arrest: a systematic review and meta-analysis. *Circ Cardiovasc Qual Outcomes.* 2010;3:63–81.

6. Christenson J, Andrusiek D, Everson-Stewart S, Kudenchuk P, Hostler D, Powell J, Callaway CW, Bishop D, Vaillancourt C, Davis D, Aufderheide TP, Idris A, Stouffer JA, Stiell I, Berg R. Chest compression fraction determines survival in patients with out-of-hospital ventricular fibrillation. *Circulation.* 2009;120:1241–1247.

7. Valenzuela TD, Roe DJ, Cretin S, Spaite DW, Larsen MP. Estimating effectiveness of cardiac arrest interventions: a logistic regression survival model. *Circulation.* 1997;96:3308–3313.

8. Chan PS, Krumholz HM, Nichol G, Nallamothu BK. Delayed time to defibrillation after in-hospital cardiac arrest. *N Engl J Med.* 2008; 358:9–17.

9. Hallstrom AP, Ornato JP, Weisfeldt M, Travers A, Christenson J, McBurnie MA, Zalenski R, Becker LB, Schron EB, Proschan M. Public-access defibrillation and survival after out-of-hospital cardiac arrest. *N Engl J Med.* 2004;351:637–646.

10. Valenzuela TD, Roe DJ, Nichol G, Clark LL, Spaite DW, Hardman RG. Outcomes of rapid defibrillation by security officers after cardiac arrest in casinos. *N Engl J Med.* 2000;343:1206–1209.

11. Agarwal DA, Hess EP, Atkinson EJ, White RD. Ventricular fibrillation in Rochester, Minnesota: experience over 18 years. *Resuscitation.* 2009; 80:1253–1258.

12. Eisenberg MS, Hallstrom AP, Copass MK, Bergner L, Short F, Pierce J. Treatment of ventricular fibrillation: emergency medical technician defibrillation and paramedic services. *JAMA.* 1984;251:1723–1726.

13. Rho RW, Page RL. The automated external defibrillator. *J Cardiovasc Electrophysiol.* 2007;18:896–899.

14. Becker LB, Pepe PE. Ensuring the effectiveness of community-wide emergency cardiac care. *Ann Emerg Med.* 22(pt 2):354–365, 1993.

15. Calle PA, Lagaert L, Vanhaute O, Buylaert WA. Do victims of an out-of-hospital cardiac arrest benefit from a training program for emergency medical dispatchers? *Resuscitation.* 1997;35:213–218.

16. Emergency medical dispatching: rapid identification and treatment of acute myocardial infarction. National Heart Attack Alert Program Coordinating Committee Access to Care Subcommittee. *Am J Emerg Med.* 1995;13:67–73.

17. Hallstrom A, Cobb L, Johnson E, Copass M. Cardiopulmonary resuscitation by chest compression alone or with mouth-to-mouth ventilation. *N Engl J Med.* 2000;342:1546–1553.

18. Culley LL, Clark JJ, Eisenberg MS, Larsen MP. Dispatcher-assisted telephone CPR: common delays and time standards for delivery. *Ann Emerg Med.* 1991;20:362–366.

19. Berdowski J, Beekhuis F, Zwinderman AH, Tijssen JG, Koster RW. Importance of the first link: description and recognition of an out-of-hospital cardiac arrest in an emergency call. *Circulation.* 2009;119: 2096–2102.

20. Kuisma M, Boyd J, Vayrynen T, Repo J, Nousila-Wiik M, Holmstrom P. Emergency call processing and survival from out-of-hospital ventricular fibrillation. *Resuscitation*. 2005;67:89–93.

21. Rea TD, Eisenberg MS, Culley LL, Becker L. Dispatcher-assisted cardiopulmonary resuscitation and survival in cardiac arrest. *Circulation*. 2001;104:2513–2516.

22. Hauff SR, Rea TD, Culley LL, Kerry F, Becker L, Eisenberg MS. Factors impeding dispatcher-assisted telephone cardiopulmonary resuscitation. *Ann Emerg Med*. 2003;42:731–737.

23. Vaillancourt C, Verma A, Trickett J, Crete D, Beaudoin T, Nesbitt L, Wells GA, Stiell IG. Evaluating the effectiveness of dispatch-assisted cardiopulmonary resuscitation instructions. *Acad Emerg Med*. 2007;14:877–883.

24. Bohm K, Rosenqvist M, Hollenberg J, Biber B, Engerstrom L, Svensson L. Dispatcher-assisted telephone-guided cardiopulmonary resuscitation: an underused lifesaving system. *Eur J Emerg Med*. 2007;14:256–259.

25. Hallstrom AP, Cobb LA, Johnson E, Copass MK. Dispatcher assisted CPR: implementation and potential benefit. A 12-year study. *Resuscitation*. 2003;57:123–129.

26. Nurmi J, Pettila V, Biber B, Kuisma M, Komulainen R, Castren M. Effect of protocol compliance to cardiac arrest identification by emergency medical dispatchers. *Resuscitation*. 2006;70:463–469.

27. Clawson J, Olola C, Heward A, Patterson B. Cardiac arrest predictability in seizure patients based on emergency medical dispatcher identification of previous seizure or epilepsy history. *Resuscitation*. 2007;75:298–304.

28. White L, Rogers J, Bloomingdale M, Fahrenbruch C, Culley L, Subido C, Eisenberg M, Rea T. Dispatcher-assisted cardiopulmonary resuscitation: risks for patients not in cardiac arrest. *Circulation.*121:91–97.

29. Sayre MR, Berg RA, Cave DM, Page RL, Potts J, White RD. Hands-only (compression-only) cardiopulmonary resuscitation: a call to action for bystander response to adults who experience out-of-hospital sudden cardiac arrest: a science advisory for the public from the American Heart Association Emergency Cardiovascular Care Committee. *Circulation*. 2008;117:2162–2167.

30. Kitamura T, Iwami T, Kawamura T, Nagao K, Tanaka H, Nadkarni VM, Berg RA, Hiraide A. Conventional and chest-compression-only cardiopulmonary resuscitation by bystanders for children who have out-of-hospital cardiac arrests: a prospective, nationwide, population-based cohort study. *Lancet*. 2010.

31. Heward A, Damiani M, Hartley-Sharpe C. Does the use of the Advanced Medical Priority Dispatch System affect cardiac arrest detection? *Emerg Med J*. 2004;21:115–118.

32. Roppolo LP, Westfall A, Pepe PE, Nobel LL, Cowan J, Kay JJ, Idris AH. Dispatcher assessments for agonal breathing improve detection of cardiac arrest. *Resuscitation*. 2009;80:769–772.

33. Bohm K, Stalhandske B, Rosenqvist M, Ulfvarson J, Hollenberg J, Svensson L. Tuition of emergency medical dispatchers in the recognition of agonal respiration increases the use of telephone assisted CPR. *Resuscitation*. 2009;80:1025–1028.

34. Clawson J, Olola C, Scott G, Heward A, Patterson B. Effect of a Medical Priority Dispatch System key question addition in the seizure/convulsion/fitting protocol to improve recognition of ineffective (agonal) breathing. *Resuscitation*. 2008;79:257–264.

35. Bahr J, Klingler H, Panzer W, Rode H, Kettler D. Skills of lay people in checking the carotid pulse. *Resuscitation*. 1997;35:23–26.

36. Brennan RT, Braslow A. Skill mastery in public CPR classes. *Am J Emerg Med*. 1998;16:653–657.

37. Chamberlain D, Smith A, Woollard M, Colquhoun M, Handley AJ, Leaves S, Kern KB. Trials of teaching methods in basic life support : comparison of simulated CPR performance after first training and at 6 months, with a note on the value of re-training. *Resuscitation*. 2002;53:179–187.

38. Eberle B, Dick WF, Schneider T, Wisser G, Doetsch S, Tzanova I. Checking the carotid pulse check: diagnostic accuracy of first responders in patients with and without a pulse. *Resuscitation*. 1996;33:107–116.

39. Frederick K, Bixby E, Orzel MN, Stewart-Brown S, Willett K. Will changing the emphasis from 'pulseless' to 'no signs of circulation' improve the recall scores for effective life support skills in children? *Resuscitation*. 2002;55:255–261.

40. Lapostolle F, Le Toumelin P, Agostinucci JM, Catineau J, Adnet F. Basic cardiac life support providers checking the carotid pulse: performance, degree of conviction, and influencing factors. *Acad Emerg Med*. 2004;11:878–880.

41. Moule P. Checking the carotid pulse: diagnostic accuracy in students of the healthcare professions. *Resuscitation*. 2000;44:195–201.

42. Nyman J, Sihvonen M. Cardiopulmonary resuscitation skills in nurses and nursing students. *Resuscitation*. 2000;47:179–184.

43. Owen CJ, Wyllie JP. Determination of heart rate in the baby at birth. *Resuscitation*. 2004;60:213–217.

44. Sarti A, Savron F, Ronfani L, Pelizzo G, Barbi E. Comparison of three sites to check the pulse and count heart rate in hypotensive infants. *Paediatr Anaesth*. 2006;16:394–398.

45. Ochoa FJ, Ramalle-Gomara E, Carpintero JM, Garcia A, Saralegui I. Competence of health professionals to check the carotid pulse. *Resuscitation*. 1998;37:173–175.

46. Mather C, O'Kelly S. The palpation of pulses. *Anaesthesia*. 1996;51:189–191.

47. Olasveengen TM, Wik L, Steen PA. Standard basic life support vs. continuous chest compressions only in out-of-hospital cardiac arrest. *Acta Anaesthesiol Scand*. 2008;52:914–919.

48. Ong ME, Ng FS, Anushia P, Tham LP, Leong BS, Ong VY, Tiah L, Lim SH, Anantharaman V. Comparison of chest compression only and standard cardiopulmonary resuscitation for out-of-hospital cardiac arrest in Singapore. *Resuscitation*. 2008;78:119–126.

49. Bohm K, Rosenqvist M, Herlitz J, Hollenberg J, Svensson L. Survival is similar after standard treatment and chest compression only in out-of-hospital bystander cardiopulmonary resuscitation. *Circulation*. 2007;116:2908–2912.

50. Iwami T, Kawamura T, Hiraide A, Berg RA, Hayashi Y, Nishiuchi T, Kajino K, Yonemoto N, Yukioka H, Sugimoto H, Kakuchi H, Sase K, Yokoyama H, Nonogi H. Effectiveness of bystander-initiated cardiac-only resuscitation for patients with out-of-hospital cardiac arrest. *Circulation*. 2007;116:2900–2907.

51. SOS-KANTO Study Group. Cardiopulmonary resuscitation by bystanders with chest compression only (SOS-KANTO): an observational study. *Lancet*. 2007;369:920–926.

52. Assar D, Chamberlain D, Colquhoun M, Donnelly P, Handley AJ, Leaves S, Kern KB. Randomised controlled trials of staged teaching for basic life support, 1: skill acquisition at bronze stage. *Resuscitation*. 2000;45:7–15.

53. Heidenreich JW, Higdon TA, Kern KB, Sanders AB, Berg RA, Niebler R, Hendrickson J, Ewy GA. Single-rescuer cardiopulmonary resuscitation: 'two quick breaths'–an oxymoron. *Resuscitation*. 2004;62:283–289.

54. Kobayashi M, Fujiwara A, Morita H, Nishimoto Y, Mishima T, Nitta M, Hayashi T, Hotta T, Hayashi Y, Hachisuka E, Sato K. A manikin-based observational study on cardiopulmonary resuscitation skills at the Osaka Senri medical rally. *Resuscitation*. 2008;78:333–339.

55. Baskett P, Nolan J, Parr M. Tidal volumes which are perceived to be adequate for resuscitation. *Resuscitation*. 1996;31:231–234.

56. Ruppert M, Reith MW, Widmann JH, Lackner CK, Kerkmann R, Schweiberer L, Peter K. Checking for breathing: evaluation of the diagnostic capability of emergency medical services personnel, physicians, medical students, and medical laypersons. *Ann Emerg Med*. 1999;34:720–729.

57. Safar P, Escarraga LA, Chang F. Upper airway obstruction in the unconscious patient. *J Appl Physiol*. 1959;14:760–764.

58. Perkins GD, Stephenson B, Hulme J, Monsieurs KG. Birmingham assessment of breathing study (BABS). *Resuscitation*. 2005;64:109–113.

59. Handley AJ, Handley JA. Performing chest compressions in a confined space. *Resuscitation*. 2004;61:55–61.

60. Andersen LO, Isbye DL, Rasmussen LS. Increasing compression depth during manikin CPR using a simple backboard. *Acta Anaesthesiol Scand*. 2007;51:747–750.

61. Perkins GD, Smith CM, Augre C, Allan M, Rogers H, Stephenson B, Thickett DR. Effects of a backboard, bed height, and operator position on compression depth during simulated resuscitation. *Intensive Care Med*. 2006;32:1632–1635.

62. Perkins GD, Kocierz L, Smith SC, McCulloch RA, Davies RP. Compression feedback devices over estimate chest compression depth when performed on a bed. *Resuscitation*. 2009;80:79–82.

63. Noordergraaf GJ, Paulussen IW, Venema A, van Berkom PF, Woerlee PH, Scheffer GJ, Noordergraaf A. The impact of compliant surfaces on in-hospital chest compressions: effects of common mattresses and a backboard. *Resuscitation*. 2009;80:546–552.

64. Delvaux AB, Trombley MT, Rivet CJ, Dykla JJ, Jensen D, Smith MR, Gilbert RJ. Design and development of a cardiopulmonary resuscitation mattress. *J Intensive Care Med.* 2009;24:195–199.

65. Perkins GD, Benny R, Giles S, Gao F, Tweed MJ. Do different mattresses affect the quality of cardiopulmonary resuscitation? *Intensive Care Med.* 2003;29:2330–2335.

66. Kundra P, Dey S, Ravishankar M. Role of dominant hand position during external cardiac compression. *Br J Anaesth.* 2000;84:491–493.

67. Nikandish R, Shahbazi S, Golabi S, Beygi N. Role of dominant versus non-dominant hand position during uninterrupted chest compression CPR by novice rescuers: a randomized double-blind crossover study. *Resuscitation.* 2008;76:256–260.

68. Shin J, Rhee JE, Kim K. Is the inter-nipple line the correct hand position for effective chest compression in adult cardiopulmonary resuscitation? *Resuscitation.* 2007;75:305–310.

69. Kusunoki S, Tanigawa K, Kondo T, Kawamoto M, Yuge O. Safety of the inter-nipple line hand position landmark for chest compression. *Resuscitation.* 2009;80:1175–1180.

70. Babbs CF, Kemeny AE, Quan W, Freeman G. A new paradigm for human resuscitation research using intelligent devices. *Resuscitation.* 2008;77:306–315.

71. Edelson DP, Abella BS, Kramer-Johansen J, Wik L, Myklebust H, Barry AM, Merchant RM, Hoek TL, Steen PA, Becker LB. Effects of compression depth and pre-shock pauses predict defibrillation failure during cardiac arrest. *Resuscitation.* 2006;71:137–145.

72. Kramer-Johansen J, Myklebust H, Wik L, Fellows B, Svensson L, Sorebo H, Steen PA. Quality of out-of-hospital cardiopulmonary resuscitation with real time automated feedback: a prospective interventional study. *Resuscitation.* 2006;71:283–292.

73. Edelson DP, Litzinger B, Arora V, Walsh D, Kim S, Lauderdale DS, Vanden Hoek TL, Becker LB, Abella BS. Improving in-hospital cardiac arrest process and outcomes with performance debriefing. *Arch Intern Med.* 2008;168:1063–1069.

74. Talley DB, Ornato JP, Clarke AM. Computer-aided characterization and optimization of the Thumper compression waveform in closed-chest CPR. *Biomed Instrum Technol.* 1990;24:283–288.

75. Handley AJ, Handley SA. Improving CPR performance using an audible feedback system suitable for incorporation into an automated external defibrillator. *Resuscitation.* 2003;57:57–62.

76. Yannopoulos D, McKnite S, Aufderheide TP, Sigurdsson G, Pirrallo RG, Benditt D, Lurie KG. Effects of incomplete chest wall decompression during cardiopulmonary resuscitation on coronary and cerebral perfusion pressures in a porcine model of cardiac arrest. *Resuscitation.* 2005;64:363–372.

77. Aufderheide TP, Pirrallo RG, Yannopoulos D, Klein JP, von Briesen C, Sparks CW, Deja KA, Kitscha DJ, Provo TA, Lurie KG. Incomplete chest wall decompression: A clinical evaluation of CPR performance by trained laypersons and an assessment of alternative manual chest compression-decompression techniques. *Resuscitation.* 2006;71:341–351.

78. Sutton RM, Niles D, Nysaether J, Abella BS, Arbogast KB, Nishisaki A, Maltese MR, Donoghue A, Bishnoi R, Helfaer MA, Myklebust H, Nadkarni V. Quantitative analysis of CPR quality during in-hospital resuscitation of older children and adolescents. *Pediatrics.* 2009;124:494–499.

79. Sutton RM, Maltese MR, Niles D, French B, Nishisaki A, Arbogast KB, Donoghue A, Berg RA, Helfaer MA, Nadkarni V. Quantitative analysis of chest compression interruptions during in-hospital resuscitation of older children and adolescents. *Resuscitation.* 2009;80:1259–1263.

80. Niles D, Nysaether J, Sutton R, Nishisaki A, Abella BS, Arbogast K, Maltese MR, Berg RA, Helfaer M, Nadkarni V. Leaning is common during in-hospital pediatric CPR, and decreased with automated corrective feedback. *Resuscitation.* 2009;80:553–557.

81. Aufderheide TP, Pirrallo RG, Yannopoulos D, Klein JP, von Briesen C, Sparks CW, Conrad CJ, Kitscha DJ, Provo TA, Lurie KG. Incomplete chest wall decompression: a clinical evaluation of CPR performance by EMS personnel and assessment of alternative manual chest compression-decompression techniques. *Resuscitation.* 2005;64:353–362.

82. Zuercher M, Hilwig RW, Ranger-Moore J, Nysaether J, Nadkarni VM, Berg MD, Kern KB, Sutton R, Berg RA. Leaning during chest compressions impairs cardiac output and left ventricular myocardial blood flow in piglet cardiac arrest. *Crit Care Med.* 2010;38:1141–1146.

83. Babbs CF, Kern KB. Optimum compression to ventilation ratios in CPR under realistic, practical conditions: a physiological and mathematical analysis. *Resuscitation.* 2002;54:147–157.

84. Kern KB, Hilwig RW, Berg RA, Ewy GA. Efficacy of chest compression-only BLS CPR in the presence of an occluded airway. *Resuscitation.* 1998;39:179–188.

85. Abella BS, Sandbo N, Vassilatos P, Alvarado JP, O'Hearn N, Wigder HN, Hoffman P, Tynus K, Vanden Hoek TL, Becker LB. Chest compression rates during cardiopulmonary resuscitation are suboptimal: a prospective study during in-hospital cardiac arrest. *Circulation.* 2005;111:428–434.

86. Wolfe JA, Maier GW, Newton JR Jr, Glower DD, Tyson GS Jr, Spratt JA, Rankin JS, Olsen CO. Physiologic determinants of coronary blood flow during external cardiac massage. *J Thorac Cardiovasc Surg.* 1988;95:523–532.

87. Maier GW, Tyson GS Jr, Olsen CO, Kernstein KH, Davis JW, Conn EH, Sabiston DC Jr, Rankin JS. The physiology of external cardiac massage: high-impulse cardiopulmonary resuscitation. *Circulation.* 1984;70:86–101.

88. Feneley MP, Maier GW, Kern KB, Gaynor JW, Gall SA Jr, Sanders AB, Raessler K, Muhlbaier LH, Rankin JS, Ewy GA. Influence of compression rate on initial success of resuscitation and 24 hour survival after prolonged manual cardiopulmonary resuscitation in dogs. *Circulation.* 1988;77:240–252.

89. Halperin HR, Tsitlik JE, Guerci AD, Mellits ED, Levin HR, Shi AY, Chandra N, Weisfeldt ML. Determinants of blood flow to vital organs during cardiopulmonary resuscitation in dogs. *Circulation.* 1986;73:539–550.

90. Handley AJ, Handley JA. The relationship between rate of chest compression and compression:relaxation ratio. *Resuscitation.* 1995;30:237–241.

91. Wik L, Kramer-Johansen J, Myklebust H, Sorebo H, Svensson L, Fellows B, Steen PA. Quality of cardiopulmonary resuscitation during out-of-hospital cardiac arrest. *JAMA.* 2005;293:299–304.

92. Abella BS, Alvarado JP, Myklebust H, Edelson DP, Barry A, O'Hearn N, Vanden Hoek TL, Becker LB. Quality of cardiopulmonary resuscitation during in-hospital cardiac arrest. *JAMA.* 2005;293:305–310.

93. Valenzuela TD, Kern KB, Clark LL, Berg RA, Berg MD, Berg DD, Hilwig RW, Otto CW, Newburn D, Ewy GA. Interruptions of chest compressions during emergency medical systems resuscitation. *Circulation.* 2005;112:1259–1265.

94. Berg RA, Hilwig RW, Berg MD, Berg DD, Samson RA, Indik JH, Kern KB. Immediate post-shock chest compressions improve outcome from prolonged ventricular fibrillation. *Resuscitation.* 2008;78:71–76.

95. Tang W, Snyder D, Wang J, Huang L, Chang YT, Sun S, Weil MH. One-shock versus three-shock defibrillation protocol significantly improves outcome in a porcine model of prolonged ventricular fibrillation cardiac arrest. *Circulation.* 2006;113:2683–2689.

96. Garza AG, Gratton MC, Salomone JA, Lindholm D, McElroy J, Archer R. Improved patient survival using a modified resuscitation protocol for out-of-hospital cardiac arrest. *Circulation.* 2009;119:2597–2605.

97. Bobrow BJ, Clark LL, Ewy GA, Chikani V, Sanders AB, Berg RA, Richman PB, Kern KB. Minimally interrupted cardiac resuscitation by emergency medical services for out-of-hospital cardiac arrest. *JAMA.* 2008;299:1158–1165.

98. Kellum MJ, Kennedy KW, Barney R, Keilhauer FA, Bellino M, Zuercher M, Ewy GA. Cardiocerebral resuscitation improves neurologically intact survival of patients with out-of-hospital cardiac arrest. *Ann Emerg Med.* 2008;52:244–252.

99. Sayre MR, Cantrell SA, White LJ, Hiestand BC, Keseg DP, Koser S. Impact of the 2005 American Heart Association cardiopulmonary resuscitation and emergency cardiovascular care guidelines on out-of-hospital cardiac arrest survival. *Prehosp Emerg Care.* 2009;13:469–477.

100. Steinmetz J, Barnung S, Nielsen SL, Risom M, Rasmussen LS. Improved survival after an out-of-hospital cardiac arrest using new guidelines. *Acta Anaesthesiol Scand.* 2008;52:908–913.

101. Aufderheide TP, Yannopoulos D, Lick CJ, Myers B, Romig LA, Stothert JC, Barnard J, Vartanian L, Pilgrim AJ, Benditt DG. Implementing the 2005 American Heart Association Guidelines Improves Outcomes after Out-of-Hospital Cardiac Arrest. *Heart Rhythm.* 2010.

102. Hinchey PR, Myers JB, Lewis R, De Maio VJ, Reyer E, Licatese D, Zalkin J, Snyder G. Improved Out-of-Hospital Cardiac Arrest Survival After the Sequential Implementation of 2005 AHA Guidelines for Compressions, Ventilations, and Induced Hypothermia: The Wake County Experience. *Ann Emerg Med.* 2010.

103. Jost D, Degrange H, Verret C, Hersan O, Banville IL, Chapman FW, Lank P, Petit JL, Fuilla C, Migliani R, Carpentier JP. DEFI 2005: a randomized controlled trial of the effect of automated external defibrillator cardiopulmonary resuscitation protocol on outcome from out-of-hospital cardiac arrest. *Circulation.* 2010;121:1614–1622.

104. Sugerman NT, Edelson DP, Leary M, Weidman EK, Herzberg DL, Vanden Hoek TL, Becker LB, Abella BS. Rescuer fatigue during actual in-hospital cardiopulmonary resuscitation with audiovisual feedback: a prospective multicenter study. *Resuscitation.* 2009;80:981–984.

105. Manders S, Geijsel FE. Alternating providers during continuous chest compressions for cardiac arrest: every minute or every two minutes? *Resuscitation.* 2009;80:1015–1018.

106. Heidenreich JW, Berg RA, Higdon TA, Ewy GA, Kern KB, Sanders AB. Rescuer fatigue: standard versus continuous chest-compression cardiopulmonary resuscitation. *Acad Emerg Med.* 2006;13:1020–1026.

107. Dorph E, Wik L, Stromme TA, Eriksen M, Steen PA. Oxygen delivery and return of spontaneous circulation with ventilation:compression ratio 2:30 versus chest compressions only CPR in pigs. *Resuscitation.* 2004; 60:309–318.

108. Berg RA, Sanders AB, Kern KB, Hilwig RW, Heidenreich JW, Porter ME, Ewy GA. Adverse hemodynamic effects of interrupting chest compressions for rescue breathing during cardiopulmonary resuscitation for ventricular fibrillation cardiac arrest. *Circulation.* 2001;104: 2465–2470.

109. Berg RA, Hilwig RW, Kern KB, Ewy GA. "Bystander" chest compressions and assisted ventilation independently improve outcome from piglet asphyxial pulseless "cardiac arrest." *Circulation.* 2000;101: 1743–1748.

110. Berg RA, Kern KB, Hilwig RW, Berg MD, Sanders AB, Otto CW, Ewy GA. Assisted ventilation does not improve outcome in a porcine model of single-rescuer bystander cardiopulmonary resuscitation. *Circulation.* 1997;95:1635–1641.

111. Berg RA, Kern KB, Hilwig RW, Ewy GA. Assisted ventilation during 'bystander' CPR in a swine acute myocardial infarction model does not improve outcome. *Circulation.* 1997;96:4364–4371.

112. Vaillancourt C, Stiell IG, Wells GA. Understanding and improving low bystander CPR rates: a systematic review of the literature. *CJEM.* 2008;10:51–65.

113. Stiell IG, Wells GA, Field B, Spaite DW, Nesbitt LP, De Maio VJ, Nichol G, Cousineau D, Blackburn J, Munkley D, Luinstra-Toohey L, Campeau T, Dagnone E, Lyver M. Advanced cardiac life support in out-of-hospital cardiac arrest. *N Engl J Med.* 2004;351:647–656.

114. Ornato JP, Hallagan LF, McMahan SB, Peeples EH, Rostafinski AG. Attitudes of BCLS instructors about mouth-to-mouth resuscitation during the AIDS epidemic. *Ann Emerg Med.* 1990;19:151–156.

115. Brenner BE, Van DC, Cheng D, Lazar EJ. Determinants of reluctance to perform CPR among residents and applicants: the impact of experience on helping behavior. *Resuscitation.* 1997;35:203–211.

116. Hew P, Brenner B, Kaufman J. Reluctance of paramedics and emergency medical technicians to perform mouth-to-mouth resuscitation. *J Emerg Med.* 1997;15:279–284.

117. Sirbaugh PE, Pepe PE, Shook JE, Kimball KT, Goldman MJ, Ward MA, Mann DM. A prospective, population-based study of the demographics, epidemiology, management, and outcome of out-of-hospital pediatric cardiopulmonary arrest. *Ann Emerg Med.* 1999;33:174–184.

118. Swor R, Khan I, Domeier R, Honeycutt L, Chu K, Compton S. CPR training and CPR performance: do CPR-trained bystanders perform CPR? *Acad Emerg Med.* 2006;13:596–601.

119. Tang W, Weil MH, Sun S, Kette D, Gazmuri RJ, O'Connell F, Bisera J. Cardiopulmonary resuscitation by precordial compression but without mechanical ventilation. *Am J Respir Crit Care Med.* 1994;150(6 pt 1):1709–1713.

120. Bobrow BJ, Zuercher M, Ewy GA, Clark L, Chikani V, Donahue D, Sanders AB, Hilwig RW, Berg RA, Kern KB. Gasping during cardiac arrest in humans is frequent and associated with improved survival. *Circulation.* 2008;118:2550–2554.

121. Clark JJ, Larsen MP, Culley LL, Graves JR, Eisenberg MS. Incidence of agonal respirations in sudden cardiac arrest. *Ann Emerg Med.* 1992;21: 1464–1467.

122. Bang A, Herlitz J, Martinell S. Interaction between emergency medical dispatcher and caller in suspected out-of-hospital cardiac arrest calls with focus on agonal breathing. A review of 100 tape recordings of true cardiac arrest cases. *Resuscitation.* 2003;56:25–34.

123. Becker LB, Berg RA, Pepe PE, Idris AH, Aufderheide TP, Barnes TA, Stratton SJ, Chandra NC. A reappraisal of mouth-to-mouth ventilation during bystander-initiated cardiopulmonary resuscitation. A statement for healthcare professionals from the Ventilation Working Group of the Basic Life Support and Pediatric Life Support Subcommittees, American Heart Association. *Resuscitation.* 1997;35:189–201.

124. Weil MH, Rackow EC, Trevino R, Grundler W, Falk JL, Griffel MI. Difference in acid-base state between venous and arterial blood during cardiopulmonary resuscitation. *N Engl J Med.* 1986;315:153–156.

125. Sanders AB, Otto CW, Kern KB, Rogers JN, Perrault P, Ewy GA. Acid-base balance in a canine model of cardiac arrest. *Ann Emerg Med.* 1988;17:667–671.

126. Steen-Hansen JE. Favourable outcome after 26 minutes of "Compression only" resuscitation: a case report. *Scand J Trauma Resusc Emerg Med.* 2010;18:19.

127. Berg RA, Hilwig RW, Kern KB, Babar I, Ewy GA. Simulated mouth-to-mouth ventilation and chest compressions (bystander cardiopulmonary resuscitation) improves outcome in a swine model of prehospital pediatric asphyxial cardiac arrest. *Crit Care Med.* 1999;27:1893–1899.

128. Iglesias JM, Lopez-Herce J, Urbano J, Solana MJ, Mencia S, Del Castillo J. Chest compressions versus ventilation plus chest compressions in a pediatric asphyxial cardiac arrest animal model. *Intensive Care Med.* 2010;36:712–716.

129. Idris AH, Becker LB, Fuerst RS, Wenzel V, Rush WJ, Melker RJ, Orban DJ. Effect of ventilation on resuscitation in an animal model of cardiac arrest. *Circulation.* 1994;90:3063–3069.

130. Guildner CW. Resuscitation: opening the airway. A comparative study of techniques for opening an airway obstructed by the tongue. *JACEP.* 1976;5:588–590.

131. Greene DG, Elam JO, Dobkin AB, Studley CL. Cinefluorographic study of hyperextension of the neck and upper airway patency. *JAMA.* 1961; 176:570–573.

132. Ruben HM, Elam JO, al. e. Investigations of pharyngeal xrays and perfomance by laymen. *Anesthesiology.* 1961;22:271–279.

133. Elam JO, Greene DG, Schneider MA, Ruben HM, Gordon AS, Hustead RF, Benson DW, Clements JA, Ruben A. Head-tilt method of oral resuscitation. *JAMA.* 1960;172:812–815.

134. Rhee P, Kuncir EJ, Johnson L, Brown C, Velmahos G, Martin M, Wang D, Salim A, Doucet J, Kennedy S, Demetriades D. Cervical spine injury is highly dependent on the mechanism of injury following blunt and penetrating assault. *J Trauma.* 2006;61:1166–1170.

135. Lowery DW, Wald MM, Browne BJ, Tigges S, Hoffman JR, Mower WR. Epidemiology of cervical spine injury victims. *Ann Emerg Med.* 2001;38:12–16.

136. Milby AH, Halpern CH, Guo W, Stein SC. Prevalence of cervical spinal injury in trauma. *Neurosurg Focus.* 2008;25:E10.

137. Mithani SK, St-Hilaire H, Brooke BS, Smith IM, Bluebond-Langner R, Rodriguez ED. Predictable patterns of intracranial and cervical spine injury in craniomaxillofacial trauma: analysis of 4786 patients. *Plast Reconstr Surg.* 2009;123:1293–1301.

138. Hackl W, Hausberger K, Sailer R, Ulmer H, Gassner R. Prevalence of cervical spine injuries in patients with facial trauma. *Oral Surg Oral Med Oral Pathol Oral Radiol Endod.* 2001;92:370–376.

139. Holly LT, Kelly DF, Counelis GJ, Blinman T, McArthur DL, Cryer HG. Cervical spine trauma associated with moderate and severe head injury: incidence, risk factors, and injury characteristics. *J Neurosurg Spine.* 2002;96:285–291.

140. Demetriades D, Charalambides K, Chahwan S, Hanpeter D, Alo K, Velmahos G, Murray J, Asensio J. Nonskeletal cervical spine injuries: epidemiology and diagnostic pitfalls. *J Trauma.* 2000;48:724–727.

141. Majernick TG, Bieniek R, Houston JB, Hughes HG. Cervical spine movement during orotracheal intubation. *Ann Emerg Med.* 1986;15: 417–420.

142. Lennarson PJ, Smith DW, Sawin PD, Todd MM, Sato Y, Traynelis VC. Cervical spinal motion during intubation: efficacy of stabilization maneuvers in the setting of complete segmental instability. *J Neurosurg Spine.* 2001;94:265–270.

143. Hastings RH, Wood PR. Head extension and laryngeal view during laryngoscopy with cervical spine stabilization maneuvers. *Anesthesiology.* 1994; 80:825–831.

144. Gerling MC, Davis DP, Hamilton RS, Morris GF, Vilke GM, Garfin SR, Hayden SR. Effects of cervical spine immobilization technique and laryngoscope blade selection on an unstable cervical spine in a cadaver model of intubation. *Ann Emerg Med.* 2000;36:293–300.

145. Wenzel V, Keller C, Idris AH, Dorges V, Lindner KH, Brimacombe JR. Effects of smaller tidal volumes during basic life support venti-

lation in patients with respiratory arrest: good ventilation, less risk? *Resuscitation.* 1999;43:25–29.

146. Dorges V, Ocker H, Hagelberg S, Wenzel V, Idris AH, Schmucker P. Smaller tidal volumes with room-air are not sufficient to ensure adequate oxygenation during bag-valve-mask ventilation. *Resuscitation.* 2000;44:37–41.

147. Dorges V, Ocker H, Hagelberg S, Wenzel V, Schmucker P. Optimisation of tidal volumes given with self-inflatable bags without additional oxygen. *Resuscitation.* 2000;43:195–199.

148. Finer NN, Barrington KJ, Al-Fadley F, Peters KL. Limitations of self-inflating resuscitators. *Pediatrics.* 1986;77:417–420.

149. Hirschman AM, Kravath RE. Venting vs ventilating. A danger of manual resuscitation bags. *Chest.* 1982;82:369–370.

150. Berg MD, Idris AH, Berg RA. Severe ventilatory compromise due to gastric distention during pediatric cardiopulmonary resuscitation. *Resuscitation.* 1998;36:71–73.

151. Garnett AR, Ornato JP, Gonzalez ER, Johnson EB. End-tidal carbon dioxide monitoring during cardiopulmonary resuscitation. *JAMA.* 1987;257:512–515.

152. Aufderheide TP, Sigurdsson G, Pirrallo RG, Yannopoulos D, McKnite S, von Briesen C, Sparks CW, Conrad CJ, Provo TA, Lurie KG. Hyperventilation-induced hypotension during cardiopulmonary resuscitation. *Circulation.* 2004;109:1960–1965.

153. Kern KB, Hilwig RW, Berg RA, Sanders AB, Ewy GA. Importance of continuous chest compressions during cardiopulmonary resuscitation: improved outcome during a simulated single lay-rescuer scenario. *Circulation.* 2002;105:645–649.

154. Wang HE, Simeone SJ, Weaver MD, Callaway CW. Interruptions in cardiopulmonary resuscitation from paramedic endotracheal intubation. *Ann Emerg Med.* 2009;54:645–652 e641.

155. Wenzel V, Idris AH, Banner MJ, Fuerst RS, Tucker KJ. The composition of gas given by mouth-to-mouth ventilation during CPR. *Chest.* 1994;106:1806–1810.

156. Ruben H. The immediate treatment of respiratory failure. *Br J Anaesth.* 1964;36:542–549.

157. Bhalla RK, Corrigan A, Roland NJ. Comparison of two face masks used to deliver early ventilation to laryngectomized patients. *Ear Nose Throat J.* 2004;83:414, 416.

158. Barnes TA. Emergency ventilation techniques and related equipment. *Respir Care.* 1992;37:673–690, discussion 690–674.

159. Johannigman JA, Branson RD, Davis K Jr, Hurst JM. Techniques of emergency ventilation: a model to evaluate tidal volume, airway pressure, and gastric insufflation. *J Trauma.* 1991;31:93–98.

160. Elam JO. Bag-valve-mask $O_2$ ventilation. In: Safar P, Elam JO, eds. *Advances in Cardiopulmonary Resuscitation: The Wolf Creek Conference on Cardiopulmonary Resuscitation.* New York, NY: Springer-Verlag, Inc.; 1977:73–79.

161. Dailey R, Young G, Simon B, Stewart R. The Airway: Emergency *Management*: C.V. Mosby; 1992.

162. Elling R, Politis J. An evaluation of emergency medical technicians' ability to use manual ventilation devices. *Ann Emerg Med.* 1983;12:765–768.

163. von Goedecke A, Bowden K, Wenzel V, Keller C, Gabrielli A. Effects of decreasing inspiratory times during simulated bag-valve-mask ventilation. *Resuscitation.* 2005;64:321–325.

164. von Goedecke A, Bowden K, Keller C, Voelckel WG, Jeske HC, Wenzel V. [Decreased inspiratory time during ventilation of an unprotected airway. Effect on stomach inflation and lung ventilation in a bench model.] *Anaesthesist.* 2005;54:117–122.

165. von Goedecke A, Paal P, Keller C, Voelckel WG, Herff H, Lindner KH, Wenzel V. [Ventilation of an unprotected airway: evaluation of a new peak-inspiratory-flow and airway-pressure-limiting bag-valve-mask.] *Anaesthesist.* 2006;55:629–634.

166. Rumball CJ, MacDonald D. The PTL, Combitube, laryngeal mask, and oral airway: a randomized prehospital comparative study of ventilatory device effectiveness and cost-effectiveness in 470 cases of cardiorespiratory arrest. *Prehosp Emerg Care.* 1997;1:1–10.

167. Comparison of arterial blood gases of laryngeal mask airway and bag-valve-mask ventilation in out-of-hospital cardiac arrests. *Circ J.* 2009;73:490–496.

168. Stone BJ, Chantler PJ, Baskett PJ. The incidence of regurgitation during cardiopulmonary resuscitation: a comparison between the bag valve mask and laryngeal mask airway. *Resuscitation.* 1998;38:3–6.

169. Atherton GL, Johnson JC. Ability of paramedics to use the Combitube in prehospital cardiac arrest. *Ann Emerg Med.* 1993;22:1263–1268.

170. Kette F, Reffo I, Giordani G, Buzzi F, Borean V, Cimarosti R, Codiglia A, Hattinger C, Mongiat A, Tararan S. The use of laryngeal tube by nurses in out-of-hospital emergencies: Preliminary experience. *Resuscitation.* 2005;66:21–25.

171. Timmermann A, Russo SG, Rosenblatt WH, Eich C, Barwing J, Roessler M, Graf BM. Intubating laryngeal mask airway for difficult out-of-hospital airway management: a prospective evaluation. *Br J Anaesth.* 2007;99:286–291.

172. Kellum MJ, Kennedy KW, Ewy GA. Cardiocerebral resuscitation improves survival of patients with out-of-hospital cardiac arrest. *Am J Med.* 2006;119:335–340.

173. Bobrow BJ, Ewy GA, Clark L, Chikani V, Berg RA, Sanders AB, Vadeboncoeur TF, Hilwig RW, Kern KB. Passive oxygen insufflation is superior to bag-valve-mask ventilation for witnessed ventricular fibrillation out-of-hospital cardiac arrest. *Ann Emerg Med.* 2009;54:656–662 e651.

174. McNelis U, Syndercombe A, Harper I, Duggan J. The effect of cricoid pressure on intubation facilitated by the gum elastic bougie. *Anaesthesia.* 2007;62:456–459.

175. Harry RM, Nolan JP. The use of cricoid pressure with the intubating laryngeal mask. *Anaesthesia.* 1999;54:656–659.

176. Noguchi T, Koga K, Shiga Y, Shigematsu A. The gum elastic bougie eases tracheal intubation while applying cricoid pressure compared to a stylet. *Can J Anaesth.* 2003;50:712–717.

177. Asai T, Murao K, Shingu K. Cricoid pressure applied after placement of laryngeal mask impedes subsequent fibreoptic tracheal intubation through mask. *Br J Anaesth.* 2000;85:256–261.

178. Snider DD, Clarke D, Finucane BT. The "BURP" maneuver worsens the glottic view when applied in combination with cricoid pressure. *Can J Anaesth.* 2005;52:100–104.

179. Smith CE, Boyer D. Cricoid pressure decreases ease of tracheal intubation using fibreoptic laryngoscopy (WuScope System). *Can J Anaesth.* 2002;49:614–619.

180. Asai T, Barclay K, Power I, Vaughan RS. Cricoid pressure impedes placement of the laryngeal mask airway and subsequent tracheal intubation through the mask. *Br J Anaesth.* 1994;72:47–51.

181. Domuracki KJ, Moule CJ, Owen H, Kostandoff G, Plummer JL. Learning on a simulator does transfer to clinical practice. *Resuscitation.* 2009;80:346–349.

182. Beavers RA, Moos DD, Cuddeford JD. Analysis of the application of cricoid pressure: implications for the clinician. *J Perianesth Nurs.* 2009;24:92–102.

183. Meek T, Gittins N, Duggan JE. Cricoid pressure: knowledge and performance amongst anaesthetic assistants. *Anaesthesia.* 1999;54:59–62.

184. Clark RK, Trethewy CE. Assessment of cricoid pressure application by emergency department staff. *Emerg Med Australas.* 2005;17:376–381.

185. Kopka A, Robinson D. The 50 ml syringe training aid should be utilized immediately before cricoid pressure application. *Eur J Emerg Med.* 2005;12:155–158.

186. Flucker CJ, Hart E, Weisz M, Griffiths R, Ruth M. The 50-millilitre syringe as an inexpensive training aid in the application of cricoid pressure. *Eur J Anaesthesiol.* 2000;17:443–447.

187. Shimabukuro A, Kawatani M, Nagao N, Inoue Y, Hayashida M, Hikawa Y. [Training in application of cricoid pressure.] *Masui.* 2006;55:742–744.

188. Schmidt A, Akeson J. Practice and knowledge of cricoid pressure in southern Sweden. *Acta Anaesthesiol Scand.* 2001;45:1210–1214.

189. Patten SP. Educating nurses about correct application of cricoid pressure. *AORN J.* 2006;84:449–461.

190. Koziol CA, Cuddeford JD, Moos DD. Assessing the force generated with application of cricoid pressure. *AORN J.* 2000;72:1018–1028, 1030.

191. Clayton TJ, Vanner RG. A novel method of measuring cricoid force. *Anaesthesia.* 2002;57:326–329.

192. Owen H, Follows V, Reynolds KJ, Burgess G, Plummer J. Learning to apply effective cricoid pressure using a part task trainer. *Anaesthesia.* 2002;57:1098–1101.

193. Kopka A, Crawford J. Cricoid pressure: a simple, yet effective biofeedback trainer. *Eur J Anaesthesiol.* 2004;21:443–447.

194. Quigley P, Jeffrey P. Cricoid pressure: assessment of performance and effect of training in emergency department staff. *Emerg Med Australas.* 2007;19:218–222.

195. The Public Access Defibrillation Trial Investigators. Public-access defibrillation and survival after out-of-hospital cardiac arrest. *N Engl J Med.* 2004;351:637–646.

196. Rea TD, Cook AJ, Stiell IG, Powell J, Bigham B, Callaway CW, Chugh S, Aufderheide TP, Morrison L, Terndrup TE, Beaudoin T, Wittwer L, Davis D, Idris A, Nichol G. Predicting survival after out-of-hospital cardiac arrest: role of the Utstein data elements. *Ann Emerg Med*. 2010;55:249–257.

197. Caffrey SL, Willoughby PJ, Pepe PE, Becker LB. Public use of automated external defibrillators. *N Engl J Med*. 2002;347:1242–1247.

198. Fries M, Tang W, Chang YT, Wang J, Castillo C, Weil MH. Microvascular blood flow during cardiopulmonary resuscitation is predictive of outcome. *Resuscitation*. 2006;71:248–253.

199. Stiell IG, Callaway C, Davis D, Terndrup T, Powell J, Cook A, Kudenchuk PJ, Daya M, Kerber R, Idris A, Morrison LJ, Aufderheide T. Resuscitation Outcomes Consortium (ROC) PRIMED cardiac arrest trial methods part 2: rationale and methodology for "Analyze Later vs. Analyze Early" protocol. *Resuscitation*. 2008;78:186–195.

200. Baker PW, Conway J, Cotton C, Ashby DT, Smyth J, Woodman RJ, Grantham H. Defibrillation or cardiopulmonary resuscitation first for patients with out-of-hospital cardiac arrests found by paramedics to be in ventricular fibrillation? A randomised control trial. *Resuscitation*. 2008;79:424–431.

201. Jacobs IG, Finn JC, Oxer HF, Jelinek GA. CPR before defibrillation in out-of-hospital cardiac arrest: a randomized trial. *Emerg Med Australas*. 2005;17:39–45.

202. Wik L, Hansen TB, Fylling F, Steen T, Vaagenes P, Auestad BH, Steen PA. Delaying defibrillation to give basic cardiopulmonary resuscitation to patients with out-of-hospital ventricular fibrillation: a randomized trial. *JAMA*. 2003;289:1389–1395.

203. Cobb LA, Fahrenbruch CE, Walsh TR, Copass MK, Olsufka M, Breskin M, Hallstrom AP. Influence of cardiopulmonary resuscitation prior to defibrillation in patients with out-of-hospital ventricular fibrillation. *JAMA*. 1999;281:1182–1188.

204. Handley AJ. Recovery Position. *Resuscitation*. 1993;26:93–95.

205. Turner S, Turner I, Chapman D, Howard P, Champion P, Hatfield J, James A, Marshall S, Barber S. A comparative study of the 1992 and 1997 recovery positions for use in the UK. *Resuscitation*. 1998;39:153–160.

206. Gunn BD, Eizenberg N, Silberstein M, McMeeken JM, Tully EA, Stillman BC, Brown DJ, Gutteridge GA. How should an unconscious person with a suspected neck injury be positioned? *Prehospital Disaster Med*. 1995;10:239–244.

207. Blake WE, Stillman BC, Eizenberg N, Briggs C, McMeeken JM. The position of the spine in the recovery position–an experimental comparison between the lateral recovery position and the modified HAINES position. *Resuscitation*. 2002;53:289–297.

208. WRITING GROUP MEMBERS, Lloyd-Jones D, Adams RJ, Brown TM, Carnethon M, Dai S, De Simone G, Ferguson TB, Ford E, Furie K, Gillespie C, Go A, Greenlund K, Haase N, Hailpern S, Ho PM, Howard V, Kissela B, Kittner S, Lackland D, Lisabeth L, Marelli A, McDermott MM, Meigs J, Mozaffarian D, Mussolino M, Nichol G, Roger VL, Rosamond W, Sacco R, Sorlie P, Stafford R, Thom T, Wasserthiel-Smoller S, Wong ND, Wylie-Rosett J. Committee obotAHAS, Stroke Statistics Subcommittee. Heart Disease and Stroke Statistics–2010 Update: A Report From the American Heart Association. *Circulation*. 2010;121:e46–e215.

209. Chiriboga D, Yarzebski J, Goldberg RJ, Gore JM, Alpert JS. Temporal trends (1975 through 1990) in the incidence and case-fatality rates of primary ventricular fibrillation complicating acute myocardial infarction: a communitywide perspective. *Circulation*. 1994;89:998–1003.

210. Anderson JL, Karagounis LA, Califf RM. Metaanalysis of five reported studies on the relation of early coronary patency grades with mortality and outcomes after acute myocardial infarction. *Am J Cardiol*. 1996;78:1–8.

211. Raitt MH, Maynard C, Wagner GS, Cerqueira MD, Selvester RH, Weaver WD. Relation between symptom duration before thrombolytic therapy and final myocardial infarct size. *Circulation*. 1996;93:48–53.

212. Douglas PS, Ginsburg GS. The evaluation of chest pain in women. *N Engl J Med*. 1996;334:1311–1315.

213. Solomon CG, Lee TH, Cook EF, Weisberg MC, Brand DA, Rouan GW, Goldman L. Comparison of clinical presentation of acute myocardial infarction in patients older than 65 years of age to younger patients: the Multicenter Chest Pain Study experience. *Am J Cardiol*. 1989;63:772–776.

214. Peberdy MA, Ornato JP. Coronary artery disease in women. *Heart Dis Stroke*. 1992;1:315–319.

215. Body R, Carley S, Wibberley C, McDowell G, Ferguson J, Mackway-Jones K. The value of symptoms and signs in the emergent diagnosis of acute coronary syndromes. *Resuscitation*. 2010;81:281–286.

216. Goodacre SW, Angelini K Arnold J, Revill S, Morris F. Clinical predictors of acute coronary syndromes in patients with undifferentiated chest pain. *QJM*. 2003;96:893–898.

217. Goodacre S, Locker T, Morris F, Campbell S. How useful are clinical features in the diagnosis of acute, undifferentiated chest pain? *Acad Emerg Med*. 2002;9:203–208.

218. Everts B, Karlson BW, Wahrborg P, Hedner T, Herlitz J. Localization of pain in suspected acute myocardial infarction in relation to final diagnosis, age and sex, and site and type of infarction. *Heart Lung*. 1996;25:430–437.

219. McSweeney JC, Cody M, O'Sullivan P, Elberson K, Moser DK, Garvin BJ. Women's early warning symptoms of acute myocardial infarction. *Circulation*. 2003;108:2619–2623.

220. Panju AA, BR Hemmelgarn, GG Guyatt, DL Simel. Is this patient having a myocardial infarction? *JAMA*. 1998;280:1256–1263.

221. Mant J, McManus RJ, Oakes RA, Delaney BC, Barton PM, Deeks JJ, Hammersley L, Davies RC, Davies MK, Hobbs FD. Systematic review and modelling of the investigation of acute and chronic chest pain presenting in primary care. *Health Technol Assess*. 2004;8:iii,1–158.

222. Berger JP, Buclin T, Haller E, Van Melle G, Yersin B. Right arm involvement and pain extension can help to differentiate coronary diseases from chest pain of other origin: a prospective emergency ward study of 278 consecutive patients admitted for chest pain. *J Intern Med*. 1990;227:165–172.

223. Jonsbu J, Rollag A, Aase O, Lippestad CT, Arnesen KE, Erikssen J, Koss A. Rapid and correct diagnosis of myocardial infarction: standardized case history and clinical examination provide important information for correct referral to monitored beds. *J Intern Med*. 1991;229:143–149.

224. Hargarten KM, Aprahamian C, Stueven H, Olson DW, Aufderheide TP, Mateer JR. Limitations of prehospital predictors of acute myocardial infarction and unstable angina. *Ann Emerg Med*. 1987;16:1325–1329.

225. Herlitz J, Hansson E, Ringvall E, Starke M, Karlson BW, Waagstein L. Predicting a life-threatening disease and death among ambulance-transported patients with chest pain or other symptoms raising suspicion of an acute coronary syndrome. *Am J Emerg Med*. 2002;20:588–594.

226. Lee TH, Pearson SD, Johnson PA, Garcia TB, Weisberg MC, Guadagnoli E, Cook EF, Goldman L. Failure of information as an intervention to modify clinical management. A time-series trial in patients with acute chest pain. *Ann Intern Med*. 1995;122:434–437.

227. Henrikson CA, Howell EE, Bush DE, Miles JS, Meininger GR, Friedlander T, Bushnell AC, Chandra-Strobos N. Chest pain relief by nitroglycerin does not predict active coronary artery disease. *Ann Intern Med*. 2003;139:979–986.

228. Lee TH, Rouan GW, Weisberg MC, Brand DA, Acampora D, Stasiulewicz C, Walshon J, Terranova G, Gottlieb L, Goldstein-Wayne B, et al. Clinical characteristics and natural history of patients with acute myocardial infarction sent home from the emergency room. *Am J Cardiol*. 1987;60:219–224.

229. Freimark D, Matetzky S, Leor J, Boyko V, Barbash IM, Behar S, Hod H. Timing of aspirin administration as a determinant of survival of patients with acute myocardial infarction treated with thrombolysis. *Am J Cardiol*. 2002;89:381–385.

230. Barbash IM, Freimark D, Gottlieb S, Hod H, Hasin Y, Battler A, Crystal E, Matetzky S, Boyko V, Mandelzweig L, Behar S, Leor J. Outcome of myocardial infarction in patients treated with aspirin is enhanced by pre-hospital administration. *Cardiology*. 2002;98:141–147.

231. Randomised trial of intravenous streptokinase, oral aspirin, both, or neither among 17,187 cases of suspected acute myocardial infarction: ISIS-2. ISIS-2 (Second International Study of Infarct Survival) Collaborative Group. *Lancet*. 1988;2:349–360.

232. Casaccia M, Bertello F, De Bernardi A, Sicuro M, Scacciatella P. Prehospital management of acute myocardial infarct in an experimental metropolitan system of medical emergencies [in Italian]. *G Ital Cardiol*. 1996;26:657–672.

233. Quan D, LoVecchio F, Clark B, Gallagher JV III. Prehospital use of aspirin rarely is associated with adverse events. *Prehosp Disaster Med*. 2004;19:362–365.

234. Verheugt FW, van der Laarse A, Funke-Kupper AJ, Sterkman LG, Galema TW, Roos JP. Effects of early intervention with low-dose

aspirin (100 mg) on infarct size, reinfarction and mortality in anterior wall acute myocardial infarction. *Am J Cardiol.* 1990;66:267–270.

235. Le May MR, So DY, Dionne R, Glover CA, Froeschl MP, Wells GA, Davies RF, Sherrard HL, Maloney J, Marquis JF, O'Brien ER, Trickett J, Poirier P, Ryan SC, Ha A, Joseph PG, Labinaz M. A citywide protocol for primary PCI in ST-segment elevation myocardial infarction. *N Engl J Med.* 2008;358:231–240.

236. Stenestrand U, Lindback J, Wallentin L. Long-term outcome of primary percutaneous coronary intervention vs prehospital and in-hospital thrombolysis for patients with ST-elevation myocardial infarction. *JAMA.* 2006;296:1749–1756.

237. Le May MR, Davies RF, Dionne R, Maloney J, Trickett J, So D, Ha A, Sherrard H, Glover C, Marquis JF, O'Brien ER, Stiell IG, Poirier P, Labinaz M. Comparison of early mortality of paramedic-diagnosed ST-segment elevation myocardial infarction with immediate transport to a designated primary percutaneous coronary intervention center to that of similar patients transported to the nearest hospital. *Am J Cardiol.* 2006;98:1329–1333.

238. Wijesinghe M, Perrin K, Ranchord A, Simmonds M, Weatherall M, Beasley R. Routine use of oxygen in the treatment of myocardial infarction: systematic review. *Heart.* 2009;95:198–202.

239. Haynes BE, Pritting J. A rural emergency medical technician with selected advanced skills. *Prehosp Emerg Care.* 1999;3:343–346.

240. Funk D, Groat C, Verdile VP. Education of paramedics regarding aspirin use. *Prehosp Emerg Care.* 2000;4:62–64.

241. Bussmann WD, Passek D, Seidel W, Kaltenbach M. Reduction of CK and CK-MB indexes of infarct size by intravenous nitroglycerin. *Circulation.* 1981;63:615–622.

242. Charvat J, Kuruvilla T, al Amad H. Beneficial effect of intravenous nitroglycerin in patients with non-Q myocardial infarction. *Cardiologia.* 1990;35:49–54.

243. Jugdutt BI, Warnica JW. Intravenous nitroglycerin therapy to limit myocardial infarct size, expansion, and complications. Effect of timing, dosage, and infarct location. *Circulation.* 1988;78:906–919.

244. Madsen JK, Chevalier B, Darius H, Rutsch W, Wojcik J, Schneider S, Allikmets K. Ischaemic events and bleeding in patients undergoing percutaneous coronary intervention with concomitant bivalirudin treatment. *EuroIntervention.* 2008;3:610–616.

245. Lloyd-Jones DM, Hong Y, Labarthe D, Mozaffarian D, Appel LJ, Van Horn L, Greenlund K, Daniels S, Nichol G, Tomaselli GF, Arnett DK, Fonarow GC, Ho PM, Lauer MS, Masoudi FA, Robertson RM, Roger V, Schwamm LH, Sorlie P, Yancy CW, Rosamond WD. Defining and setting national goals for cardiovascular health promotion and disease reduction: the American Heart Association's strategic Impact Goal through 2020 and beyond. *Circulation.* 2010;121:586–613.

246. Grotta JC, Chiu D, Lu M, Patel S, Levine SR, Tilley BC, Brott TG, Haley EC Jr, Lyden PD, Kothari R, Frankel M, Lewandowski CA, Libman R, Kwiatkowski T, Broderick JP, Marler JR, Corrigan J, Huff S, Mitsias P, Talati S, Tanne D. Agreement and variability in the interpretation of early CT changes in stroke patients qualifying for intravenous rtPA therapy. *Stroke.* 1999;30:1528–1533.

247. Ingall TJ, O'Fallon WM, Asplund K, Goldfrank LR, Hertzberg VS, Louis TA, Christianson TJ. Findings from the reanalysis of the NINDS tissue plasminogen activator for acute ischemic stroke treatment trial. *Stroke.* 2004;35:2418–2424.

248. Hacke W, Kaste M, Bluhmki E, Brozman M, Davalos A, Guidetti D, Larrue V, Lees KR, Medeghri Z, Machnig T, Schneider D, von Kummer R, Wahlgren N, Toni D. Thrombolysis with alteplase 3 to 4.5 hours after acute ischemic stroke. *N Engl J Med.* 2008;359:1317–1329.

249. Hacke W, Donnan G, Fieschi C, Kaste M, von Kummer R, Broderick JP, Brott T, Frankel M, Grotta JC, Haley EC Jr, Kwiatkowski T, Levine SR, Lewandowski C, Lu M, Lyden P, Marler JR, Patel S, Tilley BC, Albers G, Bluhmki E, Wilhelm M, Hamilton S. Association of outcome with early stroke treatment: pooled analysis of ATLANTIS, ECASS, and NINDS rt-PA stroke trials. *Lancet.* 2004;363:768–774.

250. Alberts MJ, Latchaw RE, Selman WR, Shephard T, Hadley MN, Brass LM, Koroshetz W, Marler JR, Booss J, Zorowitz RD, Croft JB, Magnis E, Mulligan D, Jagoda A, O'Connor R, Cawley CM, Connors JJ, Rose-DeRenzy JA, Emr M, Warren M, Walker MD. Recommendations for comprehensive stroke centers: a consensus statement from the Brain Attack Coalition. *Stroke.* 2005;36:1597–1616.

251. Alberts MJ, Hademenos G, Latchaw RE, Jagoda A, Marler JR, Mayberg MR, Starke RD, Todd HW, Viste KM, Girgus M, Shephard T, Emr M, Shwayder P, Walker MD. Recommendations for the establishment of primary stroke centers. Brain Attack Coalition. *JAMA.* 2000;283:3102–3109.

252. Barsan WG, Brott TG, Olinger CP, Adams HP Jr, Haley EC Jr, Levy DE. Identification and entry of the patient with acute cerebral infarction. *Ann Emerg Med.* 1988;17:1192–1195.

253. Barsan WG, Brott TG, Broderick JP, Haley EC, Levy DE, Marler JR. Time of hospital presentation in patients with acute stroke. *Arch Intern Med.* 1993;153:2558–2561.

254. Morgenstern LB, Bartholomew LK, Grotta JC, Staub L, King M, Chan W. Sustained benefit of a community and professional intervention to increase acute stroke therapy. *Arch Intern Med.* 2003;163:2198–2202.

255. Scott PA. Enhancing community delivery of tissue plasminogen activator in stroke through community-academic collaborative clinical knowledge translation. *Emerg Med Clin North Am.* 2009;27:115–136, ix.

256. Kleindorfer D, Khoury J, Broderick JP, Rademacher E, Woo D, Flaherty ML, Alwell K, Moomaw CJ, Schneider A, Pancioli A, Miller R, Kissela BM. Temporal trends in public awareness of stroke: warning signs, risk factors, and treatment. *Stroke.* 2009;40:2502–2506.

257. Smith WS, Isaacs M, Corry MD. Accuracy of paramedic identification of stroke and transient ischemic attack in the field. *Prehosp Emerg Care.* 1998;2:170–175.

258. Kidwell CS, Starkman S, Eckstein M, Weems K, Saver JL. Identifying stroke in the field. Prospective validation of the Los Angeles prehospital stroke screen (LAPSS). *Stroke.* 2000;31:71–76.

259. Smith WS, Corry MD, Fazackerley J, Isaacs SM. Improved paramedic sensitivity in identifying stroke victims in the prehospital setting. *Prehosp Emerg Care.* 1999;3:207–210.

260. Kim SK, Lee SY, Bae HJ, Lee YS, Kim SY, Kang MJ, Cha JK. Pre-hospital notification reduced the door-to-needle time for iv t-PA in acute ischaemic stroke. *Eur J Neurol.* 2009;16:1331–1335.

261. Quain DA, Parsons MW, Loudfoot AR, Spratt NJ, Evans MK, Russell ML, Royan AT, Moore AG, Miteff F, Hullick CJ, Attia J, McElduff P, Levi CR. Improving access to acute stroke therapies: a controlled trial of organised pre-hospital and emergency care. *Med J Aust.* 2008;189:429–433.

262. Abdullah AR, Smith EE, Biddinger PD, Kalenderian D, Schwamm LH. Advance hospital notification by EMS in acute stroke is associated with shorter door-to-computed tomography time and increased likelihood of administration of tissue-plasminogen activator. *Prehosp Emerg Care.* 2008;12:426–431.

263. Gropen TI, Gagliano PJ, Blake CA, Sacco RL, Kwiatkowski T, Richmond NJ, Leifer D, Libman R, Azhar S, Daley MB. Quality improvement in acute stroke: the New York State Stroke Center Designation Project. *Neurology.* 2006;67:88–93.

264. Gladstone DJ, Rodan LH, Sahlas DJ, Lee L, Murray BJ, Ween JE, Perry JR, Chenkin J, Morrison LJ, Beck S, Black SE. A citywide prehospital protocol increases access to stroke thrombolysis in Toronto. *Stroke.* 2009;40:3841–3844.

265. Langhorne P, Tong BL, Stott DJ. Association between physiological homeostasis and early recovery after stroke. *Stroke.* 2000;31:2518–2519.

266. National Center for Injury Prevention and Control Web-based Injury Statistics Query and Reporting System (WISQARS). *Centers for Disease Control and Prevention.* Available at: http://www.cdc.gov/injury/wisqars/index.html.

267. Youn CS, Choi SP, Yim HW, Park KN. Out-of-hospital cardiac arrest due to drowning: An Utstein Style report of 10 years of experience from St. Mary's Hospital. *Resuscitation.* 2009;80:778–783.

268. Suominen P, Baillie C, Korpela R, Rautanen S, Ranta S, Olkkola KT. Impact of age, submersion time and water temperature on outcome in near-drowning. *Resuscitation.* 2002;52:247–254.

269. Perkins GD. In-water resuscitation: a pilot evaluation. *Resuscitation.* 2005;65:321–324.

270. Rosen P, Stoto M, Harley J. The use of the Heimlich maneuver in near-drowning: Institute of Medicine report. *J Emerg Med.* 1995;13:397–405.

271. Watson RS, Cummings P, Quan L, Bratton S, Weiss NS. Cervical spine injuries among submersion victims. *J Trauma.* 2001;51:658–662.

272. Hwang V, Shofer FS, Durbin DR, Baren JM. Prevalence of traumatic injuries in drowning and near drowning in children and adolescents. *Arch Pediatr Adolesc Med.* 2003;157:50–53.

273. Fingerhut LA, Cox CS. Warner M International comparative analysis of injury mortality. Findings from the ICE on injury statistics. International Collaborative Effort on Injury Statistics. *Adv Data.* 1998(303):1–20.

274. Dolkas L, Stanley C, Smith AM, Vilke GM. Deaths associated with choking in San Diego county. *J Forensic Sci.* 2007;52:176–179.

275. Soroudi A, Shipp HE, Stepanski BM, Ray LU, Murrin PA, Chan TC, Davis DP, Vilke GM. Adult foreign body airway obstruction in the prehospital setting. *Prehosp Emerg Care.* 2007;11:25–29.

276. Redding JS. The choking controversy: critique of evidence on the Heimlich maneuver. *Crit Care Med.* 1979;7:475–479.

277. Vilke GM, Smith AM, Ray LU, Steen PJ, Murrin PA, Chan TC. Airway obstruction in children aged less than 5 years: the prehospital experience. *Prehosp Emerg Care.* 2004;8:196–199.

278. Ingalls TH. Heimlich versus a slap on the back. *N Engl J Med.* 1979; 300:990.

279. Heimlich HJ, Hoffmann KA, Canestri FR. Food-choking and drowning deaths prevented by external subdiaphragmatic compression. Physiological basis. *Ann Thorac Surg.* 1975;20:188–195.

280. Boussuges S, Maitrerobert P, Bost M. [Use of the Heimlich Maneuver on children in the Rhone-Alpes area.] *Arch Fr Pediatr.* 1985;42: 733–736.

281. Guildner CW, Williams D, Subitch T. Airway obstructed by foreign material: the Heimlich maneuver. *JACEP.* 1976;5:675–677.

282. Langhelle A, Sunde K, Wik L, Steen PA. Airway pressure with chest compressions versus Heimlich manoeuvre in recently dead adults with complete airway obstruction. *Resuscitation.* 2000;44:105–108.

283. Ruben H, Macnaughton FI. The treatment of food-choking. *Practitioner.* 1978;221:725–729.

284. Brauner DJ. The Heimlich maneuver: procedure of choice? *J Am Geriatr Soc.* 1987;35:78.

285. Hartrey R, Bingham RM. Pharyngeal trauma as a result of blind finger sweeps in the choking child. *J Accid Emerg Med.* 1995;12:52–54.

286. Kabbani M, Goodwin SR. Traumatic epiglottis following blind finger sweep to remove a pharyngeal foreign body. *Clin Pediatr (Phila).* 1995;34:495–497.

287. Rea TD, Stickney RE, Doherty A, Lank P. Performance of chest compressions by laypersons during the Public Access Defibrillation Trial. *Resuscitation.* 2010;81:293–296.

288. Chiang WC, Chen WJ, Chen SY, Ko PC, Lin CH, Tsai MS, Chang WT, Chen SC, Tsan CY, Ma MH. Better adherence to the guidelines during cardiopulmonary resuscitation through the provision of audio-prompts. *Resuscitation.* 2005;64:297–301.

289. Kern KB, Sanders AB, Raife J, Milander MM, Otto CW, Ewy GA. A study of chest compression rates during cardiopulmonary resuscitation in humans: the importance of rate-directed chest compressions. *Arch Intern Med.* 1992;152:145–149.

290. Berg RA, Sanders AB, Milander M, Tellez D, Liu P, Beyda D. Efficacy of audio-prompted rate guidance in improving resuscitator performance of cardiopulmonary resuscitation on children. *Acad Emerg Med.* 1994; 1:35–40.

291. Abella BS, Edelson DP, Kim S, Retzer E, Myklebust H, Barry AM, O'Hearn N, Hoek TL, Becker LB. CPR quality improvement during in-hospital cardiac arrest using a real-time audiovisual feedback system. *Resuscitation.* 2007;73:54–61.

292. Fletcher D, Galloway R, Chamberlain D, Pateman J, Bryant G, Newcombe RG. Basics in advanced life support: a role for download audit and metronomes. *Resuscitation.* 2008;78:127–134.

293. Gruben KG, Romlein J, Halperin HR, Tsitlik JE. System for mechanical measurements during ardiopulmonary resuscitation in humans. *IEEE Trans Biomed Eng.* 1990;37:204–210.

294. Nishisaki A, Nysaether J, Sutton R, Maltese M, Niles D, Donoghue A, Bishnoi R, Helfaer M, Perkins GD, Berg R, Arbogast K, Nadkarni V. Effect of mattress deflection on CPR quality assessment for older children and adolescents. *Resuscitation.* 2009;80:540–545.

KEY WORDS: cardiacarrest ■ defibrillation ■ emergency

# Part 6: Electrical Therapies
## Automated External Defibrillators, Defibrillation, Cardioversion, and Pacing
## 2010 American Heart Association Guidelines for Cardiopulmonary Resuscitation and Emergency Cardiovascular Care

Mark S. Link, Chair; Dianne L. Atkins; Rod S. Passman; Henry R. Halperin; Ricardo A. Samson; Roger D. White; Michael T. Cudnik; Marc D. Berg; Peter J. Kudenchuk; Richard E. Kerber

## Overview

This chapter presents guidelines for defibrillation with manual defibrillators and automated external defibrillators (AEDs), synchronized cardioversion, and pacing. AEDs may be used by lay rescuers and healthcare providers as part of basic life support. Manual defibrillation, cardioversion, and pacing are advanced life support therapies.

## Defibrillation Plus CPR: A Critical Combination

Early defibrillation is critical to survival from sudden cardiac arrest (SCA) for several reasons[1]: the most frequent initial rhythm in out-of-hospital witnessed SCA is ventricular fibrillation (VF),[2] the treatment for ventricular fibrillation is defibrillation,[3] the probability of successful defibrillation diminishes rapidly over time,[4] and VF tends to deteriorate to asystole over time.[1,5,6]

Several studies have documented the effects of time to defibrillation and the effects of bystander CPR on survival from SCA. For every minute that passes between collapse and defibrillation, survival rates from witnessed VF SCA decrease 7% to 10% if no CPR is provided.[1] When bystander CPR is provided, the decrease in survival rates is more gradual and averages 3% to 4% per minute from collapse to defibrillation.[1,2,5,7] CPR can double[1,3] or triple[4] survival from witnessed SCA at most intervals to defibrillation.

If bystanders provide immediate CPR, many adults in VF can survive with intact neurologic function, especially if defibrillation is performed within 5 to 10 minutes after SCA.[8,9] CPR prolongs VF, delays the onset of asystole,[10–12] and extends the window of time during which defibrillation can occur. Basic CPR alone, however, is unlikely to terminate VF and restore a perfusing rhythm.

## New Recommendations to Integrate CPR and AED Use

To treat VF SCA, rescuers must be able to rapidly integrate CPR with use of the AED. To give the victim the best chance of survival, 3 actions must occur within the first moments of a cardiac arrest[1]: activation of the emergency medical services (EMS) system,[2] provision of CPR, and operation of an AED.[3] When 2 or more rescuers are present, activation of EMS and initiation of CPR can occur simultaneously.

Delays to either the start of CPR or the start of defibrillation reduce survival from SCA. In the 1990s, some predicted that CPR could be rendered obsolete by the widespread development of community AED programs. However, Cobb[9] noted that as more of Seattle's first responders were equipped with AEDs, survival rates from SCA unexpectedly fell. This decline was attributed to reduced emphasis on CPR, and there is growing evidence to support this view. Part 5: "Adult Basic Life Support" summarizes the evidence on the importance of provision of high-quality CPR (including chest compressions of adequate rate and depth, allowing full chest recoil after each compression and minimizing interruptions in compressions).

Two critical questions about integration of CPR with defibrillation were evaluated during the 2010 International Consensus Conference on CPR and Emergency Cardiovascular Care.[13] The first question concerned whether CPR should be provided before defibrillation is attempted. The second question concerned the number of shocks to be delivered in a sequence before the rescuer resumes CPR.

### Shock First Versus CPR First

When any rescuer witnesses an out-of-hospital arrest and an AED is immediately available on-site, the rescuer should start CPR and use the AED as soon as possible. Healthcare providers who treat cardiac arrest in hospitals and other facilities with AEDs on-site should provide immediate CPR and should use the AED/defibrillator as soon as it is available. These recommendations are designed to support early CPR and early defibrillation, particularly when an AED is available within moments of the onset of SCA.

In studies in which EMS call-to-arrival intervals were 4[9] to 5[8] minutes or longer, 1 ½ to 3 minutes of CPR before defibrillation increased the rate of initial resuscitation (return of spontaneous circulation or ROSC), survival to hospital discharge,[8,9] and 1-year survival[8] when compared with immediate defibrillation

The American Heart Association requests that this document be cited as follows: Link MS, Atkins DL, Passman RS, Halperin HR, Samson RA, White RD, Cudnik MT, Berg MD, Kudenchuk PJ, Kerber RE. Part 6: electrical therapies: automated external defibrillators, defibrillation, cardioversion, and pacing: 2010 American Heart Association Guidelines for Cardiopulmonary Resuscitation and Emergency Cardiovascular Care. *Circulation.* 2010;122(suppl 3):S706–S719.

(*Circulation.* 2010;122[suppl 3]:S706–S719.)

*Circulation* is available at http://circ.ahajournals.org

DOI: 10.1161/CIRCULATIONAHA.110.970954

for VF SCA. However, in 2 randomized controlled trials,[14,15] a period of 1 ½ to 3 minutes of CPR by EMS personnel before defibrillation did not improve ROSC or survival to hospital discharge in patients with out-of-hospital VF or pulseless ventricular tachycardia (VT) compared with immediate defibrillation, regardless of EMS response interval, in systems with low overall survival. In 1 retrospective before/after study,[16] immediate CPR by EMS personnel was associated with no significant difference in survival to discharge but significantly improved neurological status at 30 days or 1 year compared with immediate defibrillation in patients with out-of-hospital VF. In a retrospective observational study,[17] probability of survival was increased if chest compressions were performed during a higher proportion of the initial CPR period as compared to a lower proportion.

When VF is present for more than a few minutes, the myocardium is depleted of oxygen and metabolic substrates. A brief period of chest compressions can deliver oxygen and energy substrates, increasing the likelihood that a shock may terminate VF (defibrillation) and a perfusing rhythm will return (ie, ROSC).[18]

When an out-of-hospital cardiac arrest is not witnessed by EMS personnel, EMS may initiate CPR while checking the ECG rhythm and preparing for defibrillation. There is insufficient evidence to determine if 1 ½ to 3 minutes of CPR should be provided prior to defibrillation. CPR should be performed while a defibrillator is being readied (Class I, LOE B). One cycle of CPR consists of 30 compressions and 2 breaths. When compressions are delivered at a rate of about 100 per minute, 5 cycles of CPR should take roughly 2 minutes (range: about 1 ½ to 3 minutes).

EMS system medical directors may consider implementing a protocol that allows EMS responders to provide CPR while preparing for defibrillation of patients found by EMS personnel to be in VF. In practice, however, CPR can be initiated while the AED is being readied.

With in-hospital SCA, there is insufficient evidence to support or refute CPR before defibrillation. However, in monitored patients, the time from VF to defibrillation should be under 3 minutes. When 2 or more rescuers are present, one rescuer should begin CPR while the other activates the emergency response system and prepares the defibrillator.

### 1-Shock Protocol Versus 3-Shock Sequence

At the time of the 2010 Consensus Conference, there were 2 new published human studies that compared a 1-shock protocol versus a 3-stacked-shock protocol for treatment of VF cardiac arrest. Evidence from these 2 well-conducted pre/post design[19,20] studies suggested significant survival benefit with the single-shock defibrillation protocol compared with 3-stacked-shock protocols. If 1 shock fails to eliminate VF, the incremental benefit of another shock is low, and resumption of CPR is likely to confer a greater value than another shock. This fact, combined with the data from animal studies documenting harmful effects from interruptions to chest compressions and human studies suggesting a survival benefit with a 1-shock protocol, indicate that it is reasonable to use 1-shock for VF, then immediate CPR (Class IIa, LOE B).

First-shock efficacy for biphasic shocks is comparable or better than 3 monophasic shocks.[21–25] Although the optimal energy level for defibrillation using any of the monophasic or biphasic waveforms has not been determined, a recommendation for higher initial energy when using a monophasic waveform was weighed by expert consensus with consideration of the potential negative effects of a high first-shock energy versus the negative effects of prolonged VF. The consensus was that rescuers using monophasic defibrillators should give an initial shock of 360 J; if VF persists after the first shock, second and subsequent shocks of 360 J should be given. This single dose for monophasic shocks is designed to simplify instructions to rescuers but is not a mandate to recall monophasic AEDs for reprogramming. If the monophasic AED being used is programmed to deliver a different first or subsequent dose, that dose is acceptable.

After shock delivery, the rescuer should not delay resumption of chest compressions to recheck the rhythm or pulse. After about 5 cycles of CPR (about 2 minutes, although this time is not firm), ideally ending with compressions, the AED should then analyze the cardiac rhythm and deliver another shock if indicated (Class I, LOE B). If a nonshockable rhythm is detected, the AED should instruct the rescuer to resume CPR immediately, beginning with chest compressions (Class I, LOE B).

Concern that chest compressions in the presence of a postshock organized rhythm might provoke recurrent VF has been expressed by 1 animal and 2 human studies,[26–28] but this has not been shown to adversely affect survival if the current algorithms are followed.[19,20]

Furthermore, in animal studies, frequent or long interruptions in precordial chest compressions for rhythm analysis[29] or rescue breathing[30,31] were associated with postresuscitation myocardial dysfunction and reduced survival rates. Data from a prospective observational study showed that interruption in chest compressions is associated with a decreased probability of successful conversion of VF to a perfusing rhythm after shock.[32] In a recent clinical observational study of out-of-hospital CPR[33] and an in-hospital study of CPR[34] by healthcare providers, chest compressions were performed only for 51%[33] to 76%[34] of total CPR time.

The rhythm analysis for a 3-shock sequence performed by commercially available AEDs can result in delays of up to 37 seconds between delivery of the first shock and delivery of the first postshock compression.[29] This delay is difficult to justify in light of the first-shock efficacy of >90% reported by current biphasic defibrillators.[28,35–39]

AED manufacturers should seek innovative methods to decrease the amount of time chest compressions are interrupted for AED operation. Training materials for lay rescuers should emphasize the importance of continued CPR until basic or advanced life support personnel take over CPR or the victim begins to move.

Shortening the interval between the last compression and the shock by even a few seconds can improve shock success (defibrillation and ROSC).[18,32,40] Thus, it is reasonable for healthcare providers to practice efficient coordination between CPR and defibrillation to minimize the hands-off interval between stopping compression and administering shock (Class IIa, LOE C). For example, when 2 rescuers are present, the rescuer operating the AED should be prepared to deliver a shock as soon as the compressor removes his or her hands from the victim's chest and all rescuers are "clear" of contact with the victim. Rescue breathing prior to the shock will increase the time from compression to shock, and thus it is reasonable to proceed immediately to shock without rescue breathing (Class IIa, LOE B).

## Defibrillation Waveforms and Energy Levels

The term *defibrillation* (shock success) is typically defined as termination of VF for at least 5 seconds following the shock.[41,42] VF frequently recurs after successful shocks, but this recurrence should not be equated with shock failure.[21,28]

Shock success using the typical definition of *defibrillation* should not be confused with resuscitation outcomes such as restoration of a perfusing rhythm (ROSC), survival to hospital admission, or survival to hospital discharge.[41,43] Since resuscitation outcomes, including survival, depend on many variables in addition to shock delivery, defibrillation programs must strive to improve patient survival, not just shock success.

Modern defibrillators are classified according to 2 types of waveforms: monophasic and biphasic. Monophasic waveform defibrillators were introduced first, but biphasic waveforms are used in almost all AEDs and manual defibrillators sold today. Energy levels vary by type of device and manufacturer.

### Monophasic Waveform Defibrillators

Monophasic waveforms deliver current of one polarity (ie, direction of current flow). Monophasic waveforms can be further categorized by the rate at which the current pulse decreases to zero. The monophasic damped sinusoidal waveform (MDS) returns to zero gradually, whereas the monophasic truncated exponential waveform (MTE) current returns abruptly (is truncated) to zero current flow.

Few monophasic waveform defibrillators are being manufactured, but many are still in use, and most use MDS waveforms. As noted above, no specific waveform characteristic (either monophasic or biphasic) is consistently associated with a greater incidence of ROSC or higher survival to hospital discharge rates after cardiac arrest.

### Biphasic Waveform Defibrillators

Data from both out-of-hospital and in-hospital studies indicate that lower-energy biphasic waveform shocks have equivalent or higher success for termination of VF than either MDS or MTE monophasic waveform shocks.[21,23,39,44-46] However, the optimal energy for first-shock biphasic waveform defibrillation has not been determined. One study[47] in which a pulsed biphasic waveform was used showed a first-shock success rate of 90%. There is no new evidence regarding the first-shock success rate with the rectilinear biphasic waveform since publication of the 2005 Guidelines. Several randomized[21,23,39] and observational studies[22,48] have shown that defibrillation with biphasic waveforms of relatively low energy ($\leq$200 J) is safe and has equivalent or higher efficacy for termination of VF than monophasic waveform shocks of equivalent or higher energy.[42,49-53]

Evidence from 3 randomized trials[21,23,39] and 3 other human studies[22,42,54] suggests that defibrillation with biphasic waveforms improves the short-term outcome of termination of VF, but no individual study has demonstrated improved survival to discharge using biphasic waveforms when compared with studies using monophasic waveforms. There is no human study to support defibrillation with a multiphasic waveform when compared with any biphasic waveform. Data from animal studies suggest that multiphasic waveforms (triphasic, quadriphasic, or higher) may defibrillate at lower energies and induce less postshock myocardial dysfunction. These results are limited by studies of only short-duration VF (approximately 30 seconds) and lack of human studies for validation of these experimental observations.

Biphasic waveforms are safe and have equivalent or higher efficacy for termination of VF when compared with monophasic waveforms. In the absence of biphasic defibrillators, monophasic defibrillators are acceptable (Class IIb, LOE B). Different biphasic waveforms have not been compared in humans with regard to efficacy. Therefore, for biphasic defibrillators, providers should use the manufacturer's recommended energy dose (120 to 200 J) (Class I, LOE B). If the manufacturer's recommended dose is not known, defibrillation at the maximal dose may be considered (Class IIb, LOE C).

In pediatric defibrillation, there are limited data regarding the lowest effective dose or the upper limit for safe defibrillation. Initial monophasic doses of 2 J/kg are effective in terminating 18% to 50% of VF[55-57] and 48% of VF using similar doses of biphasic energy.[57] However, even with higher energies (up to 9 J/kg), defibrillation has been successful with no clear adverse effects.[58-61] Thus, for pediatric patients, it is acceptable to use an initial dose of 2 to 4 J/kg (Class IIa, LOE C), but for ease of teaching an initial dose of 2 J/kg may be considered. For refractory VF, it is reasonable to increase the dose to 4 J/kg. Subsequent energy levels should be at least 4 J/kg, and higher energy levels may be considered, not to exceed 10 J/kg or the adult maximum dose (Class IIb, LOE C).

### Fixed and Escalating Energy

Commercially available biphasic AEDs provide either fixed or escalating energy levels. Multiple prospective human clinical studies[23,52,53] and retrospective studies[21,22,39,48,62,63] have failed to identify an optimal biphasic energy level for first or subsequent shocks. Human studies[50,52] have not demonstrated evidence of harm from any biphasic waveform defibrillation energy up to 360 J, with harm defined as elevated biomarker levels, ECG findings, and reduced ejection fraction. Conversely, several animal studies have shown the potential for myocardial damage with much higher energy shocks.[64-66] Therefore, it is not possible to make a definitive recommendation for the selected energy for subsequent biphasic defibrillation attempts. However, based on available evidence, we recommend that second and subsequent energy levels should be at least equivalent and higher energy levels may be considered, if available (Class IIb, LOE B).

### Current-Based Defibrillation

Modern defibrillators deliver current based on stored energy. Because it is accepted that defibrillation is accomplished by the passage of sufficient current through the heart, the concept of current-based defibrillation is appealing. Energy is a nonphysiologic descriptor of defibrillation despite its entrenchment in traditional jargon. Current-based defibrillation has been assessed[67,68] and in 1 study was superior to energy-based defibrillation with monophasic waveforms.[69] This concept merits exploration in light of the variety of biphasic waveforms available that deliver current in different ways. Peak current amplitude, average current, phasic duration, and phasic current flow need to be examined as determinants of shock efficacy. Transition to current-based defibrillation is timely and should be encouraged.

Clinical studies using MDS waveform shocks have tried to identify the range of current necessary to achieve defibrillation and cardioversion. The optimal current for ventricular defibrillation appears to be 30 to 40 A MDS.[67] Comparable information on current dose for biphasic waveform shocks is under investigation.

## Electrodes

### Electrode Placement

Data demonstrate that 4 pad positions (anterolateral, anteroposterior, anterior-left infrascapular, and anterior-right-infrascapular)[70] are equally effective to treat atrial or ventricular arrhythmias.[71–75] There are no studies directly pertaining to placement of pads/paddles for defibrillation success with the end point of ROSC. All 4 positions are equally effective in shock success.[71–74,76–82] Any of the 4 pad positions is reasonable for defibrillation (Class IIa, LOE B). For ease of placement and education, anterolateral is a reasonable default electrode placement (Class IIa, LOE C). Alternative pad positions may be considered based on individual patient characteristics.

Lateral pads/paddles should be placed under breast tissue,[83] and hirsute males should be shaved prior to application of pads.[84,85] Ten studies[65,81,86–93] indicated that larger pad/paddle size (8 to 12 cm diameter) lowers transthoracic impedance.

### Defibrillation With Implanted Cardioverter Defibrillator

If the patient has an implantable cardioverter defibrillator (ICD) that is delivering shocks (ie, the patient's muscles contract in a manner similar to that observed during external defibrillation), allow 30 to 60 seconds for the ICD to complete the treatment cycle before attaching an AED. Occasionally, the analysis and shock cycles of automatic ICDs and AEDs will conflict.[94] There is the potential for pacemaker or ICD malfunction after defibrillation when the pads are in close proximity to the device.[95,96] One study with cardioversion[95] demonstrated that positioning the pads at least 8 cm away did not produce changes in pacing thresholds or sensing measurements. Pacemaker spikes with unipolar pacing may confuse AED software and may prevent VF detection.[94] The anteroposterior and anterolateral locations are acceptable in patients with these devices. In patients with ICDs or pacemakers, pad/paddle placement should not delay defibrillation. It might be reasonable to avoid placing the pads or paddles over the device (Class IIb, LOE C).

Do not place AED electrode pads directly on top of a transdermal medication patch, (eg, patch containing nitroglycerin, nicotine, analgesics, hormone replacements, antihypertensives) because the patch may block delivery of energy from the electrode pad to the heart and may cause small burns to the skin.[97] If shock delivery will not be delayed, remove medication patches and wipe the area before attaching the electrode pad (Class IIb, LOE C).

If an unresponsive victim is lying in water or if the victim's chest is covered with water or the victim is extremely diaphoretic, it may be reasonable to remove the victim from water and briskly wipe the chest before attaching electrode pads and attempting defibrillation (Class IIb, LOE C). AEDs can be used when the victim is lying on snow or ice (Class IIb, LOE C). Attempt to remove excess chest hair by briskly removing an electrode pad (which will remove some hair) or rapidly shaving the chest in that area provided chest compressions are not interrupted and defibrillation is not delayed.

### Electrode Size

In 1993 the Association for the Advancement of Medical Instrumentation recommended a minimum electrode size of 50 cm$^2$ for individual electrodes.[98] However, advances in electrode design and chemical composition may soon require modification of this recommendation. For adult defibrillation, both handheld paddle electrodes and self-adhesive pad electrodes 8 to 12 cm in diameter perform well, although defibrillation success may be higher with electrodes 12 cm in diameter rather than with those 8 cm in diameter.[86,99] Small electrodes (4.3 cm) may be harmful and may cause myocardial necrosis.[88] When using handheld paddles and gel or pads, rescuers must ensure that the paddle is in full contact with the skin. Even smaller pads have been found to be effective[100] in VF of brief duration. Use of the smallest (pediatric) pads, however, can result in unacceptably high transthoracic impedance in larger children.[93] For adults, an electrode size of 8 to 12 cm is reasonable (Class IIa, LOE B).

### Transthoracic Impedance

The average adult human impedance is $\approx$70 to 80 $\Omega$.[67,86,101] When transthoracic impedance is too high, a low-energy shock will not generate sufficient current to achieve defibrillation.[101–103] To reduce transthoracic impedance, the defibrillator operator should use conductive materials. This is accomplished with the use of gel pads or electrode paste with paddles or through the use of self-adhesive pads. No existing data suggest that one of these modalities is better than the others in decreasing impedance.

## Automated External Defibrillators

AEDs are sophisticated, reliable computerized devices that use voice and visual prompts to guide lay rescuers and healthcare providers to safely defibrillate VF and (pulseless) rapid ventricular tachycardia (VT) SCA.[44,46,104,105] In recent clinical trials,[33,34] modified prototype AEDs recorded information about frequency and depth of chest compressions during CPR. These devices are now commercially available and can prompt rescuers to improve CPR performance.

### Lay Rescuer AED Programs

Since 1995 the American Heart Association (AHA) has recommended the development of lay rescuer AED programs to improve survival rates from out-of-hospital SCA.[106–108] These programs are also known as public access defibrillation or PAD programs. The goal of these programs is to shorten the time from onset of SCA VF/pulseless VT until CPR and shock delivery by ensuring that AEDs and trained lay rescuers are available in public areas where SCA is likely to occur. To maximize the effectiveness of these programs, the AHA has emphasized the importance of organizing, planning, training, linking with the EMS system, and establishing a process of continuous quality improvement.[109,110]

Studies of lay rescuer AED programs in airports[111] and casinos[112,113] and of first-responder programs with police officers[22,44,46,63,114–116] have shown survival rates of 41% to 74% from out-of-hospital witnessed VF SCA when immediate bystander CPR is provided and defibrillation occurs within about 3 to 5 minutes of collapse.[70,117a] Other studies[117b,118] have demonstrated decreased time intervals from collapse to delivery of the first shock when AEDs were used during adult out-of-hospital cardiac arrest. However, if no decrease in time to defibrillation is achieved, then high survival rates are not observed.[119–121]

In the large prospective randomized trial Public Access Defibrillation Trial (PAD),[122] lay rescuer CPR + AED programs in targeted public settings doubled the number of survivors from out-of-hospital VF SCA when compared with programs that provided early EMS call and early CPR. The programs included a planned response, lay rescuer training, and frequent retraining/practice. In another large population-based study, AED use prior to EMS arrival resulted in a doubling of survival.[123] In a prospective population-based study of >300 000 patients, increased penetration of AEDs resulted in increased defibrillation by bystanders and increased survival compared to historical control.[124]

Lay rescuer AED programs will have the greatest potential impact on survival from SCA if the programs are created in locations where SCA is likely to occur. In the PAD trial, programs were established at sites with a history of at least 1 out-of-hospital cardiac arrest every 2 years or where at least 1 out-of-hospital SCA was predicted during the study period (ie, sites having >250 adults over 50 years of age present for >16 hours/d).[122] Other data suggest that there is benefit when 1 out-of-hospital arrest is likely every 5 years.[125,126]

CPR and AED use by public safety first responders (traditional and nontraditional) is recommended to increase survival rates for SCA (Class I, LOE B). Establishment of AED programs in public locations where there is a reasonable likelihood of witnessed cardiac arrest (eg, airports, casinos, and sports facilities) is recommended (Class I, LOE B).

Because the improvement in survival rates in AED programs is affected by the time to CPR and to defibrillation, it is reasonable for sites that deploy AEDs to establish a response plan, train likely responders in CPR and AED use, maintain equipment, and coordinate with local EMS systems (Class IIa, LOE B).[109,110] Sites without these components are unlikely to demonstrate any improvement in survival rates.[126]

Approximately 80% of out-of-hospital cardiac arrests occur in private or residential settings.[127] One study[128] demonstrated that survival was not improved in homes of high-risk individuals equipped with AEDs compared with homes where only CPR training had been provided.

AEDs are of no value for arrest not caused by VF/pulseless VT, and they are not effective for treatment of nonshockable rhythms that may develop after termination of VF. Nonperfusing rhythms are present in most patients after shock delivery,[22,28,63,129] and in general, CPR is required until a perfusing rhythm returns. Therefore, the AED rescuer should be trained not only to recognize emergencies and use the AED, but also to provide CPR until the AED is retrieved and ready for shock delivery and immediately after shock delivery.

The mere presence of an AED does not ensure that it will be used when SCA occurs. Even in the PAD trial, in which almost 20 000 rescuers were trained to respond to SCA, lay rescuers attempted resuscitation before EMS arrival for only half of the victims of witnessed SCA, and the on-site AED was used for only 34% of the victims who experienced an arrest at locations with AED programs.[122] These findings suggest that lay rescuers need frequent practice to optimize response to emergencies.

It is reasonable for lay rescuer AED programs to implement processes of continuous quality improvement (Class IIa, LOE C). These quality improvement efforts should use both routine inspections and postevent data (from AED recordings and responder reports) to evaluate the following[110,130]:

- Performance of the emergency response plan, including accurate time intervals for key interventions (such as collapse to shock or no shock advisory to initiation of CPR), and patient outcome
- Responder performance
- AED function, including accuracy of the ECG rhythm analysis
- Battery status and function
- Electrode pad function and readiness, including expiration date

## Automated Rhythm Analysis

AEDs analyze multiple features of the surface ECG signal, including frequency, amplitude, and some integration of frequency and amplitude, such as slope or wave morphology. Filters check for QRS-like signals, radio transmission, or 50- or 60-cycle interference, as well as loose electrodes and poor electrode contact. The AHA has recommended performance goals for AED arrhythmia analysis algorithms, specifying sensitivity and specificity for various arrhythmias.[131]

AEDs have been tested extensively both in vitro against libraries of recorded cardiac rhythms and clinically in many field trials in adults[131,132] and children.[133–135] They are extremely accurate in rhythm analysis. Although AEDs are not designed to deliver synchronized shocks (ie, cardioversion for VT with pulses), AEDs will recommend a (nonsynchronized) shock for monomorphic and polymorphic VT if the rate and R-wave morphology exceed preset values.

Some devices are programmed to detect spontaneous movement by the patient or others. Prototype defibrillators were used in 2 recent clinical trials evaluating quality of CPR in the out-of-hospital and in-hospital settings, which led to the development of AEDs that prompt rescuers to improve the quality of CPR provided.[33,34]

## AED Use in Children

Cardiac arrest is less common in children than adults, and its causes are more diverse.[136–139] Although VF is not a common arrhythmia in children, it is observed in 5% to 15% of pediatric and adolescent arrests.[138,140–143] In these patients rapid defibrillation may improve outcomes.[143,144] The lowest-energy dose for effective defibrillation in infants and children is not known. The upper limit for safe defibrillation is also not known, but doses >4 J/kg (as high as 9 J/kg) have effectively defibrillated children[60,61] and pediatric animal models[145] with no significant adverse effects. Based on adult clinical data[21,39] and pediatric animal models,[145–147] biphasic shocks appear to be at least as effective as monophasic shocks and are less harmful than monophasic shocks. As noted above, it is acceptable to use an initial dose of 2 to 4 J/kg (Class IIa, LOE C), but for ease of teaching an initial dose of 2 J/kg may be considered. For refractory VF, it is reasonable to increase the dose to 4 J/kg. Subsequent energy levels should be at least 4 J/kg, and higher energy levels may be considered, not to exceed 10 J/kg or the adult maximum dose (Class IIb, LOE C).

Many AEDs can accurately detect VF in children of all ages[133–135] and differentiate shockable from nonshockable rhythms with a high degree of sensitivity and specificity.[133–135] Some AEDs are equipped with pediatric attenuator systems (eg, pad-cable systems or a key) to reduce the delivered energy to a dose suitable for children.

For children 1 to 8 years of age, it is reasonable to use a pediatric dose-attenuator system if one is available (Class IIa, LOE C).[61,148,149] If the rescuer provides CPR to a child in cardiac arrest and does not have an AED with a pediatric attenuator system, the rescuer should use a standard AED.

For infants (<1 year of age), a manual defibrillator is preferred. If a manual defibrillator is not available, an AED with pediatric attenuation is desirable. If neither is available, an AED without a dose attenuator may be used. AEDs with relatively high-energy doses have been successfully used in infants with minimal myocardial damage and good neurological outcomes (Class IIb, LOE C).[150,151]

If an AED program is established in systems or institutions that routinely provide care to children, the program should be equipped with AEDs with a pediatric attenuator system. This statement, however, should not be interpreted as a recommendation for or against AED placement in specific locations where children are present. Ideally, healthcare systems that routinely provide care to children at risk for cardiac arrest should have available manual defibrillators capable of dose adjustment.[148]

### In-Hospital Use of AEDs

At the time of the 2010 Consensus Conference, there were no published in-hospital randomized trials of AEDs versus manual defibrillators. Evidence from 1 study with historic controls,[152] 1 case series,[153] and 2 retrospective studies[117,118] indicated higher rates of survival to hospital discharge when AEDs were used to treat adult VF or pulseless VT in the hospital. However, 1 before/after study did not show an improvement in survival to discharge or ROSC when in-hospital AEDs were implemented in noncritical areas of a hospital,[154] and 1 observational study with historical controls observed no improvement in survival to discharge when comparing biphasic AEDs to standard monophasic defibrillators.[155] The Gombotz and Hanefeld studies observed a decrease in the time interval from collapse to first shock delivery as well as increased ROSC and survival.

Defibrillation may be delayed when patients develop SCA in unmonitored hospital beds and in outpatient and diagnostic facilities. In such areas, several minutes may elapse before centralized response teams arrive with the defibrillator, attach it, and deliver shocks.[156] Despite limited evidence, AEDs may be considered for the hospital setting as a way to facilitate early defibrillation (a goal of ≤3 minutes from collapse), especially in areas where staff have no rhythm recognition skills or defibrillators are used infrequently (Class IIb, LOE C).

When hospitals deploy AEDs, first-responding personnel should also receive authorization and training to use an AED, with the goal of providing the first shock for any SCA within 3 minutes of collapse. The objective is to make goals for in-hospital use of AEDs consistent with goals established in the out-of-hospital setting.[157] Early defibrillation capability should be available in ambulatory care facilities, as well as throughout hospital inpatient areas. Hospitals should monitor collapse-to–first shock intervals and resuscitation outcomes.

### Fibrillation Waveform Analysis to Predict Outcome

There is evidence that VF waveforms change over time.[158,159] Several retrospective case series, animal studies, and theoretical models suggest that it is possible to predict, with varying reliability, the success of attempted defibrillation by analyzing the VF waveform.[18,40,160–177] However, there are currently no prospective studies that have identified optimal waveforms and/or timing. The value of VF waveform analysis to guide defibrillation management is uncertain (Class IIb, LOE C).

### "Occult" Versus "False" Asystole

In certain cases of cardiac arrest, it is difficult to be certain whether the rhythm is fine VF or asystole. In 1989, Losek[178] published a retrospective review of initial shock delivery for 49 children (infants through 19 years of age) in asystole compared with no shock delivery for 41 children in asystole and found no improvement in rhythm change, ROSC, or survival in the group that received the shocks. In 1993, the Nine City High-Dose Epinephrine Study Group published an analysis of 77 asystolic patients who received initial shock compared with 117 who received standard therapy.[179] There was a worse outcome of ROSC and survival for those who received shocks. Thus, it is not useful to shock asystole (Class III, LOE B).

### Fire Hazard

Several case reports have described fires ignited by sparks from poorly applied defibrillator paddles in the presence of an oxygen-enriched atmosphere.[180–185] Fires have been reported when ventilator tubing is disconnected from the endotracheal tube and then left adjacent to the patient's head, blowing oxygen across the chest during attempted defibrillation.[181,183,185] It may be reasonable for rescuers to take precautions to minimize sparking during attempted defibrillation; try to avoid defibrillation in an oxygen-enriched atmosphere (Class IIb, LOE C).

The use of self-adhesive defibrillation pads and ensuring good pad–chest-wall contact will likely minimize the risk of sparks igniting during defibrillation. If manual paddles are used, gel pads are preferable to electrode pastes and gels, because the pastes and gels can spread between the 2 paddles, creating the potential for a spark (Class IIb, LOE C).

### Synchronized Cardioversion

*Synchronized cardioversion* is shock delivery that is timed (synchronized) with the QRS complex. This synchronization avoids shock delivery during the relative refractory portion of the cardiac cycle, when a shock could produce VF.[186] For additional information, see Part 8.3: "Management of Symptomatic Bradycardia and Tachycardia."

Synchronized cardioversion is recommended to treat supraventricular tachycardia due to reentry, atrial fibrillation, atrial flutter, and atrial tachycardia. Synchronized cardioversion is also recommended to treat monomorphic VT with pulses. Cardioversion is not effective for treatment of junctional tachycardia or multifocal atrial tachycardia.

Synchronized cardioversion must not be used for treatment of VF as the device may not sense a QRS wave and thus a shock may not be delivered. Synchronized cardioversion should also not be used for pulseless VT or polymorphic (irregular VT). These rhythms require delivery of high-energy *unsynchronized* shocks (ie, defibrillation doses). Electric therapy for VT is discussed further below. For additional information see Part 8.2: "Management of Cardiac Arrest."

### Supraventricular Tachycardias (Reentry Rhythms)

The recommended initial biphasic energy dose for cardioversion of adult atrial fibrillation is 120 to 200 J (Class IIa, LOE A).[187–191] If the initial shock fails, providers should increase the dose in a stepwise fashion. Cardioversion of adult atrial flutter and other supraventricular tachycardias generally requires less energy; an initial energy of 50 J to 100 J is often sufficient.[191] If the initial shock fails, providers should increase the dose in a stepwise fashion.[102] Adult cardioversion of atrial fibrillation with monophasic waveforms should begin at 200 J and increase in a stepwise fashion if not successful (Class IIa, LOE B).[187–189] For cardioversion of SVT in children, use an initial dose of 0.5 to 1 J/kg. If unsuccessful, increase the dose up to 2 J/kg (Class IIb, LOE C). For further information, see Part 14: "Pediatric Advanced Life Support."

### Ventricular Tachycardia

The energy dose and timing of shocks for treatment of VT with pulses are determined by the patient's condition and the morphological characteristics of the VT.[192] Pulseless VT is treated as VF (see Part 8.2: "Management of Cardiac Arrest"). Management of stable VT is summarized in Part 8.3: "Management of Symptomatic Bradycardia and Tachycardia." Unstable monomorphic (regular) VT with pulses is treated with synchronized cardioversion. Unstable polymorphic (irregular) VT with or without pulses is treated as VF using *unsynchronized* high-energy shocks (ie, defibrillation doses).

Adult monomorphic VT (regular form and rate) with a pulse responds well to monophasic or biphasic waveform cardioversion (synchronized) shocks at initial energies of 100 J. If there is no response to the first shock, it may be reasonable to increase the dose in a stepwise fashion. No studies were identified that addressed this issue. Thus, this recommendation represents expert opinion (Class IIb, LOE C).

For electric cardioversion in children the recommended starting energy dose is 0.5 to 1 J/kg. If that fails, increase the dose up to 2 J/kg (Class I, LOE C). For further information, see Part 14: "Pediatric Advanced Life Support."

Although synchronized cardioversion is preferred for treatment of an organized ventricular rhythm, for some arrhythmias synchronization is not possible. The many QRS configurations and irregular rates that comprise polymorphic ventricular

tachycardia make it difficult or impossible to reliably synchronize to a QRS complex. If there is any doubt whether monomorphic or polymorphic VT is present in the *unstable* patient, do not delay shock delivery to perform detailed rhythm analysis—provide high-energy unsynchronized shocks (ie, defibrillation doses).

The recommended shock doses for high-energy, *unsynchronized* shocks (defibrillation) with a biphasic or monophasic device are those presented earlier in this section (Defibrillation Waveforms and Energy Levels). After shock delivery, the healthcare provider should be prepared to provide immediate CPR (beginning with chest compressions) and follow the ACLS Cardiac Arrest Algorithm if pulseless arrest develops (for further information see Part 8.2: "Management of Cardiac Arrest").

### Pacing

Pacing is not recommended for patients in asystolic cardiac arrest. Randomized controlled trials[193–195] and additional studies[196–202] indicate no improvement in the rate of admission to hospital or survival to hospital discharge when paramedics or physicians attempted to provide pacing in asystolic patients in the prehospital or hospital (emergency department) setting. Pacing is not effective for asystolic cardiac arrest and may delay or interrupt the delivery of chest compressions. Pacing for patients in asystole is not recommended (Class III, LOE B).

In symptomatic bradycardia with a pulse, 2 randomized adult trials comparing transcutaneous pacing to drug therapy showed no difference in survival.[203,204] It is reasonable for healthcare providers to be prepared to initiate pacing in patients who do not respond to atropine (or second-line drugs if these do not delay definitive management) (Class IIa, LOE B). Immediate pacing might be considered if the patient is severely symptomatic (Class IIb, LOE C). If the patient does not respond to drugs or transcutaneous pacing, transvenous pacing is probably indicated (Class IIa, LOE C). For further information see Part 8.3: "Management of Symptomatic Bradycardia and Tachycardia."

### Maintaining Devices in a State of Readiness

User checklists have been developed to reduce equipment malfunction and operator errors. Failure to properly maintain the defibrillator or power supply is responsible for the majority of reported malfunctions. Many currently available defibrillators do an automated check and display readiness. Checklists are useful when designed to identify and prevent such deficiencies. It is recommended to maintain devices in a state of readiness (Class I, LOE C).

### Summary

The recommendations for electrical therapies described in this section are designed to improve survival from SCA and life-threatening arrhythmias. Whenever defibrillation is attempted, rescuers must coordinate high-quality CPR with defibrillation to minimize interruptions in chest compressions and to ensure immediate resumption of chest compressions after shock delivery. The high first-shock efficacy of newer biphasic defibrillators led to the recommendation of single shocks plus immediate CPR instead of 3-shock sequences that were recommended prior to 2005 to treat VF. Further data are needed to refine recommendations for energy levels for defibrillation and cardioversion using biphasic waveforms.

# Disclosures

## Guidelines Part 6: Electrical Therapies: Writing Group Disclosures

| Writing Group Member | Employment | Research Grant | Other Research Support | Speakers' Bureau/Honoraria | Ownership Interest | Consultant/Advisory Board | Other |
|---|---|---|---|---|---|---|---|
| Mark S. Link | Tufts Medical Center–MD | None | None | None | None | None | None |
| Dianne L. Atkins | University of Iowa: University and Medical School—Professor *Compensated works sheet editor for the Guidelines 2010 Process. Money is paid approximately 2/3 to my institution and 1/3 to directly me. My salary from my institution is not changed by this reimbursement | None | None | None | None | None | *Serving as defense expert witness |
| Rod S. Passman | Northwestern University–Associate Professor | None | None | None | None | None | None |
| Henry R. Halperin | Johns Hopkins University–Professor | †Zoll Circulation | None | None | *Surgivision Lexmed | †Zoll Circulation *Cardiac Concepts | †State of Hawaii *US Department of Justice |
| Ricardo A. Samson | University of Arizona: clinical care, teaching and research with pediatric cardiology in an academic setting-Professor | None | None | None | None | None | None |
| Roger D. White | Mayo Clinic–staff physician | None | None | None | None | None | None |
| Michael T. Cudnik | The Ohio State University Medical Center–Assistant Professor, Dept of Emergency Medicine | †Current Funding AHA Scientist Development Grant. I am the PI on this 4 year project (July 2008-June 2012) that is evaluating the impact of transport distance, transport time, and hospital level factors on survival from CA. There is no perceived conflict with this project. The money from the AHA goes to the Ohio State Research Foundation. Pending Funding R03 Small Research Grant Program, Funding Agency AHRQ. This grant is pending. It is a 1 year project designed to look at the location of current AEDs in the city of Columbus relative to the location of the out of hospital CA in order to determine the optimal location of AEDs in a community. If funded, the money will go to the Ohio State Research Foundation | None | None | None | None | None |
| Marc D. Berg | University of Arizona/University Physician's Healthcare (UPH): Attending pediatric intensivist and Board Member of UPH. UPH is a physician group of the faculty of the College of Medicine. The Board oversees three distinct entities: the physician group, the UPH managed care plan, and the operations of UPH Hospital.- Associate Prof. of Clinical Pediatrics and Member, BOD | None | None | None | None | None | None |
| Peter J. Kudenchuk | University of Washington - Medical Professor of Medicine; Contracted Associate Medical Director, King County Emergency Medical Services - Associate Medical Director | Resuscitation Outcomes Consortium (NIH) –multicenter study of resuscitation. Funds come to the University of Washington | None | *Network for Continuing Medical Education, Academy for Healthcare Education, Sanofi-Aventis, Pri-Med, Horiizon CME, with honoraria | *Sanofi-Aventis, Novartis | None | *Occasional expert witness in medical malpractice cases |

*(Continued)*

**Guidelines Part 6: Electrical Therapies: Writing Group Disclosures, *Continued***

| Writing Group Member | Employment | Research Grant | Other Research Support | Speakers' Bureau/Honoraria | Ownership Interest | Consultant/Advisory Board | Other |
|---|---|---|---|---|---|---|---|
| Richard E. Kerber | University of Iowa Hospitals and Clinics: Staff Cardiologist–Professor of Medicine | None | None | *Occasional speaker at Cardiology Grand Rounds at other hospitals. Usual honorarium is $1000 for such talks, about 3/year. The money is paid by the institution that invites me to speak, and is paid to me personally. I gave a talk several months ago to Philips Medical Co. on my hypothermia research, and provided advice on aspects of defibrillator design $1000 honorarium; one-time event I am a member of a DSMB of a clinical trial of a new Resuscitation product of Zoll. There have been 2 meetings of this DSMB in the past 2 years, & expect subsequent meetings to review/discuss the trial as data are acquired. Compensation so far about $2000 | None | *See previous comments about relationships with Philips (one-time) and Zoll (DSMB) | †I have served as an expert witness in lawsuits in the past. Occasionally such suits have involved cardiac resuscitation, although not for several years. |

This table represents the relationships of writing group members that may be perceived as actual or reasonably perceived conflicts of interest as reported on the Disclosure Questionnaire, which all members of the writing group are required to complete and submit. A relationship is considered to be "significant" if (a) the person receives $10 000 or more during any 12-month period, or 5% or more of the person's gross income; or (b) the person owns 5% or more of the voting stock or share of the entity, or owns $10 000 or more of the fair market value of the entity. A relationship is considered to be "modest" if it is less than "significant" under the preceding definition.

*Modest.

†Significant.

# References

1. Larsen MP, Eisenberg MS, Cummins RO, Hallstrom AP. Predicting survival from out-of-hospital cardiac arrest: a graphic model. *Ann Emerg Med.* 1993;22:1652–1658.
2. Valenzuela TD, Roe DJ, Cretin S, Spaite DW, Larsen MP. Estimating effectiveness of cardiac arrest interventions: a logistic regression survival model. *Circulation.* 1997;96:3308–3313.
3. Swor RA, Jackson RE, Cynar M, Sadler E, Basse E, Boji B, Rivera-Rivera EJ, Maher A, Grubb W, Jacobson R, Dalbec DL. Bystander CPR, ventricular fibrillation, and survival in witnessed, unmonitored out-of-hospital cardiac arrest. *Ann Emerg Med.* 1995;25:780–784.
4. Holmberg M, Holmberg S, Herlitz J. Incidence, duration and survival of ventricular fibrillation in out-of-hospital cardiac arrest patients in Sweden. *Resuscitation.* 2000;44:7–17.
5. Chan PS, Krumholz HM, Nichol G, Nallamothu BK. Delayed time to defibrillation after in-hospital cardiac arrest. *N Engl J Med.* 2008;358:9–17.
6. Kudenchuk PJ. Electrical therapies. In: Field JM, Kudenchuk JP, O'Conner RE, Vanden Hoek TL, Bresler MJ, Mattu A, Silvers SM, eds. *The Textbook of Emergency Cardiovascular Care and CPR.* Philadelphia, PA: Lippincott Williams & Wilkins; 2008:362–378.
7. Stiell IG, Wells GA, Field B, Spaite DW, Nesbitt LP, De Maio VJ, Nichol G, Cousineau D, Blackburn J, Munkley D, Luinstra-Toohey L, Campeau T, Dagnone E, Lyver M. Advanced cardiac life support in out-of-hospital cardiac arrest. *N Engl J Med.* 2004;351:647–656.
8. Wik L, Hansen TB, Fylling F, Steen T, Vaagenes P, Auestad BH, Steen PA. Delaying defibrillation to give basic cardiopulmonary resuscitation to patients with out-of-hospital ventricular fibrillation: a randomized trial. *JAMA.* 2003;289:1389–1395.
9. Cobb LA, Fahrenbruch CE, Walsh TR, Copass MK, Olsufka M, Breskin M, Hallstrom AP. Influence of cardiopulmonary resuscitation prior to defibrillation in patients with out-of-hospital ventricular fibrillation. *JAMA.* 1999;281:1182–1188.
10. Cummins RO, Eisenberg MS, Hallstrom AP, Litwin PE. Survival of out-of-hospital cardiac arrest with early initiation of cardiopulmonary resuscitation. *Am J Emerg Med.* 1985;3:114–119.
11. Holmberg M, Holmberg S, Herlitz J. Effect of bystander cardiopulmonary resuscitation in out-of-hospital cardiac arrest patients in Sweden. *Resuscitation.* 2000;47:59–70.
12. Waalewijn RA, Tijssen JG, Koster RW. Bystander initiated actions in out-of-hospital cardiopulmonary resuscitation: results from the Amsterdam Resuscitation Study (ARRESUST). *Resuscitation.* 2001;50:273–279.
13. Jacobs I, Sunde K, Deakin CD, Hazinski MF, Kerber RE, Koster RW, Morrison LJ, Nolan JP, Sayre MR, on behalf of Defibrillation Chapter Collaborators. Part 6: defibrillation: 2010 International Consensus on Cardiopulmonary Resuscitation and Emergency Cardiovascular Care Science with Treatment Recommendations. *Circulation.* 2010;122(suppl 2):S325–S337.
14. Baker PW, Conway J, Cotton C, Ashby DT, Smyth J, Woodman RJ, Grantham H. Defibrillation or cardiopulmonary resuscitation first for patients with out-of-hospital cardiac arrests found by paramedics to be in ventricular fibrillation? A randomised control trial. *Resuscitation.* 2008;79:424–431.
15. Jacobs IG, Finn JC, Oxer HF, Jelinek GA. CPR before defibrillation in out-of-hospital cardiac arrest: a randomized trial. *Emerg Med Australas.* 2005;17:39–45.
16. Hayakawa M, Gando S, Okamoto H, Asai Y, Uegaki S, Makise H. Shortening of cardiopulmonary resuscitation time before the defibrillation worsens the outcome in out-of-hospital VF patients. *Am J Emerg Med.* 2009;27:470–474.
17. Christenson J, Andrusiek D, Everson-Stewart S, Kudenchuk P, Hostler D, Powell J, Callaway CW, Bishop D, Vaillancourt C, Davis D, Aufderheide TP, Idris A, Stouffer JA, Stiell I, Berg R. Chest compression fraction determines survival in patients with out-of-hospital ventricular fibrillation. *Circulation.* 2009;120:1241–1247.
18. Eftestol T, Wik L, Sunde K, Steen PA. Effects of cardiopulmonary resuscitation on predictors of ventricular fibrillation defibrillation success during out-of-hospital cardiac arrest. *Circulation.* 2004;110:10–15.
19. Bobrow BJ, Clark LL, Ewy GA, Chikani V, Sanders AB, Berg RA, Richman PB, Kern KB. Minimally interrupted cardiac resuscitation by emergency medical services for out-of-hospital cardiac arrest. *JAMA.* 2008;299:1158–1165.
20. Rea TD, Helbock M, Perry S, Garcia M, Cloyd D, Becker L, Eisenberg M. Increasing use of cardiopulmonary resuscitation during out-of-hospital ventricular fibrillation arrest: survival implications of guideline changes. *Circulation.* 2006;114:2760–2765.
21. van Alem AP, Chapman FW, Lank P, Hart AA, Koster RW. A prospective, randomised and blinded comparison of first shock success of monophasic and biphasic waveforms in out-of-hospital cardiac arrest. *Resuscitation.* 2003;58:17–24.

22. Carpenter J, Rea TD, Murray JA, Kudenchuk PJ, Eisenberg MS. Defibrillation waveform and post-shock rhythm in out-of-hospital ventricular fibrillation cardiac arrest. *Resuscitation*. 2003;59:189–196.

23. Morrison LJ, Dorian P, Long J, Vermeulen M, Schwartz B, Sawadsky B, Frank J, Cameron B, Burgess R, Shield J, Bagley P, Mausz V, Brewer JE, Lerman BB. Out-of-hospital cardiac arrest rectilinear biphasic to monophasic damped sine defibrillation waveforms with advanced life support intervention trial (ORBIT). *Resuscitation*. 2005;66:149–157.

24. Kudenchuk PJ, Cobb LA, Copass MK, Olsufka M, Maynard C, Nichol G. Transthoracic incremental monophasic versus biphasic defibrillation by emergency responders (TIMBER): a randomized comparison of monophasic with biphasic waveform ascending energy defibrillation for the resuscitation of out-of-hospital cardiac arrest due to ventricular fibrillation. *Circulation*. 2006;114:2010–2018.

25. Leng CT, Paradis NA, Calkins H, Berger RD, Lardo AC, Rent KC, Halperin HR. Resuscitation after prolonged ventricular fibrillation with use of monophasic and biphasic waveform pulses for external defibrillation. *Circulation*. 2000;101:2968–2974.

26. Osorio J, Dosdall DJ, Robichaux RP Jr, Tabereaux PB, Ideker RE. In a swine model, chest compressions cause ventricular capture and, by means of a long-short sequence, ventricular fibrillation. *Circ Arrhythm Electrophysiol*. 2008;1:282–289.

27. Berdowski J, Tijssen JG, Koster RW. Chest compressions cause recurrence of ventricular fibrillation after the first successful conversion by defibrillation in out-of-hospital cardiac arrest. *Circ Arrhythm Electrophysiol*. 3:72–78.

28. Hess EP, White RD. Ventricular fibrillation is not provoked by chest compression during post-shock organized rhythms in out-of-hospital cardiac arrest. *Resuscitation*. 2005;66:7–11.

29. Yu T, Weil MH, Tang W, Sun S, Klouche K, Povoas H, Bisera J. Adverse outcomes of interrupted precordial compression during automated defibrillation. *Circulation*. 2002;106:368–372.

30. Berg RA, Sanders AB, Kern KB, Hilwig RW, Heidenreich JW, Porter ME, Ewy GA. Adverse hemodynamic effects of interrupting chest compressions for rescue breathing during cardiopulmonary resuscitation for ventricular fibrillation cardiac arrest. *Circulation*. 2001;104:2465–2470.

31. Kern KB, Hilwig RW, Berg RA, Sanders AB, Ewy GA. Importance of continuous chest compressions during cardiopulmonary resuscitation: improved outcome during a simulated single lay-rescuer scenario. *Circulation*. 2002;105:645–649.

32. Eftestol T, Sunde K, Steen PA. Effects of interrupting precordial compressions on the calculated probability of defibrillation success during out-of-hospital cardiac arrest. *Circulation*. 2002;105:2270–2273.

33. Wik L, Kramer-Johansen J, Myklebust H, Sorebo H, Svensson L, Fellows B, Steen PA. Quality of cardiopulmonary resuscitation during out-of-hospital cardiac arrest. *JAMA*. 2005;293:299–304.

34. Abella BS, Alvarado JP, Myklebust H, Edelson DP, Barry A, O'Hearn N, Vanden Hoek TL, Becker LB. Quality of cardiopulmonary resuscitation during in-hospital cardiac arrest. *JAMA*. 2005;293:305–310.

35. Bain AC, Swerdlow CD, Love CJ, Ellenbogen KA, Deering TF, Brewer JE, Augostini RS, Tchou PJ. Multicenter study of principles-based waveforms for external defibrillation. *Ann Emerg Med*. 2001;37:5–12.

36. Poole JE, White RD, Kanz KG, Hengstenberg F, Jarrard GT, Robinson JC, Santana V, McKenas DK, Rich N, Rosas S, Merritt S, Magnotto L, Gallagher JV III, Gliner BE, Jorgenson DB, Morgan CB, Dillon SM, Kronmal RA, Bardy GH. Low-energy impedance-compensating biphasic waveforms terminate ventricular fibrillation at high rates in victims of out-of-hospital cardiac arrest. LIFE Investigators. *J Cardiovasc Electrophysiol*. 1997;8:1373–1385.

37. White RD, Blackwell TH, Russell JK, Snyder DE, Jorgenson DB. Transthoracic impedance does not affect defibrillation, resuscitation or survival in patients with out-of-hospital cardiac arrest treated with a non-escalating biphasic waveform defibrillator. *Resuscitation*. 2005;64:63–69.

38. Mittal S, Ayati S, Stein KM, Knight BP, Morady F, Schwartzman D, Cavlovich D, Platia EV, Calkins H, Tchou PJ, Miller JM, Wharton JM, Sung RJ, Slotwiner DJ, Markowitz SM, Lerman BB. Comparison of a novel rectilinear biphasic waveform with a damped sine wave monophasic waveform for transthoracic ventricular defibrillation. ZOLL Investigators. *J Am Coll Cardiol*. 1999;34:1595–1601.

39. Schneider T, Martens PR, Paschen H, Kuisma M, Wolcke B, Gliner BE, Russell JK, Weaver WD, Bossaert L, Chamberlain D. Multicenter, randomized, controlled trial of 150-J biphasic shocks compared with 200- to 360-J monophasic shocks in the resuscitation of out-of-hospital

cardiac arrest victims. Optimized Response to Cardiac Arrest (ORCA) Investigators. *Circulation*. 2000;102:1780–1787.

40. Eftestol T, Sunde K, Aase SO, Husoy JH, Steen PA. Predicting outcome of defibrillation by spectral characterization and nonparametric classification of ventricular fibrillation in patients with out-of-hospital cardiac arrest. *Circulation*. 2000;102:1523–1529.

41. White RD. External defibrillation: the need for uniformity in analyzing and reporting results [editorial]. *Ann Emerg Med*. 1998;32:234–236.

42. Gliner BE, White RD. Electrocardiographic evaluation of defibrillation shocks delivered to out-of-hospital sudden cardiac arrest patients. *Resuscitation*. 1999;41:133–144.

43. Cummins RO, Chamberlain DA, Abramson NS, Allen M, Baskett PJ, Becker L, Bossaert L, Delooz HH, Dick WF, Eisenberg MS, Evans TR, Holmberg S, Kerber R, Mullie A, Ornato JP, Sandoe E, Skulberg A, Tunstall-Pedoe H, Swanson R, Thies WH. Recommended guidelines for uniform reporting of data from out-of-hospital cardiac arrest: the Utstein Style. A statement for health professionals from a task force of the American Heart Association, the European Resuscitation Council, the Heart and Stroke Foundation of Canada, and the Australian Resuscitation Council. *Circulation*. 1991;84:960–975.

44. White RD, Hankins DG, Bugliosi TF. Seven years' experience with early defibrillation by police and paramedics in an emergency medical services system. *Resuscitation*. 1998;39:145–151.

45. Cummins RO, Eisenberg MS, Bergner L, Hallstrom A, Hearne T, Murray JA. Automatic external defibrillation: evaluations of its role in the home and in emergency medical services. *Ann Emerg Med*. 1984; 13:798–801.

46. White RD, Vukov LF, Bugliosi TF. Early defibrillation by police: initial experience with measurement of critical time intervals and patient outcome. *Ann Emerg Med*. 1994;23:1009–1013.

47. Didon JP, Fontaine G, White RD, Jekova I, Schmid JJ, Cansell A. Clinical experience with a low-energy pulsed biphasic waveform in out-of-hospital cardiac arrest. *Resuscitation*. 2008;76:350–353.

48. Stothert JC, Hatcher TS, Gupton CL, Love JE, Brewer JE. Rectilinear biphasic waveform defibrillation of out-of-hospital cardiac arrest. *Prehosp Emerg Care*. 2004;8:388–392.

49. Schwarz B, Bowdle TA, Jett GK, Mair P, Lindner KH, Aldea GS, Lazzara RG, O'Grady SG, Schmitt PW, Walker RG, Chapman FW, Tacker WA. Biphasic shocks compared with monophasic damped sine wave shocks for direct ventricular defibrillation during open heart surgery. *Anesthesiology*. 2003;98:1063–1069.

50. Higgins SL, Herre JM, Epstein AE, Greer GS, Friedman PL, Gleva ML, Porterfield JG, Chapman FW, Finkel ES, Schmitt PW, Nova RC, Greene HL. A comparison of biphasic and monophasic shocks for external defibrillation. Physio-Control Biphasic Investigators. *Prehosp Emerg Care*. 2000;4:305–313.

51. Martens PR, Russell JK, Wolcke B, Paschen H, Kuisma M, Gliner BE, Weaver WD, Bossaert L, Chamberlain D, Schneider T. Optimal Response to Cardiac Arrest study: defibrillation waveform effects. *Resuscitation*. 2001;49:233–243.

52. Stiell IG, Walker RG, Nesbitt LP, Chapman FW, Cousineau D, Christenson J, Bradford P, Sookram S, Berringer R, Lank P, Wells GA. BIPHASIC Trial: a randomized comparison of fixed lower versus escalating higher energy levels for defibrillation in out-of-hospital cardiac arrest. *Circulation*. 2007;115:1511–1517.

53. Walsh SJ, McClelland AJ, Owens CG, Allen J, Anderson JM, Turner C, Adgey AA. Efficacy of distinct energy delivery protocols comparing two biphasic defibrillators for cardiac arrest. *Am J Cardiol*. 2004;94:378–380.

54. Freeman K, Hendey GW, Shalit M, Stroh G. Biphasic defibrillation does not improve outcomes compared to monophasic defibrillation in out-of-hospital cardiac arrest. *Prehosp Emerg Care*. 2008;12:152–156.

55. Berg MD, Samson RA, Meyer RJ, Clark LL, Valenzuela TD, Berg RA. Pediatric defibrillation doses often fail to terminate prolonged out-of-hospital ventricular fibrillation in children. *Resuscitation*. 2005;67:63–67.

56. Rodriguez-Nunez A, Lopez-Herce J, Garcia C, Dominguez P, Carrillo A, Bellon JM. Pediatric defibrillation after cardiac arrest: initial response and outcome. *Crit Care*. 2006;10:R113.

57. Tibballs J, Carter B, Kiraly NJ, Ragg P, Clifford M. External and internal biphasic direct current shock doses for pediatric ventricular fibrillation and pulseless ventricular tachycardia. *Pediatr Crit Care Med*. 2010. [epub ahead of print].

58. Atkins DL, Hartley LL, York DK. Accurate recognition and effective treatment of ventricular fibrillation by automated external defibrillators in adolescents. *Pediatrics*. 1998;101:393–397.

59. Rossano JW, Quan L, Kenney MA, Rea TD, Atkins DL. Energy doses for treatment of out-of-hospital pediatric ventricular fibrillation. *Resuscitation*. 2006;70:80–89.

60. Gurnett CA, Atkins DL. Successful use of a biphasic waveform automated external defibrillator in a high-risk child. *Am J Cardiol*. 2000;86:1051–1053.

61. Atkins DL, Jorgenson DB. Attenuated pediatric electrode pads for automated external defibrillator use in children. *Resuscitation*. 2005;66: 31–37.

62. Gliner BE, Jorgenson DB, Poole JE, White RD, Kanz KG, Lyster TD, Leyde KW, Powers DJ, Morgan CB, Kronmal RA, Bardy GH. Treatment of out-of-hospital cardiac arrest with a low-energy impedance-compensating biphasic waveform automatic external defibrillator. The LIFE Investigators. *Biomed Instrum Technol*. 1998;32: 631–644.

63. White RD, Russell JK. Refibrillation, resuscitation and survival in out-of-hospital sudden cardiac arrest victims treated with biphasic automated external defibrillators. *Resuscitation*. 2002;55:17–23.

64. Berg RA, Samson RA, Berg MD, Chapman FW, Hilwig RW, Banville I, Walker RG, Nova RC, Anavy N, Kern KB. Better outcome after pediatric defibrillation dosage than adult dosage in a swine model of pediatric ventricular fibrillation. *J Am Coll Cardiol*. 2005;45:786–789.

65. Killingsworth CR, Melnick SB, Chapman FW, Walker RG, Smith WM, Ideker RE, Walcott GP. Defibrillation threshold and cardiac responses using an external biphasic defibrillator with pediatric and adult adhesive patches in pediatric-sized piglets. *Resuscitation*. 2002;55:177–185.

66. Tang W, Weil MH, Sun S, Jorgenson D, Morgan C, Klouche K, Snyder D. The effects of biphasic waveform design on post-resuscitation myocardial function. *J Am Coll Cardiol*. 2004;43:1228–1235.

67. Lerman BB, DiMarco JP, Haines DE. Current-based versus energy-based ventricular defibrillation: a prospective study. *J Am Coll Cardiol*. 1988;12:1259–1264.

68. Kerber RE, McPherson D, Charbonnier F, Kieso R, Hite P. Automated impedance-based energy adjustment for defibrillation: experimental studies. *Circulation*. 1985;71:136–140.

69. Kerber RE, Kieso RA, Kienzle MG, Olshansky B, Waldo AL, Carlson MD, Wilber DJ, Aschoff AM, Birger S, Charbonnier F. Current-based transthoracic defibrillation. *Am J Cardiol*. 1996;78:1113–1118.

70. England H, Hoffman C, Hodgman T, Singh S, Homoud M, Weinstock J, Link M, Estes NA III. Effectiveness of automated external defibrillators in high schools in greater Boston. *Am J Cardiol*. 2005;95: 1484–1486.

71. Boodhoo L, Mitchell AR, Bordoli G, Lloyd G, Patel N, Sulke N. DC cardioversion of persistent atrial fibrillation: a comparison of two protocols. *Int J Cardiol*. 2007;114:16–21.

72. Brazdzionyte J, Babarskiene RM, Stanaitiene G. Anterior-posterior versus anterior-lateral electrode position for biphasic cardioversion of atrial fibrillation. *Medicina (Kaunas)*. 2006;42:994–998.

73. Chen CJ, Guo GB. External cardioversion in patients with persistent atrial fibrillation: a reappraisal of the effects of electrode pad position and transthoracic impedance on cardioversion success. *Jpn Heart J*. 2003;44:921–932.

74. Stanaitiene G, Babarskiene RM. [Impact of electrical shock waveform and paddle positions on efficacy of direct current cardioversion for atrial fibrillation]. *Medicina (Kaunas)*. 2008;44:665–672.

75. Krasteva V, Matveev M, Mudrov N, Prokopova R. Transthoracic impedance study with large self-adhesive electrodes in two conventional positions for defibrillation. *Physiol Meas*. 2006;27:1009–1022.

76. Kerber RE, Martins JB, Ferguson DW, Jensen SR, Parke JD, Kieso R, Melton J. Experimental evaluation and initial clinical application of new self-adhesive defibrillation electrodes. *Int J Cardiol*. 1985;8:57–66.

77. Garcia LA, Kerber RE. Transthoracic defibrillation: does electrode adhesive pad position alter transthoracic impedance? *Resuscitation*. 1998;37:139–143.

78. Dodd TE, Deakin CD, Petley GW, Clewlow F. External defibrillation in the left lateral position—a comparison of manual paddles with self-adhesive pads. *Resuscitation*. 2004;63:283–286.

79. Kerber RE, Jensen SR, Grayzel J, Kennedy J, Hoyt R. Elective cardioversion: influence of paddle-electrode location and size on success rates and energy requirements. *N Engl J Med*. 1981;305:658–662.

80. Mathew TP, Moore A, McIntyre M, Harbinson MT, Campbell NP, Adgey AA, Dalzell GW. Randomised comparison of electrode positions for cardioversion of atrial fibrillation. *Heart*. 1999;81:576–579.

81. Camacho MA, Lehr JL, Eisenberg SR. A three-dimensional finite element model of human transthoracic defibrillation: paddle placement and size. *IEEE Trans Biomed Eng*. 1995;42:572–578.

82. Lateef F, Lim SH, Anantharaman V, Lim CS. Changes in chest electrode impedance. *Am J Emerg Med*. 2000;18:381–384.

83. Pagan-Carlo LA, Spencer KT, Robertson CE, Dengler A, Birkett C, Kerber RE. Transthoracic defibrillation: importance of avoiding electrode placement directly on the female breast. *J Am Coll Cardiol*. 1996;27:449–452.

84. Bissing JW, Kerber RE. Effect of shaving the chest of hirsute subjects on transthoracic impedance to self-adhesive defibrillation electrode pads. *Am J Cardiol*. 2000;86:587–589.

85. Sado DM, Deakin CD, Petley GW, Clewlow F. Comparison of the effects of removal of chest hair with not doing so before external defibrillation on transthoracic impedance. *Am J Cardiol*. 2004;93: 98–100.

86. Kerber RE, Grayzel J, Hoyt R, Marcus M, Kennedy J. Transthoracic resistance in human defibrillation. Influence of body weight, chest size, serial shocks, paddle size and paddle contact pressure. *Circulation*. 1981;63:676–682.

87. Connell PN, Ewy GA, Dahl CF, Ewy MD. Transthoracic impedance to defibrillator discharge. Effect of electrode size and electrode-chest wall interface. *J Electrocardiol*. 1973;6:313-M.

88. Dahl CF, Ewy GA, Warner ED, Thomas ED. Myocardial necrosis from direct current countershock: effect of paddle electrode size and time interval between discharges. *Circulation*. 1974;50:956–961.

89. Hoyt R, Grayzel J, Kerber RE. Determinants of intracardiac current in defibrillation. Experimental studies in dogs. *Circulation*. 1981;64: 818–823.

90. Thomas ED, Ewy GA, Dahl CF, Ewy MD. Effectiveness of direct current defibrillation: role of paddle electrode size. *Am Heart J*. 1977; 93:463–467.

91. Atkins DL, Kerber RE. Pediatric defibrillation: current flow is improved by using "adult" electrode paddles. *Pediatrics*. 1994;94:90–93.

92. Atkins DL, Sirna S, Kieso R, Charbonnier F, Kerber RE. Pediatric defibrillation: importance of paddle size in determining transthoracic impedance. *Pediatrics*. 1988;82:914–918.

93. Samson RA, Atkins DL, Kerber RE. Optimal size of self-adhesive preapplied electrode pads in pediatric defibrillation. *Am J Cardiol*. 1995;75:544–545.

94. Monsieurs KG, Conraads VM, Goethals MP, Snoeck JP, Bossaert LL. Semi-automatic external defibrillation and implanted cardiac pacemakers: understanding the interactions during resuscitation. *Resuscitation*. 1995;30: 127–131.

95. Manegold JC, Israel CW, Ehrlich JR, Duray G, Pajitnev D, Wegener FT, Hohnloser SH. External cardioversion of atrial fibrillation in patients with implanted pacemaker or cardioverter-defibrillator systems: a randomized comparison of monophasic and biphasic shock energy application. *Eur Heart J*. 2007;28:1731–1738.

96. Alferness CA. Pacemaker damage due to external countershock in patients with implanted cardiac pacemakers. *Pacing Clin Electrophysiol*. 1982;5:457–458.

97. Panacek EA, Munger MA, Rutherford WF, Gardner SF. Report of nitropatch explosions complicating defibrillation. *Am J Emerg Med*. 1992;10:128–129.

98. *American National Standard: Automatic External Defibrillators and Remote Controlled Defibrillators (DF39)*. Arlington, VA: Association for the Advancement of Medical Instrumentation; 1993.

99. Stults KR, Brown DD, Cooley F, Kerber RE. Self-adhesive monitor/defibrillation pads improve prehospital defibrillation success. *Ann Emerg Med*. 1987;16:872–877.

100. Wilson RF, Sirna S, White CW, Kerber RE. Defibrillation of high-risk patients during coronary angiography using self-adhesive, preapplied electrode pads. *Am J Cardiol*. 1987;60:380–382.

101. Kerber RE, Kouba C, Martins J, Kelly K, Low R, Hoyt R, Ferguson D, Bailey L, Bennett P, Charbonnier F. Advance prediction of transthoracic impedance in human defibrillation and cardioversion: importance of impedance in determining the success of low-energy shocks. *Circulation*. 1984;70:303–308.

102. Kerber RE, Martins JB, Kienzle MG, Constantin L, Olshansky B, Hopson R, Charbonnier F. Energy, current, and success in defibrillation

and cardioversion: clinical studies using an automated impedance-based method of energy adjustment. *Circulation*. 1988;77:1038–1046.

103. Dalzell GW, Cunningham SR, Anderson J, Adgey AA. Electrode pad size, transthoracic impedance and success of external ventricular defibrillation. *Am J Cardiol*. 1989;64:741–744.

104. Cummins RO, Eisenberg M, Bergner L, Murray JA. Sensitivity, accuracy, and safety of an automatic external defibrillator. *Lancet*. 1984;2:318–320.

105. Davis EA, Mosesso VN Jr. Performance of police first responders in utilizing automated external defibrillation on victims of sudden cardiac arrest. *Prehosp Emerg Care*. 1998;2:101–107.

106. Weisfeldt ML, Kerber RE, McGoldrick RP, Moss AJ, Nichol G, Ornato JP, Palmer DG, Riegel B, Smith SCJ. American Heart Association Report on the Public Access Defibrillation Conference December 8–10, 1994. Automatic External Defibrillation Task Force. *Circulation*. 1995; 92:2740–2747.

107. Weisfeldt ML, Kerber RE, McGoldrick RP, Moss AJ, Nichol G, Ornato JP, Palmer DG, Riegel B, Smith SC Jr. Public access defibrillation. A statement for healthcare professionals from the American Heart Association Task Force on Automatic External Defibrillation. *Circulation*. 1995;92:2763.

108. Nichol G, Hallstrom AP, Ornato JP, Riegel B, Stiell IG, Valenzuela T, Wells GA, White RD, Weisfeldt ML. Potential cost-effectiveness of public access defibrillation in the United States. *Circulation*. 1998;97: 1315–1320.

109. American Heart Association in collaboration with International Liaison Committee on Resuscitation. Guidelines 2000 for Cardiopulmonary Resuscitation and Emergency Cardiovascular Care. *Circulation*. 2000; 102(suppl):I1–I384.

110. Hazinski MF, Idris AH, Kerber RE, Epstein A, Atkins D, Tang W, Lurie K. Lay rescuer automated external defibrillator ("public access defibrillation") programs: lessons learned from an international multicenter trial: advisory statement from the American Heart Association Emergency Cardiovascular Committee; the Council on Cardiopulmonary, Perioperative, and Critical Care; and the Council on Clinical Cardiology. *Circulation*. 2005;111:3336–3340.

111. Caffrey SL, Willoughby PJ, Pepe PE, Becker LB. Public use of automated external defibrillators. *N Engl J Med*. 2002;347:1242–1247.

112. Valenzuela TD, Bjerke HS, Clark LL, Hardman R, Spaite DW, Nichol G. Rapid defibrillation by nontraditional responders: the Casino Project. *Acad Emerg Med*. 1998;5:414–415.

113. Valenzuela TD, Roe DJ, Nichol G, Clark LL, Spaite DW, Hardman RG. Outcomes of rapid defibrillation by security officers after cardiac arrest in casinos. *N Engl J Med*. 2000;343:1206–1209.

114. White RD, Asplin BR, Bugliosi TF, Hankins DG. High discharge survival rate after out-of-hospital ventricular fibrillation with rapid defibrillation by police and paramedics. *Ann Emerg Med*. 1996;28: 480–485.

115. White RD. Early out-of-hospital experience with an impedance-compensating low-energy biphasic waveform automatic external defibrillator. *J Interv Card Electrophysiol*. 1997;1:203–208.

116. White RD, Bunch TJ, Hankins DG. Evolution of a community-wide early defibrillation programme experience over 13 years using police/fire personnel and paramedics as responders. *Resuscitation*. 2005; 65:279–283.

117a. Rea TD, Olsufka M, Bemis B, White L, Yin L, Becker L, Copass M, Eisenberg M, Cobb L. A population based investigation of public access defibrillation: Rose of emergency medical services care. *Resuscitation*. 2010;81:163–167.

117b. Gombotz H, Weh B, Mitterndorfer W, Rehak P. In-hospital cardiac resuscitation outside the ICU by nursing staff equipped with automated external defibrillators—the first 500 cases. *Resuscitation*. 2006;70: 416–422.

118. Hanefeld C, Lichte C, Mentges-Schroter I, Sirtl C, Mugge A. Hospital-wide first-responder automated external defibrillator programme: 1 year experience. *Resuscitation*. 2005;66:167–170.

119. Groh WJ, Newman MM, Beal PE, Fineberg NS, Zipes DP. Limited response to cardiac arrest by police equipped with automated external defibrillators: lack of survival benefit in suburban and rural Indiana—the police as responder automated defibrillation evaluation (PARADE). *Acad Emerg Med*. 2001;8:324–330.

120. de Vries W, van Alem AP, de Vos R, van Oostrom J, Koster RW. Trained first-responders with an automated external defibrillator: how do they perform in real resuscitation attempts? *Resuscitation*. 2005;64: 157–161.

121. Sayre MR, Evans J, White LJ, Brennan TD. Providing automated external defibrillators to urban police officers in addition to a fire department rapid defibrillation program is not effective. *Resuscitation*. 2005;66:189–196.

122. The Public Access Defibrillation Trial Investigators. Public-access defibrillation and survival after out-of-hospital cardiac arrest. *N Engl J Med*. 2004;351:637–646.

123. Weisfeldt ML, Sitlani CM, Ornato JP, Rea T, Aufderheide TP, Davis D, Dreyer J, Hess EP, Jui J, Maloney J, Sopko G, Powell J, Nichol G, Morrison LJ. Survival after application of automatic external defibrillators before arrival of the emergency medical system: evaluation in the resuscitation outcomes consortium population of 21 million. *J Am Coll Cardiol*. 2010;55:1713–1720.

124. Kitamura T, Iwami T, Kawamura T, Nagao K, Tanaka H, Hiraide A. Nationwide public-access defibrillation in Japan. *N Engl J Med*. 2010; 362:994–1004.

125. Cram P, Vijan S, Fendrick AM. Cost-effectiveness of automated external defibrillator deployment in selected public locations. *J Gen Intern Med*. 2003;18:745–754.

126. Folke F, Lippert FK, Nielsen SL, Gislason GH, Hansen ML, Schramm TK, Sorensen R, Fosbol EL, Andersen SS, Rasmussen S, Kober L, Torp-Pedersen C. Location of cardiac arrest in a city center: strategic placement of automated external defibrillators in public locations. *Circulation*. 2009;120:510–517.

127. Becker L, Eisenberg M, Fahrenbruch C, Cobb L. Public locations of cardiac arrest: implications for public access defibrillation. *Circulation*. 1998;97:2106–2109.

128. Bardy GH, Lee KL, Mark DB, Poole JE, Toff WD, Tonkin AM, Smith W, Dorian P, Packer DL, White RD, Longstreth WT Jr, Anderson J, Johnson G, Bischoff E, Yallop JJ, McNulty S, Ray LD, Clapp-Channing NE, Rosenberg Y, Schron EB. Home use of automated external defibrillators for sudden cardiac arrest. *N Engl J Med*. 2008;358:1793–1804.

129. Weaver WD, Cobb LA, Copass MK, Hallstrom AP. Ventricular defibrillation: a comparative trial using 175-J and 320-J shocks. *N Engl J Med*. 1982;307:1101–1106.

130. 2005 American Heart Association Guidelines for Cardiopulmonary Resuscitation and Emergency Cardiovascular Care. *Circulation*. 2005; 112(suppl):IV1–203.

131. Kerber RE, Becker LB, Bourland JD, Cummins RO, Hallstrom AP, Michos MB, Nichol G, Ornato JP, Thies WH, White RD, Zuckerman BD. Automatic external defibrillators for public access defibrillation: recommendations for specifying and reporting arrhythmia analysis algorithm performance, incorporating new waveforms, and enhancing safety. A statement for health professionals from the American Heart Association Task Force on Automatic External Defibrillation, Subcommittee on AED Safety and Efficacy. *Circulation*. 1997;95:1677–1682.

132. Dickey W, Dalzell GW, Anderson JM, Adgey AA. The accuracy of decision-making of a semi-automatic defibrillator during cardiac arrest. *Eur Heart J*. 1992;13:608–615.

133. Atkinson E, Mikysa B, Conway JA, Parker M, Christian K, Deshpande J, Knilans TK, Smith J, Walker C, Stickney RE, Hampton DR, Hazinski MF. Specificity and sensitivity of automated external defibrillator rhythm analysis in infants and children. *Ann Emerg Med*. 2003;42: 185–196.

134. Cecchin F, Jorgenson DB, Berul CI, Perry JC, Zimmerman AA, Duncan BW, Lupinetti FM, Snyder D, Lyster TD, Rosenthal GL, Cross B, Atkins DL. Is arrhythmia detection by automatic external defibrillator accurate for children? Sensitivity and specificity of an automatic external defibrillator algorithm in 696 pediatric arrhythmias. *Circulation*. 2001;103:2483–2488.

135. Atkins DL, Scott WA, Blaufox AD, Law IH, Dick M II, Geheb F, Sobh J, Brewer JE. Sensitivity and specificity of an automated external defibrillator algorithm designed for pediatric patients. *Resuscitation*. 2008; 76:168–174.

136. Kuisma M, Suominen P, Korpela R. Paediatric out-of-hospital cardiac arrests: epidemiology and outcome. *Resuscitation*. 1995;30:141–150.

137. Sirbaugh PE, Pepe PE, Shook JE, Kimball KT, Goldman MJ, Ward MA, Mann DM. A prospective, population-based study of the demographics, epidemiology, management, and outcome of out-of-hospital pediatric cardiopulmonary arrest. *Ann Emerg Med*. 1999;33:174–184.

138. Hickey RW, Cohen DM, Strausbaugh S, Dietrich AM. Pediatric patients requiring CPR in the prehospital setting. *Ann Emerg Med*. 1995;25: 495–501.

139. Atkins DL, Everson-Stewart S, Sears GK, Daya M, Osmond MH, Warden CR, Berg RA. Epidemiology and outcomes from out-of-hospital

cardiac arrest in children: the Resuscitation Outcomes Consortium Epistry–Cardiac Arrest. *Circulation*. 2009;119:1484–1491.

140. Appleton GO, Cummins RO, Larson MP, Graves JR. CPR and the single rescuer: at what age should you "call first" rather than "call fast"? *Ann Emerg Med*. 1995;25:492–494.

141. Ronco R, King W, Donley DK, Tilden SJ. Outcome and cost at a children's hospital following resuscitation for out-of-hospital cardiopulmonary arrest. *Arch Pediatr Adolesc Med*. 1995;149:210–214.

142. Losek JD, Hennes H, Glaeser P, Hendley G, Nelson DB. Prehospital care of the pulseless, nonbreathing pediatric patient. *Am J Emerg Med*. 1987;5:370–374.

143. Mogayzel C, Quan L, Graves JR, Tiedeman D, Fahrenbruch C, Herndon P. Out-of-hospital ventricular fibrillation in children and adolescents: causes and outcomes. *Ann Emerg Med*. 1995;25:484–491.

144. Safranek DJ, Eisenberg MS, Larsen MP. The epidemiology of cardiac arrest in young adults. *Ann Emerg Med*. 1992;21:1102–1106.

145. Berg RA, Chapman FW, Berg MD, Hilwig RW, Banville I, Walker RG, Nova RC, Sherrill D, Kern KB. Attenuated adult biphasic shocks compared with weight-based monophasic shocks in a swine model of prolonged pediatric ventricular fibrillation. *Resuscitation*. 2004;61: 189–197.

146. Tang W, Weil MH, Jorgenson D, Klouche K, Morgan C, Yu T, Sun S, Snyder D. Fixed-energy biphasic waveform defibrillation in a pediatric model of cardiac arrest and resuscitation. *Crit Care Med*. 2002;30: 2736–2741.

147. Clark CB, Zhang Y, Davies LR, Karlsson G, Kerber RE. Pediatric transthoracic defibrillation: biphasic versus monophasic waveforms in an experimental model. *Resuscitation*. 2001;51:159–163.

148. Samson RA, Berg RA, Bingham R, Biarent D, Coovadia A, Hazinski MF, Hickey RW, Nadkarni V, Nichol G, Tibballs J, Reis AG, Tse S, Zideman D, Potts J, Uzark K, Atkins D. Use of automated external defibrillators for children: an update: an advisory statement from the pediatric advanced life support task force, International Liaison Committee on Resuscitation. *Circulation*. 2003;107:3250–3255.

149. Jorgenson D, Morgan C, Snyder D, Griesser H, Solosko T, Chan K, Skarr T. Energy attenuator for pediatric application of an automated external defibrillator. *Crit Care Med*. 2002;30(suppl):S145–S147.

150. Bar-Cohen Y, Walsh EP, Love BA, Cecchin F. First appropriate use of automated external defibrillator in an infant. *Resuscitation*. 2005;67: 135–137.

151. Konig B, Benger J, Goldsworthy L. Automatic external defibrillation in a 6 year old. *Arch Dis Child*. 2005;90:310–311.

152. Zafari AM, Zarter SK, Heggen V, Wilson P, Taylor RA, Reddy K, Backscheider AG, Dudley SC Jr. A program encouraging early defibrillation results in improved in-hospital resuscitation efficacy. *J Am Coll Cardiol*. 2004;44:846–852.

153. Destro A, Marzaloni M, Sermasi S, Rossi F. Automatic external defibrillators in the hospital as well? *Resuscitation*. 1996;31:39–43.

154. Smith M. Service is improving everywhere . . . but what about EMS? *EMS Mag*. 2009;38:26.

155. Forcina MS, Farhat AY, O'Neil WW, Haines DE. Cardiac arrest survival after implementation of automated external defibrillator technology in the in-hospital setting. *Crit Care Med*. 2009;37:1229–1236.

156. Kaye W, Mancini ME, Richards N. Organizing and implementing a hospital-wide first-responder automated external defibrillation program: strengthening the in-hospital chain of survival. *Resuscitation*. 1995;30: 151–156.

157. Peberdy MA, Kaye W, Ornato JP, Larkin GL, Nadkarni V, Mancini ME, Berg RA, Nichol G, Lane-Trultt T. Cardiopulmonary resuscitation of adults in the hospital: a report of 14720 cardiac arrests from the National Registry of Cardiopulmonary Resuscitation. *Resuscitation*. 2003;58: 297–308.

158. Asano Y, Davidenko JM, Baxter WT, Gray RA, Jalife J. Optical mapping of drug-induced polymorphic arrhythmias and torsade de pointes in the isolated rabbit heart. *J Am Coll Cardiol*. 1997;29: 831–842.

159. Gray RA, Jalife J, Panfilov A, Baxter WT, Cabo C, Davidenko JM, Pertsov AM. Nonstationary vortexlike reentrant activity as a mechanism of polymorphic ventricular tachycardia in the isolated rabbit heart. *Circulation*. 1995;91:2454–2469.

160. Callaway CW, Sherman LD, Mosesso VN Jr, Dietrich TJ, Holt E, Clarkson MC. Scaling exponent predicts defibrillation success for out-of-hospital ventricular fibrillation cardiac arrest. *Circulation*. 2001;103: 1656–1661.

161. Weaver WD, Cobb LA, Dennis D, Ray R, Hallstrom AP, Copass MK. Amplitude of ventricular fibrillation waveform and outcome after cardiac arrest. *Ann Intern Med*. 1985;102:53–55.

162. Brown CG, Dzwonczyk R. Signal analysis of the human electrocardiogram during ventricular fibrillation: frequency and amplitude parameters as predictors of successful countershock. *Ann Emerg Med*. 1996;27: 184–188.

163. Callaham M, Braun O, Valentine W, Clark DM, Zegans C. Prehospital cardiac arrest treated by urban first-responders: profile of patient response and prediction of outcome by ventricular fibrillation waveform. *Ann Emerg Med*. 1993;22:1664–1677.

164. Strohmenger HU, Lindner KH, Brown CG. Analysis of the ventricular fibrillation ECG signal amplitude and frequency parameters as predictors of countershock success in humans. *Chest*. 1997;111:584–589.

165. Strohmenger HU, Eftestol T, Sunde K, Wenzel V, Mair M, Ulmer H, Lindner KH, Steen PA. The predictive value of ventricular fibrillation electrocardiogram signal frequency and amplitude variables in patients with out-of-hospital cardiac arrest. *Anesth Analg*. 2001;93:1428–1433.

166. Podbregar M, Kovacic M, Podbregar-Mars A, Brezocnik M. Predicting defibrillation success by 'genetic' programming in patients with out-of-hospital cardiac arrest. *Resuscitation*. 2003;57:153–159.

167. Menegazzi JJ, Callaway CW, Sherman LD, Hostler DP, Wang HE, Fertig KC, Logue ES. Ventricular fibrillation scaling exponent can guide timing of defibrillation and other therapies. *Circulation*. 2004;109: 926–931.

168. Povoas HP, Weil MH, Tang W, Bisera J, Klouche K, Barbatsis A. Predicting the success of defibrillation by electrocardiographic analysis. *Resuscitation*. 2002;53:77–82.

169. Noc M, Weil MH, Tang W, Sun S, Pernat A, Bisera J. Electrocardiographic prediction of the success of cardiac resuscitation. *Crit Care Med*. 1999;27:708–714.

170. Strohmenger HU, Lindner KH, Keller A, Lindner IM, Pfenninger EG. Spectral analysis of ventricular fibrillation and closed-chest cardiopulmonary resuscitation. *Resuscitation*. 1996;33:155–161.

171. Noc M, Weil MH, Gazmuri RJ, Sun S, Biscera J, Tang W. Ventricular fibrillation voltage as a monitor of the effectiveness of cardiopulmonary resuscitation. *J Lab Clin Med*. 1994;124:421–426.

172. Lightfoot CB, Nremt P, Callaway CW, Hsieh M, Fertig KC, Sherman LD, Menegazzi JJ. Dynamic nature of electrocardiographic waveform predicts rescue shock outcome in porcine ventricular fibrillation. *Ann Emerg Med*. 2003;42:230–241.

173. Marn-Pernat A, Weil MH, Tang W, Pernat A, Bisera J. Optimizing timing of ventricular defibrillation. *Crit Care Med*. 2001;29:2360–2365.

174. Hamprecht FA, Achleitner U, Krismer AC, Lindner KH, Wenzel V, Strohmenger HU, Thiel W, van Gunsteren WF, Amann A. Fibrillation power, an alternative method of ECG spectral analysis for prediction of countershock success in a porcine model of ventricular fibrillation. *Resuscitation*. 2001;50:287–296.

175. Amann A, Achleitner U, Antretter H, Bonatti JO, Krismer AC, Lindner KH, Rieder J, Wenzel V, Voelckel WG, Strohmenger HU. Analysing ventricular fibrillation ECG-signals and predicting defibrillation success during cardiopulmonary resuscitation employing N(alpha)-histograms. *Resuscitation*. 2001;50:77–85.

176. Brown CG, Griffith RF, Van Ligten P, Hoekstra J, Nejman G, Mitchell L, Dzwonczyk R. Median frequency—a new parameter for predicting defibrillation success rate. *Ann Emerg Med*. 1991;20:787–789.

177. Amann A, Rheinberger K, Achleitner U, Krismer AC, Lingnau W, Lindner KH, Wenzel V. The prediction of defibrillation outcome using a new combination of mean frequency and amplitude in porcine models of cardiac arrest. *Anesth Analg*. 2002;95:716–722.

178. Losek JD, Hennes H, Glaeser PW, Smith DS, Hendley G. Prehospital countershock treatment of pediatric asystole. *Am J Emerg Med*. 1989; 7:571–575.

179. Martin DR, Gavin T, Bianco J, Brown CG, Stueven H, Pepe PE, Cummins RO, Gonzalez E, Jastremski M. Initial countershock in the treatment of asystole. *Resuscitation*. 1993;26:63–68.

180. Miller PH. Potential fire hazard in defibrillation. *JAMA*. 1972;221:192.

181. Hummel RS III, Ornato JP, Weinberg SM, Clarke AM. Spark-generating properties of electrode gels used during defibrillation. A potential fire hazard. *JAMA*. 1988;260:3021–3024.

182. Fires from defibrillation during oxygen administration. *Health Devices*. 1994;23:307–309.

183. Lefever J, Smith A. Risk of fire when using defibrillation in an oxygen enriched atmosphere. *Medical Devices Agency Safety Notices*. 1995; 3:1–3.

184. Ward ME. Risk of fires when using defibrillators in an oxygen enriched atmosphere. *Resuscitation*. 1996;31:173.

185. Theodorou AA, Gutierrez JA, Berg RA. Fire attributable to a defibrillation attempt in a neonate. *Pediatrics*. 2003;112:677–679.

186. Lown B. Electrical reversion of cardiac arrhythmias. *Br Heart J*. 1967; 29:469–489.

187. Mittal S, Ayati S, Stein KM, Schwartzman D, Cavlovich D, Tchou PJ, Markowitz SM, Slotwiner DJ, Scheiner MA, Lerman BB. Transthoracic cardioversion of atrial fibrillation: comparison of rectilinear biphasic versus damped sine wave monophasic shocks. *Circulation*. 2000;101: 1282–1287.

188. Page RL, Kerber RE, Russell JK, Trouton T, Waktare J, Gallik D, Olgin JE, Ricard P, Dalzell GW, Reddy R, Lazzara R, Lee K, Carlson M, Halperin B, Bardy GH. Biphasic versus monophasic shock waveform for conversion of atrial fibrillation: the results of an international randomized, double-blind multicenter trial. *J Am Coll Cardiol*. 2002;39: 1956–1963.

189. Scholten M, Szili-Torok T, Klootwijk P, Jordaens L. Comparison of monophasic and biphasic shocks for transthoracic cardioversion of atrial fibrillation. *Heart*. 2003;89:1032–1034.

190. Glover BM, Walsh SJ, McCann CJ, Moore MJ, Manoharan G, Dalzell GW, McAllister A, McClements B, McEneaney DJ, Trouton TG, Mathew TP, Adgey AA. Biphasic energy selection for transthoracic cardioversion of atrial fibrillation. The BEST AF Trial. *Heart*. 2008;94: 884–887.

191. Reisinger J, Gstrein C, Winter T, Zeindlhofer E, Hollinger K, Mori M, Schiller A, Winter A, Geiger H, Siostrzonek P. Optimization of initial energy for cardioversion of atrial tachyarrhythmias with biphasic shocks. *Am J Emerg Med*. 2010;28:159–165.

192. Kerber RE, Kienzle MG, Olshansky B, Waldo AL, Wilber D, Carlson MD, Aschoff AM, Birger S, Fugatt L, Walsh S. Ventricular tachycardia rate and morphology determine energy and current requirements for transthoracic cardioversion. *Circulation*. 1992;85:158–163.

193. Hedges JR, Syverud SA, Dalsey WC, Feero S, Easter R, Shultz B. Prehospital trial of emergency transcutaneous cardiac pacing. *Circulation*. 1987;76:1337–1343.

194. Barthell E, Troiano P, Olson D, Stueven HA, Hendley G. Prehospital external cardiac pacing: a prospective, controlled clinical trial. *Ann Emerg Med*. 1988;17:1221–1226.

195. Cummins RO, Graves JR, Larsen MP, Hallstrom AP, Hearne TR, Ciliberti J, Nicola RM, Horan S. Out-of-hospital transcutaneous pacing by emergency medical technicians in patients with asystolic cardiac arrest. *N Engl J Med*. 1993;328:1377–1382.

196. Ornato JP, Peberdy MA. The mystery of bradyasystole during cardiac arrest. *Ann Emerg Med*. 1996;27:576–587.

197. Niemann JT, Adomian GE, Garner D, Rosborough JP. Endocardial and transcutaneous cardiac pacing, calcium chloride, and epinephrine in postcountershock asystole and bradycardias. *Crit Care Med*. 1985;13: 699–704.

198. Quan L, Graves JR, Kinder DR, Horan S, Cummins RO. Transcutaneous cardiac pacing in the treatment of out-of-hospital pediatric cardiac arrests. *Ann Emerg Med*. 1992;21:905–909.

199. Dalsey WC, Syverud SA, Hedges JR. Emergency department use of transcutaneous pacing for cardiac arrests. *Crit Care Med*. 1985;13: 399–401.

200. Knowlton AA, Falk RH. External cardiac pacing during in-hospital cardiac arrest. *Am J Cardiol*. 1986;57:1295–1298.

201. Ornato JP, Carveth WL, Windle JR. Pacemaker insertion for prehospital bradyasystolic cardiac arrest. *Ann Emerg Med*. 1984;13:101–103.

202. White JD. Transthoracic pacing in cardiac asystole. *Am J Emerg Med*. 1983;1:264–266.

203. Smith I, Monk TG, White PF. Comparison of transesophageal atrial pacing with anticholinergic drugs for the treatment of intraoperative bradycardia. *Anesth Analg*. 1994;78:245–252.

204. Morrison LJ, Long J, Vermeulen M, Schwartz B, Sawadsky B, Frank J, Cameron B, Burgess R, Shield J, Bagley P, Mausz V, Brewer JE, Dorian P. A randomized controlled feasibility trial comparing safety and effectiveness of prehospital pacing versus conventional treatment: "PrePACE." *Resuscitation*. 2008;76:341–349.

KEY WORDS: arrhythmia ■ automatic external defibrillator ■ cardioversion ■ ventricular fibrillation

# Part 7: CPR Techniques and Devices
## 2010 American Heart Association Guidelines for Cardiopulmonary Resuscitation and Emergency Cardiovascular Care

Diana M. Cave, Chair; Raul J. Gazmuri; Charles W. Otto; Vinay M. Nadkarni; Adam Cheng; Steven C. Brooks; Mohamud Daya; Robert M. Sutton; Richard Branson; Mary Fran Hazinski

Over the past 25 years a variety of alternatives to conventional manual CPR have been developed in an effort to enhance perfusion during attempted resuscitation from cardiac arrest and to improve survival. Compared with conventional CPR, these techniques and devices typically require more personnel, training, and equipment, or they apply to a specific setting. Application of these devices has the potential to delay or interrupt CPR, so rescuers should be trained to minimize any interruption of chest compressions or defibrillation and should be retrained as needed. Efficacy for some techniques and devices has been reported in selected settings and patient conditions; however, no alternative technique or device in routine use has consistently been shown to be superior to conventional CPR for out-of-hospital basic life support. In this section, no class of recommendation is made when there is insufficient evidence of benefit or harm, particularly if human data are extremely limited. For those devices assigned a 2005 Class of Recommendation other than Indeterminate, Classes of Recommendation were assigned when possible using the same criteria applied throughout this document (see Part 1: "Executive Summary" and Part 2: "Evidence Evaluation").

Whenever these devices are used, providers should monitor for evidence of benefit versus harm. The experts are aware of several clinical trials of the devices listed below that are under way and/or recently concluded, so readers are encouraged to monitor for the publication of additional trial results in peer-reviewed journals and AHA scientific advisory statements.

## CPR Techniques

### High-Frequency Chest Compressions
High-frequency chest compression (typically at a frequency >120 per minute) has been studied as a technique for improving resuscitation from cardiac arrest.[1] The sparse human data have demonstrated mixed results. One clinical trial including 9 patients[2] and another including 23 patients[3] showed that a compression frequency of 120 per minute improved hemodynamics compared to conventional chest compressions; no change in clinical outcome was reported. These *2010 AHA Guidelines for CPR and ECC* recommend compressions at a rate of at least 100/ min. There is insufficient evidence to recommend the routine use of high-frequency chest compressions for cardiac arrest. However, high-frequency chest compressions may be considered by adequately trained rescue personnel as an alternative (Class IIb, LOE C).

### Open-Chest CPR
In open-chest CPR the heart is accessed through a thoracotomy (typically created through the 5th left intercostal space) and compression is performed using the thumb and fingers, or with the palm and extended fingers against the sternum. Use of this technique generates forward blood flow and coronary perfusion pressure that typically exceed those generated by closed chest compressions.

There are few human studies comparing open-chest CPR to conventional CPR in cardiac arrest and no prospective randomized trials. Several studies of open-chest CPR have demonstrated improved coronary perfusion pressure and/or return of spontaneous circulation (ROSC) for both the in-hospital (eg, following cardiac surgery)[4–6] and out-of-hospital environments.[7–10]

Several small case series of cardiac arrest patients treated with thoracotomy and open-chest CPR after blunt[11,12] or penetrating trauma[12–14] reported survivors with mild or no neurological deficit.

There is insufficient evidence of benefit or harm to recommend the routine use of open-chest CPR. However, open-chest CPR can be useful if cardiac arrest develops during surgery when the chest or abdomen is already open, or in the early postoperative period after cardiothoracic surgery (Class IIa, LOE C). A resuscitative thoracotomy to facilitate open-chest CPR may be considered in very select circumstances of adults and children with out-of-hospital cardiac arrest from penetrating trauma with short transport times to a trauma facility (Class IIb, LOE C).[15,16]

The American Heart Association requests that this document be cited as follows: Cave DM, Gazmuri RJ, Otto CW, Nadkarni VM, Cheng A, Brooks SC, Daya M, Sutton RM, Branson R, Hazinski MF. Part 7: CPR techniques and devices: 2010 American Heart Association Guidelines for Cardiopulmonary Resuscitation and Emergency Cardiovascular Care. *Circulation.* 2010;122(suppl 3):S720–S728.

**(*Circulation.* 2010;122[suppl 3]:S720–S728.)**

*Circulation* is available at http://circ.ahajournals.org                    DOI: 10.1161/CIRCULATIONAHA.110.970970

## Interposed Abdominal Compression-CPR

The interposed abdominal compression (IAC)-CPR is a 3-rescuer technique (an abdominal compressor plus the chest compressor and the rescuer providing ventilations) that includes conventional chest compressions combined with alternating abdominal compressions. The dedicated rescuer who provides manual abdominal compressions will compress the abdomen midway between the xiphoid and the umbilicus during the relaxation phase of chest compression. Hand position, depth, rhythm, and rate of abdominal compressions are similar to those for chest compressions and the force required is similar to that used to palpate the abdominal aorta. In most reports, an endotracheal tube is placed before or shortly after initiation of IAC-CPR. IAC-CPR increases diastolic aortic pressure and venous return, resulting in improved coronary perfusion pressure and blood flow to other vital organs.

In 2 randomized in-hospital trials, IAC-CPR performed by trained rescuers improved short-term survival[17] and survival to hospital discharge[18] compared with conventional CPR for adult cardiac arrest. The data from these studies were combined in 2 positive meta-analyses.[19,20] However, 1 randomized controlled trial of adult out-of-hospital cardiac arrest[21] did not show any survival advantage to IAC-CPR. Although there were no complications reported in adults,[19] 1 pediatric case report[22] documented traumatic pancreatitis following IAC-CPR.

IAC-CPR may be considered during in-hospital resuscitation when sufficient personnel trained in its use are available (Class IIb, LOE B). There is insufficient evidence to recommend for or against the use of IAC-CPR in the out-of-hospital setting or in children.

## "Cough" CPR

"Cough" CPR describes the use of forceful voluntary coughs every 1 to 3 seconds in conscious patients shortly after the onset of a witnessed nonperfusing cardiac rhythm in a controlled environment such as the cardiac catheterization laboratory. Coughing episodically increases the intrathoracic pressure and can generate systemic blood pressures higher than those usually generated by conventional chest compressions,[23,24] allowing patients to maintain consciousness[23–26] for a brief arrhythmic interval (up to 92 seconds documented in humans).[25]

"Cough" CPR has been reported exclusively in awake, monitored patients (predominantly in the cardiac catheterization laboratory) when arrhythmic cardiac arrest can be anticipated, the patient remains conscious and can be instructed before and coached during the event, and cardiac activity can be promptly restored.[23–33] However, not all victims are able to produce hemodynamically effective coughs.[27]

"Cough" CPR is not useful for unresponsive victims and should not be taught to lay rescuers. "Cough" CPR may be considered in settings such as the cardiac catheterization laboratory for conscious, supine, and monitored patients if the patient can be instructed and coached to cough forcefully every 1 to 3 seconds during the initial seconds of an arrhythmic cardiac arrest. It should not delay definitive treatment (Class IIb, LOE C).

## Prone CPR

When the patient cannot be placed in the supine position, it may be reasonable for rescuers to provide CPR with the patient in the prone position, particularly in hospitalized patients with an advanced airway in place (Class IIb, LOE C).[34–37]

## Precordial Thump

This section is new to the 2010 Guidelines and is based on the conclusions reached by the 2010 ILCOR evidence evaluation process.[38]

A precordial thump has been reported to convert ventricular tachyarrhythmias in 1 study with concurrent controls,[39] single-patient case reports, and small case series.[40–44] However, 2 larger case series found that the precordial thump was ineffective in 79 (98.8%) of 80 cases[45] and in 153 (98.7%) of 155 cases of malignant ventricular arrhythmias.[46] Case reports and case series[47–49] have documented complications associated with precordial thump including sternal fracture, osteomyelitis, stroke, and triggering of malignant arrhythmias in adults and children.

The precordial thump should not be used for unwitnessed out-of-hospital cardiac arrest (Class III, LOE C). The precordial thump may be considered for patients with witnessed, monitored, unstable ventricular tachycardia including pulseless VT if a defibrillator is not immediately ready for use (Class IIb, LOE C), but it should not delay CPR and shock delivery. There is insufficient evidence to recommend for or against the use of the precordial thump for witnessed onset of asystole.

## Percussion Pacing

Percussion (eg, fist) pacing refers to the use of regular, rhythmic and forceful percussion of the chest with the rescuer's fist in an attempt to pace the myocardium. There is little evidence supporting fist or percussion pacing in cardiac arrest based on 6 single-patient case reports[50–55] and a moderate-sized case series.[56] There is insufficient evidence to recommend percussion pacing during typical attempted resuscitation from cardiac arrest.

# CPR Devices

## Devices to Assist Ventilation

### *Automatic and Mechanical Transport Ventilators*

*Automatic Transport Ventilators*
There are very few studies evaluating the use of automatic transport ventilators (ATVs) during attempted resuscitation in patients with endotracheal intubation. During prolonged resuscitation efforts, the use of an ATV (pneumatically powered and time- or pressure-cycled) may provide ventilation and oxygenation similar to that possible with the use of a manual resuscitation bag, while allowing the Emergency Medical Services (EMS) team to perform other tasks (Class IIb, LOE C[57,58]). Disadvantages of ATVs include the need for an oxygen source and a power source. Thus, providers should always have a bag-mask device available for manual backup.

For additional information regarding support of airway and ventilation in the adult, see ACLS Part 8.1 in these Guidelines.

### Manually Triggered, Oxygen-Powered, Flow-Limited Resuscitators

In a study of 104 anesthetized nonarrest patients without an advanced airway in place (ie, no endotracheal tube; patients were ventilated through a mask), patients ventilated by firefighters with manually triggered, oxygen-powered, flow-limited resuscitators had less gastric inflation than those ventilated with a bag-mask device.[59] Manually triggered, oxygen-powered, flow-limited resuscitators may be considered for the management of patients who do not have an advanced airway in place and for whom a mask is being used for ventilation during CPR (Class IIb, LOE C). Rescuers should avoid using the automatic mode of the oxygen-powered, flow-limited resuscitator during CPR because it may generate high positive end-expiratory pressure (PEEP) that may impede venous return during chest compressions and compromise forward blood flow (Class III, LOE C[60]).

## Devices to Support Circulation

### Active Compression-Decompression CPR

Active compression-decompression CPR (ACD-CPR) is performed with a device that includes a suction cup to actively lift the anterior chest during decompression. The application of external negative suction during the decompression phase of CPR creates negative intrathoracic pressure and thus potentially enhances venous return to the heart. When used, the device is positioned at midsternum on the chest.

Results from the use of ACD-CPR have been mixed. In several studies[61-66] ACD-CPR improved ROSC and short-term survival compared with conventional CPR. Of these studies, 3 showed improvement in neurologically intact survival.[61,64,65] In contrast, 1 Cochrane meta-analysis of 10 studies involving both in-hospital arrest (826 patients) and out-of-hospital arrest (4162 patients)[67] and several other controlled trials[68-74] comparing ACD-CPR to conventional CPR showed no difference in ROSC or survival. The meta-analysis[67] did not find any increase in ACD-CPR–related complications.

There is insufficient evidence to recommend for or against the routine use of ACD-CPR. ACD-CPR may be considered for use when providers are adequately trained and monitored (Class IIb, LOE B).

### Phased Thoracic-Abdominal Compression-Decompression CPR With a Handheld Device

Phased thoracic-abdominal compression-decompression CPR (PTACD-CPR) combines the concepts of IAC-CPR and ACD-CPR. A handheld device alternates chest compression and abdominal decompression with chest decompression and abdominal compression. Evidence from 1 prospective randomized clinical study of adults in cardiac arrest[75] demonstrated no improvement in survival to hospital discharge with use of PTACD-CPR during out-of-hospital cardiac arrest.

There is insufficient evidence to support or refute the use of PTACD-CPR for the treatment of cardiac arrest.

### Impedance Threshold Device

The impedance threshold device (ITD) is a pressure-sensitive valve that is attached to an endotracheal tube, supraglottic airway, or face mask. The ITD limits air entry into the lungs during the decompression phase of CPR, creating negative intrathoracic pressure and improving venous return to the heart and cardiac output during CPR. It does so without impeding positive pressure ventilation or passive exhalation.

Originally, the ITD was used with a cuffed endotracheal tube during bag-tube ventilation and ACD-CPR.[76-78] The ITD and ACD-CPR devices are thought to act synergistically to enhance venous return. During ACD-CPR with or without the ITD, 1 randomized study[76] found no difference in survival, whereas another randomized study[79] found that the addition of an ITD improved short-term survival (24-hour survival and survival to ICU admission).

The ITD also has been used during conventional CPR with an endotracheal tube or with a face mask, if a tight seal is maintained.[77,80,81] During conventional CPR with and without the ITD, 1 randomized trial[80] reported no difference in overall survival; however, 1 prospective cohort study[82] reported improved survival to emergency department (ED) admission with the use of the ITD. One meta-analysis of pooled data from both conventional CPR and ACD-CPR randomized trials[83] demonstrated improved ROSC and short-term survival associated with the use of an ITD in the management of adult out-of-hospital cardiac arrest patients but no significant improvement in either survival to hospital discharge or neurologically intact survival to discharge.

Three cohort studies with historic controls that implemented 2005 Guidelines plus ITD demonstrated improved survival to hospital discharge for out-of-hospital cardiac arrest.[84-86] It was not possible to determine the relative contribution of the ITD to the improved outcome. The use of the ITD may be considered by trained personnel as a CPR adjunct in adult cardiac arrest (Class IIb, LOE B).

### Mechanical Piston Devices

A mechanical piston device consists of a compressed gas- or electric-powered plunger mounted on a backboard; it is used to depress the sternum. Some incorporate a suction cup in the piston device while others do not. In 3 studies[87-89] the use of a mechanical piston device for CPR improved end-tidal $CO_2$ and mean arterial pressure during adult cardiac arrest resuscitation. However, compared with manual CPR, no improvement in short- and long-term survival in adult patients was demonstrated.[87,90] Initiation and removal of the mechanical piston device were noted to increase interruptions in CPR.[91]

The Lund University Cardiac Arrest System (LUCAS) is a gas- (oxygen or air) or electric-powered piston device that produces a consistent chest compression rate and depth. It incorporates a suction cup attached to the sternum that returns the sternum to the starting position. There are no randomized control trials comparing the device with conventional CPR in human cardiac arrests. One case series with concurrent controls[92] showed no benefit over conventional CPR for out-of-hospital witnessed cardiac arrest. Additional case series have reported variable success with the device.[93–98] One feasibility study reported successful deployment during diagnostic and interventional procedures.[99]

There is insufficient evidence to support or refute the routine use of mechanical piston devices in the treatment of cardiac arrest. Mechanical piston devices may be considered for use by properly trained personnel in specific settings for the treatment of adult cardiac arrest in circumstances (eg, during diagnostic and interventional procedures) that make manual resuscitation difficult (Class IIb, LOE C). Rescuers should attempt to limit substantial interruptions in CPR during deployment. The device should be programmed to deliver high-quality CPR, ensuring an adequate compression depth of at least 2 inches (5 cm)—this may require conversion from a percent of chest depth, a rate of at least 100 compressions per minute, and a compression duration of approximately 50% of the cycle length.

### Load-Distributing Band CPR or Vest CPR

The load-distributing band (LDB) is a circumferential chest compression device composed of a pneumatically or electrically actuated constricting band and backboard. Case series have demonstrated improved hemodynamics,[100] ROSC,[101,102] and survival to hospital discharge with use of the LDB for cardiac arrest.[102] In a study using concurrent controls,[103] the use of LDB-CPR was associated with lower odds of 30-day survival (odds ratio 0.4). One multicenter prospective randomized controlled trial[104,104A] comparing LDB-CPR (Autopulse device) to manual CPR for out-of-hospital cardiac arrest demonstrated no improvement in 4-hour survival and worse neurologic outcome when the device was used. These results raised concerns about possible harm with use of this device. Further studies are required to determine whether site-specific factors[105] and experience with deployment of the device[106] could influence its efficacy.

The LDB may be considered for use by properly trained personnel in specific settings for the treatment of cardiac arrest (Class IIb, LOE B). However, there is insufficient evidence to support the routine use of the LDB in the treatment of cardiac arrest.

## Extracorporeal Techniques and Invasive Perfusion Devices

### Extracorporeal CPR

For the purpose of these Guidelines, extracorporeal membrane oxygenation (ECMO) and cardiopulmonary bypass are considered together as different forms of extracorporeal CPR (ECPR; an alternative term may be extracorporeal life support or ECLS) when either is used for resuscitation for cardiac arrest. Both are sophisticated

techniques for circulating blood outside the body with or without extracorporeal oxygenation, with the goal of supporting the body's circulation in the absence of an adequately functioning cardiac pump. The initiation of ECPR and the management of a patient on ECPR require highly trained personnel and specialized equipment.

Although there are no data from randomized studies to support the routine use of ECPR, in case series and observational studies the use of ECPR for in-hospital[107,108] and out-of-hospital[109–111] cardiac arrest has been associated with improved survival when compared with conventional CPR in patients <75 years old with potentially correctable conditions. However, supportive studies consisted of small numbers of patients, and some had unbalanced comparison groups with respect to age, witnessed arrest, bystander CPR, and the quality of conventional CPR.

There are no randomized studies that compare ECPR with conventional CPR for patients in cardiac arrest. However, data from several case series have demonstrated the feasibility and safety of ECPR in highly specialized centers.[108,110,111] Observational studies of adults in both the in-hospital[107] and out-of-hospital[109] settings have demonstrated an association between ECPR use and improved survival when compared with conventional CPR in patients with potentially correctable conditions. These studies had small numbers of patients, and some had unbalanced comparison groups with respect to age, witness status, bystander CPR, and the quality of conventional CPR. Please refer to the Pediatrics section for discussion and specific recommendations related to the pediatric population (See Part 14: "Pediatric Advanced Life Support").

There is insufficient evidence to recommend the routine use of ECPR for patients in cardiac arrest. However, in settings where ECPR is readily available, it may be considered when the time without blood flow is brief and the condition leading to the cardiac arrest is reversible (eg, accidental hypothermia drug intoxication) or amenable to heart transplantation (eg, myocarditis) or revascularization (eg, acute myocardial infarction) (Class IIb, LOE C).

## Summary

A variety of CPR techniques and devices may improve hemodynamics or short-term survival when used by well-trained providers in selected patients. All of these techniques and devices have the potential to delay chest compressions and defibrillation. In order to prevent delays and maximize efficiency, initial training, ongoing monitoring, and retraining programs should be offered to providers on a frequent and ongoing basis. To date, no adjunct has consistently been shown to be superior to standard conventional (manual) CPR for out-of-hospital basic life support, and no device other than a defibrillator has consistently improved long-term survival from out-of-hospital cardiac arrest.

# Disclosures

## Guidelines Part 7: CPR Techniques and Devices: Writing Group Disclosures

| Writing Group Member | Employment | Research Grant | Other Research Support | Speakers' Bureau/Honoraria | Ownership Interest | Consultant/Advisory Board | Other |
|---|---|---|---|---|---|---|---|
| Diana M. Cave | Legacy Health System, Emanuel Hospital, Emergency Services–RN, MSN; Portland Com. College–Institute for Health Prof.-Faculty/Instructor | None | None | None | None | None | None |
| Raul Gazmuri | North Chicago VA Medical Center–Section Chief, Critical Care and Professor of Medicine | †Volume-Controlled Manual Ventilation during Resuscitation from Cardiac Arrest. Funded by Dessinier Corporation. Funds come to my institution (Rosalind Franklin UniversityRFU) Vitamin-C Preserves Myocardial Distensibility during Resuscitation from CA. Funded by Maribor University, Slovenia. Funds come to my institution (RFU) | None | None | †Patent titled "Facilitation of Resuscitation from Cardiac Arrest by Erythropoietin" (pending) | None | None |
| Charles W. Otto | University of Arizona–Professor | None | None | None | None | None | None |
| Vinay M. Nadkarni | University of Pennsylvania/The Children's Hospital of Philadelphia–Attending Physician, Departement of Anesthesia, Critical Care and Pediatrics | None | None | None | None | None | *Voluntary (Unpaid) member of Data Safety Monitoring Committee for Automated CPR device trial |
| Adam Cheng | British Columbia Children's Hospital: University Affiliated–Director, Pediatric Simulation Program | †American Heart Association RFP - educational grant. Money comes to my institution, and is distributed to our group of collaborative pediatric hospitals | None | None | None | None | None |
| Steven C. Brooks | University of Toronto–Clinician-Scientist | †PI-1. Univ.of Toronto Faculty of Medicine New Staff Grant. 01/07/2009–01/07/2010 A pilot study to explore missed opportunities for public access defibrillation in OHCA and to determine the potential impact of emergency medical dispatchers. Role: PI $10,000 unrestricted grant administered through the research institute 2. University of Toronto Connaught New Staff Matching Grant 2009–2010. 04/05/2009–03/05/2011 Development of Centres of Excellence to Improve Outcomes after OHCAt: A Pilot Study. Role: PI $23,700 unrestricted grant administered through the research institute 3. Ontario Ministry of Health and Long Term Care and the Sunnybrook Medical Services Alternative Funding Plan Association. 04/22/2009–04/21/2010 2008–2009 Alternative Funding Plan Phase III Innovation Fund Project Funding. Project: "Inventing the Future of Post Cardiac Arrest Care: Collaborative Development of Standardized Patient Care Pathways at Sunnybrook Health Sciences Centre." Role: PI $100,000 unrestricted grant administered through the research institute Co-Investigator 1. National Institutes of Health Slutsky AS (PI) 01/09/2004–01/09/2009 From Bench to Bedside to Curbside. Clinical Research Consortium to improve Resuscitation. Role: Co-Investigator $2, 454, 201 US 2. Canadian Institute of Health Research Slutsky AS (PI) 01/04/2005–01/10/2010 Epistry component of the Resuscitation Outcomes Consortium. Role: Co-Investigator $500,001 3. Laerdal Foundation for Acute Medicine Morrison LJ (PI) 01/12/2007–01/12/2010 Centre Grant Program for knowledge translation projects in post resuscitation care. Role: Co-Investigator $150,000 4. Heart and Stroke Foundation of Canada. Morrison LJ & Dorian P (Co-PI's) 01/12/2007–01/12/2009 Operating Grant in the Area of Resuscitation and Knowledge Transfer for the Strategies in Post-Arrest Care (SPARC) project. Role: Co-Investigator $200,000 | None | None | None | None | None |

*(Continued)*

**Guidelines Part 7: CPR Techniques and Devices: Writing Group Disclosures,** *Continued*

| Writing Group Member | Employment | Research Grant | Other Research Support | Speakers' Bureau/Honoraria | Ownership Interest | Consultant/Advisory Board | Other |
|---|---|---|---|---|---|---|---|
| Mohamud Daya | Oregon Health & Science University: Attending Physician–Associate Professor of Emergency Medicine | †PI Resuscitation Outcomes Consoritum - Portland Site, NHLBI, grant is awarded directly to the insitution (OHSU) | None | *Lectures at local, regional and national meetings, income is directly to me, last lectures CPR update at the Timberline EMS conference, there was no honorarium but conference paid for my lodging Stroke Update in Corvallis at Samaritan Health, Honorarium fee was 500 dollars Advanced 12 lead ECG diagnostic algoritms, Lecutre for Philips Healthcare at EMS today, honoarium for 2 lectures was 1000 dollars | *Stock held in the following health care companies; Johnson and Johnson - 250 shares Amgen - 100 shares Roche - 100 shares | *Philips Health Care - Consultant on 12 lead ECG diagnostic algorithms and resuscitation products, no reimbursement for this activity | †I am an EMS medical director for 2 fire departments and one 911 agency, this is a private contract and the money comes directly to me, this is independent of my employment at OHSU which is at an 80% FTE level, my EMS activities are 20% FTE |
| Robert M. Sutton | The Children's Hospital of Philadelphia–Critical Care Attending | *Unrestricted Research Grant Support through a Center of Excellence Grant from the Laerdal Found | None | None | None | None | |
| Richard Branson | University of Cincinnati-Associate Professor | None | †SeQual. Sponsor of laboratory study of the use of oxygen concentrators in conjunction with mechanical ventilators for military and mass casualty scenarios. $40,000. All monies are paid to the Univ. I have no financial interest in the company and do not receive any personal income | †Cardinal - makers of ICU and home care ventilators. I am paid directly for speaking. Newport Medical makers of ICU and home care ventilators. I am paid directly for speaking. *IKARIA - manufactures and distributes inhaled nitric oxide. I am paid directly | None | *Bayer Pharmaceuticals. Treatment of ventilator associated pneumonia | *KIngs Daughters Hospital Ashland KY. Paid directly to me |
| Mary Fran Hazinski | Vanderbilt University School of Nursing—Professor; American Heart Association– Senior Science Editor †Significant AHA compensation for my editing responsibilities-writing and editing of the 2010 AHA Guidelines for CPR and ECC | None | None | None | None | None | None |

This table represents the relationships of writing group members that may be perceived as actual or reasonably perceived conflicts of interest as reported on the Disclosure Questionnaire, which all members of the writing group are required to complete and submit. A relationship is considered to be "significant" if (a) the person receives $10 000 or more during any 12-month period, or 5% or more of the person's gross income; or (b) the person owns 5% or more of the voting stock or share of the entity, or owns $10 000 or more of the fair market value of the entity. A relationship is considered to be "modest" if it is less than "significant" under the preceding definition.

*Modest.

†Significant.

# References

1. Ornato JP, Gonzalez ER, Garnett AR, Levine RL, McClung BK. Effect of cardiopulmonary resuscitation compression rate on end-tidal carbon dioxide concentration and arterial pressure in man. *Crit Care Med.* 1988;16:241–245.

2. Swenson RD, Weaver WD, Niskanen RA, Martin J, Dahlberg S. Hemodynamics in humans during conventional and experimental methods of cardiopulmonary resuscitation. *Circulation.* 1988;78:630–639.

3. Kern KB, Sanders AB, Raife J, Milander MM, Otto CW, Ewy GA. A study of chest compression rates during cardiopulmonary resuscitation in humans: the importance of rate-directed chest compressions. *Arch Intern Med.* 1992;152:145–149.

4. Raman J, Saldanha RF, Branch JM, Esmore DS, Spratt PM, Farnsworth AE, Harrison GA, Chang VP, Shanahan MX. Open cardiac compression in the postoperative cardiac intensive care unit. *Anaesth Intensive Care.* 1989;17:129–135.

5. Anthi A, Tzelepis GE, Alivizatos P, Michalis A, Palatianos GM, Geroulanos S. Unexpected cardiac arrest after cardiac surgery: incidence, predisposing causes, and outcome of open chest cardiopulmonary resuscitation. *Chest.* 1998;113:15–19.

6. Pottle A, Bullock I, Thomas J, Scott L. Survival to discharge following Open Chest Cardiac Compression (OCCC): a 4-year retrospective audit in a cardiothoracic specialist centre–Royal Brompton and Harefield NHS Trust, United Kingdom. *Resuscitation.* 2002;52:269–272.

7. Takino M, Okada Y. The optimum timing of resuscitative thoracotomy for non-traumatic out-of-hospital cardiac arrest. *Resuscitation.* 1993;26:69–74.

8. Boczar ME, Howard MA, Rivers EP, Martin GB, Horst HM, Lewandowski C, Tomlanovich MC, Nowak RM. A technique revisited: hemodynamic comparison of closed- and open-chest cardiac massage during human cardiopulmonary resuscitation. *Crit Care Med.* 1995;23:498–503.

9. Hachimi-Idrissi S, Leeman J, Hubloue Y, Huyghens L, Corne L. Open chest cardiopulmonary resuscitation in out-of-hospital cardiac arrest. *Resuscitation*. 1997;35:151–156.

10. Calinas-Correia J, Phair I. Physiological variables during open chest cardiopulmonary resuscitation: results from a small series. *J Accid Emerg Med*. 2000;17:201–204.

11. Fialka C, Sebok C, Kemetzhofer P, Kwasny O, Sterz F, Vecsei V. Open-chest cardiopulmonary resuscitation after cardiac arrest in cases of blunt chest or abdominal trauma: a consecutive series of 38 cases. *J Trauma*. 2004;57:809–814.

12. Powell DW, Moore EE, Cothren CC, Ciesla DJ, Burch JM, Moore JB, Johnson JL. Is emergency department resuscitative thoracotomy futile care for the critically injured patient requiring prehospital cardiopulmonary resuscitation? *J Am Coll Surg*. 2004;199:211–215.

13. Sheppard FR, Cothren CC, Moore EE, Orfanakis A, Ciesla DJ, Johnson JL, Burch JM. Emergency department resuscitative thoracotomy for nontorso injuries. *Surgery*. 2006;139:574–576.

14. Seamon MJ, Fisher CA, Gaughan JP, Kulp H, Dempsey DT, Goldberg AJ. Emergency department thoracotomy: survival of the least expected. *World J Surg*. 2008;32:604–612.

15. Powell RW, Gill EA, Jurkovich GJ, Ramenofsky ML. Resuscitative thoracotomy in children and adolescents. *Am Surg*. 1988;54:188–191.

16. Rothenberg SS, Moore EE, Moore FA, Baxter BT, Moore JB, Cleveland HC. Emergency Department thoracotomy in children–a critical analysis. *J Trauma*. 1989;29:1322–1325.

17. Sack JB, Kesselbrenner MB, Jarrad A. Interposed abdominal compression-cardiopulmonary resuscitation and resuscitation outcome during asystole and electromechanical dissociation. *Circulation*. 1992; 86:1692–1700.

18. Sack JB, Kesselbrenner MB, Bregman D. Survival from in-hospital cardiac arrest with interposed abdominal counterpulsation during cardiopulmonary resuscitation. *JAMA*. 1992;267:379–385.

19. Babbs CF. Interposed abdominal compression CPR: a comprehensive evidence based review. *Resuscitation*. 2003;59:71–82.

20. Babbs CF. Simplified meta-analysis of clinical trials in resuscitation. *Resuscitation*. 2003;57:245–255.

21. Mateer JR, Stueven HA, Thompson BM, Aprahamian C, Darin JC. Pre-hospital IAC-CPR versus standard CPR: paramedic resuscitation of cardiac arrests. *Am J Emerg Med*. 1985;3:143–146.

22. Waldman PJ, Walters BL, Grunau CF. Pancreatic injury associated with interposed abdominal compressions in pediatric cardiopulmonary resuscitation. *Am J Emerg Med*. 1984;2:510–512.

23. Miller B, Cohen A, Serio A, Bettock D. Hemodynamics of cough cardiopulmonary resuscitation in a patient with sustained torsades de pointes/ventricular flutter. *J Emerg Med*. 1994;12:627–632.

24. Keeble W, Tymchak WJ. Triggering of the Bezold Jarisch Reflex by reperfusion during primary PCI with maintenance of consciousness by cough CPR: a case report and review of pathophysiology. *J Invasive Cardiol*. 2008;20:E239–E242.

25. Niemann JT, Rosborough J, Hausknecht M, Brown D, Criley JM. Cough-CPR: documentation of systemic perfusion in man and in an experimental model: a "window" to the mechanism of blood flow in external CPR. *Crit Care Med*. 1980;8:141–146.

26. Saba SE, David SW. Sustained consciousness during ventricular fibrillation: case report of cough cardiopulmonary resuscitation. *Cathet Cardiovasc Diagn*. 1996;37:47–48.

27. Criley JM, Blaufuss AH, Kissel GL. Cough-induced cardiac compression: self-administered form of cardiopulmonary resuscitation. *JAMA*. 1976;236:1246–1250.

28. Wei JY, Greene HL, Weisfeldt ML. Cough-facilitated conversion of ventricular tachycardia. *Am J Cardiol*. 1980;45:174–176.

29. Caldwell G, Millar G, Quinn E, Vincent R, Chamberlain DA. Simple mechanical methods for cardioversion: defence of the precordial thump and cough version. *Br Med J (Clin Res Ed)*. 1985;291:627–630.

30. Miller B, Lesnefsky E, Heyborne T, Schmidt B, Freeman K, Breckinridge S, Kelley K, Mann D, Reiter M. Cough-cardiopulmonary resuscitation in the cardiac catheterization laboratory: hemodynamics during an episode of prolonged hypotensive ventricular tachycardia. *Cathet Cardiovasc Diagn*. 1989;18:168–171.

31. Rieser MJ. The use of cough-CPR in patients with acute myocardial infarction. *J Emerg Med*. 1992;10:291–293.

32. Petelenz T, Iwinski J, Chlebowczyk J, Czyz Z, Flak Z, Fiutowski L, Zaorski K, Zeman S. Self-administered cough cardiopulmonary resuscitation (c-CPR) in patients threatened by MAS events of cardiovascular origin. *Wiad Lek*. 1998;51(7–8):326–336.

33. Girsky MJ, Criley JM. Images in cardiovascular medicine. Cough cardiopulmonary resuscitation revisited. *Circulation*. 2006;114:e530–531.

34. Mazer SP, Weisfeldt M, Bai D, Cardinale C, Arora R, Ma C, Sciacca RR, Chong D, Rabbani LE. Reverse CPR: a pilot study of CPR in the prone position. *Resuscitation*. 2003;57:279–285.

35. Sun WZ, Huang FY, Kung KL, Fan SZ, Chen TL. Successful cardiopulmonary resuscitation of two patients in the prone position using reversed precordial compression. *Anesthesiology*. 1992;77:202–204.

36. Tobias JD, Mencio GA, Atwood R, Gurwitz GS. Intraoperative cardiopulmonary resuscitation in the prone position. *J Pediatr Surg*. 1994;29: 1537–1538.

37. Brown J, Rogers J, Soar J. Cardiac arrest during surgery and ventilation in the prone position: a case report and systematic review. *Resuscitation*. 2001;50:233–238.

38. Shuster M, Lim SH, Deakin CD, Kleinman ME, Koster RW, Morrison LJ, Nolan JP, Sayre MR; on behalf of the CPR Techniques and Devices Collaborators. Part 7: CPR techniques and devices: 2010 International Consensus on Cardiopulmonary Resuscitation and Emergency Cardiovascular Care Science with Treatment Recommendations. *Circulation*. 2010;122(suppl 2):S338–S344.

39. Pellis T, Kette F, Lovisa D, Franceschino E, Magagnin L, Mercante WP, Kohl P. Utility of pre-cordial thump for treatment of out of hospital cardiac arrest: a prospective study. *Resuscitation*. 2009;80:17–23.

40. Bornemann C, Scherf D. Electrocardiogram of the month. Paroxysmal ventricular tachycardia abolished by a blow to the precordium. *Dis Chest*. 1969;56:83–84.

41. Dale KM, Lertsburapa K, Kluger J, White CM. Moxifloxacin and torsade de pointes. *Ann Pharmacother*. 2007;41:336–340.

42. De Maio VJ, Stiell IG, Spaite DW, Ward RE, Lyver MB, Field BJ III, Munkley DP, Wells GA. CPR-only survivors of out-of-hospital cardiac arrest: implications for out-of-hospital care and cardiac arrest research methodology. *Ann Emerg Med*. 2001;37:602–608.

43. Pennington JE, Taylor J, Lown B. Chest thump for reverting ventricular tachycardia. *N Engl J Med*. 1970;283:1192–1195.

44. Rahner E, Zeh E. Die Regularisierung von Kammertachykardien durch präkordialen Faustschlag. ("The Regularization of Ventricular Tachycardias by Precordial Thumping.") *Med Welt*. 1978;29: 1659–1663.

45. Amir O, Schliamser JE, Nemer S, Arie M. Ineffectiveness of precordial thump for cardioversion of malignant ventricular tachyarrhythmias. *Pacing Clin Electrophysiol*. 2007;30:153–156.

46. Haman L, Parizek P, Vojacek J. Precordial thump efficacy in termination of induced ventricular arrhythmias. *Resuscitation*. 2009;80: 14–16.

47. Ahmar W, Morley P, Marasco S, Chan W, Aggarwal A. Sternal fracture and osteomyelitis: an unusual complication of a precordial thump. *Resuscitation*. 2007;75:540–542.

48. Miller J, Tresch D, Horwitz L, Thompson BM, Aprahamian C, Darin JC. The precordial thump. *Ann Emerg Med*. 1984;13(9 Pt 2):791–794.

49. Muller GI, Ulmer HE, Bauer JA. Complications of chest thump for termination of supraventricular tachycardia in children. *Eur J Pediatr*. 1992;151:12–14.

50. Chan L, Reid C, Taylor B. Effect of three emergency pacing modalities on cardiac output in cardiac arrest due to ventricular asystole. *Resuscitation*. 2002;52:117–119.

51. Dowdle JR. Ventricular standstill and cardiac percussion. *Resuscitation*. 1996;32:31–32.

52. Eich C, Bleckmann A, Schwarz SK. Percussion pacing–an almost forgotten procedure for haemodynamically unstable bradycardias? A report of three case studies and review of the literature. *Br J Anaesth*. 2007; 98:429–433.

53. Eich C, Bleckmann A, Paul T. Percussion pacing in a three-year-old girl with complete heart block during cardiac catheterization. *Br J Anaesth*. 2005;95:465–467.

54. Iseri LT, Allen BJ, Baron K, Brodsky MA. Fist pacing, a forgotten procedure in bradyasystolic cardiac arrest. *Am Heart J*. 1987;113: 1545–1550.

55. Tucker KJ, Shaburihvili TS, Gedevanishvili AT. Manual external (fist) pacing during high-degree atrioventricular block: a lifesaving intervention. *Am J Emerg Med*. 1995;13:53–54.

56. Zeh E, Rahner E. [The manual extrathoracal stimulation of the heart. Technique and effect of the precordial thump (author's transl)]. *Z Kardiol*. 1978;67:299–304.

57. Weiss SJ, Ernst AA, Jones R, Ong M, Filbrun T, Augustin C, Barnum M, Nick TG. Automatic transport ventilator versus bag valve in the EMS setting: a prospective, randomized trial. *South Med J*. 2005;98:970–976.

58. Johannigman JA, Branson RD, Johnson DJ, Davis K Jr, Hurst JM. Out-of-hospital ventilation: bag–valve device vs transport ventilator. *Acad Emerg Med*. 1995;2:719–724.

59. Noordergraaf GJ, van Dun PJ, Kramer BP, Schors MP, Hornman HP, de Jong W, Noordergraaf A. Can first responders achieve and maintain normocapnia when sequentially ventilating with a bag-valve device and two oxygen-driven resuscitators? A controlled clinical trial in 104 patients. *Eur J Anaesthesiol*. 2004;21:367–372.

60. Hevesi ZG, Thrush DN, Downs JB, Smith RA. Cardiopulmonary resuscitation: effect of CPAP on gas exchange during chest compressions. *Anesthesiology*. 1999;90:1078–1083.

61. Cohen TJ, Goldner BG, Maccaro PC, Ardito AP, Trazzera S, Cohen MB, Dibs SR. A comparison of active compression-decompression cardiopulmonary resuscitation with standard cardiopulmonary resuscitation for cardiac arrests occurring in the hospital. *N Engl J Med*. 1993;329:1918–1921.

62. Lurie KG, Shultz JJ, Callaham ML, Schwab TM, Gisch T, Rector T, Frascone RJ, Long L. Evaluation of active compression-decompression CPR in victims of out-of-hospital cardiac arrest. *JAMA*. 1994;271:1405–1411.

63. Tucker KJ, Galli F, Savitt MA, Kahsai D, Bresnahan L, Redberg RF. Active compression-decompression resuscitation: effect on resuscitation success after in-hospital cardiac arrest. *J Am Coll Cardiol*. 1994;24:201–209.

64. Plaisance P, Adnet F, Vicaut E, Hennequin B, Magne P, Prudhomme C, Lambert Y, Cantineau JP, Leopold C, Ferracci C, Gizzi M, Payen D. Benefit of active compression-decompression cardiopulmonary resuscitation as a prehospital advanced cardiac life support: a randomized multicenter study. *Circulation*. 1997;95:955–961.

65. Plaisance P, Lurie KG, Vicaut E, Adnet F, Petit JL, Epain D, Ecollan P, Gruat R, Cavagna P, Biens J, Payen D. A comparison of standard cardiopulmonary resuscitation and active compression-decompression resuscitation for out-of-hospital cardiac arrest. French Active Compression-Decompression Cardiopulmonary Resuscitation Study Group. *N Engl J Med*. 1999;341:569–575.

66. He Q, Wan Z, Wang L. [Random control trial of the efficacy of cardiopump on pre-hospital cardiac arrest]. *Zhongguo Wei Zhong Bing Ji Jiu Yi Xue*. 2003;15:292–294.

67. Lafuente-Lafuente C, Melero-Bascones M. Active chest compression-decompression for cardiopulmonary resuscitation. *Cochrane Database Syst Rev*. 2004;:CD002751.

68. Mauer D, Schneider T, Dick W, Withelm A, Elich D, Mauer M. Active compression-decompression resuscitation: a prospective, randomized study in a two-tiered EMS system with physicians in the field. *Resuscitation*. 1996;33:125–134.

69. Stiell IG, Hebert PC, Wells GA, Laupacis A, Vandemheen K, Dreyer JF, Eisenhauer MA, Gibson J, Higginson LA, Kirby AS, Mahon JL, Maloney JP, Weitzman BN. The Ontario trial of active compression-decompression cardiopulmonary resuscitation for in-hospital and pre-hospital cardiac arrest. *JAMA*. 1996;275:1417–1423.

70. Goralski M, Villeger JL, Cami G, Linassier P, Guilles-Des-Buttes P, Fabbri P, Venot P, Tazarourte K, Cami M. Evaluation of active compression-decompression cardiopulmonary resuscitation in out-of-hospital cardiac arrest. *Reanimation Urgences*. 1998;7:543–550.

71. Skogvoll E, Wik L. Active compression-decompression cardiopulmonary resuscitation: a population-based, prospective randomised clinical trial in out-of-hospital cardiac arrest. *Resuscitation*. 1999;42:163–172.

72. Schwab TM, Callaham ML, Madsen CD, Utecht TA. A randomized clinical trial of active compression-decompression CPR vs standard CPR in out-of-hospital cardiac arrest in two cities. *JAMA*. 1995;273:1261–1268.

73. Luiz T, Ellinger K, Denz C. Active compression-decompression cardiopulmonary resuscitation does not improve survival in patients with prehospital cardiac arrest in a physician-manned emergency medical system. *J Cardiothorac Vasc Anesth*. 1996;10:178–186.

74. Nolan J, Smith G, Evans R, McCusker K, Lubas P, Parr M, Baskett P. The United Kingdom pre-hospital study of active compression-decompression resuscitation. *Resuscitation*. 1998;37:119–125.

75. Arntz HR, Agrawal R, Richter H, Schmidt S, Rescheleit T, Menges M, Burbach H, Schroder J, Schultheiss HP. Phased chest and abdominal compression-decompression versus conventional cardiopulmonary

76. Plaisance P, Lurie KG, Payen D. Inspiratory impedance during active compression-decompression cardiopulmonary resuscitation: a randomized evaluation in patients in cardiac arrest. *Circulation*. 2000;101:989–994.

77. Plaisance P, Soleil C, Lurie KG, Vicaut E, Ducros L, Payen D. Use of an inspiratory impedance threshold device on a facemask and endotracheal tube to reduce intrathoracic pressures during the decompression phase of active compression-decompression cardiopulmonary resuscitation. *Crit Care Med*. 2005;33:990–994.

78. Wolcke BB, Mauer DK, Schoefmann MF, Teichmann H, Provo TA, Lindner KH, Dick WF, Aeppli D, Lurie KG. Comparison of standard cardiopulmonary resuscitation versus the combination of active compression-decompression cardiopulmonary resuscitation and an inspiratory impedance threshold device for out-of-hospital cardiac arrest. *Circulation*. 2003;108:2201–2205.

79. Plaisance P, Lurie KG, Vicaut E, Martin D, Gueugniaud PY, Petit JL, Payen D. Evaluation of an impedance threshold device in patients receiving active compression-decompression cardiopulmonary resuscitation for out of hospital cardiac arrest. *Resuscitation*. 2004;61:265–271.

80. Aufderheide TP, Pirrallo RG, Provo TA, Lurie KG. Clinical evaluation of an inspiratory impedance threshold device during standard cardiopulmonary resuscitation in patients with out-of-hospital cardiac arrest. *Crit Care Med*. 2005;33:734–740.

81. Pirrallo RG, Aufderheide TP, Provo TA, Lurie KG. Effect of an inspiratory impedance threshold device on hemodynamics during conventional manual cardiopulmonary resuscitation. *Resuscitation*. 2005;66:13–20.

82. Thayne RC, Thomas DC, Neville JD, Van Dellen A. Use of an impedance threshold device improves short-term outcomes following out-of-hospital cardiac arrest. *Resuscitation*. 2005;67:103–108.

83. Cabrini L, Beccaria P, Landoni G, Biondi-Zoccai GG, Sheiban I, Cristofolini M, Fochi O, Maj G, Zangrillo A. Impact of impedance threshold devices on cardiopulmonary resuscitation: a systematic review and meta-analysis of randomized controlled studies. *Crit Care Med*. 2008;36:1625–1632.

84. Aufderheide T, Alexander C, Lick C, Myers B, Romig L, Vartanian L, Stothert J, McKnite S, Matsuura T, Yannopoulos D, Lurie K. From laboratory science to six emergency medical services systems: new understanding of the physiology of cardiopulmonary resuscitation increase survival rates after cardiac arrest. *Crit Care Med*. 2008;36(11[Suppl.]):S397–S404.

85. Aufderheide TP, Yannopoulos D, Lick CJ, Myers B, Romig LA, Stothert JC, Barnard J, Vartanian L, Pilgrim AJ, Benditt DG. Implementing the 2005 American Heart Association Guidelines improves outcomes after out-of-hospital cardiac arrest. April 26, 2010. doi:10.1016/j.hrthm.2010.04.022. Available at: http://www.heartrhythmjournal.com/article/PIIS1547527110003078/fulltext.

86. Hinchey PR, Myers JB, Lewis R, De Maio VJ, Reyer E, Licatese D, Zalkin J, Snyder G. Improved out-of-hospital cardiac arrest survival after the sequential implementation of 2005 AHA guidelines for compressions, ventilations, and induced hypothermia: the Wake County experience. *Ann Emerg Med*. 2010. April 1, 2010. doi:10.1016/j.annemergmed.2010.01.036. Available at: http://www.annemergmed.com/article/S0196-0644(10)00116-2/fulltext.

87. Dickinson ET, Verdile VP, Schneider RM, Salluzzo RF. Effectiveness of mechanical versus manual chest compressions in out-of-hospital cardiac arrest resuscitation: a pilot study. *Am J Emerg Med*. 1998;16:289–292.

88. McDonald JL. Systolic and mean arterial pressures during manual and mechanical CPR in humans. *Ann Emerg Med*. 1982;11:292–295.

89. Ward KR, Menegazzi JJ, Zelenak RR, Sullivan RJ, McSwain NE Jr. A comparison of chest compressions between mechanical and manual CPR by monitoring end-tidal PCO2 during human cardiac arrest. *Ann Emerg Med*. 1993;22:669–674.

90. Taylor GJ, Rubin R, Tucker M, Greene HL, Rudikoff MT, Weisfeldt ML. External cardiac compression: a randomized comparison of mechanical and manual techniques. *JAMA*. 1978;240:644–646.

91. Wang HC, Chiang WC, Chen SY, Ke YL, Chi CL, Yang CW, Lin PC, Ko PC, Wang YC, Tsai TC, Huang CH, Hsiung KH, Ma MH, Chen SC, Chen WJ, Lin FY. Video-recording and time-motion analyses of manual versus mechanical cardiopulmonary resuscitation during ambulance transport. *Resuscitation*. 2007;74:453–460.

92. Axelsson C, Nestin J, Svensson L, Axelsson AB, Herlitz J. Clinical consequences of the introduction of mechanical chest compression in the EMS system for treatment of out-of-hospital cardiac arrest-a pilot study. *Resuscitation*. 2006;71:47–55.

93. Steen S, Liao Q, Pierre L, Paskevicius A, Sjoberg T. Evaluation of LUCAS, a new device for automatic mechanical compression and active decompression resuscitation. *Resuscitation*. 2002;55:285–299.

94. Steen S, Sjoberg T, Olsson P, Young M. Treatment of out-of-hospital cardiac arrest with LUCAS, a new device for automatic mechanical compression and active decompression resuscitation. *Resuscitation*. 2005;67:25–30.

95. Larsen AI, Hjornevik AS, Ellingsen CL, Nilsen DW. Cardiac arrest with continuous mechanical chest compression during percutaneous coronary intervention: a report on the use of the LUCAS device. *Resuscitation*. 2007;75:454–459.

96. Deakin CD, O'Neill JF, Tabor T. Does compression-only cardiopulmonary resuscitation generate adequate passive ventilation during cardiac arrest? *Resuscitation*. 2007;75:53–59.

97. Bonnemeier H, Olivecrona G, Simonis G, Gotberg M, Weitz G, Iblher P, Gerling I, Schunkert H. Automated continuous chest compression for in-hospital cardiopulmonary resuscitation of patients with pulseless electrical activity: a report of five cases. *Int J Cardiol*. 2009;136: e39–e50.

98. Wagner H, Terkelsen CJ, Friberg H, Harnek J, Kern K, Lassen JF, Olivecrona GK. Cardiac arrest in the catheterisation laboratory: a 5-year experience of using mechanical chest compressions to facilitate PCI during prolonged resuscitation efforts. *Resuscitation*. 2009.

99. Wirth S, Korner M, Treitl M, Linsenmaier U, Leidel BA, Jaschkowitz T, Reiser MF, Kanz KG. Computed tomography during cardiopulmonary resuscitation using automated chest compression devices: an initial study. *Eur Radiol*. 2009;19:1857–1866.

100. Timerman S, Cardoso LF, Ramires JA, Halperin H. Improved hemodynamic performance with a novel chest compression device during treatment of in-hospital cardiac arrest. *Resuscitation*. 2004;61:273–280.

101. Casner M, Andersen D, Isaacs SM. The impact of a new CPR assist device on rate of return of spontaneous circulation in out-of-hospital cardiac arrest. *Prehosp Emerg Care*. 2005;9:61–67.

102. Ong ME, Ornato JP, Edwards DP, Dhindsa HS, Best AM, Ines CS, Hickey S, Clark B, Williams DC, Powell RG, Overton JL, Peberdy MA. Use of an automated, load-distributing band chest compression device for out-of-hospital cardiac arrest resuscitation. *JAMA*. 2006;295: 2629–2637.

103. Steinmetz J, Barnung S, Nielsen SL, Risom M, Rasmussen LS. Improved survival after an out-of-hospital cardiac arrest using new guidelines. *Acta Anaesthesiol Scand*. 2008;52:908–913.

104. Hallstrom A, Rea TD, Sayre MR, Christenson J, Anton AR, Mosesso VN Jr, Van Ottingham L, Olsufka M, Pennington S, White LJ, Yahn S, Husar J, Morris MF, Cobb LA. Manual chest compression vs use of an automated chest compression device during resuscitation following out-of-hospital cardiac arrest: a randomized trial. *JAMA*. 2006;295: 2620–2628.

104A. Hallstrom A, Rea TD, Sayre MR, Christenson J, Cobb LA, Mosesso VN Jr, Anton AR. The ASPIRE trial investigators respond to inhomogenity and temporal effects assertion. *Am J Emerg Med*. August 16, 2010. doi:10.1016/j.ajem.2010.07.001. Available at: http://www.ajem-journal.com/article/S0735-6757(10)00307-4/fulltext.

105. Paradis N, Young G, Lemeshow S, Brewer J, Halperin H. Inhomogeneity and temporal effects in ASPIRE - An Exception from Consent Trial Terminated Early. *Am J Emerg Med*. In Press.

106. Tomte O, Sunde K, Lorem T, Auestad B, Souders C, Jensen J, Wik L. Advanced life support performance with manual and mechanical chest compressions in a randomized, multicentre manikin study. *Resuscitation*. 2009;80:1152–1157.

107. Chen YS, Lin JW, Yu HY, Ko WJ, Jerng JS, Chang WT, Chen WJ, Huang SC, Chi NH, Wang CH, Chen LC, Tsai PR, Wang SS, Hwang JJ, Lin FY. Cardiopulmonary resuscitation with assisted extracorporeal life-support versus conventional cardiopulmonary resuscitation in adults with in-hospital cardiac arrest: an observational study and propensity analysis. *Lancet*. 2008;372:554–561.

108. Athanasuleas CL, Buckberg GD, Allen BS, Beyersdorf F, Kirsh MM. Sudden cardiac death: directing the scope of resuscitation towards the heart and brain. *Resuscitation*. 2006;70:44–51.

109. Tanno K, Itoh Y, Takeyama Y, Nara S, Mori K, Asai Y. Utstein style study of cardiopulmonary bypass after cardiac arrest. *Am J Emerg Med*. 2008;26:649–654.

110. Chen YS, Yu HY, Huang SC, Lin JW, Chi NH, Wang CH, Wang SS, Lin FY, Ko WJ. Extracorporeal membrane oxygenation support can extend the duration of cardiopulmonary resuscitation. *Crit Care Med*. 2008;36:2529–2535.

111. Nagao K, Kikushima K, Watanabe K, Tachibana E, Tominaga Y, Tada K, Ishii M, Chiba N, Kasai A, Soga T, Matsuzaki M, Nishikawa K, Tateda Y, Ikeda H, Yagi T. Early induction of hypothermia during cardiac arrest improves neurological outcomes in patients with out-of-hospital cardiac arrest who undergo emergency cardiopulmonary bypass and percutaneous coronary intervention. *Circ J*. 2010;74:77–85.

KEY WORDS: cardiac arrest ■ cardiopulmonary resuscitation ■ emergency ■ ventricular fibrillation

# Part 8: Adult Advanced Cardiovascular Life Support

## 2010 American Heart Association Guidelines for Cardiopulmonary Resuscitation and Emergency Cardiovascular Care

Robert W. Neumar, Chair; Charles W. Otto; Mark S. Link; Steven L. Kronick;
Michael Shuster; Clifton W. Callaway; Peter J. Kudenchuk; Joseph P. Ornato; Bryan McNally;
Scott M. Silvers; Rod S. Passman; Roger D. White; Erik P. Hess; Wanchun Tang;
Daniel Davis; Elizabeth Sinz; Laurie J. Morrison

Advanced cardiovascular life support (ACLS) impacts multiple key links in the chain of survival that include interventions to prevent cardiac arrest, treat cardiac arrest, and improve outcomes of patients who achieve return of spontaneous circulation (ROSC) after cardiac arrest. ACLS interventions aimed at preventing cardiac arrest include airway management, ventilation support, and treatment of bradyarrhythmias and tachyarrhythmias. For the treatment of cardiac arrest, ACLS interventions build on the basic life support (BLS) foundation of immediate recognition and activation of the emergency response system, early CPR, and rapid defibrillation to further increase the likelihood of ROSC with drug therapy, advanced airway management, and physiologic monitoring. Following ROSC, survival and neurologic outcome can be improved with integrated post–cardiac arrest care.

Part 8 presents the 2010 Adult ACLS Guidelines: 8.1: "Adjuncts for Airway Control and Ventilation"; 8.2: "Management of Cardiac Arrest"; and 8.3: "Management of Symptomatic Bradycardia and Tachycardia." Post–cardiac arrest interventions are addressed in Part 9: "Post–Cardiac Arrest Care."

Key changes from the 2005 ACLS Guidelines include

- Continuous quantitative waveform capnography is recommended for confirmation and monitoring of endotracheal tube placement.
- Cardiac arrest algorithms are simplified and redesigned to emphasize the importance of high-quality CPR (including chest compressions of adequate rate and depth, allowing complete chest recoil after each compression, minimizing interruptions in chest compressions and avoiding excessive ventilation).
- Atropine is no longer recommended for routine use in the management of pulseless electrical activity (PEA)/asystole.
- There is an increased emphasis on physiologic monitoring to optimize CPR quality and detect ROSC.
- Chronotropic drug infusions are recommended as an alternative to pacing in symptomatic and unstable bradycardia.

- Adenosine is recommended as a safe and potentially effective therapy in the initial management of stable undifferentiated regular monomorphic wide-complex tachycardia.

## Part 8.1: Adjuncts for Airway Control and Ventilation

### Overview of Airway Management

This section highlights recommendations for the support of ventilation and oxygenation during CPR and the peri-arrest period. The purpose of ventilation during CPR is to maintain adequate oxygenation and sufficient elimination of carbon dioxide. However, research has not identified the optimal tidal volume, respiratory rate, and inspired oxygen concentration required during resuscitation from cardiac arrest.

Both ventilation and chest compressions are thought to be important for victims of prolonged ventricular fibrillation (VF) cardiac arrest and for all victims with other presenting rhythms. Because both systemic and pulmonary perfusion are substantially reduced during CPR, normal ventilation-perfusion relationships can be maintained with a minute ventilation that is much lower than normal. During CPR with an advanced airway in place, a lower rate of rescue breathing is needed to avoid hyperventilation.

### Ventilation and Oxygen Administration During CPR

During low blood flow states such as CPR, oxygen delivery to the heart and brain is limited by blood flow rather than by arterial oxygen content.[1,2] Therefore, rescue breaths are less important than chest compressions during the first few minutes of resuscitation from witnessed VF cardiac arrest and could reduce CPR efficacy due to interruption in chest compressions and the increase in intrathoracic pressure that accompanies positive-pressure ventilation. Thus, during the first few minutes of witnessed cardiac arrest a lone rescuer should not interrupt chest

---

The American Heart Association requests that this document be cited as follows: Neumar RW, Otto CW, Link MS, Kronick SL, Shuster M, Callaway CW, Kudenchuk PJ, Ornato JP, McNally B, Silvers SM, Passman RS, White RD, Hess EP, Tang W, Davis D, Sinz E, Morrison LJ. Part 8: adult advanced cardiovascular life support: 2010 American Heart Association Guidelines for Cardiopulmonary Resuscitation and Emergency Cardiovascular Care. *Circulation.* 2010;122(suppl 3):S729–S767.

(*Circulation.* **2010;122[suppl 3]:S729–S767.**)

*Circulation* **is available at http://circ.ahajournals.org**          DOI: 10.1161/CIRCULATIONAHA.110.970988

compressions for ventilation. Advanced airway placement in cardiac arrest should not delay initial CPR and defibrillation for VF cardiac arrest (Class I, LOE C).

## Oxygen During CPR

### Oxygen Administration During CPR

The optimal inspired oxygen concentration during adult CPR has not been established in human or animal studies. In addition, it is unknown whether 100% inspired oxygen ($F_{IO_2}=1.0$) is beneficial or whether titrated oxygen is better. Although prolonged exposure to 100% inspired oxygen ($F_{IO_2}=1.0$) has potential toxicity, there is insufficient evidence to indicate that this occurs during brief periods of adult CPR.[3–5] Empirical use of 100% inspired oxygen during CPR optimizes arterial oxyhemoglobin content and in turn oxygen delivery; therefore, use of 100% inspired oxygen ($F_{IO_2}=1.0$) as soon as it becomes available is reasonable during resuscitation from cardiac arrest (Class IIa, LOE C). Management of oxygen after ROSC is discussed in Part 9: "Post-Cardiac Arrest Care."

### Passive Oxygen Delivery During CPR

Positive-pressure ventilation has been a mainstay of CPR but recently has come under scrutiny because of the potential for increased intrathoracic pressure to interfere with circulation due to reduced venous return to the heart. In the out-of-hospital setting, passive oxygen delivery via mask with an opened airway during the first 6 minutes of CPR provided by emergency medical services (EMS) personnel was part of a protocol of bundled care interventions (including continuous chest compressions) that resulted in improved survival.[6–8] When passive oxygen delivery using a fenestrated tracheal tube (Boussignac tube) during uninterrupted physician-managed CPR was compared with standard CPR, there was no difference in oxygenation, ROSC, or survival to hospital admission.[9,10] Chest compressions cause air to be expelled from the chest and oxygen to be drawn into the chest passively due to the elastic recoil of the chest. In theory, because ventilation requirements are lower than normal during cardiac arrest, oxygen supplied by passive delivery is likely to be sufficient for several minutes after onset of cardiac arrest with a patent upper airway.[2] **At this time there is insufficient evidence to support the removal of ventilations from CPR performed by ACLS providers.**

## Bag-Mask Ventilation

Bag-mask ventilation is an acceptable method of providing ventilation and oxygenation during CPR but is a challenging skill that requires practice for continuing competency. All healthcare providers should be familiar with the use of the bag-mask device.[11,12] Use of bag-mask ventilation is not recommended for a lone provider. When ventilations are performed by a lone provider, mouth-to-mouth or mouth-to-mask are more efficient. When a second provider is available, bag-mask ventilation may be used by a trained and experienced provider. But bag-mask ventilation is most effective when performed by 2 trained and experienced providers. One provider opens the airway and seals the mask to the face while the other squeezes the bag. Bag-mask ventilation is particularly helpful when

placement of an advanced airway is delayed or unsuccessful. The desirable components of a bag-mask device are listed in Part 5: "Adult Basic Life Support."

The provider should use an adult (1 to 2 L) bag and the provider should deliver approximately 600 mL of tidal volume sufficient to produce chest rise over 1 second.[13] This volume of ventilation is adequate for oxygenation and minimizes the risk of gastric inflation. The provider should be sure to open the airway adequately with a head tilt–chin lift, lifting the jaw against the mask and holding the mask against the face, creating a tight seal. During CPR give 2 breaths (each 1 second) during a brief (about 3 to 4 seconds) pause after every 30 chest compressions.

Bag-mask ventilation can produce gastric inflation with complications, including regurgitation, aspiration, and pneumonia. Gastric inflation can elevate the diaphragm, restrict lung movement, and decrease respiratory system compliance.[14–16]

## Airway Adjuncts

### Cricoid Pressure

Cricoid pressure in nonarrest patients may offer some measure of protection to the airway from aspiration and gastric insufflation during bag-mask ventilation.[17–20] However, it also may impede ventilation and interfere with placement of a supraglottic airway or intubation.[21–27] The role of cricoid pressure during out-of-hospital cardiac arrest and in-hospital cardiac arrest has not been studied. If cricoid pressure is used in special circumstances during cardiac arrest, the pressure should be adjusted, relaxed, or released if it impedes ventilation or advanced airway placement. The routine use of cricoid pressure in cardiac arrest is not recommended (Class III, LOE C).

### Oropharyngeal Airways

Although studies have not specifically considered the use of oropharyngeal airways in patients with cardiac arrest, airways may aid in the delivery of adequate ventilation with a bag-mask device by preventing the tongue from occluding the airway. Incorrect insertion of an oropharyngeal airway can displace the tongue into the hypopharynx, causing airway obstruction. To facilitate delivery of ventilations with a bag-mask device, oropharyngeal airways can be used in unconscious (unresponsive) patients with no cough or gag reflex and should be inserted only by persons trained in their use (Class IIa, LOE C).

### Nasopharyngeal Airways

Nasopharyngeal airways are useful in patients with airway obstruction or those at risk for developing airway obstruction, particularly when conditions such as a clenched jaw prevent placement of an oral airway. Nasopharyngeal airways are better tolerated than oral airways in patients who are not deeply unconscious. Airway bleeding can occur in up to 30% of patients following insertion of a nasopharyngeal airway.[28] Two case reports of inadvertent intracranial placement of a nasopharyngeal airway in patients with basilar skull fractures[29,30] suggest that nasopharyngeal airways should be used with caution in patients with severe craniofacial injury.

As with all adjunctive equipment, safe use of the nasopharyngeal airway requires adequate training, practice, and retraining. No studies have specifically examined the use of nasopharyngeal airways in cardiac arrest patients. To facilitate delivery of ventilations with a bag-mask device, the nasopharyngeal airway can be used in patients with an obstructed airway. In the presence of known or suspected basal skull fracture or severe coagulopathy, an oral airway is preferred (Class IIa, LOE C).

## Advanced Airways

Ventilation with a bag and mask or with a bag through an advanced airway (eg, endotracheal tube or supraglottic airway) is acceptable during CPR. All healthcare providers should be trained in delivering effective oxygenation and ventilation with a bag and mask. Because there are times when ventilation with a bag-mask device is inadequate, ideally ACLS providers also should be trained and experienced in insertion of an advanced airway.

Providers must be aware of the risks and benefits of insertion of an advanced airway during a resuscitation attempt. Such risks are affected by the patient's condition and the provider's expertise in airway control. There are no studies directly addressing the timing of advanced airway placement and outcome during resuscitation from cardiac arrest. Although insertion of an endotracheal tube can be accomplished during ongoing chest compressions, intubation frequently is associated with interruption of compressions for many seconds. Placement of a supraglottic airway is a reasonable alternative to endotracheal intubation and can be done successfully without interrupting chest compressions.

The provider should weigh the need for minimally interrupted compressions against the need for insertion of an endotracheal tube or supraglottic airway. There is inadequate evidence to define the optimal timing of advanced airway placement in relation to other interventions during resuscitation from cardiac arrest. In a registry study of 25 006 in-hospital cardiac arrests, earlier time to invasive airway (<5 minutes) was not associated with improved ROSC but was associated with improved 24-hour survival.[31] In an urban out-of-hospital setting, intubation that was achieved in <12 minutes was associated with better survival than intubation achieved in ≥13 minutes.[32]

In out-of-hospital urban and rural settings, patients intubated during resuscitation had a better survival rate than patients who were not intubated,[33] whereas in an in-hospital setting, patients who required intubation during CPR had a worse survival rate.[34] A recent study[8] found that delayed endotracheal intubation combined with passive oxygen delivery and minimally interrupted chest compressions was associated with improved neurologically intact survival after out-of-hospital cardiac arrest in patients with adult witnessed VF/pulseless VT. If advanced airway placement will interrupt chest compressions, providers may consider deferring insertion of the airway until the patient fails to respond to initial CPR and defibrillation attempts or demonstrates ROSC (Class IIb, LOE C).

For a patient with perfusing rhythm who requires intubation, pulse oximetry and electrocardiographic (ECG) status should be monitored continuously during airway placement. Intubation attempts should be interrupted to provide oxygenation and ventilation as needed.

To use advanced airways effectively, healthcare providers must maintain their knowledge and skills through frequent practice. It may be helpful for providers to master one primary method of airway control. Providers should have a second (backup) strategy for airway management and ventilation if they are unable to establish the first-choice airway adjunct. Bag-mask ventilation may serve as that backup strategy.

Once an advanced airway is inserted, providers should immediately perform a thorough assessment to ensure that it is properly positioned. This assessment should not interrupt chest compressions. Assessment by physical examination consists of visualizing chest expansion bilaterally and listening over the epigastrium (breath sounds should not be heard) and the lung fields bilaterally (breath sounds should be equal and adequate). A device also should be used to confirm correct placement (see the section "Endotracheal Intubation" below).

Continuous waveform capnography is recommended in addition to clinical assessment as the most reliable method of confirming and monitoring correct placement of an endotracheal tube (Class I, LOE A). Providers should observe a persistent capnographic waveform with ventilation to confirm and monitor endotracheal tube placement in the field, in the transport vehicle, on arrival at the hospital, and after any patient transfer to reduce the risk of unrecognized tube misplacement or displacement.

The use of capnography to confirm and monitor correct placement of supraglottic airways has not been studied, and its utility will depend on airway design. However, effective ventilation through a supraglottic airway device should result in a capnograph waveform during CPR and after ROSC.

Once an advanced airway is in place, the 2 providers should no longer deliver cycles of CPR (ie, compressions interrupted by pauses for ventilation) unless ventilation is inadequate when compressions are not paused. Instead the compressing provider should give continuous chest compressions at a rate of at least 100 per minute, without pauses for ventilation. The provider delivering ventilation should provide 1 breath every 6 to 8 seconds (8 to 10 breaths per minute). Providers should avoid delivering an excessive ventilation rate because doing so can compromise venous return and cardiac output during CPR. The 2 providers should change compressor and ventilator roles approximately every 2 minutes to prevent compressor fatigue and deterioration in quality and rate of chest compressions. When multiple providers are present, they should rotate the compressor role about every 2 minutes.

### Supraglottic Airways

Supraglottic airways are devices designed to maintain an open airway and facilitate ventilation. Unlike endotracheal intubation, intubation with a supraglottic airway does not require visualization of the glottis, so both initial training and maintenance of skills are easier. Also, because direct visualization is not necessary, a supraglottic airway is inserted without interrupting compressions. Supraglottic airways that have been studied in cardiac arrest are the laryngeal mask airway (LMA), the esophageal-tracheal tube (Combitube) and the laryngeal tube

(Laryngeal Tube or King LT). When prehospital providers are trained in the use of advanced supraglottic airways such as the esophageal-tracheal tube, laryngeal tube, and the laryngeal mask airway, they appear to be able to use these devices safely and can provide ventilation that is as effective as that provided with a bag and mask or an endotracheal tube.[12,35–41]

Advanced airway interventions are technically complicated. Failure can occur; thus maintenance of skills through frequent experience or practice is essential.[42] It is important to remember that there is no evidence that advanced airway measures improve survival rates in the setting of out-of-hospital cardiac arrest. During CPR performed by providers trained in its use, the supraglottic airway is a reasonable alternative to bag-mask ventilation (Class IIa, LOE B) and endotracheal intubation (Class IIa, LOE A).

### Esophageal-Tracheal Tube

The advantages of the esophageal-tracheal tube (Combitube) are similar to the advantages of the endotracheal tube when either is compared with bag-mask ventilation: isolation of the airway, reduced risk of aspiration, and more reliable ventilation. The advantages of the esophageal-tracheal tube over the endotracheal tube are related chiefly to ease of training.[12,43] Ventilation and oxygenation with the esophageal-tracheal tube compare favorably with those achieved with the endotracheal tube.[44]

In several controlled clinical trials involving both in-hospital and out-of-hospital resuscitation of adults, providers with all levels of experience were able to insert the esophageal-tracheal tube and deliver ventilation comparable to that achieved with endotracheal intubation.[35,45–48] In a retrospective study no difference in outcome was observed in patients treated with the esophageal-tracheal tube compared with those treated with endotracheal intubation.[38] The esophageal-tracheal tube is reported to provide successful ventilation during CPR in 62% to 100% of patients.[35,45–49] For healthcare professionals trained in its use, the esophageal-tracheal tube is an acceptable alternative to both bag-mask ventilation (Class IIa, LOE C) or endotracheal intubation (Class IIa, LOE A) for airway management in cardiac arrest.

Fatal complications may occur with use of the esophageal-tracheal tube if the position of the distal lumen of the esophageal-tracheal tube in the esophagus or trachea is identified incorrectly. For this reason, confirmation of tube placement is essential. Other possible complications related to the use of the esophageal-tracheal tube are esophageal trauma, including lacerations, bruising, and subcutaneous emphysema.[45,50,51]

### Laryngeal Tube

The advantages of the laryngeal tube (Laryngeal Tube or King LT) are similar to those of the esophageal-tracheal tube; however, the laryngeal tube is more compact and less complicated to insert (unlike the esophageal-tracheal tube, the laryngeal tube can only go into the esophagus). At this time there are limited data published on the use of the laryngeal tube in cardiac arrest.[40,41,52,53] In one case series assessing 40 out-of-hospital cardiac arrest patients, insertion of the laryngeal tube by trained paramedics was successful and ventilation was effective in 85% of patients.[41] For 3 patients, ventilation was ineffective because of cuff rupture; for 3 other patients, ventilation was ineffective because of massive regurgitation and aspiration before laryngeal tube placement.

Another out-of-hospital assessment of 157 attempts at laryngeal tube placement revealed a 97% success rate in a mixed population of cardiac arrest and noncardiac arrest patients.[40] For healthcare professionals trained in its use, the laryngeal tube may be considered as an alternative to bag-mask ventilation (Class IIb, LOE C) or endotracheal intubation for airway management in cardiac arrest (Class IIb, LOE C).

### Laryngeal Mask Airway

The laryngeal mask airway provides a more secure and reliable means of ventilation than the face mask.[54,55] Although the laryngeal mask airway does not ensure absolute protection against aspiration, studies have shown that regurgitation is less likely with the laryngeal mask airway than with the bag-mask device and that aspiration is uncommon. When compared with the endotracheal tube, the laryngeal mask airway provides equivalent ventilation[49,55]; successful ventilation during CPR has been reported in 72% to 97% of patients.[36,37,44,56–58]

Because insertion of the laryngeal mask airway does not require laryngoscopy and visualization of the vocal cords, training in its placement and use is simpler than that for endotracheal intubation. The laryngeal mask airway also may have advantages over the endotracheal tube when access to the patient is limited,[59,60] there is a possibility of unstable neck injury,[61] or appropriate positioning of the patient for endotracheal intubation is impossible.

Results from studies in anesthetized patients comparing the laryngeal mask airway with endotracheal intubation, as well as additional studies comparing it with other airways or ventilation techniques support the use of the laryngeal mask airway for airway control in a variety of settings by nurses, respiratory therapists, and EMS personnel, many of whom had not previously used this device.[12,39,44,55,62–65]

After successful insertion, a small proportion of patients cannot be ventilated with the laryngeal mask airway.[12,44,55] With this in mind, it is important for providers to have an alternative strategy for airway management. Providers who insert the laryngeal mask airway should receive adequate initial training and then should practice insertion of the device regularly. Success rates and the occurrence of complications should be monitored closely. For healthcare professionals trained in its use, the laryngeal mask airway is an acceptable alternative to bag-mask ventilation (Class IIa, LOE B) or endotracheal intubation (Class IIa, LOE C) for airway management in cardiac arrest.

### Endotracheal Intubation

The endotracheal tube was once considered the optimal method of managing the airway during cardiac arrest. However, intubation attempts by unskilled providers can produce complications, such as trauma to the oropharynx, interruption of compressions and ventilations for unacceptably long periods, and hypoxemia from prolonged intubation attempts or failure to recognize tube misplacement or displacement. It is now clear that the incidence of complications is unacceptably high when intubation is performed by inexperienced providers or monitoring of tube placement is inadequate. The optimal method of managing the airway during cardiac arrest will vary based on provider experience, characteristics of the

EMS or healthcare system, and the patient's condition. Frequent experience or frequent retraining is recommended for providers who perform endotracheal intubation (Class I, LOE B).[31,66] EMS systems that perform prehospital intubation should provide a program of ongoing quality improvement to minimize complications (Class IIa, LOE B).

No prospective randomized clinical trials have performed a direct comparison of bag-mask ventilation versus endotracheal intubation in adult victims of cardiac arrest. One prospective, randomized controlled trial in an EMS system with short out-of-hospital transport intervals[67] showed no survival advantage for endotracheal intubation over bag-mask ventilation in children; providers in this study had limited training and experience in intubation.

The endotracheal tube keeps the airway patent, permits suctioning of airway secretions, enables delivery of a high concentration of oxygen, provides an alternative route for the administration of some drugs, facilitates delivery of a selected tidal volume, and, with use of a cuff, may protect the airway from aspiration.

Indications for emergency endotracheal intubation are (1) the inability of the provider to ventilate the unconscious patient adequately with a bag and mask and (2) the absence of airway protective reflexes (coma or cardiac arrest). The provider must have appropriate training and experience in endotracheal intubation.

During CPR providers should minimize the number and duration of interruptions in chest compressions, with a goal to limit interruptions to no more than 10 seconds. Interruptions for supraglottic airway placement should not be necessary at all, whereas interruptions for endotracheal intubation can be minimized if the intubating provider is prepared to begin the intubation attempt—ie, insert the laryngoscope blade with the tube ready at hand—as soon as the compressing provider pauses compressions. Compressions should be interrupted only for the time required by the intubating provider to visualize the vocal cords and insert the tube; this is ideally less than 10 seconds. The compressing provider should be prepared to resume chest compressions immediately after the tube is passed through the vocal cords. If the initial intubation attempt is unsuccessful, a second attempt may be reasonable, but early consideration should be given to using a supraglottic airway.

In retrospective studies, endotracheal intubation has been associated with a 6% to 25% incidence of unrecognized tube misplacement or displacement.[68–72] This may reflect inadequate initial training or lack of experience on the part of the provider who performed intubation, or it may have resulted from displacement of a correctly positioned tube when the patient was moved. The risk of tube misplacement, displacement, or obstruction is high,[67,70] especially when the patient is moved.[73] Thus, even when the endotracheal tube is seen to pass through the vocal cords and tube position is verified by chest expansion and auscultation during positive-pressure ventilation, providers should obtain additional confirmation of placement using waveform capnography or an exhaled $CO_2$ or esophageal detector device (EDD).[74]

The provider should use both clinical assessment and confirmation devices to verify tube placement immediately after insertion and again when the patient is moved. However, no single confirmation technique is completely reliable.[75,76] Continuous waveform capnography is recommended in addition to clinical assessment as the most reliable method of confirming and monitoring correct placement of an endotracheal tube (Class I, LOE A).

If waveform capnography is not available, an EDD or nonwaveform exhaled $CO_2$ monitor in addition to clinical assessment is reasonable (Class IIa, LOE B). Techniques to confirm endotracheal tube placement are further discussed below.

*Clinical Assessment to Confirm Tube Placement*
Providers should perform a thorough assessment of endotracheal tube position immediately after placement. This assessment should not require interruption of chest compressions. Assessment by physical examination consists of visualizing chest expansion bilaterally and listening over the epigastrium (breath sounds should not be heard) and the lung fields bilaterally (breath sounds should be equal and adequate). A device should also be used to confirm correct placement in the trachea (see below). If there is doubt about correct tube placement, use the laryngoscope to visualize the tube passing through the vocal cords. If still in doubt, remove the tube and provide bag-mask ventilation until the tube can be replaced.

*Use of Devices to Confirm Tube Placement*
Providers should always use both clinical assessment and devices to confirm endotracheal tube location immediately after placement and throughout the resuscitation. Two studies of patients in cardiac arrest[72,77] demonstrated 100% sensitivity and 100% specificity for waveform capnography in identifying correct endotracheal tube placement in victims of cardiac arrest. However, 3 studies demonstrated 64% sensitivity and 100% specificity when waveform capnography was first used for victims with prolonged resuscitation and transport times.[78–80] All confirmation devices should be considered adjuncts to other confirmation techniques.

*Exhaled $CO_2$ Detectors.* Detection of exhaled $CO_2$ is one of several independent methods of confirming endotracheal tube position. Studies of waveform capnography to verify endotracheal tube position in victims of cardiac arrest have shown 100% sensitivity and 100% specificity in identifying correct endotracheal tube placement.[72,77,81–88] Continuous waveform capnography is recommended in addition to clinical assessment as the most reliable method of confirming and monitoring correct placement of an endotracheal tube (Class I, LOE A).

Given the simplicity of colorimetric and nonwaveform exhaled $CO_2$ detectors, these methods can be used in addition to clinical assessment as the initial method for confirming correct tube placement in a patient in cardiac arrest when waveform capnography is not available (Class IIa, LOE B). However, studies of colorimetric exhaled $CO_2$ detectors[89–94] and nonwaveform $PETCO_2$ capnometers[77,89,90,95] indicate that the accuracy of these devices does not exceed that of auscultation and direct visualization for confirming the tracheal position of an endotracheal tube in victims of cardiac arrest.

When exhaled $CO_2$ is detected (positive reading for $CO_2$) in cardiac arrest, it is usually a reliable indicator of tube position in the trachea. False-positive readings (ie, $CO_2$ is detected but the tube is located in the esophagus) have been observed in animals after ingestion of large amounts of carbonated liquids before the arrest; however, the waveform does not continue during subsequent breaths.[96]

False-negative readings (defined in this context as failure to detect $CO_2$ despite tube placement in the trachea) may be present during cardiac arrest for several reasons. The most common is that blood flow and delivery of $CO_2$ to the lungs is low. False-negative results also have been reported in association with pulmonary embolus because pulmonary blood flow and delivery of $CO_2$ to the lungs are reduced. If the detector is contaminated with gastric contents or acidic drugs (eg, endotracheally administered epinephrine), a color-imetric device may display a constant color rather than breath-to-breath color change. In addition, elimination and detection of $CO_2$ can be drastically reduced with severe airway obstruction (eg, status asthmaticus) and pulmonary edema.[93,97,98] For these reasons, if $CO_2$ is not detected, we recommend that a second method be used to confirm endo-tracheal tube placement, such as direct visualization or the esophageal detector device.

Use of $CO_2$-detecting devices to determine the correct placement of other advanced airways (eg, Combitube, laryn-geal mask airway) has not been studied; their utility will depend on airway design. However, effective ventilation through a supraglottic airway device should result in capno-graph waveform during CPR and after ROSC.

*Esophageal Detector Devices.* The EDD consists of a bulb that is compressed and attached to the endotracheal tube. If the tube is in the esophagus (positive result for an EDD), the suction created by the EDD will collapse the lumen of the esophagus or pull the esophageal tissue against the tip of the tube, and the bulb will not re-expand. The EDD may also consist of a syringe that is attached to the endotracheal tube; the provider attempts to pull the barrel of the syringe. If the tube is in the esophagus, it will not be possible to pull the barrel (aspirate air) with the syringe.

However, studies of the syringe aspiration EDD[79,99] and the self-inflating bulb EDD[78-80] indicate that the accuracy of these devices does not exceed that of auscultation and direct visualization for confirming the tracheal position of an endotracheal tube in victims of cardiac arrest. Given the simplicity of the EDD, it can be used as the initial method for confirming correct tube placement in addition to clinical assessment in the victim of cardiac arrest when waveform capnography is not available (Class IIa, LOE B).

The EDD may yield misleading results in patients with morbid obesity, late pregnancy, or status asthmaticus, or when there are copious endotracheal secretions,[100,101] because the trachea tends to collapse in the presence of these condi-tions. There is no evidence that the EDD is accurate for the continued monitoring of endotracheal tube placement.

*Thoracic Impedance.* Transthoracic impedance is slightly but significantly higher during inspiration than during exhala-tion.[102] Air is a poor electric conductor. Preliminary studies suggest that changes in thoracic impedance, as measured

through standard defibrillation pads, may distinguish tracheal from esophageal intubations.[103-105]

There are 2 published reports involving 6 patients where ventilation-induced changes in thoracic impedance disap-peared after esophageal intubation.[106,107] There is little evi-dence for the use of thoracic impedance in diagnosing adequacy of ventilation during CPR. Treatment decisions should not be based solely on thoracic impedance measure-ments until further study has confirmed its utility and accu-racy in this population.

*Postintubation Airway Management*
After inserting and confirming correct placement of an endotracheal tube, the provider should record the depth of the tube as marked at the front teeth or gums and secure it. There is significant potential for endotracheal tube move-ment with head flexion and extension[108-110] and when the patient is moved from one location to another.[111,112] Continuous monitoring of endotracheal tube placement with waveform capnography is recommended as discussed above. The endotracheal tube should be secured with tape or a commercial device (Class I, LOE C). Devices and tape should be applied in a manner that avoids compression of the front and sides of the neck, which may impair venous return from the brain.

One out-of-hospital study[113] and 2 studies in an intensive-care setting[114,115] indicate that backboards, commercial de-vices for securing the endotracheal tube, and other strategies provide equivalent methods for preventing inadvertent tube displacement when compared with traditional methods of securing the tube (tape). These devices may be considered during patient transport (Class IIb, LOE C). After tube confirmation and fixation, obtain a chest x-ray (when feasi-ble) to confirm that the end of the endotracheal tube is properly positioned above the carina.

*Ventilation After Advanced Airway Placement*
Except for respiratory rate, it is unknown whether monitoring ventilatory parameters (eg, minute ventilation, peak pressure) during CPR will influence outcome. However, positive-pressure ventilation increases intrathoracic pressure and may reduce venous return and cardiac output, especially in pa-tients with hypovolemia or obstructive airway disease. Ven-tilation at high respiratory rates (>25 breaths per minute) is common during resuscitation from cardiac arrest.[116,117] In animal models, slower ventilation rates (6 to 12 breaths per minute) are associated with improved hemodynamic param-eters and short-term survival.[116,118-124]

Because cardiac output is lower than normal during cardiac arrest, the need for ventilation is reduced. Follow-ing placement of an advanced airway, the provider deliv-ering ventilations should perform 1 breath every 6 to 8 seconds (8 to 10 breaths per minute) without pausing in applying chest compressions (unless ventilation is inade-quate when compressions are not paused) (Class IIb, LOE C). Monitoring respiratory rate coupled with real-time feedback during CPR may result in better compliance with ventilation guidelines.[125]

### Automatic Transport Ventilators

In both out-of-hospital and in-hospital settings, automatic transport ventilators (ATVs) can be useful for ventilation of adult patients in noncardiac arrest who have an advanced airway in place (Class IIb, LOE C). There are very few studies evaluating the use of ATVs attached to advanced airways during ongoing resuscitative efforts. During prolonged resuscitative efforts the use of an ATV (pneumatically powered and time- or pressure-cycled) may allow the EMS team to perform other tasks while providing adequate ventilation and oxygenation (Class IIb, LOE C).[126,127] Providers should always have a bag-mask device available for backup.

### Suction Devices

Both portable and installed suction devices should be available for resuscitation emergencies. Portable units should provide adequate vacuum and flow for pharyngeal suction. The suction device should be fitted with large-bore, nonkinking suction tubing and semirigid pharyngeal tips. Several sterile suction catheters of various sizes should be available for suctioning the lumen of the advanced airway, along with a nonbreakable collection bottle and sterile water for cleaning tubes and catheters. The installed suction unit should be powerful enough to provide an airflow of >40 L/min at the end of the delivery tube and a vacuum of >300 mm Hg when the tube is clamped. The amount of suction should be adjustable for use in children and intubated patients.

### Summary

All basic and advanced healthcare providers should be able to provide ventilation with a bag-mask device during CPR or when the patient demonstrates cardiorespiratory compromise. Airway control with an advanced airway, which may include an endotracheal tube or a supraglottic airway device, is a fundamental ACLS skill. Prolonged interruptions in chest compressions should be avoided during advanced airway placement. All providers should be able to confirm and monitor correct placement of advanced airways; this key skill is required to ensure the safe and effective use of these devices. Training, frequency of use, and monitoring of success and complications are more important than the choice of a specific advanced airway device for use during CPR.

## Part 8.2: Management of Cardiac Arrest

### Overview

This section details the general care of a patient in cardiac arrest and provides an overview of the 2010 ACLS Adult Cardiac Arrest Algorithms (Figures 1 and 2). Cardiac arrest can be caused by 4 rhythms: ventricular fibrillation (VF), pulseless ventricular tachycardia (VT), pulseless electric activity (PEA), and asystole. VF represents disorganized electric activity, whereas pulseless VT represents organized electric activity of the ventricular myocardium. Neither of these rhythms generates significant forward blood flow. PEA encompasses a heterogeneous group of organized electric rhythms that are associated with either absence of mechanical ventricular activity or mechanical ventricular activity that is insufficient to generate a clinically detectable pulse. Asystole (perhaps better described as ventricular asystole) represents absence of detectable ventricular electric activity with or without atrial electric activity.

Survival from these cardiac arrest rhythms requires both basic life support (BLS) and a system of advanced cardiovascular life support (ACLS) with integrated post–cardiac arrest care. The foundation of successful ACLS is high-quality CPR, and, for VF/pulseless VT, attempted defibrillation within minutes of collapse. For victims of witnessed VF arrest, early CPR and rapid defibrillation can significantly increase the chance for survival to hospital discharge.[128–133] In comparison, other ACLS therapies such as some medications and advanced airways, although associated with an increased rate of ROSC, have not been shown to increase the rate of survival to hospital discharge.[31,33,134–138] The majority of clinical trials testing these ACLS interventions, however, preceded the recently renewed emphasis on high-quality CPR and advances in post–cardiac arrest care (see Part 9: "Post–Cardiac Arrest Care"). Therefore, it remains to be determined if improved rates of ROSC achieved with ACLS interventions might better translate into improved long-term outcomes when combined with higher-quality CPR and post–cardiac arrest interventions such as therapeutic hypothermia and early percutaneous coronary intervention (PCI).

The 2010 ACLS Adult Cardiac Arrest Algorithms (Figures 1 and 2) are presented in the traditional box-and-line format and a new circular format. The 2 formats are provided to facilitate learning and memorization of the treatment recommendations discussed below. Overall these algorithms have been simplified and redesigned to emphasize the importance of high-quality CPR that is fundamental to the management of all cardiac arrest rhythms. Periodic pauses in CPR should be as brief as possible and only as necessary to assess rhythm, shock VF/VT, perform a pulse check when an organized rhythm is detected, or place an advanced airway. Monitoring and optimizing quality of CPR on the basis of either mechanical parameters (chest compression rate and depth, adequacy of relaxation, and minimization of pauses) or, when feasible, physiologic parameters (partial pressure of end-tidal $CO_2$ [$P_{ETCO_2}$], arterial pressure during the relaxation phase of chest compressions, or central venous oxygen saturation [$S_{cvO_2}$]) are encouraged (see "Monitoring During CPR" below). In the absence of an advanced airway, a synchronized compression–ventilation ratio of 30:2 is recommended at a compression rate of at least 100 per minute. After placement of a supraglottic airway or an endotracheal tube, the provider performing chest compressions should deliver at least 100 compressions per minute continuously without pauses for ventilation. The provider delivering ventilations should give 1 breath every 6 to 8 seconds (8 to 10 breaths per minute) and should be particularly careful to avoid delivering an excessive number of ventilations (see Part 8.1: "Adjuncts for Airway Control and Ventilation").

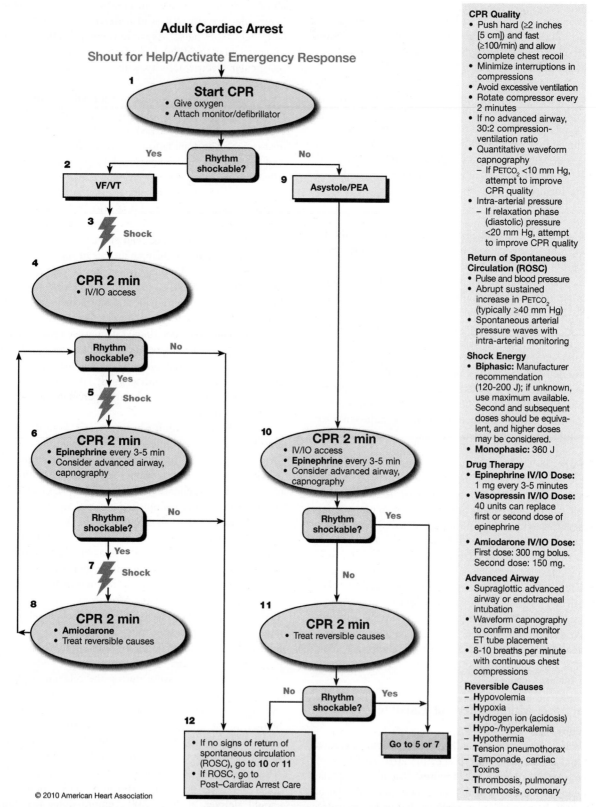

**Figure 1.** ACLS Cardiac Arrest Algorithm.

In addition to high-quality CPR, the only rhythm-specific therapy proven to increase survival to hospital discharge is defibrillation of VF/pulseless VT. Therefore, this intervention is included as an integral part of the CPR cycle when the rhythm check reveals VF/pulseless VT. Other ACLS inter-ventions during cardiac arrest may be associated with an increased rate of ROSC but have not yet been proven to increase survival to hospital discharge. Therefore, they are recommended as considerations and should be performed without compromising quality of CPR or timely defibril-

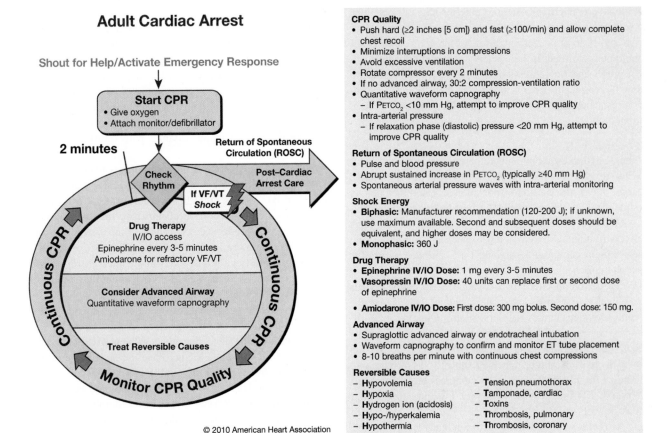

**Figure 2.** ACLS Cardiac Arrest Circular Algorithm.

lation. In other words, vascular access, drug delivery, and advanced airway placement should not cause significant interruptions in chest compression or delay defibrillation. There is insufficient evidence to recommend a specific timing or sequence (order) of drug administration and advanced airway placement during cardiac arrest. In most cases the timing and sequence of these secondary interventions will depend on the number of providers participating in the resuscitation and their skill levels. Timing and sequence will also be affected by whether vascular access has been established or an advanced airway placed before cardiac arrest.

Understanding the importance of diagnosing and treating the underlying cause is fundamental to management of all cardiac arrest rhythms. During management of cardiac arrest the provider should consider the H's and T's to identify and treat any factor that may have caused the arrest or may be complicating the resuscitative effort (Table 1).

It is common for the arrest rhythm to evolve during the course of resuscitation. In such cases management should shift smoothly to the appropriate rhythm-based strategy. In particular, providers should be prepared to deliver a timely shock when a patient who presented with asystole or PEA is found to be in VF/pulseless VT during a rhythm check. There is no evidence that the resuscitation strategy for a new cardiac arrest rhythm should necessarily be altered based on the characteristics of the previous rhythm. Medications administered during resuscitation should be monitored and total doses tabulated to avoid potential toxicity.

If the patient achieves ROSC, it is important to begin post–cardiac arrest care immediately to avoid rearrest and optimize the patient's chance of long-term survival with good neurologic function (see Part 9). Finally, the reality is that the majority of resuscitative efforts do not result in ROSC. Criteria for ending unsuccessful resuscitative efforts are addressed briefly below (see "When Should Resuscitative Efforts Stop?") and in more detail in Part 3: "Ethics."

## Rhythm-Based Management of Cardiac Arrest

In most cases of witnessed and unwitnessed cardiac arrest the first provider should start CPR with chest compressions and the second provider should get or turn on the defibrillator, place the adhesive pads or paddles, and check the rhythm. Paddles and electrode pads should be placed on the exposed chest in an anterior-lateral position. Acceptable alternative

**Table 1.    Treatable Causes of Cardiac Arrest: The H's and T's**

| H's | T's |
| --- | --- |
| Hypoxia | Toxins |
| Hypovolemia | Tamponade (cardiac) |
| Hydrogen ion (acidosis) | Tension pneumothorax |
| Hypo-/hyperkalemia | Thrombosis, pulmonary |
| Hypothermia | Thrombosis, coronary |

For further explanation of the H's and T's, see Part 12: "Special Resuscitation Situations."

positions are anterior-posterior, anterior-left infrascapular, and anterior-right infrascapular. Rhythm checks should be brief, and if an organized rhythm is observed, a pulse check should be performed. If there is any doubt about the presence of a pulse, chest compressions should be resumed immediately. If a cardiac monitor is attached to the patient at the time of arrest, the rhythm can be diagnosed before CPR is initiated.

### VF/Pulseless VT

When a rhythm check by an automated external defibrillator (AED) reveals VF/VT, the AED will typically prompt to charge, "clear" the victim for shock delivery, and then deliver a shock, all of which should be performed as quickly as possible. CPR should be resumed immediately after shock delivery (without a rhythm or pulse check and beginning with chest compressions) and continue for 2 minutes before the next rhythm check.

When a rhythm check by a manual defibrillator reveals VF/VT, the first provider should resume CPR while the second provider charges the defibrillator. Once the defibrillator is charged, CPR is paused to "clear" the patient for shock delivery. After the patient is "clear," the second provider gives a single shock as quickly as possible to minimize the interruption in chest compressions ("hands-off interval"). The first provider resumes CPR immediately after shock delivery (without a rhythm or pulse check and beginning with chest compressions) and continues for 2 minutes. After 2 minutes of CPR the sequence is repeated, beginning with a rhythm check.

The provider giving chest compressions should switch at every 2-minute cycle to minimize fatigue. CPR quality should be monitored based on mechanical or physiologic parameters (see "Monitoring During CPR" below).

### Defibrillation Strategies

#### Waveform and Energy

If a biphasic defibrillator is available, providers should use the manufacturer's recommended energy dose (120 to 200 J) for terminating VF (Class I, LOE B). If the provider is unaware of the effective dose range, the provider may use the maximal dose (Class IIb, LOE C). Second and subsequent energy levels should be at least equivalent, and higher energy levels may be considered if available (Class IIb, LOE B). If a monophasic defibrillator is used, providers should deliver an initial shock of 360 J and use that dose for all subsequent shocks. If VF is terminated by a shock but then recurs later in the arrest, deliver subsequent shocks at the previously successful energy level.

#### Automatic Versus Manual Modes for Multimodal Defibrillators

Use of a multimodal defibrillator in manual mode may reduce the duration of interruption of CPR required for rhythm analysis compared with automatic mode but could increase the frequency of inappropriate shock.[139,140] Current evidence indicates that the benefit of using a multimodal defibrillator in manual instead of automatic mode during cardiac arrest is uncertain (Class IIb, LOE C).

#### CPR Before Defibrillation

During treatment of VF/pulseless VT healthcare providers must ensure that coordination between CPR and shock delivery is efficient. When VF is present for more than a few minutes, the myocardium is depleted of oxygen and metabolic substrates. A brief period of chest compressions can deliver oxygen and energy substrates and "unload" the volume-overloaded right ventricle, increasing the likelihood that a perfusing rhythm will return after shock delivery.[141]

Performing CPR while a defibrillator is readied for use is strongly recommended for all patients in cardiac arrest (Class I, LOE B). Analyses of VF waveform characteristics predictive of shock success have documented that the shorter the time interval between the last chest compression and shock delivery, the more likely the shock will be successful.[141] A reduction of even a few seconds in the interval from pausing compressions to shock delivery can increase the probability of shock success.[142]

The value of intentionally delaying defibrillation to perform CPR is less clear. One randomized controlled trial (RCT)[143] and one clinical trial[144] involving adults with out-of-hospital cardiac arrest not witnessed by EMS personnel showed that survival was improved by a period of CPR performed before the first defibrillation shock when the EMS response interval was >4 to 5 minutes. But 2 RCTs[145,146] demonstrated no improvement in ROSC or survival to hospital discharge in patients with out-of-hospital VF or pulseless VT who received CPR from EMS personnel for 1.5 to 3 minutes before defibrillation, regardless of EMS response interval. At this time the benefit of delaying defibrillation to perform CPR before defibrillation is unclear (Class IIb, LOE B).

#### VF Waveform Analysis to Predict Defibrillation Success

Retrospective analysis of VF waveforms in multiple clinical studies suggests that it is possible to predict the success of defibrillation from the fibrillation waveform with varying reliability.[141,147–166] No prospective human studies have specifically evaluated whether treatment altered by predicting success of defibrillation can improve successful defibrillation, rate of ROSC, or survival from cardiac arrest. The value of VF waveform analysis to guide management of defibrillation in adults with in-hospital and out-of-hospital cardiac arrest is uncertain (Class IIb, LOE C).

### Drug Therapy in VF/Pulseless VT

When VF/pulseless VT persists after at least 1 shock and a 2-minute CPR period, a vasopressor can be given with the primary goal of increasing myocardial blood flow during CPR and achieving ROSC (see "Medications for Arrest Rhythms" below for dosing) (Class IIb, LOE A). The peak effect of an intravenous (IV)/intraosseous (IO) vasopressor given as a bolus dose during CPR is delayed for at least 1 to 2 minutes. The optimal timing of vasopressor administration during the 2-minute period of uninterrupted CPR has not been established. If a shock fails to generate a perfusing rhythm, then giving a vasopressor soon after the shock will optimize the potential impact of increased myocardial blood flow before the next shock. However, if a shock results in a perfusing rhythm, a bolus dose of vasopressor at any time during the subsequent 2-minute period of CPR (before rhythm check) could theoretically have detrimental effects on cardiovascular stability. This may be avoided by using physiologic monitoring such as quantitative waveform capnography, intra-arterial pressure monitoring, and continuous central venous oxygen saturation monitoring to detect ROSC during chest compressions.[93,167–177] However, adding an additional pause for rhythm and pulse check after shock delivery but before vasopressor therapy will decrease myocardial perfusion during the critical postshock period and could reduce the chance of achieving ROSC.

Amiodarone is the first-line antiarrhythmic agent given during cardiac arrest because it has been clinically demonstrated to improve the rate of ROSC and hospital admission in adults with refractory VF/pulseless VT. Amiodarone may be considered when VF/VT is unresponsive to CPR, defibrillation, and vasopressor therapy (Class IIb, LOE A). If amiodarone is unavailable, lidocaine may be considered, but in clinical studies lidocaine has not been demonstrated to improve rates of ROSC and hospital admission compared with amiodarone (Class IIb, LOE B). Magnesium sulfate should be considered only for torsades de pointes associated with a long QT interval (Class IIb, LOE B).

### Treating Potentially Reversible Causes of VF/Pulseless VT
The importance of diagnosing and treating the underlying cause of VF/pulseless VT is fundamental to the management of all cardiac arrest rhythms. As always, the provider should recall the H's and T's to identify a factor that may have caused the arrest or may be complicating the resuscitative effort (see Table 1 and Part 12: "Special Resuscitation Situations"). In the case of refractory VF/pulseless VT, acute coronary ischemia or myocardial infarction should be considered as a potential etiology. Reperfusion strategies such as coronary angiography and PCI during CPR or emergency cardiopulmonary bypass have been demonstrated to be feasible in a number of case studies and case series but have not been evaluated for their effectiveness in RCTs.[178–187] Fibrinolytic therapy administered during CPR for acute coronary occlusion has not been shown to improve outcome.[188]

### ROSC After VF/Pulseless VT
If the patient has ROSC, post–cardiac arrest care should be started (Part 9). Of particular importance are treatment of hypoxemia and hypotension, early diagnosis and treatment of ST-elevation myocardial infarction (STEMI) (Class I, LOE B) and therapeutic hypothermia in comatose patients (Class I, LOE B).

## PEA/Asystole
When a rhythm check by an AED reveals a nonshockable rhythm, CPR should be resumed immediately, beginning with chest compressions, and should continue for 2 minutes before the rhythm check is repeated. When a rhythm check using a manual defibrillator or cardiac monitor reveals *an organized rhythm*, a pulse check is performed. If a pulse is detected, post–cardiac arrest care should be initiated immediately (see

Part 9). If the rhythm is asystole or the pulse is absent (eg, PEA), CPR should be resumed immediately, beginning with chest compressions, and should continue for 2 minutes before the rhythm check is repeated. The provider performing chest compressions should switch every 2 minutes. CPR quality should be monitored on the basis of mechanical or physiologic parameters (see "Monitoring During CPR" below).

### Drug Therapy for PEA/Asystole
A vasopressor can be given as soon as feasible with the primary goal of increasing myocardial and cerebral blood flow during CPR and achieving ROSC (see "Vasopressors" below for dosing) (Class IIb, LOE A). Available evidence suggests that the routine use of atropine during PEA or asystole is unlikely to have a therapeutic benefit (Class IIb, LOE B). For this reason atropine has been removed from the cardiac arrest algorithm.

### Treating Potentially Reversible Causes of PEA/Asystole
PEA is often caused by reversible conditions and can be treated successfully if those conditions are identified and corrected. During each 2-minute period of CPR the provider should recall the H's and T's to identify factors that may have caused the arrest or may be complicating the resuscitative effort (see Table 1 and Part 12: "Special Resuscitation Situations"). Given the potential association of PEA with hypoxemia, placement of an advanced airway is theoretically more important than during VF/pulseless VT and might be necessary to achieve adequate oxygenation or ventilation. PEA caused by severe volume loss or sepsis will potentially benefit from administration of empirical IV/IO crystalloid. A patient with PEA caused by severe blood loss will potentially benefit from a blood transfusion. When pulmonary embolism is presumed or known to be the cause of cardiac arrest, empirical fibrinolytic therapy can be considered (Class IIa, LOE B; see Part 12). Finally, if tension pneumothorax is clinically suspected as the cause of PEA, initial management includes needle decompression. If available, echocardiography can be used to guide management of PEA because it provides useful information about intravascular volume status (assessing ventricular volume), cardiac tamponade, mass lesions (tumor, clot), left ventricular contractility, and regional wall motion.[189] See Part 12 for management of toxicological causes of cardiac arrest.

Asystole is commonly the end-stage rhythm that follows prolonged VF or PEA, and for this reason the prognosis is generally much worse.

### ROSC After PEA/Asystole
If the patient has ROSC, post–cardiac arrest care should be initiated (see Part 9). Of particular importance is treatment of hypoxemia and hypotension and early diagnosis and treatment of the underlying cause of cardiac arrest. Therapeutic hypothermia may be considered when the patient is comatose (Class IIb, LOE C).

## Monitoring During CPR

### Mechanical Parameters
CPR quality can be improved by using a number of nonphysiologic techniques that help the provider adhere to recom-

mended CPR parameters such as rate and depth of compression and rate of ventilation. The most simple are auditory or visual metronomes to guide providers in performing the recommended rate of chest compressions or ventilations. More sophisticated devices actually monitor chest compression rate, depth, relaxation, and pauses in real time and provide visual and auditory feedback. When recorded, this information can also be useful in providing feedback to the entire team of providers after the resuscitation has ended. This type of CPR quality monitoring is discussed in more detail in Part 5: "Adult Basic Life Support" and Part 16: "Education, Implementation and Teams."

### Physiologic Parameters

In humans cardiac arrest is the most critically ill condition, yet it is typically monitored by rhythm assessment using selected electocardiographic (ECG) leads and pulse checks as the only physiologic parameters to guide therapy. Animal and human studies indicate that monitoring of $PETCO_2$, coronary perfusion pressure (CPP), and central venous oxygen saturation ($ScvO_2$) provides valuable information on both the patient's condition and response to therapy. Most importantly, $PETCO_2$, CPP, and $ScvO_2$ correlate with cardiac output and myocardial blood flow during CPR, and threshold values below which ROSC is rarely achieved have been reported.[168,190–195] Furthermore, an abrupt increase in any of these parameters is a sensitive indicator of ROSC that can be monitored without interrupting chest compressions.[91,93,167–175,177,196–201] Although no clinical study has examined whether titrating resuscitative efforts to these or other physiologic parameters improves outcome, it is reasonable to consider using these parameters when feasible to optimize chest compressions and guide vasopressor therapy during cardiac arrest (Class IIb, LOE C).

### Pulse

Clinicians frequently try to palpate arterial pulses during chest compressions to assess the effectiveness of compressions. No studies have shown the validity or clinical utility of checking pulses during ongoing CPR. Because there are no valves in the inferior vena cava, retrograde blood flow into the venous system may produce femoral vein pulsations.[202] Thus, palpation of a pulse in the femoral triangle may indicate venous rather than arterial blood flow. Carotid pulsations during CPR do not indicate the efficacy of myocardial or cerebral perfusion during CPR. Palpation of a pulse when chest compressions are paused is a reliable indicator of ROSC but is potentially less sensitive than other physiologic measures discussed below.

Healthcare providers also may take too long to check for a pulse[203,204] and have difficulty determining if a pulse is present or absent.[203–205] There is no evidence, however, that checking for breathing, coughing, or movement is superior for detection of circulation.[206] Because delays in chest compressions should be minimized, the healthcare provider should take no more than 10 seconds to check for a pulse, and if it is not felt within that time period chest compressions should be started.[205,207]

### End-Tidal CO₂

End-tidal $CO_2$ is the concentration of carbon dioxide in exhaled air at the end of expiration. It is typically expressed as a partial pressure in mm Hg ($PETCO_2$). Because $CO_2$ is a trace gas in atmospheric air, $CO_2$ detected by capnography in exhaled air is produced in the body and delivered to the lungs by circulating blood. Under normal conditions $PETCO_2$ is in the range of 35 to 40 mm Hg. During untreated cardiac arrest $CO_2$ continues to be produced in the body, but there is no $CO_2$ delivery to the lungs. Under these conditions $PETCO_2$ will approach zero with continued ventilation. With initiation of CPR, cardiac output is the major determinant of $CO_2$ delivery to the lungs. If ventilation is relatively constant, $PETCO_2$ correlates well with cardiac output during CPR. The correlation between $PETCO_2$ and cardiac output during CPR can be transiently altered by giving IV sodium bicarbonate.[208] This is explained by the fact that the bicarbonate is converted to water and $CO_2$, causing a transient increase in delivery of $CO_2$ to the lungs. Therefore, a transient rise in $PETCO_2$ after sodium bicarbonate therapy is expected and should not be misinterpreted as an improvement in quality of CPR or a sign of ROSC. Animal and human studies have also shown that $PETCO_2$ correlates with CPP and cerebral perfusion pressure during CPR.[209,210] The correlation of $PETCO_2$ with CPP during CPR can be altered by vasopressor therapy, especially at high doses (ie, >1 mg of epinephrine).[211–214] Vasopressors cause increased afterload, which will increase blood pressure and myocardial blood flow during CPR but will also decrease cardiac output. Therefore, a small decrease in $PETCO_2$ after vasopressor therapy may occur but should not be misinterpreted as a decrease in CPR quality.

Persistently low $PETCO_2$ values (<10 mm Hg) during CPR in intubated patients suggest that ROSC is unlikely.[171,173,174,190,191,215,216] Similar data using quantitative monitoring of $PETCO_2$ are not available for patients with a supraglottic airway or those receiving bag-mask ventilation during CPR. One study using colorimetic end-tidal $CO_2$ detection in nonintubated patients during CPR found that low end-tidal $CO_2$ was not a reliable predictor of failure to achieve ROSC.[217] An air leak during bag-mask ventilation or ventilation with a supraglottic airway could result in lower measured $PETCO_2$ values. Although a $PETCO_2$ value of <10 mm Hg in intubated patients indicates that cardiac output is inadequate to achieve ROSC, a specific target $PETCO_2$ value that optimizes the chance of ROSC has not been established. Monitoring $PETCO_2$ trends during CPR has the potential to guide individual optimization of compression depth and rate and to detect fatigue in the provider performing compressions.[201,218,219] In addition, an abrupt sustained increase in $PETCO_2$ during CPR is an indicator of ROSC.[91,177,196,198–201] Therefore, it is reasonable to consider using quantitative waveform capnography in intubated patients to monitor CPR quality, optimize chest compressions, and detect ROSC during chest compressions or when rhythm check reveals an organized rhythm (Class IIb, LOE C). If $PETCO_2$ is <10 mm Hg, it is reasonable to consider trying to improve CPR quality by optimizing chest compression parameters (Class IIb, LOE C). If $PETCO_2$ abruptly increases to a normal value (35 to 40 mm Hg), it is reasonable to consider that this is an indicator of ROSC (Class IIa, LOE B). The value of using quantitative waveform capnography in nonintubated patients to monitor and optimize CPR quality and detect ROSC is uncertain (Class IIb, LOE C).

### Coronary Perfusion Pressure and Arterial Relaxation Pressure
CPP (coronary perfusion pressure=aortic relaxation ["diastolic"] pressure minus right atrial relaxation ["diastolic"] pressure) during CPR correlates with both myocardial blood flow and ROSC.[168,192,220] Relaxation pressure during CPR is the trough of the pressure waveform during the relaxation phase of chest compressions and is analogous to diastolic pressure when the heart is beating. Increased CPP correlates with improved 24-hour survival rates in animal studies[193] and is associated with improved myocardial blood flow and ROSC in animal studies of epinephrine, vasopressin, and angiotensin II.[193–195] In one human study ROSC did not occur unless a CPP ≥15 mm Hg was achieved during CPR.[168] However, monitoring of CPP during CPR is rarely available clinically because measurement and calculation require simultaneous recording of aortic and central venous pressure.

A reasonable surrogate for CPP during CPR is arterial relaxation ("diastolic") pressure, which can be measured using a radial, brachial, or femoral artery catheter. These closely approximate aortic relaxation pressures during CPR in humans.[211,221] The same study that identified a CPP threshold of ≥15 mm Hg for ROSC also reported that ROSC was not achieved if aortic relaxation "diastolic" pressure did not exceed 17 mm Hg during CPR.[168] A specific target arterial relaxation pressure that optimizes the chance of ROSC has not been established. It is reasonable to consider using arterial relaxation "diastolic" pressure to monitor CPR quality, optimize chest compressions, and guide vasopressor therapy. (Class IIb, LOE C). If the arterial relaxation "diastolic" pressure is <20 mm Hg, it is reasonable to consider trying to improve quality of CPR by optimizing chest compression parameters or giving a vasopressor or both (Class IIb, LOE C). Arterial pressure monitoring can also be used to detect ROSC during chest compressions or when a rhythm check reveals an organized rhythm (Class IIb, LOE C).

### Central Venous Oxygen Saturation
When oxygen consumption, arterial oxygen saturation ($SaO_2$), and hemoglobin are constant, changes in $ScvO_2$ reflect changes in oxygen delivery by means of changes in cardiac output. $ScvO_2$ can be measured continuously using oximetric tipped central venous catheters placed in the superior vena cava. $ScvO_2$ values normally range from 60% to 80%. During cardiac arrest and CPR these values range from 25% to 35%, indicating the inadequacy of blood flow produced during CPR. In one clinical study the failure to achieve $ScvO_2$ of 30% during CPR was associated with failure to achieve ROSC.[169] $ScvO_2$ also helps to rapidly detect ROSC without interrupting chest compressions to check rhythm and pulse. When available, continuous $ScvO_2$ monitoring is a potentially useful indicator of cardiac output and

oxygen delivery during CPR. Therefore, when in place before cardiac arrest, it is reasonable to consider using continuous $ScvO_2$ measurement to monitor quality of CPR, optimize chest compressions, and detect ROSC during chest compressions or when rhythm check reveals an organized rhythm (Class IIb, LOE C). If $ScvO_2$ is <30%, it is reasonable to consider trying to improve the quality of CPR by optimizing chest compression parameters (Class IIb, LOE C).

### Pulse Oximetry
During cardiac arrest, pulse oximetry typically does not provide a reliable signal because pulsatile blood flow is inadequate in peripheral tissue beds. But the presence of a plethysmograph waveform on pulse oximetry is potentially valuable in detecting ROSC, and pulse oximetry is useful to ensure appropriate oxygenation after ROSC.

### Arterial Blood Gases
Arterial blood gas monitoring during CPR is not a reliable indicator of the severity of tissue hypoxemia, hypercarbia (and therefore adequacy of ventilation during CPR), or tissue acidosis.[222] Routine measurement of arterial blood gases during CPR has uncertain value (Class IIb, LOE C).

### Echocardiography
No studies specifically examine the impact of echocardiography on patient outcomes in cardiac arrest. However, a number of studies suggest that transthoracic and transesophageal echocardiography have potential utility in diagnosing treatable causes of cardiac arrest such as cardiac tamponade, pulmonary embolism, ischemia, and aortic dissection.[223–227] In addition, 3 prospective studies[228–230] found that absence of cardiac motion on sonography during resuscitation of patients in cardiac arrest was highly predictive of inability to achieve ROSC: of the 341 patients from the 3 studies, 218 had no detectable cardiac activity and only 2 of these had ROSC (no data on survival-to-hospital discharge were reported). Transthoracic or transesophageal echocardiography may be considered to diagnose treatable causes of cardiac arrest and guide treatment decisions (Class IIb, LOE C).

## Access for Parenteral Medications During Cardiac Arrest

### Timing of IV/IO Access
During cardiac arrest, provision of high-quality CPR and rapid defibrillation are of primary importance and drug administration is of secondary importance. After beginning CPR and attempting defibrillation for identified VF or pulseless VT, providers can establish IV or IO access. This should be performed without interrupting chest compressions. The primary purpose of IV/IO access during cardiac arrest is to provide drug therapy. Two clinical studies[134,136] reported data suggesting worsened survival for every minute that antiarrhythmic drug delivery was delayed (measured from time of dispatch). However, this finding was potentially biased by a concomitant delay in onset of other ACLS interventions. In one study[136] the interval from first shock to administration of an antiarrhythmic drug was a significant predictor of survival.

One animal study[231] reported lower CPP when delivery of a vasopressor was delayed. Time to drug administration was also a predictor of ROSC in a retrospective analysis of swine cardiac arrest.[232] Thus, although time to drug treatment appears to have importance, there is insufficient evidence to specify exact time parameters or the precise sequence with which drugs should be administered during cardiac arrest.

### Peripheral IV Drug Delivery

If a resuscitation drug is administered by a peripheral venous route, it should be administered by bolus injection and followed with a 20-mL bolus of IV fluid to facilitate the drug flow from the extremity into the central circulation.[233] Briefly elevating the extremity during and after drug administration theoretically may also recruit the benefit of gravity to facilitate delivery to the central circulation but has not been systematically studied.

### IO Drug Delivery

IO cannulation provides access to a noncollapsible venous plexus, enabling drug delivery similar to that achieved by peripheral venous access at comparable doses. Two prospective trials in children[234] and adults[235] and 6 other studies[236–242] suggest that IO access can be established efficiently; is safe and effective for fluid resuscitation, drug delivery, and blood sampling for laboratory evaluation; and is attainable in all age groups. However, many of these studies were conducted during normal perfusion states or hypovolemic shock or in animal models of cardiac arrest. Although virtually all ACLS drugs have been given intraosseously in the clinical setting without known ill effects, there is little information on the efficacy and effectiveness of such administration in clinical cardiac arrest during ongoing CPR. It is reasonable for providers to establish IO access if IV access is not readily available (Class IIa, LOE C). Commercially available kits can facilitate IO access in adults.

### Central IV Drug Delivery

The appropriately trained provider may consider placement of a central line (internal jugular or subclavian) during cardiac arrest, unless there are contraindications (Class IIb, LOE C). The primary advantage of a central line is that peak drug concentrations are higher and drug circulation times shorter compared with drugs administered through a peripheral IV catheter.[243–245] In addition, a central line extending into the superior vena cava can be used to monitor $ScvO_2$ and estimate CPP during CPR, both of which are predictive of ROSC.[168,169] However, central line placement can interrupt CPR. Central venous catheterization is a relative (but not absolute) contraindication for fibrinolytic therapy in patients with acute coronary syndromes.

### Endotracheal Drug Delivery

One study in children,[246] 5 studies in adults,[247–251] and multiple animal studies[252–254] have shown that lidocaine,[248,255] epinephrine,[256] atropine,[257] naloxone, and vasopressin[254] are absorbed via the trachea. There are no data

regarding endotracheal administration of amiodarone. Administration of resuscitation drugs into the trachea results in lower blood concentrations than when the same dose is given intravascularly. Furthermore, the results of recent animal studies[258,259] suggest that the lower epinephrine concentrations achieved when the drug is delivered endotracheally may produce transient $\beta$-adrenergic effects, resulting in vasodilation. These effects can be detrimental, causing hypotension, lower CPP and flow, and reduced potential for ROSC. Thus, although endotracheal administration of some resuscitation drugs is possible, IV or IO drug administration is preferred because it will provide more predictable drug delivery and pharmacologic effect.

In one nonrandomized cohort study of out-of-hospital cardiac arrest in adults[260] using a randomized control, IV administration of atropine and epinephrine was associated with a higher rate of ROSC and survival to hospital admission than administration by the endotracheal route. Five percent of those who received IV drugs survived to hospital discharge, but no patient survived in the group receiving drugs by the endotracheal route.

If IV or IO access cannot be established, epinephrine, vasopressin, and lidocaine may be administered by the endotracheal route during cardiac arrest (Class IIb, LOE B). The optimal endotracheal dose of most drugs is unknown, but typically the dose given by the endotracheal route is 2 to 2½ times the recommended IV dose. In 2 animal CPR studies the equipotent epinephrine dose given endotracheally was approximately 3 to 10 times higher than the IV dose.[261,262] Providers should dilute the recommended dose in 5 to 10 mL of sterile water or normal saline and inject the drug directly into the endotracheal tube.[256] Studies with epinephrine[263] and lidocaine[251] showed that dilution with sterile water instead of 0.9% saline may achieve better drug absorption.

## Advanced Airway

There is inadequate evidence to define the optimal timing of advanced airway placement in relation to other interventions during resuscitation from cardiac arrest. There are no prospective studies that directly address the relationship between timing or type of advanced airway placement during CPR and outcomes. In an urban out-of-hospital setting, intubation in <12 minutes has been associated with a better rate of survival than intubation in ≥13 minutes.[32] In a registry study of 25 006 in-hospital cardiac arrests, earlier time to advanced airway (<5 minutes) was not associated with increased ROSC but was associated with improved 24-hour survival.[31] In out-of-hospital urban and rural settings, patients intubated during resuscitation had better survival rates than patients who were not intubated.[33] In an in-hospital setting patients requiring intubation during CPR had worse survival rates.[34] A recent study[8] found that delayed endotracheal intubation combined with passive oxygen delivery and minimally interrupted chest compressions was associated with improved neurologically intact survival after out-of-hospital cardiac arrest in patients with witnessed VF/VT.

Advantages of advanced airway placement include elimination of the need for pauses in chest compressions for ventilation, potentially improved ventilation and oxygenation, reduction in the risk of aspiration, and ability to use quantitative waveform capnography to monitor quality of CPR, optimize chest compressions, and detect ROSC during chest compressions or when a rhythm check reveals an organized rhythm. The primary disadvantages are interruptions in chest compression during placement and the risk of unrecognized esophageal intubation.

When an advanced airway (eg, endotracheal tube or supraglottic airway) is placed, 2 providers no longer deliver cycles of compressions interrupted with pauses for ventilation. Instead, the provider performing compressions should deliver at least 100 compressions per minute continuously without pauses for ventilation. The provider delivering ventilations should give 1 breath every 6 to 8 seconds (8 to 10 breaths per minute) and should be careful to avoid delivering an excessive number of ventilations.

## When Should Resuscitative Efforts Stop?

The final decision to stop can never rest on a single parameter, such as duration of resuscitative efforts. Rather, clinical judgment and respect for human dignity must enter into decision making. In the out-of-hospital setting, cessation of resuscitative efforts in adults should follow system-specific criteria under direct medical control. There are limited clinical data to guide this decision in neonatal and pediatric out-of-hospital or in-hospital cardiac arrest. A more detailed discussion is provided in Part 3: "Ethics."

## Medications for Arrest Rhythms

The primary goal of pharmacologic therapy during cardiac arrest is to facilitate restoration and maintenance of a perfusing spontaneous rhythm. Toward this goal, ACLS drug therapy during CPR is often associated with increased rates of ROSC and hospital admission but not increased rates of long-term survival with good neurologic outcome. One study[138] randomized patients to IV or no IV medications during management of adult out-of-hospital cardiac arrest. The study demonstrated higher rates of ROSC in the IV group (40% IV versus 25% no IV [odds ratio (OR) 1.99; 95% confidence interval (CI) 1.48 to 2.67]), but there was no statistical difference in survival to hospital discharge (10.5% IV versus 9.2% no IV [OR 1.16; 95% CI 0.74 to 1.82]) or survival with favorable neurologic outcome (9.8% IV versus 8.1% no IV [OR 1.24; 95% CI 0.77 to 1.98]). This study was not adequately powered to detect clinically important differences in long-term outcomes. Evidence from one nonrandomized trial[137] found that the addition of ACLS interventions including IV drugs in a previously optimized BLS system with rapid defibrillation resulted in an increased rate of ROSC (18.0% with ACLS versus 12.9% before ACLS, $P<0.001$) and hospital admission (14.6% with ACLS versus 10.9% before ACLS, $P<0.001$) but no statistical difference in survival to hospital discharge (5.1% with ACLS versus 5.0% before ACLS). Whether optimized high-quality CPR and advances in post–cardiac arrest care will enable the increased rates of ROSC with ACLS medications to be translated into increased long-term survival remains to be determined.

## Vasopressors

To date no placebo-controlled trials have shown that administration of any vasopressor agent at any stage during management of VF, pulseless VT, PEA, or asystole increases the rate of neurologically intact survival to hospital discharge. There is evidence, however, that the use of vasopressor agents is associated with an increased rate of ROSC.

### Epinephrine

Epinephrine hydrochloride produces beneficial effects in patients during cardiac arrest, primarily because of its α-adrenergic receptor-stimulating (ie, vasoconstrictor) properties.[264] The α-adrenergic effects of epinephrine can increase CPP and cerebral perfusion pressure during CPR.[265] The value and safety of the β-adrenergic effects of epinephrine are controversial because they may increase myocardial work and reduce subendocardial perfusion.[266]

There are no RCTs that adequately compare epinephrine with placebo in treatment of and outcomes related to out-of-hospital cardiac arrest. A retrospective study[267] compared epinephrine to no epinephrine for sustained VF and PEA/asystole and found improved ROSC with epinephrine but no difference in survival between the treatment groups. A meta-analysis and other studies have found improved ROSC, but none have demonstrated a survival benefit of high-dose epinephrine versus standard-dose epinephrine in cardiac arrest.[135,268–272]

It is reasonable to consider administering a 1 mg dose of IV/IO epinephrine every 3 to 5 minutes during adult cardiac arrest (Class IIb, LOE A). Higher doses may be indicated to treat specific problems, such as a β-blocker or calcium channel blocker overdose. Higher doses can also be considered if guided by hemodynamic monitoring such as arterial relaxation "diastolic" pressure or CPP. If IV/IO access is delayed or cannot be established, epinephrine may be given endotracheally at a dose of 2 to 2.5 mg.

### Vasopressin

Vasopressin is a nonadrenergic peripheral vasoconstrictor that also causes coronary and renal vasoconstriction.[273] Three RCTs and a meta-analysis of the trials[274–277] demonstrated no difference in outcomes (ROSC, survival to discharge, or neurologic outcome) with vasopressin (40 units IV) versus epinephrine (1 mg) as a first-line vasopressor in cardiac arrest. Two RCTs[278,279] demonstrated no difference in outcomes (ROSC, survival to discharge, or neurologic) when comparing epinephrine in combination with vasopressin versus epinephrine alone in cardiac arrest. One RCT found that repeated doses of vasopressin during cardiac arrest did not improve survival rates compared with repeated doses of epinephrine.[280]

Because the effects of vasopressin have not been shown to differ from those of epinephrine in cardiac arrest, 1 dose of vasopressin 40 units IV/IO may replace either the first or second dose of epinephrine in the treatment of cardiac arrest (Class IIb, LOE A).

### Other Vasopressors

There are no alternative vasopressors (norepinephrine, phenylephrine) with proven survival benefit compared with epinephrine.[268,281,282]

## Antiarrhythmics

There is no evidence that any antiarrhythmic drug given routinely during human cardiac arrest increases survival to hospital discharge. Amiodarone, however, has been shown to increase short-term survival to hospital admission when compared with placebo or lidocaine.

### Amiodarone

IV amiodarone affects sodium, potassium, and calcium channels and has $\alpha$- and $\beta$-adrenergic blocking properties. It can be considered for treatment of VF or pulseless VT unresponsive to shock delivery, CPR, and a vasopressor. In blinded randomized controlled clinical trials in adults with refractory VF/pulseless VT in the out-of-hospital setting,[134,136] paramedic administration of amiodarone (300 mg[134] or 5 mg/kg[136]) improved hospital admission rates when compared with administration of placebo[134] or 1.5 mg/kg of lidocaine.[136] Additional studies[283–287] documented consistent improvement in termination of arrhythmias when amiodarone was given to humans or animals with VF or hemodynamically unstable VT. A higher incidence of bradycardia and hypotension was reported for amiodarone in one out-of-hospital study.[134] A canine study[288] noted that administration of a vasoconstrictor before amiodarone prevented hypotension. The adverse hemodynamic effects of the IV formulation of amiodarone are attributed to vasoactive solvents (polysorbate 80 and benzyl alcohol). When administered in the absence of these solvents, an analysis of the combined data of 4 prospective clinical trials of patients with VT (some hemodynamically unstable) showed that amiodarone produced no more hypotension than lidocaine.[286] A formulation of IV amiodarone without these vasoactive solvents was approved for use in the United States.

Amiodarone may be considered for VF or pulseless VT unresponsive to CPR, defibrillation, and a vasopressor therapy (Class IIb, LOE B). An initial dose of 300 mg IV/IO can be followed by 1 dose of 150 mg IV/IO. Although anecdotally administered IO without known adverse effects, there is limited experience with amiodarone given by this route.

### Lidocaine

A retrospective review[289] demonstrated an association between improved hospital admission rates and use of lidocaine (compared with standard treatment) in patients with out-of-hospital VF cardiac arrest. But there is inadequate evidence to recommend the use of lidocaine in patients who have refractory VT/VF, defined as VT/VF not terminated by defibrillation or that continues to recur after defibrillation during out-of-hospital cardiac arrest or inhospital cardiac arrest.

Lidocaine is an alternative antiarrhythmic of long-standing and widespread familiarity with fewer immediate side effects than may be encountered with other antiarrhythmics. Lidocaine, however, has no proven short- or long-term efficacy in cardiac arrest. Lidocaine may be considered if amiodarone is not available (Class IIb, LOE B). The initial dose is 1 to 1.5 mg/kg IV. If VF/pulseless VT persists, additional doses of 0.5 to 0.75 mg/kg IV push may be administered at 5- to 10-minute intervals to a maximum dose of 3 mg/kg.

### Magnesium Sulfate

Two observational studies[290,291] showed that IV magnesium sulfate can facilitate termination of torsades de pointes (irregular/polymorphic VT associated with prolonged QT interval). Magnesium sulfate is not likely to be effective in terminating irregular/polymorphic VT in patients with a normal QT interval.[291]

A number of doses of magnesium sulfate have been used clinically, and an optimal dosing regimen has not been established. When VF/pulseless VT cardiac arrest is associated with torsades de pointes, providers may administer an IV/IO bolus of magnesium sulfate at a dose of 1 to 2 g diluted in 10 mL $D_5W$ (Class IIb, LOE C). See Part 8.3: "Management of Symptomatic Bradycardia and Tachycardia" for additional information about management of torsades de pointes not associated with cardiac arrest.

Three RCTs[292–294] did not identify a significant benefit from use of magnesium compared with placebo among patients with VF arrest in the prehospital, intensive care unit, and emergency department setting, respectively. Thus, routine administration of magnesium sulfate in cardiac arrest is not recommended (Class III, LOE A) unless torsades de pointes is present.

## Interventions Not Recommended for Routine Use During Cardiac Arrest

### Atropine

Atropine sulfate reverses cholinergic-mediated decreases in heart rate and atrioventricular nodal conduction. No prospective controlled clinical trials have examined the use of atropine in asystole or bradycardic PEA cardiac arrest. Lower-level clinical studies provide conflicting evidence of the benefit of routine use of atropine in cardiac arrest.[34,295–304] There is no evidence that atropine has detrimental effects during bradycardic or asystolic cardiac arrest. Available evidence suggests that routine use of atropine during PEA or asystole is unlikely to have a therapeutic benefit (Class IIb, LOE B). For this reason atropine has been removed from the cardiac arrest algorithm.

### Sodium Bicarbonate

Tissue acidosis and resulting acidemia during cardiac arrest and resuscitation are dynamic processes resulting from no blood flow during arrest and low blood flow during CPR. These processes are affected by the duration of cardiac arrest, level of blood flow, and arterial oxygen content during CPR. Restoration of oxygen content with appropriate ventilation with oxygen, support of some tissue perfusion and some cardiac output with high-quality chest compressions, then rapid ROSC are the mainstays of restoring acid-base balance during cardiac arrest.

Two studies demonstrated[305,306] increased ROSC, hospital admission, and survival to hospital discharge associated with use of bicarbonate. However, the majority of studies showed no benefit[307–309] or found a relationship with poor outcome.[304,310–312]

There are few data to support therapy with buffers during cardiac arrest. There is no evidence that bicarbonate improves the likelihood of defibrillation or survival rates in animals with VF cardiac arrest. A wide variety of adverse effects have been linked to administration of bicarbonate during cardiac arrest. Bicarbonate may compromise CPP by reducing systemic vascular resistance.[313] It can create extracellular alkalosis that will shift the oxyhemoglobin saturation curve and inhibit oxygen release. It can produce hypernatremia and therefore hyperosmolarity. It produces excess $CO_2$, which freely diffuses into myocardial and cerebral cells and may paradoxically contribute to intracellular acidosis.[314] It can exacerbate central venous acidosis and may inactivate simultaneously administered catecholamines.

In some special resuscitation situations, such as preexisting metabolic acidosis, hyperkalemia, or tricyclic antidepressant overdose, bicarbonate can be beneficial (see Part 12: "Cardiac Arrest in Special Situations"). However, routine use of sodium bicarbonate is not recommended for patients in cardiac arrest (Class III, LOE B). When bicarbonate is used for special situations, an initial dose of 1 mEq/kg is typical. Whenever possible, bicarbonate therapy should be guided by the bicarbonate concentration or calculated base deficit obtained from blood gas analysis or laboratory measurement. To minimize the risk of iatrogenically induced alkalosis, providers should not attempt complete correction of the calculated base deficit. Other non–$CO_2$-generating buffers such as carbicarb, THAM, or tribonate have shown potential for minimizing some adverse effects of sodium bicarbonate, including $CO_2$ generation, hyperosmolarity, hypernatremia, hypoglycemia, intracellular acidosis, myocardial acidosis, and "overshoot" alkalosis.[315–317] But clinical experience is greatly limited and outcome studies are lacking.

### Calcium
Studies of calcium during cardiac arrest have found variable results on ROSC, and no trial has found a beneficial effect on survival either in or out of hospital.[301,304,318–323] Routine administration of calcium for treatment of in-hospital and out-of-hospital cardiac arrest is not recommended (Class III, LOE B).

### Fibrinolysis
Fibrinolytic therapy was proposed for use during cardiac arrest to treat both coronary thrombosis (acute coronary syndrome) with presumably complete occlusion of a proximal coronary artery and major life-threatening pulmonary embolism. Ongoing CPR is not an absolute contraindication to fibrinolysis. Initial studies were promising[324–330] and suggested benefit from fibrinolytic therapy in the treatment of victims of cardiopulmonary arrest unresponsive to standard therapy. But 2 large clinical trials[188,331] failed to show any

improvement in outcome with fibrinolytic therapy during CPR. One of these showed an increased risk of intracranial bleeding associated with the routine use of fibrinolytics during cardiac arrest.[188]

Fibrinolytic therapy should not be routinely used in cardiac arrest (Class III, LOE B). When pulmonary embolism is presumed or known to be the cause of cardiac arrest, empirical fibrinolytic therapy can be considered (Class IIa, LOE B; see Part 12).

### IV Fluids
No published human study directly compares the outcome of routine IV fluid administration to no fluid administration during CPR. Most human and animal studies of fluid infusion during CPR did not have a control group,[332–343] and 2 animal studies showed that normothermic fluid infusion during CPR caused a decrease in CPP.[344–346] In addition to normothermic fluid, hypertonic and chilled fluids have been studied in animal and small human studies without a survival benefit.[332,334,336–338,341–343] If cardiac arrest is associated with extreme volume losses, hypovolemic arrest should be suspected. These patients present with signs of circulatory shock advancing to PEA. In these settings intravascular volume should be promptly restored.

### Pacing
Electric pacing is generally not effective in cardiac arrest, and no studies have observed a survival benefit from pacing in cardiac arrest.[347–350] Existing evidence suggests that pacing by transcutaneous, transvenous, or transmyocardial means in cardiac arrest does not improve the likelihood of ROSC or survival outcome regardless of the timing of pacing administration (early or delayed in established asystole), location of arrest (in-hospital or out-of-hospital), or primary cardiac rhythm (asystole, PEA) targeted for treatment. Electric pacing is not recommended for routine use in cardiac arrest (Class III, LOE B).

### Precordial Thump
The potential utility of precordial thump in cardiac arrest has not been well studied. When hemodynamically unstable ventricular tachyarrhythmias were induced during electrophysiological testing, initial administration of a precordial thump appeared to be safe but rarely effective in terminating ventricular arrhythmias.[351] In a prospective observational study of patients with out-of-hospital cardiac arrest, precordial thump was associated with ROSC when administered promptly to patients with responder-witnessed asystolic arrest. When administered for VF/VT or PEA arrest it was ineffective but resulted in no apparent harm.[352] In 3 case series[353–355] VF or pulseless VT was converted to a perfusing rhythm by a precordial thump. Conversely, other case series documented deterioration in cardiac rhythm, such as rate acceleration of VT, conversion of VT to VF, or development of complete AV block or asystole following the thump.[354,356–361]

The precordial thump may be considered for termination of witnessed monitored unstable ventricular tachyarrhythmias when a defibrillator is not immediately ready for use (Class IIb, LOE B), but should not delay CPR and shock delivery. There is insufficient evidence to recommend for or against the use of the precordial thump for witnessed onset of asystole, and there is insufficient evidence to recommend percussion pacing during typical attempted resuscitation from cardiac arrest.

## Summary

Intervention to prevent cardiac arrest in critically ill patients is ideal. When cardiac arrest occurs, high-quality CPR is fundamental to the success of any subsequent ACLS intervention. During resuscitation healthcare providers must perform chest compressions of adequate rate and depth, allow complete recoil of the chest after each compression, minimize interruptions in chest compressions, and avoid excessive ventilation, especially with an advanced airway. Quality of CPR should be continuously monitored. Physiologic monitoring may prove useful to optimize resuscitative efforts. For patients in VF/pulseless VT, shocks should be delivered promptly with minimal interruptions in chest compressions. The increased rates of ROSC associated with ACLS drug therapy have yet to be translated into long-term survival benefits. However, improved quality of CPR, advances in post–cardiac arrest care, and improved overall implementation through comprehensive systems of care may provide a pathway to optimize the outcomes of cardiac arrest patients treated with ACLS interventions.

## Part 8.3: Management of Symptomatic Bradycardia and Tachycardia

### Overview

This section highlights recommendations for management of patients with acute symptomatic arrhythmias. Electrocardiographic (ECG) and rhythm information should be interpreted within the context of total patient assessment. Errors in diagnosis and treatment are likely to occur if advanced cardiovascular life support (ACLS) providers base treatment decisions solely on rhythm interpretation and neglect clinical evaluation. Providers must evaluate the patient's symptoms and clinical signs, including ventilation, oxygenation, heart rate, blood pressure, level of consciousness, and signs of inadequate organ perfusion.

*Unstable* and *symptomatic* are terms typically used to describe the condition of patients with arrhythmias. Generally, *unstable* refers to a condition in which vital organ function is acutely impaired or cardiac arrest is ongoing or imminent. When an arrhythmia causes a patient to be unstable, immediate intervention is indicated. *Symptomatic* implies that an arrhythmia is causing symptoms, such as palpitations, lightheadedness, or dyspnea, but the patient is stable and not in imminent danger. In such cases more time is available to decide on the most appropriate intervention. In both unstable and symptomatic cases the provider must

make an assessment as to whether it is the arrhythmia that is causing the patient to be unstable or symptomatic. For example, a patient in septic shock with sinus tachycardia of 140 beats per minute is unstable; however, the arrhythmia is a physiologic compensation rather than the cause of instability. Therefore, electric cardioversion will not improve this patient's condition. Additionally, if a patient with respiratory failure and severe hypoxemia becomes hypotensive and develops a bradycardia, the bradycardia is not the primary cause of instability. Treating the bradycardia without treating the hypoxemia is unlikely to improve the patient's condition. It is critically important to determine the cause of the patient's instability in order to properly direct treatment. In general, sinus tachycardia is a response to other factors and, thus, it rarely (if ever) is the cause of instability in and of itself.

The *2010 AHA Guidlines for CPR and ECC* emphasize the importance of clinical evaluation and highlight principles of therapy with algorithms that have been refined and streamlined since publication of the *2005 AHA Guidelines for CPR and ECC.*[362] The key principles of arrhythmia recognition and management in adults are as follows:

If bradycardia produces signs and symptoms of instability (eg, acutely altered mental status, ischemic chest discomfort, acute heart failure, hypotension, or other signs of shock that persist despite adequate airway and breathing), the initial treatment is atropine (Class IIa, LOE B). If bradycardia is unresponsive to atropine, intravenous (IV) infusion of β-adrenergic agonists with rate-accelerating effects (dopamine, epinephrine) or transcutaneous pacing (TCP) can be effective (Class IIa, LOE B) while the patient is prepared for emergent transvenous temporary pacing if required.

If the tachycardic patient is unstable with severe signs and symptoms related to a suspected arrhythmia (eg, acute altered mental status, ischemic chest discomfort, acute heart failure, hypotension, or other signs of shock), immediate cardioversion should be performed (with prior sedation in the conscious patient) (Class I, LOE B). In select cases of regular narrow-complex tachycardia with unstable signs or symptoms, a trial of adenosine before cardioversion is reasonable to consider (Class IIb, LOE C).

If the patient with tachycardia is stable, determine if the patient has a narrow-complex or wide-complex tachycardia, whether the rhythm is regular or irregular, and for wide complexes whether the QRS morphology is monomorphic or polymorphic. Therapy is then tailored accordingly (Table 2).

Know when to call for expert consultation regarding complicated rhythm interpretation, drugs, or management decisions.

A comprehensive presentation of the evaluation and management of bradyarrhythmias and tachyarrhythmias is beyond the scope of the *2010 AHA Guidelines for CPR and ECC.* The following selected rhythm scenarios are meant to aid with the management of periarrest rhythm disorders. If cardiac arrest develops at any time, see the ACLS Cardiac Arrest Algorithms in Part 8.2: "Management of Cardiac Arrest."

**Table 2.    IV Drugs Used for Tachycardia**

| Drug | Characteristics | Indication(s) | Dosing | Side Effects | Precautions or Special Considerations |
|---|---|---|---|---|---|
| Intravenous Drugs Used to Treat Supraventricular Tachyarrhythmias | | | | | |
| Adenosine | Endogenous purine nucleoside; briefly depresses sinus node rate and AV node conduction; vasodilator | • Stable, narrow-complex regular tachycardias<br>• Unstable narrow-complex regular tachycardias while preparations are made for electrical cardioversion<br>• Stable, regular, monomorphic, wide complex tachycardia as a therapeutic and diagnostic maneuver | 6 mg IV as a rapid IV push followed by a 20 mL saline flush; repeat if required as 12 mg IV push | Hypotension, bronchospasm, chest discomfort | Contraindicated in patients with asthma; may precipitate atrial fibrillation, which may be very rapid in patients with WPW; thus a defibrillator should be readily available; reduce dose in post–cardiac transplant patients, those taking dipyridamole or carbamazepine and when administered via a central vein |
| Diltiazem, Verapamil | Non-dihydropyridine calcium channel blockers; slow AV node conduction and increase AV node refractoriness; vasodilators, negative inotropes | • Stable, narrow-complex tachycardias if rhythm remains uncontrolled or unconverted by adenosine or vagal maneuvers or if SVT is recurrent<br>• Control ventricular rate in patients with atrial fibrillation or atrial flutter | Diltiazem: Initial dose 15 to 20 mg (0.25 mg/kg) IV over 2 minutes; additional 20 to 25 mg (0.35 mg/kg) IV in 15 minutes if needed; 5 to 15 mg/h IV maintenance infusion (titrated to AF heart rate if given for rate control)<br>Verapamil: Initial dose 2.5 to 5 mg IV given over 2 minutes; may repeat as 5 to 10 mg every 15 to 30 minutes to total dose of 20 to 30 mg | Hypotension, bradycardia, precipitation of heart failure | Should only be given to patients with narrow-complex tachycardias (regular or irregular). Avoid in patients with heart failure and pre-excited AF or flutter or rhythms consistent with VT |
| Atenolol, Esmolol, Metoprolol, Propranolol | β-Blockers; reduce effects of circulating catecholamines; reduce heart rate, AV node conduction and blood pressure; negative inotropes | • Stable, narrow-complex tachycardias if rhythm remains uncontrolled or unconverted by adenosine or vagal maneuvers or if SVT is recurrent<br>• Control ventricular rate in patients with atrial fibrillation or atrial flutter<br>• Certain forms of polymorphic VT (associated with acute ischemia, familial LQTS, catecholaminergic) | Atenolol (β1 specific blocker) 5 mg IV over 5 minutes; repeat 5 mg in 10 minutes if arrhythmia persists or recurs<br>Esmolol (β1 specific blocker with 2- to 9-minute half-life) IV loading dose 500 mcg/kg (0.5 mg/kg) over 1 minute, followed by an infusion of 50 mcg/kg per minute (0.05 mg/kg per minute); if response is inadequate, infuse second loading bolus of 0.5 mg/kg over 1 minute and increase maintenance infusion to 100 mcg/kg (0.1 mg/kg) per minute; increment; increase in this manner if required to maximum infusion rate of 300 mcg/kg [0.3 mg/kg] per minute<br>Metoprolol (β1 specific blocker) 5 mg over 1 to 2 minutes repeated as required every 5 minutes to maximum dose of 15 mg<br>Propranolol (nonselective β-blocker) 0.5 to 1 mg over 1 minute, repeated up to a total dose of 0.1 mg/kg if required | Hypotension, bradycardia, precipitation of heart failure | Avoid in patients with asthma, obstructive airway disease, decompensated heart failure and pre-excited artrial fibrillation or flutter |
| Procainamide | Sodium and potassium channel blocker | • Pre-excited atrial fibrillation | 20 to 50 mg/min until arrhythmia suppressed, hypotension ensues, or QRS prolonged by 50%, or total cumulative dose of 17 mg/kg; or 100 mg every 5 minutes until arrhythmia is controlled or other conditions described above are met | Bradycardia, hypotension, torsades de pointes | Avoid in patients with QT prolongation and CHF |

*(Continued)*

**Table 2.** **Continued**

| Drug | Characteristics | Indication(s) | Dosing | Side Effects | Precautions or Special Considerations |
|------|-----------------|---------------|--------|--------------|---------------------------------------|
| Amiodarone | Multichannel blocker (sodium, potassium, calcium channel, and noncompetitive $\alpha/\beta$-blocker) | • Stable irregular narrow complex tachycardia (atrial fibrillation)<br>• Stable regular narrow-complex tachycardia<br>• To control rapid ventricular rate due to accessory pathway conduction in pre-excited atrial arrhythmias | 150 mg given over 10 minutes and repeated if necessary, followed by a 1 mg/min infusion for 6 hours, followed by 0.5 mg/min. Total dose over 24 hours should not exceed 2.2 g. | Bradycardia, hypotension, phlebitis | |
| Digoxin | Cardiac glycoside with positive inotropic effects; slows AV node conduction by enhancing parasympathetic tone; slow onset of action | • Stable, narrow-complex regular tachycardias if rhythm remains uncontrolled or unconverted by adenosine or vagal maneuvers or if SVT is recurrent<br>• Control ventricular rate in patients with atrial fibrillation or atrial flutter | 8 to 12 mcg/kg total loading dose, half of which is administered initially over 5 minutes, and remaining portion as 25% fractions at 4- to 8- hour intervals | Bradycardia | Slow onset of action and relative low potency renders it less useful for treatment of acute arrhythmias |
| **Intravenous Drugs Used to Treat Ventricular Tachyarrhythmias** | | | | | |
| Procainamide | Sodium and potassium channel blocker | • Hemodynamically stable monomorphic VT | 20 to 50 mg/min until arrhythmia suppressed, hypotension ensues, or QRS prolonged by 50%, or total cumulative dose of 17 mg/kg; or 100 mg every 5 minutes until arrhythmia is controlled or other conditions described above are met | Bradycardia, hypotension, torsades de pointes | Avoid in patients with QT prolongation and CHF |
| Amiodarone | Multichannel blocker (sodium, potassium, calcium channel, $\alpha$- and noncompetitive $\beta$-blocker) | • Hemodynamically stable monomorphic VT<br>• Polymorphic VT with normal QT interval | 150 mg given over 10 minutes and repeated if necessary, followed by a 1 mg/min infusion for 6 hours, followed by 0.5 mg/min. Total dose over 24 hours should not exceed 2.2 g. | Bradycardia, hypotension, phlebitis | |
| Sotalol | Potassium channel blocker and nonselective $\beta$-blocker | • Hemodynamically stable monomorphic VT | In clinical studies 1.5 mg/kg infused over 5 minutes; however, US package labeling recommends any dose of the drug should be infused slowly over a period of 5 hours | Bradycardia, hypotension, torsades de pointes | Avoid in patients with QT prolongation and CHF |
| Lidocaine | Relatively weak sodium channel blocker | • Hemodynamically stable monomorphic VT | Initial dose range from 1 to 1.5 mg/kg IV; repeated if required at 0.5 to 0.75 mg/kg IV every 5 to 10 minutes up to maximum cumulative dose of 3 mg/kg; 1 to 4 mg/min (30 to 50 mcg/kg per minute) maintenance infusion | Slurred speech, altered consciousness, seizures, bradycardia | |
| Magnesium | Cofactor in variety of cell processes including control of sodium and potassium transport | • Polymorphic VT associated with QT prolongation (torsades de pointes) | 1 to 2 g IV over 15 minutes | Hypotension, CNS toxicity, respiratory depression | Follow magnesium levels if frequent or prolonged dosing required, particularly in patients with impaired renal function |

## Bradycardia

This section summarizes the management of bradyarrhythmias. Following the overview of bradyarrhythmias and summary of the initial evaluation and treatment of bradycardia, drugs used in the treatment of bradycardia are presented. See the Bradycardia Algorithm, Figure 3. Box numbers in the text refer to the numbered boxes in the algorithm.

### Evaluation

Bradycardia is defined as a heart rate of <60 beats per minute. However, when bradycardia is the cause of symptoms, the rate is generally <50 beats per minute, which is the working definition of bradycardia used here (Figure 3, **Box 1**). A slow heart rate may be physiologically normal for some patients, whereas a heart rate of >50 beats per minute may be inadequate for others. The Bradycardia Algorithm focuses on management of clinically significant bradycardia (ie, bradycardia that is inappropriate for the clinical condition).

Because hypoxemia is a common cause of bradycardia, initial evaluation of any patient with bradycardia should focus on signs of increased work of breathing (tachypnea, intercostal retractions, suprasternal retractions, paradoxical abdominal breathing) and oxyhemoglobin saturation as determined by pulse oximetry (Figure 3, **Box 2**). If oxygenation is

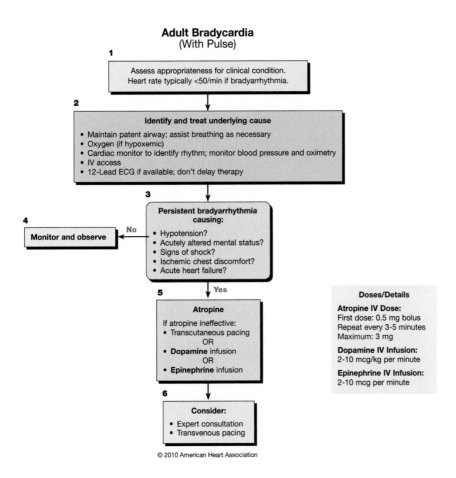

**Figure 3.** Bradycardia Algorithm.

inadequate or the patient shows signs of increased work of breathing, provide supplementary oxygen. Attach a monitor to the patient, evaluate blood pressure, and establish IV access. If possible, obtain a 12-lead ECG to better define the rhythm. While initiating treatment, evaluate the patient's clinical status and identify potentially reversible causes.

The provider must identify signs and symptoms of poor perfusion and determine if those signs are likely to be caused by the bradycardia (Figure 3, **Box 3**). If the signs and symptoms are not due to bradycardia, the provider should reassess the underlying cause of the patient's symptoms. Remember that signs and symptoms of bradycardia may be mild; asymptomatic or minimally symptomatic patients do not necessarily require treatment (Figure 3, **Box 4**) unless there is suspicion that the rhythm is likely to progress to symptoms or become life-threatening (eg, Mobitz type II second-degree AV block in the setting of acute myocardial infarction [AMI]). If the bradycardia is suspected to be the cause of acute altered mental status, ischemic chest discomfort, acute heart failure, hypotension, or other signs of shock, the patient should receive immediate treatment.

Atrioventricular (AV) blocks are classified as first-, second-, and third-degree. Blocks may be caused by medications or electrolyte disturbances, as well as structural problems resulting from AMI or other myocardial diseases. A first-degree AV block is defined by a prolonged PR interval (>0.20 second) and is generally benign. Second-degree AV block is divided into Mobitz types I and II. In Mobitz type I block, the block is at the AV node; the block is often transient and asymptomatic. In

Mobitz type II block, the block is usually below the AV node within the His-Purkinje system; this block is often symptomatic, with the potential to progress to complete (third-degree) AV block. Third-degree AV block may occur at the AV node, bundle of His, or bundle branches. When third-degree AV block is present, no impulses pass between the atria and ventricles. Third-degree AV block can be permanent or transient, depending on the underlying cause.

### Therapy (Figure 3, Box 5)

*Atropine*

Atropine remains the first-line drug for acute symptomatic bradycardia (Class IIa, LOE B). Clinical trials in adults[363–367] showed that IV atropine improved heart rate, symptoms, and signs associated with bradycardia. Atropine sulfate reverses cholinergic-mediated decreases in heart rate and should be considered a temporizing measure while awaiting a transcutaneous or transvenous pacemaker for patients with symptomatic sinus bradycardia, conduction block at the level of the AV node, or sinus arrest.[367]

The recommended atropine dose for bradycardia is 0.5 mg IV every 3 to 5 minutes to a maximum total dose of 3 mg. Doses of atropine sulfate of <0.5 mg may paradoxically result in further slowing of the heart rate.[368] Atropine administration should not delay implementation of external pacing for patients with poor perfusion.

Use atropine cautiously in the presence of acute coronary ischemia or MI; increased heart rate may worsen ischemia or increase infarction size. Atropine will likely be ineffective in patients who have undergone cardiac transplantation because the transplanted heart lacks vagal innervation. One small uncontrolled study documented paradoxical slowing of the heart rate and high-degree AV block when atropine was administered to patients after cardiac transplantation.[369]

Avoid relying on atropine in type II second-degree or third-degree AV block or in patients with third-degree AV block with a new wide-QRS complex where the location of block is likely to be in non-nodal tissue (such as in the bundle of His or more distal conduction system). These bradyarrhythmias are not likely to be responsive to reversal of cholinergic effects by atropine and are preferably treated with TCP or β-adrenergic support as temporizing measures while the patient is prepared for transvenous pacing (Figure 3, **Box 6**).

### Pacing

TCP may be useful for the treatment of symptomatic bradycardias. There are limited studies comparing TCP with drug therapy for the treatment of symptomatic bradycardia. A randomized controlled trial in which atropine and glycopyrrolate were compared with TCP showed few differences in outcome and survival, although the TCP group obtained a more consistent heart rate.[363] In a study evaluating the feasibility of treatment with dopamine as compared with TCP, no differences were observed between treatment groups in survival to hospital discharge.[370] TCP is, at best, a temporizing measure. TCP is painful in conscious patients, and, whether effective or not (achieving inconsistent capture), the patient should be prepared for transvenous pacing and expert consultation should be obtained. It is reasonable for healthcare providers to initiate TCP in unstable patients who do not respond to atropine (Class IIa, LOE B). Immediate pacing might be considered in unstable patients with high-degree AV block when IV access is not available (Class IIb, LOE C). If the patient does not respond to drugs or TCP, transvenous pacing is probably indicated (Class IIa, LOE C) (Figure 3, **Box 6**).

### Alternative Drugs to Consider

Although not first-line agents for treatment of symptomatic bradycardia, dopamine, epinephrine, and isoproterenol are alternatives when a bradyarrhythmia is unresponsive to or inappropriate for treatment with atropine, or as a temporizing measure while awaiting the availability of a pacemaker. Alternative drugs may also be appropriate in special circumstances such as the overdose of a β-blocker or calcium channel blocker.

*Dopamine.* Dopamine hydrochloride is a catecholamine with both α- and β-adrenergic actions. It can be titrated to more selectively target heart rate or vasoconstriction. At lower doses dopamine has a more selective effect on inotropy and heart rate; at higher doses (>10 mcg/kg per minute), it also has vasoconstrictive effects. Dopamine infusion may be used for patients with symptomatic bradycardia, particularly if associated with hypotension, in whom atropine may be inappropriate or after atropine fails (Class IIb, LOE B). Begin dopamine infusion at 2 to 10 mcg/kg per minute and titrate to patient response.[370] Use of vasoconstrictors requires that the recipient be assessed for adequate intravascular volume and volume status supported as needed.

*Epinephrine.* Epinephrine is a catecholamine with α- and β-adrenergic actions. Epinephrine infusion may be used for patients with symptomatic bradycardia, particularly if associated with hypotension, for whom atropine may be inappropriate or after atropine fails (Class IIb, LOE B). Begin the infusion at 2 to 10 mcg/min and titrate to patient response. Use of vasoconstrictors requires that the recipient be assessed for adequate intravascular volume and volume status supported as needed.

*Isoproterenol.* Isoproterenol is a β-adrenergic agent with β-1 and β-2 effects, resulting in an increase in heart rate and vasodilation. The recommended adult dose is 2 to 10 mcg/min by IV infusion, titrated according to heart rate and rhythm response.

## Tachycardia

This section summarizes the management of a wide variety of tachyarrhythmias. Following the overview of tachyarrhythmias and summary of the initial evaluation and treatment of tachycardia, common antiarrhythmic drugs used in the treatment of tachycardia are presented. See the Tachycardia Algorithm, Figure 4. Box numbers in the text refer to the numbered boxes in the algorithm.

### Classification of Tachyarrhythmias

Tachycardias can be classified in several ways, based on the appearance of the QRS complex, heart rate, and regularity. ACLS professionals should be able to recognize and differentiate between sinus tachycardia, narrow-complex supraventricular tachycardia (SVT), and wide-complex tachycardia. Because ACLS providers may be unable to distinguish between supraventricular and ventricular rhythms, they should be aware that most wide-complex (broad-complex) tachycardias are *ventricular* in origin.

- Narrow–QRS-complex (SVT) tachycardias (QRS <0.12 second), in order of frequency
  - Sinus tachycardia
  - Atrial fibrillation
  - Atrial flutter
  - AV nodal reentry
  - Accessory pathway–mediated tachycardia
  - Atrial tachycardia (including automatic and reentry forms)
  - Multifocal atrial tachycardia (MAT)
  - Junctional tachycardia (rare in adults)
- Wide–QRS-complex tachycardias (QRS ≥0.12 second)
  - Ventricular tachycardia (VT) and ventricular fibrillation (VF)
  - SVT with aberrancy
  - Pre-excited tachycardias (Wolff-Parkinson-White [WPW] syndrome)
  - Ventricular paced rhythms

Irregular narrow-complex tachycardias are likely atrial fibrillation or MAT; occasionally atrial flutter is irregular. The management of atrial fibrillation and flutter is discussed in the section "Irregular Tachycardias" below.

### Initial Evaluation and Treatment of Tachyarrhythmias

Tachycardia is defined as an arrhythmia with a rate of >100 beats per minute, although, as with defining bradycardia, the

## Adult Tachycardia
### (With Pulse)

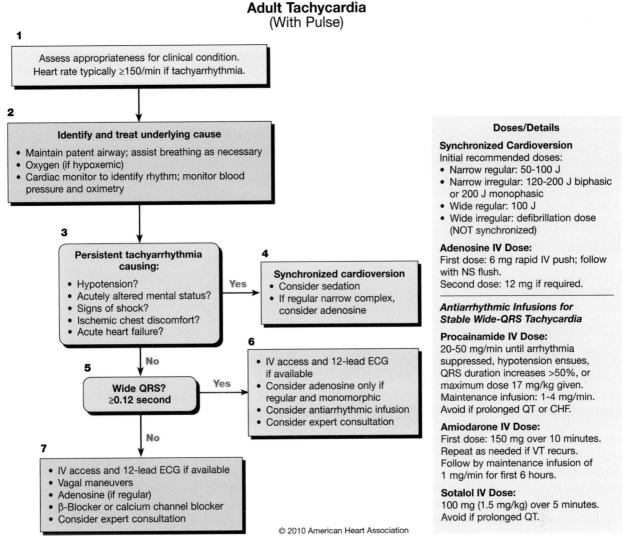

**Doses/Details**

**Synchronized Cardioversion**
Initial recommended doses:
- Narrow regular: 50-100 J
- Narrow irregular: 120-200 J biphasic or 200 J monophasic
- Wide regular: 100 J
- Wide irregular: defibrillation dose (NOT synchronized)

**Adenosine IV Dose:**
First dose: 6 mg rapid IV push; follow with NS flush.
Second dose: 12 mg if required.

*Antiarrhythmic Infusions for Stable Wide-QRS Tachycardia*

**Procainamide IV Dose:**
20-50 mg/min until arrhythmia suppressed, hypotension ensues, QRS duration increases >50%, or maximum dose 17 mg/kg given. Maintenance infusion: 1-4 mg/min. Avoid if prolonged QT or CHF.

**Amiodarone IV Dose:**
First dose: 150 mg over 10 minutes. Repeat as needed if VT recurs. Follow by maintenance infusion of 1 mg/min for first 6 hours.

**Sotalol IV Dose:**
100 mg (1.5 mg/kg) over 5 minutes. Avoid if prolonged QT.

© 2010 American Heart Association

**Figure 4.** Tachycardia Algorithm.

rate of a tachycardia takes on clinical significance at its greater extremes and is more likely attributable to an arrhythmia rate of ≥150 beats per minute (Figure 4, **Box 1**). A rapid heart rate is an appropriate response to a physiologic stress (eg, fever, dehydration) or other underlying conditions. When encountering patients with tachycardia, efforts should be made to determine whether the tachycardia is the primary cause of the presenting symptoms or secondary to an underlying condition that is causing both the presenting symptoms and the faster heart rate. Many experts suggest that when a heart rate is <150 beats per minute, it is unlikely that symptoms of instability are caused primarily by the tachycardia unless there is impaired ventricular function.

The evaluation and management of tachyarrhythmias is depicted in the ACLS Tachycardia With Pulse Algorithm (Figure 4). Box numbers in the text refer to numbered boxes in this algorithm. If cardiac arrest develops at any time, see the ACLS Cardiac Arrest Algorithms in Part 8.2: "Management of Cardiac Arrest."

Because hypoxemia is a common cause of tachycardia, initial evaluation of any patient with tachycardia should focus on signs of increased work of breathing (tachypnea, intercostal retractions, suprasternal retractions, paradoxical abdominal breathing) and oxyhemoglobin saturation as determined by pulse oximetry (Figure 4, **Box 2**). If oxygenation is inadequate or the patient shows signs of increased work of breathing, provide supplementary oxygen. Attach a monitor to the patient, evaluate blood pressure, and establish IV access. If available, obtain a 12-lead ECG to better define the rhythm, but this should not delay immediate cardioversion if the patient is unstable. While initiating treatment, evaluate the patient's clinical status and identify potential reversible causes of the tachycardia.

If signs and symptoms persist despite provision of supplementary oxygen and support of airway and ventilation, the provider should assess the patient's degree of instability and determine if the instability is related to the tachycardia (Figure 4, **Box 3**). If the patient demonstrates rate-related cardiovascular compromise with signs and symptoms such as acute altered mental status, ischemic chest discomfort, acute heart failure, hypotension, or other signs of shock suspected to be due to a tachyarrhythmia, proceed to immediate synchronized cardioversion (Figure 4, **Box 4**). However, with ventricular rates <150 beats per minute in the absence of ventricular dysfunction, it is more likely that the tachycardia is secondary to the underlying condition rather than the cause of the instability. If not hypotensive, the patient with a regular narrow-complex SVT (likely due to suspected reentry, paroxysmal supraventricular tachycardia, as described below) may be treated with adenosine while preparations are made for synchronized cardioversion (Class IIb, LOE C).

If the patient with tachycardia is stable (ie, no serious signs related to the tachycardia), the provider has time to obtain a 12-lead ECG, evaluate the rhythm, determine if the width of the QRS complex is ≥0.12 second (Figure 4, **Box 5**), and determine treatment options. Stable patients may await expert consultation because treatment has the potential for harm.

### Cardioversion
If possible, establish IV access before cardioversion and administer sedation if the patient is conscious. Do not delay cardioversion if the patient is extremely unstable. For further information about defibrillation and cardioversion, see Part 6: "Electrical Therapies."

#### Synchronized Cardioversion and Unsynchronized Shocks (Figure 4, Box 4)
Synchronized cardioversion is shock delivery that is timed (synchronized) with the QRS complex. This synchronization avoids shock delivery during the relative refractory period of the cardiac cycle when a shock could produce VF.[371] If cardioversion is needed and it is impossible to synchronize a shock, use high-energy unsynchronized shocks (defibrillation doses).

Synchronized cardioversion is recommended to treat (1) unstable SVT, (2) unstable atrial fibrillation, (3) unstable atrial flutter, and (4) unstable monomorphic (regular) VT. Shock can terminate these tachyarrhythmias by interrupting the underlying reentrant pathway that is responsible for them.

#### Waveform and Energy
The recommended initial biphasic energy dose for cardioversion of atrial fibrillation is 120 to 200 J (Class IIa, LOE A).[372–376] If the initial shock fails, providers should increase the dose in a stepwise fashion.

Cardioversion of atrial flutter and other SVTs generally requires less energy; an initial energy of 50 J to 100 J is often sufficient.[376] If the initial 50-J shock fails, the provider should increase the dose in a stepwise fashion.[377] Cardioversion with monophasic waveforms should begin at 200 J and increase in stepwise fashion if not successful (Class IIa, LOE B).[372–374]

Monomorphic VT (regular form and rate) with a pulse responds well to monophasic or biphasic waveform cardioversion (synchronized) shocks at initial energies of 100 J. If there is no response to the first shock, it may be reasonable to increase the dose in a stepwise fashion. No studies were identified that addressed this issue. Thus, this recommendation represents expert opinion (Class IIb, LOE C).

Arrhythmias with a polymorphic QRS appearance (such as torsades de pointes) will usually not permit synchronization. Thus, if a patient has polymorphic VT, treat the rhythm as VF and deliver high-energy *unsynchronized* shocks (ie, defibril-

lation doses). If there is any doubt whether monomorphic or polymorphic VT is present in the *unstable* patient, do not delay shock delivery to perform detailed rhythm analysis: provide high-energy unsynchronized shocks (ie, defibrillation doses). Use the ACLS Cardiac Arrest Algorithm (see Part 8.2: "Management of Cardiac Arrest").

### Regular Narrow-Complex Tachycardia
#### Sinus Tachycardia
Sinus tachycardia is common and usually results from a physiologic stimulus, such as fever, anemia, or hypotension/shock. Sinus tachycardia is defined as a heart rate >100 beats per minute. The upper rate of sinus tachycardia is age-related (calculated as approximately 220 beats per minute, minus the patient's age in years) and may be useful in judging whether an apparent sinus tachycardia falls within the expected range for a patient's age. If judged to be sinus tachycardia, no specific drug treatment is required. Instead, therapy is directed toward identification and treatment of the underlying cause. When cardiac function is poor, cardiac output can be dependent on a rapid heart rate. In such compensatory tachycardias, stroke volume is limited, so "normalizing" the heart rate can be detrimental.

#### Supraventricular Tachycardia (Reentry SVT)
*Evaluation.* Most SVTs are regular tachycardias that are caused by reentry, an abnormal rhythm circuit that allows a wave of depolarization to repeatedly travel in a circle in cardiac tissue. The rhythm is considered to be of supraventricular origin if the QRS complex is narrow (<120 milliseconds or <0.12 second) or if the QRS complex is wide (broad) and preexisting bundle branch block or rate-dependent aberrancy is *known* to be present. Reentry circuits resulting in SVT can occur in atrial myocardium (resulting in atrial fibrillation, atrial flutter, and some forms of atrial tachycardia). The reentry circuit may also reside in whole or in part in the AV node itself. This results in AV nodal reentry tachycardia (AVNRT) if both limbs of the reentry circuit involve AV nodal tissue. Alternatively, it may result in AV reentry tachycardia (AVRT) if one limb of the reentry circuit involves an accessory pathway and the other involves the AV node. The characteristic abrupt onset and termination of each of the latter groups of reentrant tachyarrhythmias (AVNRT and AVRT) led to the original name, paroxysmal supraventricular tachycardia (PSVT). This subgroup of reentry arrhythmias, due to either AVNRT or AVRT, is characterized by abrupt onset and termination and a regular rate that exceeds the typical upper limits of sinus tachycardia at rest (usually >150 beats per minute) and, in the case of an AVNRT, often presents without readily identifiable P waves on the ECG.

Distinguishing the forms of reentrant SVTs that are based in atrial myocardium (such as atrial fibrillation) versus those with a reentry circuit partly or wholly based in the AV node itself (PSVT) is important because each will respond differently to therapies aimed at impeding conduction through the AV node. The ventricular rate of reentry arrhythmias based in atrial myocardium will be slowed but not terminated by drugs that slow conduction through the AV node. Conversely, reentry arrhythmias for which at least one limb of the circuit resides in the AV node (PSVT attributable to AVNRT or AVRT) can be terminated by such drugs.

Yet another group of SVTs is referred to as automatic tachycardias. These arrhythmias are not due to a circulating circuit but to an excited automatic focus. Unlike the abrupt pattern of reentry, the characteristic onset and termination of these tachyarrhythmias are more gradual and analogous to how the sinus node behaves in gradually accelerating and slowing heart rate. These automatic arrhythmias include ectopic atrial tachycardia, MAT, and junctional tachycardia. These arrhythmias can be difficult to treat, are not responsive to cardioversion, and are usually controlled acutely with drugs that slow conduction through the AV node and thereby slow ventricular rate.

### Therapy

**Vagal Maneuvers.** Vagal maneuvers and adenosine are the preferred initial therapeutic choices for the termination of stable PSVT (Figure 4, **Box 7**). Vagal maneuvers alone (Valsalva maneuver or carotid sinus massage) will terminate up to 25% of PSVTs.[378–380] For other SVTs, vagal maneuvers and adenosine may transiently slow the ventricular rate and potentially assist rhythm diagnosis but will not usually terminate such arrhythmias.

**Adenosine.** If PSVT does not respond to vagal maneuvers, give 6 mg of IV adenosine as a rapid IV push through a large (eg, antecubital) vein followed by a 20 mL saline flush (Class I, LOE B). If the rhythm does not convert within 1 to 2 minutes, give a 12 mg rapid IV push using the method above. Because of the possibility of initiating atrial fibrillation with rapid ventricular rates in a patient with WPW, a defibrillator should be available when adenosine is administered to any patient in whom WPW is a consideration. As with vagal maneuvers, the effect of adenosine on other SVTs (such as atrial fibrillation or flutter) is to transiently slow ventricular rate (which may be useful diagnostically) but not afford their termination or meaningful lasting rate control.

A number of studies[381–398] support the use of adenosine in the treatment of stable PSVT. Although 2 randomized clinical trials[383,386] documented a similar PSVT conversion rate between adenosine and calcium channel blockers, adenosine was more rapid and had fewer severe side effects than verapamil. Amiodarone as well as other antiarrhythmic agents can be useful in the termination of PSVT, but the onset of action of amiodarone is slower than that of adenosine,[399] and the potential proarrhythmic risks of these agents favor the use of safer treatment alternatives.

Adenosine is safe and effective in pregnancy.[400] However, adenosine does have several important drug interactions. Larger doses may be required for patients with a significant blood level of theophylline, caffeine, or theobromine. The initial dose should be reduced to 3 mg in patients taking dipyridamole or carbamazepine, those with transplanted hearts, or if given by central venous access. Side effects with adenosine are common but transient; flushing, dyspnea, and chest discomfort are the most frequently observed.[401] Adenosine should not be given to patients with asthma.

After conversion, monitor the patient for recurrence and treat any recurrence of PSVT with adenosine or a longer-acting AV nodal blocking agent (eg, diltiazem or β-blocker). If adenosine or vagal maneuvers disclose another form of SVT (such as atrial fibrillation or flutter), treatment with a longer-acting AV nodal blocking agent should be considered to afford more lasting control of ventricular rate.

**Calcium Channel Blockers and β-Blockers.** If adenosine or vagal maneuvers fail to convert PSVT (Figure 4, **Box 7**), PSVT recurs after such treatment, or these treatments disclose a different form of SVT (such as atrial fibrillation or flutter), it is reasonable to use longer-acting AV nodal blocking agents, such as the nondihydropyridine calcium channel blockers (verapamil and diltiazem) (Class IIa, LOE B) or β-blockers (Class IIa, LOE C). These drugs act primarily on nodal tissue either to terminate the reentry PSVTs that depend on conduction through the AV node or to slow the ventricular response to other SVTs by blocking conduction through the AV node. The alternate mechanism of action and longer duration of these drugs may result in more sustained termination of PSVT or afford more sustained rate control of atrial arrhythmias (such as atrial fibrillation or flutter). A number of studies have established the effectiveness of verapamil[381,383,384,386,394, 398,402–405] and diltiazem[402,406,407] in converting PSVT to normal sinus rhythm.

For verapamil, give a 2.5 mg to 5 mg IV bolus over 2 minutes (over 3 minutes in older patients). If there is no therapeutic response and no drug-induced adverse event, repeated doses of 5 mg to 10 mg may be administered every 15 to 30 minutes to a total dose of 20 mg. An alternative dosing regimen is to give a 5 mg bolus every 15 minutes to a total dose of 30 mg. Verapamil should be given *only* to patients with narrow-complex reentry SVT or arrhythmias known with certainty to be of supraventricular origin. Verapamil should not be given to patients with wide-complex tachycardias. It should not be given to patients with impaired ventricular function or heart failure.

For diltiazem, give a dose of 15 mg to 20 mg (0.25 mg/kg) IV over 2 minutes; if needed, in 15 minutes give an additional IV dose of 20 mg to 25 mg (0.35 mg/kg). The maintenance infusion dose is 5 mg/hour to 15 mg/hour, titrated to heart rate.

A wide variety of IV β-blockers are available for treatment of supraventricular tachyarrhythmias. These include metoprolol, atenolol, propranolol, esmolol, and labetolol (the latter more commonly used for acute management of hypertension than for arrhythmias). In principle these agents exert their effect by antagonizing sympathetic tone in nodal tissue, resulting in slowing of conduction. Like calcium channel blockers, they also have negative inotropic effects and further reduce cardiac output in patients with heart failure. More detailed information is provided below. Side effects of β-blockers can include bradycardias, AV conduction delays, and hypotension. β-blockers should be used with caution in patients with obstructive pulmonary disease or congestive heart failure.

Caution is advised when encountering pre-excited atrial fibrillation or flutter that conducts to the ventricles via both the AV node and an accessory pathway. Treatment with an AV nodal blocking agent (including adenosine, calcium blockers, β-blockers, or digoxin) is unlikely to slow the ventricular rate and in some instances may accelerate the ventricular response. Therefore, AV nodal blocking drugs should not be used for pre-excited atrial fibrillation or flutter (Class III, LOE C).

Caution is also advised to avoid the combination of AV nodal blocking agents that have a longer duration of action. For example, the short elimination half-life of adenosine affords follow-up treatment, if required, with a calcium channel blocker or β-blocker. Conversely the longer half-life of a calcium channel or β-blocker means their effects will overlap; profound bradycardia can develop if they are given serially.

Although antiarrhythmic medications (eg, amiodarone, procainamide, or sotalol) can also be used to treat SVTs, the higher toxicity and risk for proarrhythmia make these medications less desirable alternatives to the described AV nodal blocking agents. A possible exception is in patients with pre-excited atrial arrhythmias; the typical AV nodal blocking drugs are contraindicated in these patients and rate control may be achieved with antiarrhythmic medications. Importantly, use of these agents for atrial-based SVTs, such as atrial fibrillation and flutter can result in their termination, which may be undesirable in the absence of precautions to prevent the thromboembolic complications that may result from such conversion.

### Wide-Complex Tachycardia (Figure 4, Boxes 5, 6, and 7)

*Evaluation*

The first step in the management of any tachycardia is to determine if the patient's condition is stable or unstable (Figure 4, **Box 3**). An unstable patient with a wide-complex tachycardia should be presumed to have VT and immediate cardioversion should be performed (Figure 4, **Box 4** and see above). Precordial thump may be considered for patients with witnessed, monitored, unstable ventricular tachycardia if a defibrillator is not immediately ready for use (Class IIb, LOE C).

If the patient is stable, the second step in management is to obtain a 12-lead ECG (Figure 4, **Boxes 6 and 7**) to evaluate the rhythm. At this point the provider should consider the need to obtain expert consultation. If the patient becomes unstable at any time, proceed with synchronized cardioversion or unsynchronized defibrillation should the arrhythmia deteriorate to VF or be due to a polymorphic VT.

Wide-complex tachycardias are defined as those with a QRS ≥0.12 second. The most common forms of wide-complex tachycardia are

- VT or VF
- SVT with aberrancy
- Pre-excited tachycardias (associated with or mediated by an accessory pathway)
- Ventricular paced rhythms

The third step in management of a tachycardia is to determine if the rhythm is regular or irregular. A *regular* wide-complex tachycardia is likely to be VT or SVT with aberrancy. An *irregular* wide-complex tachycardia may be atrial fibrillation with aberrancy, pre-excited atrial fibrillation (ie, atrial fibrillation using an accessory pathway for antegrade conduction), or polymorphic VT/torsades de pointes. Providers should consider the need for expert consultation when treating wide-complex tachycardias.

*Therapy for Regular Wide-Complex Tachycardias*

In patients with stable undifferentiated wide-QRS complex tachycardia, a reasonable approach is to try to identify the wide-complex tachycardia as SVT or VT and treat based on the algorithm for that rhythm.

If the etiology of the rhythm cannot be determined, the rate is regular, and the QRS is monomorphic, recent evidence suggests that IV adenosine is relatively safe for both treatment and diagnosis[47] (Class IIb, LOE B). However, adenosine should **not** be given for unstable or for ***irregular or polymorphic*** wide-complex tachycardias, as it may cause degeneration of the arrhythmia to VF (Class III, LOE C). If the wide-complex tachycardia proves to be SVT with aberrancy, it will likely be transiently slowed or converted by adenosine to sinus rhythm; if due to VT there will be no effect on rhythm (except in rare cases of idiopathic VT), and the brevity of the transient adenosine effect should be reasonably tolerated hemodynamically. Because close attention to these varying responses may help to diagnose the underlying rhythm, whenever possible, continuous ECG recording is strongly encouraged to provide such written documentation. This documentation can be invaluable in helping to establish a firm rhythm diagnosis even if after the fact. Typically, adenosine is administered in a manner similar to treatment of PSVT: as a 6 mg rapid IV push; providers may follow the first dose with a 12 mg bolus and a second 12 mg bolus if the rate fails to convert. When adenosine is given for undifferentiated wide-complex tachycardia, a defibrillator should be available.

Depending on the underlying rhythm, the response to adenosine challenge can be variable. Some studies[408–412] showed that adenosine converted an undifferentiated wide-complex tachycardia to sinus rhythm. Another study[413] showed poor rates of conversion to sinus rhythm in patients known to have VT. The following adverse effects were reported in patients with pre-excited atrial fibrillation treated with adenosine: conversion to atrial fibrillation with a rapid ventricular response in one patient later found to have preexcitation, conversion to VF in one patient with known WPW,[414] conversion to VF in 4 patients with pre-excited atrial fibrillation,[415] conversion to VF in 2 patients with WPW,[416] and a single case of VF in a patient with VT.[417]

Verapamil is contraindicated for wide-complex tachycardias unless known to be of supraventricular origin (Class III, LOE B). Adverse effects when the rhythm was due to VT were shown in 5 small case series.[414–418] Profound hypotension was reported in 11 of 25 patients known to have VT treated with verapamil.[418]

For patients who are stable with likely VT, IV antiarrhythmic drugs or elective cardioversion is the preferred treatment strategy. If IV antiarrhythmics are administered, procainamide (Class IIa, LOE B), amiodarone (Class IIb, LOE B), or sotalol (Class IIb, LOE B) can be considered. Procainamide and sotalol should be avoided in patients with prolonged QT. If one of these antiarrhythmic agents is given, a second agent should not be given without expert consultation (Class III, LOE B). If antiarrhythmic therapy is unsuccessful, cardioversion or expert consultation should be considered (Class IIa, LOE C).

One randomized comparison found procainamide (10 mg/kg) to be superior to lidocaine (1.5 mg/kg) for termination of hemodynamically stable monomorphic VT.[419] Procainamide can be administered at a rate of 20 to 50 mg/min until the arrhythmia is suppressed, hypotension ensues, QRS duration increases >50%, or the maximum dose of 17 mg/kg is given. Maintenance infusion is 1 to 4 mg/min. Procainamide should be avoided in patients with prolonged QT and congestive heart failure.

IV sotalol (100 mg IV over 5 minutes) was found to be more effective than lidocaine (100 mg IV over 5 minutes) when administered to patients with spontaneous hemodynamically stable sustained monomorphic VT in a double-blind randomized trial within a hospital setting.[420] In a separate study of 109 patients with a history of spontaneous and inducible sustained ventricular tachyarrhythmias, infusing 1.5 mg/kg of sotalol over ≤5 minutes was found to be relatively safe and effective, causing hypotension in only 2 patients, both of whom responded to IV fluid.[421] Package insert recommends slow infusion, but the literature supports more rapid infusion of 1.5 mg/kg over 5 minutes or less. Sotalol should be avoided in patients with a prolonged QT interval.

Amiodarone is also effective in preventing recurrent monomorphic VT or treating refractory ventricular arrhythmias[286,422–424] in patients with coronary artery disease and poor ventricular function. It is given 150 mg IV over 10 minutes; dosing should be repeated as needed to a maximum dose of 2.2 g IV per 24 hours. Higher doses (300 mg) were associated with an increased frequency of hypotension, although some reports[422,424] attributed the hypotension to the vasoactive solvents that are not present in a new form of the drug recently approved for use in the US.

By comparison, lidocaine is less effective in terminating VT than procainamide, sotalol, and amiodarone,[286,419,420] and when given to patients with or without a history of MI with spontaneous sustained stable VT in the hospital setting.[413,425,426] Lidocaine has been reported to variably terminate VT when administered intramuscularly to patients with AMI and VT in the out-of-hospital setting.[427,428] Thus, while occasionally effective, lidocaine should be considered second-line antiarrhythmic therapy for monomorphic VT. Lidocaine can be administered at a dose of 1 to 1.5 mg/kg IV bolus. Maintenance infusion is 1 to 4 mg/min (30 to 50 mcg/kg per minute).

## Irregular Tachycardias

### Atrial Fibrillation and Flutter

#### Evaluation
An irregular narrow-complex or wide-complex tachycardia is most likely atrial fibrillation (with or without aberrant conduction) with an uncontrolled ventricular response. Other diagnostic possibilities include MAT or sinus rhythm/tachycardia with frequent atrial premature beats. When there is doubt about the rhythm diagnosis and the patient is stable, a 12-lead ECG with expert consultation is recommended.

#### Therapy
General management of atrial fibrillation should focus on control of the rapid ventricular rate (rate control), conversion of hemodynamically unstable atrial fibrillation to sinus rhythm (rhythm control), or both. Patients with an atrial fibrillation duration of >48 hours are at increased risk for cardioembolic events, although shorter durations of atrial fibrillation do not exclude the possibility of such events. Electric or pharmacologic cardioversion (conversion to normal sinus rhythm) should *not be attempted* in these patients unless the patient is unstable. An alternative strategy is to perform cardioversion following anticoagulation with heparin *and* performance of transesophageal echocardiography to ensure the absence of a left atrial thrombus; see the ACC/AHA Guidelines for Management of Patients with Atrial Fibrillation.[429]

#### Rate Control
Patients who are hemodynamically unstable should receive prompt electric cardioversion. More stable patients require ventricular rate control as directed by patient symptoms and hemodynamics. IV β-blockers and nondihydropyridine calcium channel blockers such as diltiazem[430–433] are the drugs of choice for acute rate control in most individuals with atrial fibrillation and rapid ventricular response (Class IIa, LOE A). Digoxin[434–436] and amiodarone[437,438] may be used for rate control in patients with congestive heart failure; however, the potential risk of conversion to sinus rhythm with amiodarone should be considered before treating with this agent.

A wide-complex irregular rhythm should be considered pre-excited atrial fibrillation. Expert consultation is advised. Avoid AV nodal blocking agents such as adenosine, calcium channel blockers, digoxin, and possibly β-blockers in patients with pre-excitation atrial fibrillation because these drugs may cause a paradoxical increase in the ventricular response. Typically, patients with pre-excited atrial fibrillation present with very rapid heart rates and require emergent electric cardioversion. When electric cardioversion is not feasible or effective, or atrial fibrillation is recurrent, use of rhythm control agents (discussed below) may be useful for both rate control and stabilization of the rhythm.

#### Rhythm Control
A variety of agents have been shown to be effective in terminating atrial fibrillation (pharmacologic or chemical cardioversion), although success between them varies and not all are available as parenteral formulations. Expert consultation is recommended.

### Polymorphic (Irregular) VT
Polymorphic (irregular) VT requires immediate defibrillation with the same strategy used for VF.

Pharmacologic treatment to prevent recurrent polymorphic VT should be directed by the underlying cause of VT and the presence or absence of a long QT interval during sinus rhythm.

If a long QT interval is observed during sinus rhythm (ie, the VT is torsades de pointes), the first step is to stop medications known to prolong the QT interval. Correct electrolyte imbalance and other acute precipitants (eg, drug overdose or poisoning: see Part 12.7: "Cardiac Arrest Associated With Toxic Ingestions"). Although magnesium is commonly used to treat torsades de pointes VT (polymorphic VT associated with long QT interval), it is supported by only 2 observational studies[107,170] that showed effectiveness in patients with prolonged QT interval. One adult case series[439] showed that isoproterenol or ventricular pacing can be effective in terminating torsades de pointes associated with bradycardia and drug-induced QT prolongation. Polymorphic VT associated with familial long QT syndrome may be treated with IV magnesium, pacing, and/or β-blockers; isoproterenol should be avoided. Polymorphic VT associated with acquired long QT syndrome may be treated with IV magnesium. The addition of pacing or IV isoproterenol may be considered when polymorphic VT is accompanied by bradycardia or appears to be precipitated by pauses in rhythm.

In the absence of a prolonged QT interval, the most common cause of polymorphic VT is myocardial ischemia. In this situation IV amiodarone and β-blockers may reduce the frequency of arrhythmia recurrence (Class IIb, LOE C). Myocardial ischemia should be treated with β-blockers and consideration be given to expeditious cardiac catheterization with revascularization. Magnesium is unlikely to be effective in preventing polymorphic VT in patients with a normal QT interval (Class IIb, LOE C),[107] but amiodarone may be effective (Class IIb, LOE C).[440]

Other causes of polymorphic VT apart from ischemia and long QT syndrome are catecholaminergic VT (which may be responsive to β-blockers) and Brugada syndrome (which may be responsive to isoproterenol).

## Summary

The goal of therapy for bradycardia or tachycardia is to rapidly identify and treat patients who are hemodynamically unstable or symptomatic due to the arrhythmia. Drugs or, when appropriate, pacing may be used to control unstable or symptomatic bradycardia. Cardioversion or drugs or both may be used to control unstable or symptomatic tachycardia. ACLS providers should closely monitor stable patients pending expert consultation and should be prepared to aggressively treat those with evidence of decompensation.

# Disclosures

## Guidelines Part 8: ACLS Writing Group Disclosures

| Writing Group Member | Employment | Research Grant | Other Research Support | Speakers' Bureau/ Honoraria | Ownership Interest | Consultant/ Advisory Board | Other |
|---|---|---|---|---|---|---|---|
| Robert W. Neumar | University of Pennsylvania–Associate Professor of Emergency Medicine | None | None | None | None | None | None |
| Charles W. Otto | University of Arizona–Professor | None | None | None | None | None | None |
| Mark S. Link | Tufts Medical Center–Physician | None | None | None | None | None | None |
| Steven L. Kronick | University of Michigan–Assistant Professor | None | None | None | None | None | None |
| Michael Shuster | Self-employed–emergency physician | None | None | None | None | None | None |
| Clifton W. Callaway | University of Pittsburgh School of Medicine–Associate Professor; UPMC Health System—Physician *American Heart Association-Work Sheet Editor for 2010 Guidelines. My effort on this project is paid to University of Pittsburgh as a "contracted services agreement," and not paid directly to me | †Grants to University of Pittsburgh: NHLBI-Resuscitation Outcomes Consortium HRSA-Development and Dissemination of Program Tools for Uncontrolled Donation After Cardiac Death (UDCD) | *Loan of an Arctic Sun cooling device (without disposables) to human physiology laboratory for experiments on hypothermia by Medivance, Inc. | None | †Co-inventor on patent about ventricular fibrillation waveform analysis, licensed by University of Pittsburgh to Medtronic ERS, Inc. | None | None |
| Peter J. Kudenchuk | University of Washington–Professor of Medicine | †Resuscitation Outcomes Consortium (NIH/NHLBI) | None | Network for Continuing Medical Education, Academy for Healthcare Education, Sanofi-Aventis, with honoraria | Sanofi-Aventis, Novartis | None | None |
| Joseph P. Ornato | Richmond Ambulance Authority–Medical Director; Virginia Commonwealth University-Prof & Chmn, Emergency Medicine | †Consultant and Cardiac Co-Chairman, NIH Resuscitation Outcomes Consortium Principal Investigator, VCU site for NIH Neurological Emergency Treatment Trials Network | None | *Hospital grand rounds presentations funded by ZOLL Circulation *Occasional hospital grand rounds supported by unrestricted educational grants from Squibb/Sanofi, ZOLL | None | *ZOLL Circulation Science Advisory Board (UNPAID, only receive travel reimbursement) | None |

(*Continued*)

**Guidelines Part 8: ACLS Writing Group Disclosures, *Continued***

| Writing Group Member | Employment | Research Grant | Other Research Support | Speakers' Bureau/ Honoraria | Ownership Interest | Consultant/ Advisory Board | Other |
|---|---|---|---|---|---|---|---|
| Bryan McNally | Emory University– Assistant Professor of Emergency Medicine | †Center for Disease Control and Prevention, CARES-Cardiac Arrest Registry to Enhance Survival, Money comes to Emory University School of Medicine as part of a cooperative agreement through American Association of Medical Colleges | None | None | None | None | None |
| Scott M. Silvers | Mayo Clinic–Chair, Department of Emergency Medicine | None | None | None | None | None | None |
| Rod S. Passman | Northwestern University–Associate Professor | None | None | None | None | *Steering Committee member for Medtronic Crystal AF study | None |
| Roger D. White | Mayo Clinic–staff physician | None | None | None | None | None | None |
| Erik P. Hess | Mayo Clinic–Senior Associate Consultant | None | None | None | None | None | None |
| Wanchun Tang | Weil Institute of Critical Care Medicine–Professor and president | None | None | *47th Weil Critical Care Symposium: $1,500 | None | None | None |
| Daniel Davis | UC San Diego–Faculty physician | †Zoll Medical (Air Medical Advanced Monitoring Strategies) | *Bispectral EEG Analyzer (Zoll Medical) | *Continuous Renal Replacement Therapy Conference 2009 Hospital Medicine National and Regional Meeting 2009 Grand Rounds Redding Medical Center | None | †Cardinal Health (Development of a Prehospital Ventilator) | *Derek White Law Firm John Anderson Law Firm Otorowski Johnston Diamond & Golden Law Firm |
| Elizabeth Sinz | Penn State Hershey Medical Center–Professor of Anesthesiology and Neurosurgery; AHA: Paid Consultant Associate Science Editor | None | None | None | None | None | None |
| Laurie J. Morrison | St Michaels Hosp. Clinician Scientist | None | None | None | None | None | None |

This table represents the relationships of writing group members that may be perceived as actual or reasonably perceived conflicts of interest as reported on the Disclosure Questionnaire, which all members of the writing group are required to complete and submit. A relationship is considered to be "significant" if (a) the person receives $10 000 or more during any 12-month period, or 5% or more of the person's gross income; or (b) the person owns 5% or more of the voting stock or share of the entity, or owns $10 000 or more of the fair market value of the entity. A relationship is considered to be "modest" if it is less than "significant" under the preceding definition.

*Modest.

†Significant.

# References

1. Ornato JP, Garnett AR, Glauser FL. Relationship between cardiac output and the end-tidal carbon dioxide tension. *Ann Emerg Med*. 1990; 19:1104–1106.

2. Chandra NC, Gruben KG, Tsitlik JE, Brower R, Guerci AD, Halperin HH, Weisfeldt ML, Permutt S. Observations of ventilation during resuscitation in a canine model. *Circulation*. 1994;90:3070–3075.

3. Liu Y, Rosenthal RE, Haywood Y, Miljkovic-Lolic M, Vanderhoek JY, Fiskum G. Normoxic ventilation after cardiac arrest reduces oxidation of brain lipids and improves neurological outcome. *Stroke*. 1998;29: 1679–1686.

4. Zwemer CF, Whitesall SE, D'Alecy LG. Cardiopulmonary-cerebral resuscitation with 100% oxygen exacerbates neurological dysfunction following nine minutes of normothermic cardiac arrest in dogs. *Resuscitation*. 1994;27:159–170.

5. Lipinski CA, Hicks SD, Callaway CW. Normoxic ventilation during resuscitation and outcome from asphyxial cardiac arrest in rats. *Resuscitation*. 1999;42:221–229.

6. Kellum MJ, Kennedy KW, Ewy GA. Cardiocerebral resuscitation improves survival of patients with out-of-hospital cardiac arrest. *Am J Med*. 2006;119:335–340.

7. Kellum MJ, Kennedy KW, Barney R, Keilhauer FA, Bellino M, Zuercher M, Ewy GA. Cardiocerebral resuscitation improves neurologically intact survival of patients with out-of-hospital cardiac arrest. *Ann Emerg Med*. 2008;52:244–252.

8. Bobrow BJ, Ewy GA, Clark L, Chikani V, Berg RA, Sanders AB, Vadeboncoeur TF, Hilwig RW, Kern KB. Passive oxygen insufflation is superior to bag-valve-mask ventilation for witnessed ventricular fibrillation out-of-hospital cardiac arrest. *Ann Emerg Med*. 2009;54: 656–662.

9. Saissy JM, Boussignac G, Cheptel E, Rouvin B, Fontaine D, Bargues L, Levecque JP, Michel A, Brochard L. Efficacy of continuous insufflation of oxygen combined with active cardiac compression-decompression during out-of-hospital cardiorespiratory arrest. *Anesthesiology*. 2000;92: 1523–1530.

10. Bertrand C, Hemery F, Carli P, Goldstein P, Espesson C, Ruttimann M, Macher JM, Raffy B, Fuster P, Dolveck F, Rozenberg A, Lecarpentier E, Duvaldestin P, Saissy JM, Boussignac G, Brochard L. Constant flow insufflation of oxygen as the sole mode of ventilation during out-of-hospital cardiac arrest. *Intensive Care Med*. 2006;32:843–851.

11. Bailey AR, Hett DA. The laryngeal mask airway in resuscitation. *Resuscitation*. 1994;28:107–110.

12. Dorges V, Wenzel V, Knacke P, Gerlach K. Comparison of different airway management strategies to ventilate apneic, nonpreoxygenated patients. *Crit Care Med*. 2003;31:800–804.

13. Dorges V, Ocker H, Hagelberg S, Wenzel V, Idris AH, Schmucker P. Smaller tidal volumes with room-air are not sufficient to ensure adequate oxygenation during bag-valve-mask ventilation. *Resuscitation*. 2000;44:37–41.

14. Doerges V, Sauer C, Ocker H, Wenzel V, Schmucker P. Airway management during cardiopulmonary resuscitation—a comparative study of bag-valve-mask, laryngeal mask airway and combitube in a bench model. *Resuscitation*. 1999;41:63–69.

15. Weiler N, Heinrichs W, Dick W. Assessment of pulmonary mechanics and gastric inflation pressure during mask ventilation. *Prehosp Disaster Med*. 1995;10:101–105.

16. Ocker H, Wenzel V, Schmucker P, Dorges V. Effectiveness of various airway management techniques in a bench model simulating a cardiac arrest patient. *J Emerg Med*. 2001;20:7–12.

17. Petito SP, Russell WJ. The prevention of gastric inflation—a neglected benefit of cricoid pressure. *Anaesth Intensive Care*. 1988;16:139–143.

18. Lawes EG, Campbell I, Mercer D. Inflation pressure, gastric insufflation and rapid sequence induction. *Br J Anaesth*. 1987;59:315–318.

19. Salem MR, Wong AY, Mani M, Sellick BA. Efficacy of cricoid pressure in preventing gastric inflation during bag-mask ventilation in pediatric patients. *Anesthesiology*. 1974;40:96–98.

20. Moynihan RJ, Brock-Utne JG, Archer JH, Feld LH, Kreitzman TR. The effect of cricoid pressure on preventing gastric insufflation in infants and children. *Anesthesiology*. 1993;78:652–656.

21. Asai T, Goy RW, Liu EH. Cricoid pressure prevents placement of the laryngeal tube and laryngeal tube-suction II. *Br J Anaesth*. 2007;99: 282–285.

22. Turgeon AF, Nicole PC, Trepanier CA, Marcoux S, Lessard MR. Cricoid pressure does not increase the rate of failed intubation by direct laryngoscopy in adults. *Anesthesiology*. 2005;102:315–319.

23. Allman KG. The effect of cricoid pressure application on airway patency. *J Clin Anesth*. 1995;7:197–199.

24. Brimacombe J, White A, Berry A. Effect of cricoid pressure on ease of insertion of the laryngeal mask airway. *Br J Anaesth*. 1993;71:800–802.

25. McNelis U, Syndercombe A, Harper I, Duggan J. The effect of cricoid pressure on intubation facilitated by the gum elastic bougie. *Anaesthesia*. 2007;62:456–459.

26. Hartsilver EL, Vanner RG. Airway obstruction with cricoid pressure. *Anaesthesia*. 2000;55:208–211.

27. Hocking G, Roberts FL, Thew ME. Airway obstruction with cricoid pressure and lateral tilt. *Anaesthesia*. 2001;56:825–828.

28. Stoneham MD. The nasopharyngeal airway. Assessment of position by fibreoptic laryngoscopy. *Anaesthesia*. 1993;48:575–580.

29. Schade K, Borzotta A, Michaels A. Intracranial malposition of nasopharyngeal airway. *J Trauma*. 2000;49:967–968.

30. Muzzi DA, Losasso TJ, Cucchiara RF. Complication from a nasopharyngeal airway in a patient with a basilar skull fracture. *Anesthesiology*. 1991;74:366–368.

31. Wong ML, Carey S, Mader TJ, Wang HE. Time to invasive airway placement and resuscitation outcomes after inhospital cardiopulmonary arrest. *Resuscitation*. 2010;81:182–186.

32. Shy BD, Rea TD, Becker LJ, Eisenberg MS. Time to intubation and survival in prehospital cardiac arrest. *Prehosp Emerg Care*. 2004;8: 394–399.

33. Jennings PA, Cameron P, Walker T, Bernard S, Smith K. Out-of-hospital cardiac arrest in Victoria: rural and urban outcomes. *Med J Aust*. 2006;185:135–139.

34. Dumot JA, Burval DJ, Sprung J, Waters JH, Mraovic B, Karafa MT, Mascha EJ, Bourke DL. Outcome of adult cardiopulmonary resuscitations at a tertiary referral center including results of "limited" resuscitations. *Arch Intern Med*. 2001;161:1751–1758.

35. Rabitsch W, Schellongowski P, Staudinger T, Hofbauer R, Dufek V, Eder B, Raab H, Thell R, Schuster E, Frass M. Comparison of a conventional tracheal airway with the Combitube in an urban emergency medical services system run by physicians. *Resuscitation*. 2003;57: 27–32.

36. Rumball CJ, MacDonald D. The PTL, Combitube, laryngeal mask, and oral airway: a randomized prehospital comparative study of ventilatory device effectiveness and cost-effectiveness in 470 cases of cardiorespiratory arrest. *Prehosp Emerg Care*. 1997;1:1–10.

37. Verghese C, Prior-Willeard PF, Baskett PJ. Immediate management of the airway during cardiopulmonary resuscitation in a hospital without a resident anaesthesiologist. *Eur J Emerg Med*. 1994;1:123–125.

38. Cady CE, Weaver MD, Pirrallo RG, Wang HE. Effect of emergency medical technician-placed Combitubes on outcomes after out-of-hospital cardiopulmonary arrest. *Prehosp Emerg Care*. 2009;13: 495–499.

39. Comparison of arterial blood gases of laryngeal mask airway and bag-valve-mask ventilation in out-of-hospital cardiac arrests. *Circ J*. 2009; 73:490–496.

40. Schalk R, Byhahn C, Fausel F, Egner A, Oberndorfer D, Walcher F, Latasch L. Out-of-hospital airway management by paramedics and emergency physicians using laryngeal tubes. *Resuscitation*. 2010;81: 323–326.

41. Heuer JF, Barwing J, Eich C, Quintel M, Crozier TA, Roessler M. Initial ventilation through laryngeal tube instead of face mask in out-of-hospital cardiopulmonary arrest is effective and safe. *Eur J Emerg Med*. 2010;17:10–15.

42. Vertongen VM, Ramsay MP, Herbison P. Skills retention for insertion of the Combitube and laryngeal mask airway. *Emerg Med*. 2003;15: 459–464.

43. Lefrancois DP, Dufour DG. Use of the esophageal tracheal combitube by basic emergency medical technicians. *Resuscitation*. 2002;52:77–83.

44. Tanigawa K, Shigematsu A. Choice of airway devices for 12,020 cases of nontraumatic cardiac arrest in Japan. *Prehosp Emerg Care*. 1998;2: 96–100.

45. Atherton GL, Johnson JC. Ability of paramedics to use the Combitube in prehospital cardiac arrest. *Ann Emerg Med*. 1993;22:1263–1268.

46. Rumball C, Macdonald D, Barber P, Wong H, Smecher C. Endotracheal intubation and esophageal tracheal Combitube insertion by regular ambulance attendants: a comparative trial. *Prehosp Emerg Care*. 2004; 8:15–22.

47. Staudinger T, Brugger S, Roggla M, Rintelen C, Atherton GL, Johnson JC, Frass M. [Comparison of the Combitube with the endotracheal tube

in cardiopulmonary resuscitation in the prehospital phase]. *Wien Klin Wochenschr.* 1994;106:412–415.

48. Frass M, Frenzer R, Rauscha F, Schuster E, Glogar D. Ventilation with the esophageal tracheal combitube in cardiopulmonary resuscitation: promptness and effectiveness. *Chest.* 1988;93:781–784.

49. Samarkandi AH, Seraj MA, el Dawlatly A, Mastan M, Bakhamees HB. The role of laryngeal mask airway in cardiopulmonary resuscitation. *Resuscitation.* 1994;28:103–106.

50. Rabitsch W, Krafft P, Lackner FX, Frenzer R, Hofbauer R, Sherif C, Frass M. Evaluation of the oesophageal-tracheal double-lumen tube (Combitube) during general anaesthesia. *Wien Klin Wochenschr.* 2004; 116:90–93.

51. Vézina D, Lessard MR, Bussieres J, Topping C, Trepanier CA. Complications associated with the use of the Esophageal-Tracheal Combitube. *Can J Anaesth.* 1998;45:76–80.

52. Wiese CH, Semmel T, Muller JU, Bahr J, Ocker H, Graf BM. The use of the laryngeal tube disposable (LT-D) by paramedics during out-of-hospital resuscitation—an observational study concerning ERC guidelines 2005. *Resuscitation.* 2009;80:194–198.

53. Kette F, Reffo I, Giordani G, Buzzi F, Borean V, Cimarosti R, Codiglia A, Hattinger C, Mongiat A, Tararan S. The use of laryngeal tube by nurses in out-of-hospital emergencies: preliminary experience. *Resuscitation.* 2005; 66:21–25.

54. Stone BJ, Chantler PJ, Baskett PJ. The incidence of regurgitation during cardiopulmonary resuscitation: a comparison between the bag valve mask and laryngeal mask airway. *Resuscitation.* 1998;38:3–6.

55. The use of the laryngeal mask airway by nurses during cardiopulmonary resuscitation: results of a multicentre trial. *Anaesthesia.* 1994;49:3–7.

56. Grantham H, Phillips G, Gilligan JE. The laryngeal mask in prehospital emergency care. *Emerg Med.* 1994;6:193–197.

57. Kokkinis K. The use of the laryngeal mask airway in CPR. *Resuscitation.* 1994;27:9–12.

58. Leach A, Alexander CA, Stone B. The laryngeal mask in cardiopulmonary resuscitation in a district general hospital: a preliminary communication. *Resuscitation.* 1993;25:245–248.

59. Flaishon R, Sotman A, Ben-Abraham R, Rudick V, Varssano D, Weinbroum AA. Antichemical protective gear prolongs time to successful airway management: a randomized, crossover study in humans. *Anesthesiology.* 2004;100:260–266.

60. Goldik Z, Bornstein J, Eden A, Ben-Abraham R. Airway management by physicians wearing anti-chemical warfare gear: comparison between laryngeal mask airway and endotracheal intubation. *Eur J Anaesthesiol.* 2002;19:166–169.

61. Pennant JH, Pace NA, Gajraj NM. Role of the laryngeal mask airway in the immobile cervical spine. *J Clin Anesth.* 1993;5:226–230.

62. Davies PR, Tighe SQ, Greenslade GL, Evans GH. Laryngeal mask airway and tracheal tube insertion by unskilled personnel. *Lancet.* 1990; 336:977–979.

63. Reinhart DJ, Simmons G. Comparison of placement of the laryngeal mask airway with endotracheal tube by paramedics and respiratory therapists. *Ann Emerg Med.* 1994;24:260–263.

64. Pennant JH, Walker MB. Comparison of the endotracheal tube and laryngeal mask in airway management by paramedical personnel. *Anesth Analg.* 1992;74:531–534.

65. Yardy N, Hancox D, Strang T. A comparison of two airway aids for emergency use by unskilled personnel: the Combitube and laryngeal mask. *Anaesthesia.* 1999;54:181–183.

66. Warner KJ, Carlbom D, Cooke CR, Bulger EM, Copass MK, Sharar SR. Paramedic training for proficient prehospital endotracheal intubation. *Prehosp Emerg Care.* 2010;14:103–108.

67. Gausche M, Lewis RJ. Out-of-hospital endotracheal intubation of children. *JAMA.* 2000;283:2790–2792.

68. Jones JH, Murphy MP, Dickson RL, Somerville GG, Brizendine EJ. Emergency physician-verified out-of-hospital intubation: miss rates by paramedics. *Acad Emerg Med.* 2004;11:707–709.

69. Sayre MR, Sakles JC, Mistler AF, Evans JL, Kramer AT, Pancioli AM. Field trial of endotracheal intubation by basic EMTs. *Ann Emerg Med.* 1998;31:228–233.

70. Katz SH, Falk JL. Misplaced endotracheal tubes by paramedics in an urban emergency medical services system. *Ann Emerg Med.* 2001;37: 32–37.

71. Jemmett ME, Kendal KM, Fourre MW, Burton JH. Unrecognized misplacement of endotracheal tubes in a mixed urban to rural emergency medical services setting. *Acad Emerg Med.* 2003;10:961–965.

72. Silvestri S, Ralls GA, Krauss B, Thundiyil J, Rothrock SG, Senn A, Carter E, Falk J. The effectiveness of out-of-hospital use of continuous end-tidal carbon dioxide monitoring on the rate of unrecognized misplaced intubation within a regional emergency medical services system. *Ann Emerg Med.* 2005;45:497–503.

73. Beyer AJd, Land G, Zaritsky A. Nonphysician transport of intubated pediatric patients: a system evaluation. *Crit Care Med.* 1992;20: 961–966.

74. White SJ, Slovis CM. Inadvertent esophageal intubation in the field: reliance on a fool's "gold standard." *Acad Emerg Med.* 1997;4:89–91.

75. Andersen KH, Schultz-Lebahn T. Oesophageal intubation can be undetected by auscultation of the chest. *Acta Anaesthesiol Scand.* 1994;38: 580–582.

76. Kelly JJ, Eynon CA, Kaplan JL, de Garavilla L, Dalsey WC. Use of tube condensation as an indicator of endotracheal tube placement. *Ann Emerg Med.* 1998;31:575–578.

77. Grmec S. Comparison of three different methods to confirm tracheal tube placement in emergency intubation. *Intensive Care Med.* 2002;28: 701–704.

78. Takeda T, Tanigawa K, Tanaka H, Hayashi Y, Goto E, Tanaka K. The assessment of three methods to verify tracheal tube placement in the emergency setting. *Resuscitation.* 2003;56:153–157.

79. Tanigawa K, Takeda T, Goto E, Tanaka K. The efficacy of esophageal detector devices in verifying tracheal tube placement: a randomized cross-over study of out-of-hospital cardiac arrest patients. *Anesth Analg.* 2001;92:375–378.

80. Tanigawa K, Takeda T, Goto E, Tanaka K. Accuracy and reliability of the self-inflating bulb to verify tracheal intubation in out-of-hospital cardiac arrest patients. *Anesthesiology.* 2000;93:1432–1436.

81. Trikha A, Singh C, Rewari V, Arora MK. Evaluation of the SCOTI device for confirming blind nasal intubation. *Anaesthesia.* 1999;54: 347–349.

82. Tong YL, Sun M, Tang WH, Xia JY. The tracheal detecting-bulb: a new device to distinguish tracheal from esophageal intubation. *Acta Anaesthesiol Sin.* 2002;40:159–163.

83. Zaleski L, Abello D, Gold MI. The esophageal detector device. Does it work? *Anesthesiology.* 1993;79:244–247.

84. Holland R, Webb RK, Runciman WB. The Australian Incident Monitoring Study. Oesophageal intubation: an analysis of 2000 incident reports. *Anaesth Intensive Care.* 1993;21:608–610.

85. Ko FY, Hsieh KS, Yu CK. Detection of airway CO2 partial pressure to avoid esophageal intubation. *Zhonghua Min Guo Xiao Er Ke Yi Xue Hui Za Zhi.* 1993;34:91–97.

86. Linko K, Paloheimo M, Tammisto T. Capnography for detection of accidental oesophageal intubation. *Acta Anaesthesiol Scand.* 1983;27: 199–202.

87. Wayne MA, Friedland E. Prehospital use of succinylcholine: a 20-year review. *Prehosp Emerg Care.* 1999;3:107–109.

88. Williamson JA, Webb RK, Cockings J, Morgan C. The Australian Incident Monitoring Study. The capnograph: applications and limitations—an analysis of 2000 incident reports. *Anaesth Intensive Care.* 1993;21:551–557.

89. Li J. Capnography alone is imperfect for endotracheal tube placement confirmation during emergency intubation. *J Emerg Med.* 2001;20: 223–229.

90. Anton WR, Gordon RW, Jordan TM, Posner KL, Cheney FW. A disposable end-tidal CO2 detector to verify endotracheal intubation. *Ann Emerg Med.* 1991;20:271–275.

91. Bhende MS, Thompson AE. Evaluation of an end-tidal CO2 detector during pediatric cardiopulmonary resuscitation. *Pediatrics.* 1995;95: 395–399.

92. MacLeod BA, Heller MB, Gerard J, Yealy DM, Menegazzi JJ. Verification of endotracheal tube placement with colorimetric end-tidal CO2 detection. *Ann Emerg Med.* 1991;20:267–270.

93. Ornato JP, Shipley JB, Racht EM, Slovis CM, Wrenn KD, Pepe PE, Almeida SL, Ginger VF, Fotre TV. Multicenter study of a portable, hand-size, colorimetric end-tidal carbon dioxide detection device. *Ann Emerg Med.* 1992;21:518–523.

94. Varon AJ, Morrina J, Civetta JM. Clinical utility of a colorimetric end-tidal CO2 detector in cardiopulmonary resuscitation and emergency intubation. *J Clin Monit.* 1991;7:289–293.

95. Bozeman WP, Hexter D, Liang HK, Kelen GD. Esophageal detector device versus detection of end-tidal carbon dioxide level in emergency intubation. *Ann Emerg Med.* 1996;27:595–599.

96. Sum Ping ST, Mehta MP, Symreng T. Accuracy of the FEF CO2 detector in the assessment of endotracheal tube placement. *Anesth Analg*. 1992;74:415–419.

97. Ward KR, Yealy DM. End-tidal carbon dioxide monitoring in emergency medicine. Part 2: clinical applications. *Acad Emerg Med*. 1998;5:637–646.

98. Tobias JD, Meyer DJ. Noninvasive monitoring of carbon dioxide during respiratory failure in toddlers and infants: end-tidal versus transcutaneous carbon dioxide. *Anesth Analg*. 1997;85:55–58.

99. Pelucio M, Halligan L, Dhindsa H. Out-of-hospital experience with the syringe esophageal detector device. *Acad Emerg Med*. 1997;4:563–568.

100. Baraka A, Khoury PJ, Siddik SS, Salem MR, Joseph NJ. Efficacy of the self-inflating bulb in differentiating esophageal from tracheal intubation in the parturient undergoing cesarean section. *Anesth Analg*. 1997;84:533–537.

101. Davis DP, Stephen KA, Vilke GM. Inaccuracy in endotracheal tube verification using a Toomey syringe. *J Emerg Med*. 1999;17:35–38.

102. Ewy GA, Hellman DA, McClung S, Taren D. Influence of ventilation phase on transthoracic impedance and defibrillation effectiveness. *Crit Care Med*. 1980;8:164–166.

103. Mehta KH, Turley A, Peyrasse P, Janes J, Hall JE. An assessment of the ability of impedance respirometry to distinguish oesophageal from tracheal intubation. *Anaesthesia*. 2002;57:1090–1093.

104. Yao YX, Jiang Z, Lu XH, He JH, Ma XX, Zhu JH. [A clinical study of impedance graph in verifying tracheal intubation]. *Zhonghua Yi Xue Za Zhi*. 2007;87:898–901.

105. Absolom M, Roberts R, Bahlmann UB, Hall JE, Armstrong T, Turley A. The use of impedance respirometry to confirm tracheal intubation in children. *Anaesthesia*. 2006;61:1145–1148.

106. Pytte M, Olasveengen TM, Steen PA, Sunde K. Misplaced and dislodged endotracheal tubes may be detected by the defibrillator during cardiopulmonary resuscitation. *Acta Anaesthesiol Scand*. 2007;51:770–772.

107. Kramer-Johansen J, Wik L, Steen PA. Advanced cardiac life support before and after tracheal intubation—direct measurements of quality. *Resuscitation*. 2006;68:61–69.

108. Yap SJ, Morris RW, Pybus DA. Alterations in endotracheal tube position during general anaesthesia. *Anaesth Intensive Care*. 1994;22:586–588.

109. Sugiyama K, Yokoyama K. Displacement of the endotracheal tube caused by change of head position in pediatric anesthesia: evaluation by fiberoptic bronchoscopy. *Anesth Analg*. 1996;82:251–253.

110. King HK. A new device: Tube Securer. An endotracheal tube holder with integrated bite-block. *Acta Anaesthesiol Sin*. 1997;35:257–259.

111. Falk JL, Sayre MR. Confirmation of airway placement. *Prehosp Emerg Care*. 1999;3:273–278.

112. Wang HE, Kupas DF, Paris PM, Bates RR, Yealy DM. Preliminary experience with a prospective, multi-centered evaluation of out-of-hospital endotracheal intubation. *Resuscitation*. 2003;58:49–58.

113. Kupas DF, Kauffman KF, Wang HE. Effect of airway-securing method on prehospital endotracheal tube dislodgment. *Prehosp Emerg Care*. 2010;14:26–30.

114. Levy H, Griego L. A comparative study of oral endotracheal tube securing methods. *Chest*. 1993;104:1537–1540.

115. Tasota FJ, Hoffman LA, Zullo TG, Jamison G. Evaluation of two methods used to stabilize oral endotracheal tubes. *Heart Lung*. 1987;16:140–146.

116. Aufderheide TP, Sigurdsson G, Pirrallo RG, Yannopoulos D, McKnite S, von Briesen C, Sparks CW, Conrad CJ, Provo TA, Lurie KG. Hyperventilation-induced hypotension during cardiopulmonary resuscitation. *Circulation*. 2004;109:1960–1965.

117. O'Neill JF, Deakin CD. Do we hyperventilate cardiac arrest patients? *Resuscitation*. 2007;73:82–85.

118. Berg RA, Kern KB, Sanders AB, Otto CW, Hilwig RW, Ewy GA. Bystander cardiopulmonary resuscitation. Is ventilation necessary? *Circulation*. 1993;88:1907–1915.

119. Berg RA, Sanders AB, Kern KB, Hilwig RW, Heidenreich JW, Porter ME, Ewy GA. Adverse hemodynamic effects of interrupting chest compressions for rescue breathing during cardiopulmonary resuscitation for ventricular fibrillation cardiac arrest. *Circulation*. 2001;104:2465–2470.

120. Dorph E, Wik L, Steen PA. Effectiveness of ventilation-compression ratios 1:5 and 2:15 in simulated single rescuer paediatric resuscitation. *Resuscitation*. 2002;54:259–264.

121. Hwang SO, Kim SH, Kim H, Jang YS, Zhao PG, Lee KH, Choi HJ, Shin TY. Comparison of 15:1, 15:2, and 30:2 compression-to-ventilation ratios for cardiopulmonary resuscitation in a canine model of a simulated, witnessed cardiac arrest. *Acad Emerg Med*. 2008;15:183–189.

122. Yannopoulos D, Sigurdsson G, McKnite S, Benditt D, Lurie KG. Reducing ventilation frequency combined with an inspiratory impedance device improves CPR efficiency in swine model of cardiac arrest. *Resuscitation*. 2004;61:75–82.

123. Yannopoulos D, Tang W, Roussos C, Aufderheide TP, Idris AH, Lurie KG. Reducing ventilation frequency during cardiopulmonary resuscitation in a porcine model of cardiac arrest. *Respir Care*. 2005;50:628–635.

124. Yannopoulos D, Aufderheide TP, Gabrielli A, Beiser DG, McKnite SH, Pirrallo RG, Wigginton J, Becker L, Vanden Hoek T, Tang W, Nadkarni VM, Klein JP, Idris AH, Lurie KG. Clinical and hemodynamic comparison of 15:2 and 30:2 compression-to-ventilation ratios for cardiopulmonary resuscitation. *Crit Care Med*. 2006;34:1444–1449.

125. Abella BS, Edelson DP, Kim S, Retzer E, Myklebust H, Barry AM, O'Hearn N, Hoek TL, Becker LB. CPR quality improvement during in-hospital cardiac arrest using a real-time audiovisual feedback system. *Resuscitation*. 2007;73:54–61.

126. Weiss SJ, Ernst AA, Jones R, Ong M, Filbrun T, Augustin C, Barnum M, Nick TG. Automatic transport ventilator versus bag valve in the EMS setting: a prospective, randomized trial. *South Med J*. 2005;98:970–976.

127. Johannigman JA, Branson RD, Johnson DJ, Davis K Jr, Hurst JM. Out-of-hospital ventilation: bag-valve device vs transport ventilator. *Acad Emerg Med*. 1995;2:719–724.

128. Rea TD, Cook AJ, Stiell IG, Powell J, Bigham B, Callaway CW, Chugh S, Aufderheide TP, Morrison L, Terndrup TE, Beaudoin T, Wittwer L, Davis D, Idris A, Nichol G. Predicting survival after out-of-hospital cardiac arrest: role of the Utstein data elements. *Ann Emerg Med*. 2010;55:249–257.

129. Sasson C, Rogers MA, Dahl J, Kellermann AL. Predictors of survival from out-of-hospital cardiac arrest: a systematic review and meta-analysis. *Circ Cardiovasc Qual Outcomes*. 2010;3:63–81.

130. Agarwal DA, Hess EP, Atkinson EJ, White RD. Ventricular fibrillation in Rochester, Minnesota: experience over 18 years. *Resuscitation*. 2009;80:1253–1258.

131. Chan PS, Nichol G, Krumholz HM, Spertus JA, Nallamothu BK. Hospital variation in time to defibrillation after in-hospital cardiac arrest. *Arch Intern Med*. 2009;169:1265–1273.

132. Caffrey SL, Willoughby PJ, Pepe PE, Becker LB. Public use of automated external defibrillators. *N Engl J Med*. 2002;347:1242–1247.

133. Valenzuela TD, Roe DJ, Nichol G, Clark LL, Spaite DW, Hardman RG. Outcomes of rapid defibrillation by security officers after cardiac arrest in casinos. *N Engl J Med*. 2000;343:1206–1209.

134. Kudenchuk PJ, Cobb LA, Copass MK, Cummins RO, Doherty AM, Fahrenbruch CE, Hallstrom AP, Murray WA, Olsufka M, Walsh T. Amiodarone for resuscitation after out-of-hospital cardiac arrest due to ventricular fibrillation. *N Engl J Med*. 1999;341:871–878.

135. Vandycke C, Martens P. High dose versus standard dose epinephrine in cardiac arrest—a meta-analysis. *Resuscitation*. 2000;45:161–166.

136. Dorian P, Cass D, Schwartz B, Cooper R, Gelaznikas R, Barr A. Amiodarone as compared with lidocaine for shock-resistant ventricular fibrillation. *N Engl J Med*. 2002;346:884–890.

137. Stiell IG, Wells GA, Field B, Spaite DW, Nesbitt LP, De Maio VJ, Nichol G, Cousineau D, Blackburn J, Munkley D, Luinstra-Toohey L, Campeau T, Dagnone E, Lyver M. Advanced cardiac life support in out-of-hospital cardiac arrest. *N Engl J Med*. 2004;351:647–656.

138. Olasveengen TM, Sunde K, Brunborg C, Thowsen J, Steen PA, Wik L. Intravenous drug administration during out-of-hospital cardiac arrest: a randomized trial. *JAMA*. 2009;302:2222–2229.

139. Pytte M, Pedersen TE, Ottem J, Rokvam AS, Sunde K. Comparison of hands-off time during CPR with manual and semi-automatic defibrillation in a manikin model. *Resuscitation*. 2007;73:131–136.

140. Kramer-Johansen J, Edelson DP, Abella BS, Becker LB, Wik L, Steen PA. Pauses in chest compression and inappropriate shocks: a comparison of manual and semi-automatic defibrillation attempts. *Resuscitation*. 2007;73:212–220.

141. Eftestol T, Wik L, Sunde K, Steen PA. Effects of cardiopulmonary resuscitation on predictors of ventricular fibrillation defibrillation success during out-of-hospital cardiac arrest. *Circulation*. 2004;110:10–15.

142. Eftestol T, Sunde K, Steen PA. Effects of interrupting precordial compressions on the calculated probability of defibrillation success during out-of-hospital cardiac arrest. *Circulation.* 2002;105:2270–2273.

143. Wik L, Hansen TB, Fylling F, Steen T, Vaagenes P, Auestad BH, Steen PA. Delaying defibrillation to give basic cardiopulmonary resuscitation to patients with out-of-hospital ventricular fibrillation: a randomized trial. *JAMA.* 2003;289:1389–1395.

144. Cobb LA, Fahrenbruch CE, Walsh TR, Copass MK, Olsufka M, Breskin M, Hallstrom AP. Influence of cardiopulmonary resuscitation prior to defibrillation in patients with out-of-hospital ventricular fibrillation. *JAMA.* 1999;281:1182–1188.

145. Baker PW, Conway J, Cotton C, Ashby DT, Smyth J, Woodman RJ, Grantham H. Defibrillation or cardiopulmonary resuscitation first for patients with out-of-hospital cardiac arrests found by paramedics to be in ventricular fibrillation? A randomised control trial. *Resuscitation.* 2008; 79:424–431.

146. Jacobs IG, Finn JC, Oxer HF, Jelinek GA. CPR before defibrillation in out-of-hospital cardiac arrest: a randomized trial. *Emerg Med Australas.* 2005;17:39–45.

147. Box MS, Watson JN, Addison PS, Clegg GR, Robertson CE. Shock outcome prediction before and after CPR: a comparative study of manual and automated active compression-decompression CPR. *Resuscitation.* 2008;78:265–274.

148. Brown CG, Dzwonczyk R, Martin DR. Physiologic measurement of the ventricular fibrillation ECG signal: estimating the duration of ventricular fibrillation. *Ann Emerg Med.* 1993;22:70–74.

149. Callaway CW, Sherman LD, Mosesso VN Jr, Dietrich TJ, Holt E, Clarkson MC. Scaling exponent predicts defibrillation success for out-of-hospital ventricular fibrillation cardiac arrest. *Circulation.* 2001;103: 1656–1661.

150. Eftestol T, Sunde K, Aase SO, Husoy JH, Steen PA. Predicting outcome of defibrillation by spectral characterization and nonparametric classification of ventricular fibrillation in patients with out-of-hospital cardiac arrest. *Circulation.* 2000;102:1523–1529.

151. Eftestol T, Losert H, Kramer-Johansen J, Wik L, Sterz F, Steen PA. Independent evaluation of a defibrillation outcome predictor for out-of-hospital cardiac arrested patients. *Resuscitation.* 2005;67:55–61.

152. Gundersen K, Kvaloy JT, Kramer-Johansen J, Olasveengen TM, Eilevstjonn J, Eftestol T. Using within-patient correlation to improve the accuracy of shock outcome prediction for cardiac arrest. *Resuscitation.* 2008;78:46–51.

153. Gunderson EP. Breast-feeding and diabetes: long-term impact on mothers and their infants. *Curr Diab Rep.* 2008;8:279–286.

154. Gundersen K, Kvaloy JT, Kramer-Johansen J, Steen PA, Eftestol T. Development of the probability of return of spontaneous circulation in intervals without chest compressions during out-of-hospital cardiac arrest: an observational study. *BMC Med.* 2009;7:6.

155. Jekova I, Mougeolle F, Valance A. Defibrillation shock success estimation by a set of six parameters derived from the electrocardiogram. *Physiol Meas.* 2004;25:1179–1188.

156. Neurauter A, Eftestol T, Kramer-Johansen J, Abella BS, Sunde K, Wenzel V, Lindner KH, Eilevstjonn J, Myklebust H, Steen PA, Strohmenger HU. Prediction of countershock success using single features from multiple ventricular fibrillation frequency bands and feature combinations using neural networks. *Resuscitation.* 2007;73:253–263.

157. Olasveengen TM, Eftestol T, Gundersen K, Wik L, Sunde K. Acute ischemic heart disease alters ventricular fibrillation waveform characteristics in out of hospital cardiac arrest. *Resuscitation.* 2009;80: 412–417.

158. Ristagno G, Gullo A, Berlot G, Lucangelo U, Geheb E, Bisera J. Prediction of successful defibrillation in human victims of out-of-hospital cardiac arrest: a retrospective electrocardiographic analysis. *Anaesth Intensive Care.* 2008;36:46–50.

159. Russell ME, Friedman MI, Mascioli SR, Stolz LE. Off-label use: an industry perspective on expanding use beyond approved indications. *J Interv Cardiol.* 2006;19:432–438.

160. Snyder DE, White RD, Jorgenson DB. Outcome prediction for guidance of initial resuscitation protocol: shock first or CPR first. *Resuscitation.* 2007;72:45–51.

161. Watson JN, Uchaipichat N, Addison PS, Clegg GR, Robertson CE, Eftestol T, Steen PA. Improved prediction of defibrillation success for out-of-hospital VF cardiac arrest using wavelet transform methods. *Resuscitation.* 2004;63:269–275.

162. Watson JN, Addison PS, Clegg GR, Steen PA, Robertson CE. Practical issues in the evaluation of methods for the prediction of shock outcome

163. Weaver WD, Cobb LA, Dennis D, Ray R, Hallstrom AP, Copass MK. Amplitude of ventricular fibrillation waveform and outcome after cardiac arrest. *Ann Intern Med.* 1985;102:53–55.

164. Yang Z, Lu W, Harrison RG, Eftestol T, Steen PA. A probabilistic neural network as the predictive classifier of out-of-hospital defibrillation outcomes. *Resuscitation.* 2005;64:31–36.

165. Jagric T, Marhl M, Stajer D, Kocjancic ST, Podbregar M, Perc M. Irregularity test for very short electrocardiogram (ECG) signals as a method for predicting a successful defibrillation in patients with ventricular fibrillation. *Transl Res.* 2007;149:145–151.

166. Strohmenger HU, Lindner KH, Brown CG. Analysis of the ventricular fibrillation ECG signal amplitude and frequency parameters as predictors of countershock success in humans. *Chest.* 1997;111:584–589.

167. Callaham M, Barton C. Prediction of outcome of cardiopulmonary resuscitation from end-tidal carbon dioxide concentration. *Crit Care Med.* 1990;18:358–362.

168. Paradis NA, Martin GB, Rivers EP, Goetting MG, Appleton TJ, Feingold M, Nowak RM. Coronary perfusion pressure and the return of spontaneous circulation in human cardiopulmonary resuscitation. *JAMA.* 1990;263:1106–1113.

169. Rivers EP, Martin GB, Smithline H, Rady MY, Schultz CH, Goetting MG, Appleton TJ, Nowak RM. The clinical implications of continuous central venous oxygen saturation during human CPR. *Ann Emerg Med.* 1992;21:1094–1101.

170. Cantineau JP, Lambert Y, Merckx P, Reynaud P, Porte F, Bertrand C, Duvaldestin P. End-tidal carbon dioxide during cardiopulmonary resuscitation in humans presenting mostly with asystole: a predictor of outcome. *Crit Care Med.* 1996;24:791–796.

171. Grmec S, Kupnik D. Does the Mainz Emergency Evaluation Scoring (MEES) in combination with capnometry (MEESc) help in the prognosis of outcome from cardiopulmonary resuscitation in a prehospital setting? *Resuscitation.* 2003;58:89–96.

172. Grmec S, Lah K, Tusek-Bunc K. Difference in end-tidal CO2 between asphyxia cardiac arrest and ventricular fibrillation/pulseless ventricular tachycardia cardiac arrest in the prehospital setting. *Crit Care.* 2003;7: R139–R144.

173. Grmec S, Klemen P. Does the end-tidal carbon dioxide (EtCO2) concentration have prognostic value during out-of-hospital cardiac arrest? *Eur J Emerg Med.* 2001;8:263–269.

174. Kolar M, Krizmaric M, Klemen P, Grmec S. Partial pressure of end-tidal carbon dioxide successful predicts cardiopulmonary resuscitation in the field: a prospective observational study. *Crit Care.* 2008;12:R115.

175. Steedman DJ, Robertson CE. Measurement of end-tidal carbon dioxide concentration during cardiopulmonary resuscitation. *Arch Emerg Med.* 1990;7:129–134.

176. Grmec S, Mally S. Timeliness of administration of vasopressors in CPR. *Crit Care.* 2009;13:401.

177. Pokorna M, Necas E, Kratochvil J, Skripsky R, Andrlik M, Franek O. A sudden increase in partial pressure end-tidal carbon dioxide (P(ET)CO(2)) at the moment of return of spontaneous circulation. *J Emerg Med.* 2009;38:614–621.

178. Agostoni P, Cornelis K, Vermeersch P. Successful percutaneous treatment of an intraprocedural left main stent thrombosis with the support of an automatic mechanical chest compression device. *Int J Cardiol.* 2008;124:e19–e21.

179. Grogaard HK, Wik L, Eriksen M, Brekke M, Sunde K. Continuous mechanical chest compressions during cardiac arrest to facilitate restoration of coronary circulation with percutaneous coronary intervention. *J Am Coll Cardiol.* 2007;50:1093–1094.

180. Steen S, Sjoberg T, Olsson P, Young M. Treatment of out-of-hospital cardiac arrest with LUCAS, a new device for automatic mechanical compression and active decompression resuscitation. *Resuscitation.* 2005;67:25–30.

181. Larsen AI, Hjornevik AS, Ellingsen CL, Nilsen DW. Cardiac arrest with continuous mechanical chest compression during percutaneous coronary intervention. A report on the use of the LUCAS device. *Resuscitation.* 2007;75:454–459.

182. Wagner H, Terkelsen CJ, Friberg H, Harnek J, Kern K, Lassen JF, Olivecrona GK. Cardiac arrest in the catheterisation laboratory: a 5-year experience of using mechanical chest compressions to facilitate PCI during prolonged resuscitation efforts. *Resuscitation.* 2010;81:383–387.

success in out-of-hospital cardiac arrest patients. *Resuscitation.* 2006; 68:51–59.

183. Criley JM, Blaufuss AH, Kissel GL. Cough-induced cardiac compression: self-administered form of cardiopulmonary resuscitation. *JAMA*. 1976;236:1246–1250.

184. Criley JM, Blaufuss AH, Kissel GL. Self-administered cardiopulmonary resuscitation by cough-induced cardiac compression. *Trans Am Clin Climatol Assoc*. 1976;87:138–146.

185. Miller B, Lesnefsky E, Heyborne T, Schmidt B, Freeman K, Breckinridge S, Kelley K, Mann D, Reiter M. Cough-cardiopulmonary resuscitation in the cardiac catheterization laboratory: hemodynamics during an episode of prolonged hypotensive ventricular tachycardia. *Cathet Cardiovasc Diagn*. 1989;18:168–171.

186. Keeble W, Tymchak WJ. Triggering of the Bezold Jarisch Reflex by reperfusion during primary PCI with maintenance of consciousness by cough CPR: a case report and review of pathophysiology. *J Invasive Cardiol*. 2008;20:E239–E242.

187. Saba SE, David SW. Sustained consciousness during ventricular fibrillation: case report of cough cardiopulmonary resuscitation. *Cathet Cardiovasc Diagn*. 1996;37:47–48.

188. Bottiger BW, Arntz HR, Chamberlain DA, Bluhmki E, Belmans A, Danays T, Carli PA, Adgey JA, Bode C, Wenzel V. Thrombolysis during resuscitation for out-of-hospital cardiac arrest. *N Engl J Med*. 2008;359:2651–2662.

189. Porter TR, Ornato JP, Guard CS, Roy VG, Burns CA, Nixon JV. Transesophageal echocardiography to assess mitral valve function and flow during cardiopulmonary resuscitation. *Am J Cardiol*. 1992;70:1056–1060.

190. Levine RL, Wayne MA, Miller CC. End-tidal carbon dioxide and outcome of out-of-hospital cardiac arrest. *N Engl J Med*. 1997;337:301–306.

191. Wayne MA, Levine RL, Miller CC. Use of end-tidal carbon dioxide to predict outcome in prehospital cardiac arrest. *Ann Emerg Med*. 1995;25:762–767.

192. Halperin HR, Tsitlik JE, Gelfand M, Weisfeldt ML, Gruben KG, Levin HR, Rayburn BK, Chandra NC, Scott CJ, Kreps BJ, Siu CO, Guerci AD. A preliminary study of cardiopulmonary resuscitation by circumferential compression of the chest with use of a pneumatic vest. *N Engl J Med*. 1993;329:762–768.

193. Kern KB, Ewy GA, Voorhees WD, Babbs CF, Tacker WA. Myocardial perfusion pressure: a predictor of 24-hour survival during prolonged cardiac arrest in dogs. *Resuscitation*. 1988;16:241–250.

194. Lindner KH, Prengel AW, Pfenninger EG, Lindner IM, Strohmenger HU, Georgieff M, Lurie KG. Vasopressin improves vital organ blood flow during closed-chest cardiopulmonary resuscitation in pigs. *Circulation*. 1995;91:215–221.

195. Little CM, Angelos MG, Paradis NA. Compared to angiotensin II, epinephrine is associated with high myocardial blood flow following return of spontaneous circulation after cardiac arrest. *Resuscitation*. 2003;59:353–359.

196. Sehra R, Underwood K, Checchia P. End tidal CO2 is a quantitative measure of cardiac arrest. *Pacing Clin Electrophysiol*. 2003;26:515–517.

197. Grmec S, Krizmaric M, Mally S, Kozelj A, Spindler M, Lesnik B. Utstein style analysis of out-of-hospital cardiac arrest—bystander CPR and end expired carbon dioxide. *Resuscitation*. 2007;72:404–414.

198. Entholzner E, Felber A, Mielke L, Hargasser S, Breinbauer B, Hundelshausen VB, Hipp R. Assessment of end-tidal CO2 measurement in reanimation. *Anasthesiol Intensivmed Notfallmed Schmerzther*. 1992;27:473–476.

199. Garnett AR, Ornato JP, Gonzalez ER, Johnson EB. End-tidal carbon dioxide monitoring during cardiopulmonary resuscitation. *JAMA*. 1987;257:512–515.

200. Bhende MS, Karasic DG, Karasic RB. End-tidal carbon dioxide changes during cardiopulmonary resuscitation after experimental asphyxial cardiac arrest. *Am J Emerg Med*. 1996;14:349–350.

201. Falk JL, Rackow EC, Weil MH. End-tidal carbon dioxide concentration during cardiopulmonary resuscitation. *N Engl J Med*. 1988;318:607–611.

202. Connick M, Berg RA. Femoral venous pulsations during open-chest cardiac massage. *Ann Emerg Med*. 1994;24:1176–1179.

203. Eberle B, Dick WF, Schneider T, Wisser G, Doetsch S, Tzanova I. Checking the carotid pulse check: diagnostic accuracy of first responders in patients with and without a pulse. *Resuscitation*. 1996;33:107–116.

204. Moule P. Checking the carotid pulse: diagnostic accuracy in students of the healthcare professions. *Resuscitation*. 2000;44:195–201.

205. Ochoa FJ, Ramalle-Gomara E, Carpintero JM, Garcia A, Saralegui I. Competence of health professionals to check the carotid pulse. *Resuscitation*. 1998;37:173–175.

206. Perkins GD, Stephenson B, Hulme J, Monsieurs KG. Birmingham assessment of breathing study (BABS). *Resuscitation*. 2005;64:109–113.

207. Mather C, O'Kelly S. The palpation of pulses. *Anaesthesia*. 1996;51:189–191.

208. Okamoto H, Hoka S, Kawasaki T, Okuyama T, Takahashi S. Changes in end-tidal carbon dioxide tension following sodium bicarbonate administration: correlation with cardiac output and haemoglobin concentration. *Acta Anaesthesiol Scand*. 1995;39:79–84.

209. Lewis LM, Stothert J, Standeven J, Chandel B, Kurtz M, Fortney J. Correlation of end-tidal CO2 to cerebral perfusion during CPR. *Ann Emerg Med*. 1992;21:1131–1134.

210. Sanders A, Atlas M, Ewy G, Kern K, Bragg S. Expired pCO2 as an index of coronary perfusion pressure. *Am J Emerg Med*. 1985;3:147–149.

211. Gonzalez ER, Ornato JP, Garnett AR, Levine RL, Young DS, Racht EM. Dose-dependent vasopressor response to epinephrine during CPR in human beings. *Ann Emerg Med*. 1989;18:920–926.

212. Chase PB, Kern KB, Sanders AB, Otto CW, Ewy GA. Effects of graded doses of epinephrine on both noninvasive and invasive measures of myocardial perfusion and blood flow during cardiopulmonary resuscitation. *Crit Care Med*. 1993;21:413–419.

213. Cantineau JP, Merckx P, Lambert Y, Sorkine M, Bertrand C, Duvaldestin P. Effect of epinephrine on end-tidal carbon dioxide pressure during prehospital cardiopulmonary resuscitation. *Am J Emerg Med*. 1994;12:267–270.

214. Callaham M, Barton C, Matthay M. Effect of epinephrine on the ability of end-tidal carbon dioxide readings to predict initial resuscitation from cardiac arrest. *Crit Care Med*. 1992;20:337–343.

215. Ahrens T, Schallom L, Bettorf K, Ellner S, Hurt G, O'Mara V, Ludwig J, George W, Marino T, Shannon W. End-tidal carbon dioxide measurements as a prognostic indicator of outcome in cardiac arrest. *Am J Crit Care*. 2001;10:391–398.

216. Sanders AB, Kern KB, Otto CW, Milander MM, Ewy GA. End-tidal carbon dioxide monitoring during cardiopulmonary resuscitation: a prognostic indicator for survival. *JAMA*. 1989;262:1347–1351.

217. Nakatani K, Yukioka H, Fujimori M, Maeda C, Noguchi H, Ishihara S, Yamanaka I, Tase C. Utility of colorimetric end-tidal carbon dioxide detector for monitoring during prehospital cardiopulmonary resuscitation. *Am J Emerg Med*. 1999;17:203–206.

218. Ward KR, Menegazzi JJ, Zelenak RR, Sullivan RJ, McSwain NE Jr. A comparison of chest compressions between mechanical and manual CPR by monitoring end-tidal PCO2 during human cardiac arrest. *Ann Emerg Med*. 1993;22:669–674.

219. Kalenda Z. The capnogram as a guide to the efficacy of cardiac massage. *Resuscitation*. 1978;6:259–263.

220. Niemann JT, Criley JM, Rosborough JP, Niskanen RA, Alferness C. Predictive indices of successful cardiac resuscitation after prolonged arrest and experimental cardiopulmonary resuscitation. *Ann Emerg Med*. 1985;14:521–528.

221. Rivers EP, Lozon J, Enriquez E, Havstad SV, Martin GB, Lewandowski CA, Goetting MG, Rosenberg JA, Paradis NA, Nowak RM. Simultaneous radial, femoral, and aortic arterial pressures during human cardiopulmonary resuscitation. *Crit Care Med*. 1993;21:878–883.

222. Weil MH, Rackow EC, Trevino R, Grundler W, Falk JL, Griffel MI. Difference in acid-base state between venous and arterial blood during cardiopulmonary resuscitation. *N Engl J Med*. 1986;315:153–156.

223. Memtsoudis SG, Rosenberger P, Loffler M, Eltzschig HK, Mizuguchi A, Shernan SK, Fox JA. The usefulness of transesophageal echocardiography during intraoperative cardiac arrest in noncardiac surgery. *Anesth Analg*. 2006;102:1653–1657.

224. van der Wouw PA, Koster RW, Delemarre BJ, de Vos R, Lampe-Schoenmaeckers AJ, Lie KI. Diagnostic accuracy of transesophageal echocardiography during cardiopulmonary resuscitation. *J Am Coll Cardiol*. 1997;30:780–783.

225. Comess KA, DeRook FA, Russell ML, Tognazzi-Evans TA, Beach KW. The incidence of pulmonary embolism in unexplained sudden cardiac arrest with pulseless electrical activity. *Am J Med*. 2000;109:351–356.

226. Niendorff DF, Rassias AJ, Palac R, Beach ML, Costa S, Greenberg M. Rapid cardiac ultrasound of inpatients suffering PEA arrest performed by nonexpert sonographers. *Resuscitation*. 2005;67:81–87.

227. Tayal VS, Kline JA. Emergency echocardiography to detect pericardial effusion in patients in PEA and near-PEA states. *Resuscitation.* 2003; 59:315–318.

228. Salen P, O'Connor R, Sierzenski P, Passarello B, Pancu D, Melanson S, Arcona S, Reed J, Heller M. Can cardiac sonography and capnography be used independently and in combination to predict resuscitation outcomes? *Acad Emerg Med.* 2001;8:610–615.

229. Blaivas M, Fox JC. Outcome in cardiac arrest patients found to have cardiac standstill on the bedside emergency department echocardiogram. *Acad Emerg Med.* 2001;8:616–621.

230. Salen P, Melniker L, Chooljian C, Rose JS, Alteveer J, Reed J, Heller M. Does the presence or absence of sonographically identified cardiac activity predict resuscitation outcomes of cardiac arrest patients? *Am J Emerg Med.* 2005;23:459–462.

231. Wenzel V, Lindner KH, Krismer AC, Miller EA, Voelckel WG, Lingnau W. Repeated administration of vasopressin but not epinephrine maintains coronary perfusion pressure after early and late administration during prolonged cardiopulmonary resuscitation in pigs. *Circulation.* 1999;99:1379–1384.

232. Rittenberger JC, Menegazzi JJ, Callaway CW. Association of delay to first intervention with return of spontaneous circulation in a swine model of cardiac arrest. *Resuscitation.* 2007;73:154–160.

233. Emerman CL, Pinchak AC, Hancock D, Hagen JF. The effect of bolus injection on circulation times during cardiac arrest. *Am J Emerg Med.* 1990;8:190–193.

234. Banerjee S, Singhi SC, Singh S, Singh M. The intraosseous route is a suitable alternative to intravenous route for fluid resuscitation in severely dehydrated children. *Indian Pediatr.* 1994;31:1511–1520.

235. Brickman KR, Krupp K, Rega P, Alexander J, Guinness M. Typing and screening of blood from intraosseous access. *Ann Emerg Med.* 1992;21: 414–417.

236. Fiser RT, Walker WM, Seibert JJ, McCarthy R, Fiser DH. Tibial length following intraosseous infusion: a prospective, radiographic analysis. *Pediatr Emerg Care.* 1997;13:186–188.

237. Ummenhofer W, Frei FJ, Urwyler A, Drewe J. Are laboratory values in bone marrow aspirate predictable for venous blood in paediatric patients? *Resuscitation.* 1994;27:123–128.

238. Glaeser PW, Hellmich TR, Szewczuga D, Losek JD, Smith DS. Five-year experience in prehospital intraosseous infusions in children and adults. *Ann Emerg Med.* 1993;22:1119–1124.

239. Guy J, Haley K, Zuspan SJ. Use of intraosseous infusion in the pediatric trauma patient. *J Pediatr Surg.* 1993;28:158–161.

240. Macnab A, Christenson J, Findlay J, Horwood B, Johnson D, Jones L, Phillips K, Pollack C Jr, Robinson DJ, Rumball C, Stair T, Tiffany B, Whelan M. A new system for sternal intraosseous infusion in adults. *Prehosp Emerg Care.* 2000;4:173–177.

241. Ellemunter H, Simma B, Trawoger R, Maurer H. Intraosseous lines in preterm and full term neonates. *Arch Dis Child Fetal Neonatal Ed.* 1999;80:F74–F75.

242. Mader TJ, Kellogg AR, Walterscheid JK, Lodding CC, Sherman LD. A randomized comparison of cardiocerebral and cardiopulmonary resuscitation using a swine model of prolonged ventricular fibrillation. *Resuscitation.* 2010;81:596–602.

243. Barsan WG, Levy RC, Weir H. Lidocaine levels during CPR: differences after peripheral venous, central venous, and intracardiac injections. *Ann Emerg Med.* 1981;10:73–78.

244. Kuhn GJ, White BC, Swetnam RE, Mumey JF, Rydesky MF, Tintinalli JE, Krome RL, Hoehner PJ. Peripheral vs central circulation times during CPR: a pilot study. *Ann Emerg Med.* 1981;10:417–419.

245. Emerman CL, Pinchak AC, Hancock D, Hagen JF. Effect of injection site on circulation times during cardiac arrest. *Crit Care Med.* 1988;16: 1138–1141.

246. Howard RF, Bingham RM. Endotracheal compared with intravenous administration of atropine. *Arch Dis Child.* 1990;65:449–450.

247. Lee PL, Chung YT, Lee BY, Yeh CY, Lin SY, Chao CC. The optimal dose of atropine via the endotracheal route. *Ma Zui Xue Za Zhi.* 1989; 27:35–38.

248. Prengel AW, Lindner KH, Hahnel J, Ahnefeld FW. Endotracheal and endobronchial lidocaine administration: effects on plasma lidocaine concentration and blood gases. *Crit Care Med.* 1991;19:911–915.

249. Schmidbauer S, Kneifel HA, Hallfeldt KK. Endobronchial application of high dose epinephrine in out of hospital cardiopulmonary resuscitation. *Resuscitation.* 2000;47:89.

250. Raymondos K, Panning B, Leuwer M, Brechelt G, Korte T, Niehaus M, Tebbenjohanns J, Piepenbrock S. Absorption and hemodynamic effects

251. Hahnel JH, Lindner KH, Schurmann C, Prengel A, Ahnefeld FW. Plasma lidocaine levels and PaO2 with endobronchial administration: dilution with normal saline or distilled water? *Ann Emerg Med.* 1990; 19:1314–1317.

252. Brown LK, Diamond J. The efficacy of lidocaine in ventricular fibrillation due to coronary artery ligation: endotracheal vs intravenous use. *Proc West Pharmacol Soc.* 1982;25:43–45.

253. Jasani MS, Nadkarni VM, Finkelstein MS, Hofmann WT, Salzman SK. Inspiratory-cycle instillation of endotracheal epinephrine in porcine arrest. *Acad Emerg Med.* 1994;1:340–345.

254. Wenzel V, Lindner KH, Prengel AW, Lurie KG, Strohmenger HU. Endobronchial vasopressin improves survival during cardiopulmonary resuscitation in pigs. *Anesthesiology.* 1997;86:1375–1381.

255. Prengel AW, Rembecki M, Wenzel V, Steinbach G. A comparison of the endotracheal tube and the laryngeal mask airway as a route for endobronchial lidocaine administration. *Anesth Analg.* 2001;92: 1505–1509.

256. Jasani MS, Nadkarni VM, Finkelstein MS, Mandell GA, Salzman SK, Norman ME. Effects of different techniques of endotracheal epinephrine administration in pediatric porcine hypoxic-hypercarbic cardiopulmonary arrest. *Crit Care Med.* 1994;22:1174–1180.

257. Johnston C. Endotracheal drug delivery. *Pediatr Emerg Care.* 1992;8: 94–97.

258. Efrati O, Ben-Abraham R, Barak A, Modan-Moses D, Augarten A, Manisterski Y, Barzilay Z, Paret G. Endobronchial adrenaline: should it be reconsidered? Dose response and haemodynamic effect in dogs. *Resuscitation.* 2003;59:117–122.

259. Elizur A, Ben-Abraham R, Manisterski Y, Barak A, Efrati O, Lotan D, Barzilay Z, Paret G. Tracheal epinephrine or norepinephrine preceded by beta blockade in a dog model. Can beta blockade bestow any benefits? *Resuscitation.* 2003;59:271–276.

260. Niemann JT, Stratton SJ, Cruz B, Lewis RJ. Endotracheal drug administration during out-of-hospital resuscitation: where are the survivors? *Resuscitation.* 2002;53:153–157.

261. Schuttler J, Bartsch A, Ebeling BJ, Hornchen U, Kulka P, Suhling B, Stoeckel H. [Endobronchial administration of adrenaline in preclinical cardiopulmonary resuscitation]. *Anasth Intensivther Notfallmed.* 1987; 22:63–68.

262. Hornchen U, Schuttler J, Stoeckel H, Eichelkraut W, Hahn N. Endobronchial instillation of epinephrine during cardiopulmonary resuscitation. *Crit Care Med.* 1987;15:1037–1039.

263. Naganobu K, Hasebe Y, Uchiyama Y, Hagio M, Ogawa H. A comparison of distilled water and normal saline as diluents for endobronchial administration of epinephrine in the dog. *Anesth Analg.* 2000;91: 317–321.

264. Yakaitis RW, Otto CW, Blitt CD. Relative importance of $\alpha$ and $\beta$ adrenergic receptors during resuscitation. *Crit Care Med.* 1979;7: 293–296.

265. Michael JR, Guerci AD, Koehler RC, Shi AY, Tsitlik J, Chandra N, Niedermeyer E, Rogers MC, Traystman RJ, Weisfeldt ML. Mechanisms by which epinephrine augments cerebral and myocardial perfusion during cardiopulmonary resuscitation in dogs. *Circulation.* 1984;69: 822–835.

266. Ditchey RV, Lindenfeld J. Failure of epinephrine to improve the balance between myocardial oxygen supply and demand during closed-chest resuscitation in dogs. *Circulation.* 1988;78:382–389.

267. Herlitz J, Ekstrom L, Wennerblom B, Axelsson A, Bang A, Holmberg S. Adrenaline in out-of-hospital ventricular fibrillation. Does it make any difference? *Resuscitation.* 1995;29:195–201.

268. Callaham M, Madsen CD, Barton CW, Saunders CE, Pointer J. A randomized clinical trial of high-dose epinephrine and norepinephrine vs standard-dose epinephrine in prehospital cardiac arrest. *JAMA.* 1992; 268:2667–2672.

269. Gueugniaud PY, Mols P, Goldstein P, Pham E, Dubien PY, Deweerdt C, Vergnion M, Petit P, Carli P. A comparison of repeated high doses and repeated standard doses of epinephrine for cardiac arrest outside the hospital. European Epinephrine Study Group. *N Engl J Med.* 1998;339: 1595–1601.

270. Choux C, Gueugniaud PY, Barbieux A, Pham E, Lae C, Dubien PY, Petit P. Standard doses versus repeated high doses of epinephrine in cardiac arrest outside the hospital. *Resuscitation.* 1995;29:3–9.

271. Brown CG, Martin DR, Pepe PE, Stueven H, Cummins RO, Gonzalez E, Jastremski M. A comparison of standard-dose and high-dose epineph-

rine in cardiac arrest outside the hospital. The Multicenter High-Dose Epinephrine Study Group. *N Engl J Med.* 1992;327:1051–1055.

272. Stiell IG, Hebert PC, Weitzman BN, Wells GA, Raman S, Stark RM, Higginson LA, Ahuja J, Dickinson GE. High-dose epinephrine in adult cardiac arrest. *N Engl J Med.* 1992;327:1045–1050.

273. Lindner KH, Strohmenger HU, Ensinger H, Hetzel WD, Ahnefeld FW, Georgieff M. Stress hormone response during and after cardiopulmonary resuscitation. *Anesthesiology.* 1992;77:662–668.

274. Lindner A, Zierz S. [Differential sciatica pain diagnosis from the neurologic viewpoint]. *Med Klin (Munich).* 1997;92:335–343.

275. Wenzel V, Krismer AC, Arntz HR, Sitter H, Stadlbauer KH, Lindner KH. A comparison of vasopressin and epinephrine for out-of-hospital cardiopulmonary resuscitation. *N Engl J Med.* 2004;350:105–113.

276. Stiell IG, Hebert PC, Wells GA, Vandemheen KL, Tang AS, Higginson LA, Dreyer JF, Clement C, Battram E, Watpool I, Mason S, Klassen T, Weitzman BN. Vasopressin versus epinephrine for inhospital cardiac arrest: a randomised controlled trial. *Lancet.* 2001;358:105–109.

277. Aung K, Htay T. Vasopressin for cardiac arrest: a systematic review and meta-analysis. *Arch Intern Med.* 2005;165:17–24.

278. Callaway CW, Hostler D, Doshi AA, Pinchalk M, Roth RN, Lubin J, Newman DH, Kelly LJ. Usefulness of vasopressin administered with epinephrine during out-of-hospital cardiac arrest. *Am J Cardiol.* 2006; 98:1316–1321.

279. Gueugniaud PY, David JS, Chanzy E, Hubert H, Dubien PY, Mauriaucourt P, Braganca C, Billeres X, Clotteau-Lambert MP, Fuster P, Thiercelin D, Debaty G, Ricard-Hibon A, Roux P, Espesson C, Querellou E, Ducros L, Ecollan P, Halbout L, Savary D, Guillaumee F, Maupoint R, Capelle P, Bracq C, Dreyfus P, Nouguier P, Gache A, Meurisse C, Boulanger B, Lae C, Metzger J, Raphael V, Beruben A, Wenzel V, Guinhouya C, Vilhelm C, Marret E. Vasopressin and epinephrine vs. epinephrine alone in cardiopulmonary resuscitation. *N Engl J Med.* 2008;359:21–30.

280. Mukoyama T, Kinoshita K, Nagao K, Tanjoh K. Reduced effectiveness of vasopressin in repeated doses for patients undergoing prolonged cardiopulmonary resuscitation. *Resuscitation.* 2009;80:755–761.

281. Lindner KH, Brinkmann A, Pfenninger EG, Lurie KG, Goertz A, Lindner IM. Effect of vasopressin on hemodynamic variables, organ blood flow, and acid-base status in a pig model of cardiopulmonary resuscitation. *Anesth Analg.* 1993;77:427–435.

282. Silfvast T, Saarnivaara L, Kinnunen A, Erosuo J, Nick L, Pesonen P, Luomanmaki K. Comparison of adrenaline and phenylephrine in out-of-hospital cardiopulmonary resuscitation: a double-blind study. *Acta Anaesthesiol Scand.* 1985;29:610–613.

283. Skrifvars MB, Kuisma M, Boyd J, Maatta T, Repo J, Rosenberg PH, Castren M. The use of undiluted amiodarone in the management of out-of-hospital cardiac arrest. *Acta Anaesthesiol Scand.* 2004;48: 582–587.

284. Petrovic T, Adnet F, Lapandry C. Successful resuscitation of ventricular fibrillation after low-dose amiodarone. *Ann Emerg Med.* 1998;32: 518–519.

285. Levine JH, Massumi A, Scheinman MM, Winkle RA, Platia EV, Chilson DA, Gomes A, Woosley RL. Intravenous amiodarone for recurrent sustained hypotensive ventricular tachyarrhythmias. Intravenous Amiodarone Multicenter Trial Group. *J Am Coll Cardiol.* 1996; 27:67–75.

286. Somberg JC, Bailin SJ, Haffajee CI, Paladino WP, Kerin NZ, Bridges D, Timar S, Molnar J. Intravenous lidocaine versus intravenous amiodarone (in a new aqueous formulation) for incessant ventricular tachycardia. *Am J Cardiol.* 2002;90:853–859.

287. Somberg JC, Timar S, Bailin SJ, Lakatos F, Haffajee CI, Tarjan J, Paladino WP, Sarosi I, Kerin NZ, Borbola J, Bridges DE, Molnar J. Lack of a hypotensive effect with rapid administration of a new aqueous formulation of intravenous amiodarone. *Am J Cardiol.* 2004;93: 576–581.

288. Paiva EF, Perondi MB, Kern KB, Berg RA, Timerman S, Cardoso LF, Ramirez JA. Effect of amiodarone on haemodynamics during cardiopulmonary resuscitation in a canine model of resistant ventricular fibrillation. *Resuscitation.* 2003;58:203–208.

289. Herlitz J, Ekstrom L, Wennerblom B, Axelsson A, Bang A, Lindkvist J, Persson NG, Holmberg S. Lidocaine in out-of-hospital ventricular fibrillation. Does it improve survival? *Resuscitation.* 1997;33:199–205.

290. Manz M, Pfeiffer D, Jung W, Lueritz B. Intravenous treatment with magnesium in recurrent persistent ventricular tachycardia. *New Trends in Arrhythmias.* 1991;7:437–442.

291. Tzivoni D, Banai S, Schuger C, Benhorin J, Keren A, Gottlieb S, Stern S. Treatment of torsade de pointes with magnesium sulfate. *Circulation.* 1988;77:392–397.

292. Allegra J, Lavery R, Cody R, Birnbaum G, Brennan J, Hartman A, Horowitz M, Nashed A, Yablonski M. Magnesium sulfate in the treatment of refractory ventricular fibrillation in the prehospital setting. *Resuscitation.* 2001;49:245–249.

293. Thel MC, Armstrong AL, McNulty SE, Califf RM, O'Connor CM. Randomised trial of magnesium in in-hospital cardiac arrest. Duke Internal Medicine Housestaff. *Lancet.* 1997;350:1272–1276.

294. Fatovich DM, Prentice DA, Dobb GJ. Magnesium in cardiac arrest (the magic trial). *Resuscitation.* 1997;35:237–241.

295. Brown DC, Lewis AJ, Criley JM. Asystole and its treatment: the possible role of the parasympathetic nervous system in cardiac arrest. *JACEP.* 1979;8:448–452.

296. Sorensen M, Engbaek J, Viby-Mogensen J, Guldager H, Molke Jensen F. Bradycardia and cardiac asystole following a single injection of suxamethonium. *Acta Anaesthesiol Scand.* 1984;28:232–235.

297. Lovstad RZ, Granhus G, Hetland S. Bradycardia and asystolic cardiac arrest during spinal anaesthesia: a report of five cases. *Acta Anaesthesiol Scand.* 2000;44:48–52.

298. Stueven HA, Tonsfeldt DJ, Thompson BM, Whitcomb J, Kastenson E, Aprahamian C. Atropine in asystole: human studies. *Ann Emerg Med.* 1984;13:815–817.

299. Coon GA, Clinton JE, Ruiz E. Use of atropine for brady-asystolic prehospital cardiac arrest. *Ann Emerg Med.* 1981;10:462–467.

300. Tortolani AJ, Risucci DA, Powell SR, Dixon R. In-hospital cardiopulmonary resuscitation during asystole. Therapeutic factors associated with 24-hour survival. *Chest.* 1989;96:622–626.

301. Stiell IG, Wells GA, Hebert PC, Laupacis A, Weitzman BN. Association of drug therapy with survival in cardiac arrest: limited role of advanced cardiac life support drugs. *Acad Emerg Med.* 1995;2:264–273.

302. Engdahl J, Bang A, Lindqvist J, Herlitz J. Can we define patients with no and those with some chance of survival when found in asystole out of hospital? *Am J Cardiol.* 2000;86:610–614.

303. Engdahl J, Bang A, Lindqvist J, Herlitz J. Factors affecting short- and long-term prognosis among 1069 patients with out-of-hospital cardiac arrest and pulseless electrical activity. *Resuscitation.* 2001;51:17–25.

304. van Walraven C, Stiell IG, Wells GA, Hebert PC, Vandemheen K. Do advanced cardiac life support drugs increase resuscitation rates from in-hospital cardiac arrest? The OTAC Study Group. *Ann Emerg Med.* 1998;32:544–553.

305. Bar-Joseph G, Abramson NS, Kelsey SF, Mashiach T, Craig MT, Safar P. Improved resuscitation outcome in emergency medical systems with increased usage of sodium bicarbonate during cardiopulmonary resuscitation. *Acta Anaesthesiol Scand.* 2005;49:6–15.

306. Weaver WD, Fahrenbruch CE, Johnson DD, Hallstrom AP, Cobb LA, Copass MK. Effect of epinephrine and lidocaine therapy on outcome after cardiac arrest due to ventricular fibrillation. *Circulation.* 1990;82: 2027–2034.

307. Dybvik T, Strand T, Steen PA. Buffer therapy during out-of-hospital cardiopulmonary resuscitation. *Resuscitation.* 1995;29:89–95.

308. Vukmir RB, Katz L. Sodium bicarbonate improves outcome in prolonged prehospital cardiac arrest. *Am J Emerg Med.* 2006;24:156–161.

309. Aufderheide TP, Martin DR, Olson DW, Aprahamian C, Woo JW, Hendley GE, Hargarten KM, Thompson B. Prehospital bicarbonate use in cardiac arrest: a 3-year experience. *Am J Emerg Med.* 1992;10:4–7.

310. Skovron ML, Goldberg E, Suljaga-Petchel K. Factors predicting survival for six months after cardiopulmonary resuscitation: multivariate analysis of a prospective study. *Mt Sinai J Med.* 1985;52:271–275.

311. Delooz HH, Lewi PJ. Are inter-center differences in EMS-management and sodium-bicarbonate administration important for the outcome of CPR? The Cerebral Resuscitation Study Group. *Resuscitation.* 1989; 17 suppl:S161–S172; discussion S199–S206.

312. Roberts D, Landolfo K, Light R, Dobson K. Early predictors of mortality for hospitalized patients suffering cardiopulmonary arrest. *Chest.* 1990;97:413–419.

313. Kette F, Weil MH, Gazmuri RJ. Buffer solutions may compromise cardiac resuscitation by reducing coronary perfusion presssure. *JAMA.* 1991;266:2121–2126.

314. Graf H, Leach W, Arieff AI. Evidence for a detrimental effect of bicarbonate therapy in hypoxic lactic acidosis. *Science.* 1985;227: 754–756.

315. Katz LM, Wang Y, Rockoff S, Bouldin TW. Low-dose Carbicarb improves cerebral outcome after asphyxial cardiac arrest in rats. *Ann Emerg Med*. 2002;39:359–365.

316. Sun S, Weil MH, Tang W, Fukui M. Effects of buffer agents on postresuscitation myocardial dysfunction. *Crit Care Med*. 1996;24: 2035–2041.

317. Blecic S, De Backer D, Deleuze M, Vachiery JL, Vincent JL. Correction of metabolic acidosis in experimental CPR: a comparative study of sodium bicarbonate, carbicarb, and dextrose. *Ann Emerg Med*. 1991;20: 235–238.

318. Stueven HA, Thompson BM, Aprahamian C, Tonsfeldt DJ. Calcium chloride: reassessment of use in asystole. *Ann Emerg Med*. 1984;13: 820–822.

319. Stueven HA, Thompson B, Aprahamian C, Tonsfeldt DJ, Kastenson EH. The effectiveness of calcium chloride in refractory electromechanical dissociation. *Ann Emerg Med*. 1985;14:626–629.

320. Stueven HA, Thompson B, Aprahamian C, Tonsfeldt DJ, Kastenson EH. Lack of effectiveness of calcium chloride in refractory asystole. *Ann Emerg Med*. 1985;14:630–632.

321. Gando S, Tedo I, Tujinaga H, Kubota M. Variation in serum ionized calcium on cardiopulmonary resuscitation. *J Anesth*. 1988;2:154–160.

322. Stueven H, Thompson BM, Aprahamian C, Darin JC. Use of calcium in prehospital cardiac arrest. *Ann Emerg Med*. 1983;12:136–139.

323. Harrison EE, Amey BD. The use of calcium in cardiac resuscitation. *Am J Emerg Med*. 1983;1:267–273.

324. Bottiger BW, Bode C, Kern S, Gries A, Gust R, Glatzer R, Bauer H, Motsch J, Martin E. Efficacy and safety of thrombolytic therapy after initially unsuccessful cardiopulmonary resuscitation: a prospective clinical trial. *Lancet*. 2001;357:1583–1585.

325. Kurkciyan I, Meron G, Sterz F, Janata K, Domanovits H, Holzer M, Berzlanovich A, Bankl HC, Laggner AN. Pulmonary embolism as a cause of cardiac arrest: presentation and outcome. *Arch Intern Med*. 2000;160:1529–1535.

326. Janata K, Holzer M, Kurkciyan I, Losert H, Riedmuller E, Pikula B, Laggner AN, Laczika K. Major bleeding complications in cardiopulmonary resuscitation: the place of thrombolytic therapy in cardiac arrest due to massive pulmonary embolism. *Resuscitation*. 2003;57:49–55.

327. Lederer W, Lichtenberger C, Pechlaner C, Kroesen G, Baubin M. Recombinant tissue plasminogen activator during cardiopulmonary resuscitation in 108 patients with out-of-hospital cardiac arrest. *Resuscitation*. 2001;50:71–76.

328. Bozeman WP, Kleiner DM, Ferguson KL. Empiric tenecteplase is associated with increased return of spontaneous circulation and short term survival in cardiac arrest patients unresponsive to standard interventions. *Resuscitation*. 2006;69:399–406.

329. Stadlbauer KH, Krismer AC, Arntz HR, Mayr VD, Lienhart HG, Bottiger BW, Jahn B, Lindner KH, Wenzel V. Effects of thrombolysis during out-of-hospital cardiopulmonary resuscitation. *Am J Cardiol*. 2006;97:305–308.

330. Fatovich DM, Dobb GJ, Clugston RA. A pilot randomised trial of thrombolysis in cardiac arrest (the TICA trial). *Resuscitation*. 2004;61: 309–313.

331. Abu-Laban RB, Christenson JM, Innes GD, van Beek CA, Wanger KP, McKnight RD, MacPhail IA, Puskaric J, Sadowski RP, Singer J, Schechter MT, Wood VM. Tissue plasminogen activator in cardiac arrest with pulseless electrical activity. *N Engl J Med*. 2002;346: 1522–1528.

332. Bender R, Breil M, Heister U, Dahmen A, Hoeft A, Krep H, Fischer M. Hypertonic saline during CPR: feasibility and safety of a new protocol of fluid management during resuscitation. *Resuscitation*. 2007;72: 74–81.

333. Breil M, Krep H, Sinn D, Hagendorff A, Dahmen A, Eichelkraut W, Hoeft A, Fischer M. Hypertonic saline improves myocardial blood flow during CPR, but is not enhanced further by the addition of hydroxy ethyl starch. *Resuscitation*. 2003;56:307–317.

334. Bruel C, Parienti JJ, Marie W, Arrot X, Daubin C, Du Cheyron D, Massetti M, Charbonneau P. Mild hypothermia during advanced life support: a preliminary study in out-of-hospital cardiac arrest. *Crit Care*. 2008;12:R31.

335. D'Alecy LG, Lundy EF, Barton KJ, Zelenock GB. Dextrose containing intravenous fluid impairs outcome and increases death after eight minutes of cardiac arrest and resuscitation in dogs. *Surgery*. 1986;100: 505–511.

336. Fischer M, Dahmen A, Standop J, Hagendorff A, Hoeft A, Krep H. Effects of hypertonic saline on myocardial blood flow in a porcine model of prolonged cardiac arrest. *Resuscitation*. 2002;54:269–280.

337. Kamarainen A, Virkkunen I, Tenhunen J, Yli-Hankala A, Silfvast T. Prehospital induction of therapeutic hypothermia during CPR: a pilot study. *Resuscitation*. 2008;76:360–363.

338. Krep H, Breil M, Sinn D, Hagendorff A, Hoeft A, Fischer M. Effects of hypertonic versus isotonic infusion therapy on regional cerebral blood flow after experimental cardiac arrest cardiopulmonary resuscitation in pigs. *Resuscitation*. 2004;63:73–83.

339. Longstreth WT Jr, Copass MK, Dennis LK, Rauch-Matthews ME, Stark MS, Cobb LA. Intravenous glucose after out-of-hospital cardiopulmonary arrest: a community-based randomized trial. *Neurology*. 1993;43: 2534–2541.

340. Miclescu A, Basu S, Wiklund L. Methylene blue added to a hypertonic-hyperoncotic solution increases short-term survival in experimental cardiac arrest. *Crit Care Med*. 2006;34:2806–2813.

341. Nordmark J, Rubertsson S. Induction of mild hypothermia with infusion of cold (4 degrees C) fluid during ongoing experimental CPR. *Resuscitation*. 2005;66:357–365.

342. Nozari A, Safar P, Stezoski SW, Wu X, Kostelnik S, Radovsky A, Tisherman S, Kochanek PM. Critical time window for intra-arrest cooling with cold saline flush in a dog model of cardiopulmonary resuscitation. *Circulation*. 2006;113:2690–2696.

343. Ujhelyi MR, Winecoff AP, Schur M, Frede T, Bottorff MB, Gabel M, Markel ML. Influence of hypertonic saline solution infusion on defibrillation efficacy. *Chest*. 1996;110:784–790.

344. Ditchey RV, Lindenfeld J. Potential adverse effects of volume loading on perfusion of vital organs during closed-chest resuscitation. *Circulation*. 1984;69:181–189.

345. Voorhees WD, Ralston SH, Kougias C, Schmitz PM. Fluid loading with whole blood or Ringer's lactate solution during CPR in dogs. *Resuscitation*. 1987;15:113–123.

346. Yannopoulos D, Zviman M, Castro V, Kolandaivelu A, Ranjan R, Wilson RF, Halperin HR. Intra-cardiopulmonary resuscitation hypothermia with and without volume loading in an ischemic model of cardiac arrest. *Circulation*. 2009;120:1426–1435.

347. Barthell E, Troiano P, Olson D, Stueven HA, Hendley G. Prehospital external cardiac pacing: a prospective, controlled clinical trial. *Ann Emerg Med*. 1988;17:1221–1226.

348. Cummins RO, Graves JR, Larsen MP, Hallstrom AP, Hearne TR, Ciliberti J, Nicola RM, Horan S. Out-of-hospital transcutaneous pacing by emergency medical technicians in patients with asystolic cardiac arrest. *N Engl J Med*. 1993;328:1377–1382.

349. Hedges JR, Syverud SA, Dalsey WC, Feero S, Easter R, Shultz B. Prehospital trial of emergency transcutaneous cardiac pacing. *Circulation*. 1987;76:1337–1343.

350. White JD, Brown CG. Immediate transthoracic pacing for cardiac asystole in an emergency department setting. *Am J Emerg Med*. 1985; 3:125–128.

351. Haman L, Parizek P, Vojacek J. Precordial thump efficacy in termination of induced ventricular arrhythmias. *Resuscitation*. 2009;80: 14–16.

352. Pellis T, Kette F, Lovisa D, Franceschino E, Magagnin L, Mercante WP, Kohl P. Utility of pre-cordial thump for treatment of out of hospital cardiac arrest: a prospective study. *Resuscitation*. 2009;80:17–23.

353. Befeler B. Mechanical stimulation of the heart: its therapeutic value in tachyarrhythmias. *Chest*. 1978;73:832–838.

354. Volkmann H, Klumbies A, Kuhnert H, Paliege R, Dannberg G, Siegert K. [Terminating ventricular tachycardias by mechanical heart stimulation with precordial thumps]. *Z Kardiol*. 1990;79:717–724.

355. Caldwell G, Millar G, Quinn E, Vincent R, Chamberlain DA. Simple mechanical methods for cardioversion: defence of the precordial thump and cough version. *BMJ (Clin Res Ed)*. 1985;291:627–630.

356. Morgera T, Baldi N, Chersevani D, Medugno G, Camerini F. Chest thump and ventricular tachycardia. *Pacing Clin Electrophysiol*. 1979;2: 69–75.

357. Rahner E, Zeh E. Die Regularisierung von Kammertachykardien durch präkordialen Faustschlag. [Regulation of ventricular tachycardia with precordial fist blow]. *Med Welt*. 1978;29:1659–1663.

358. Gertsch M, Hottinger S, Hess T. Serial chest thumps for the treatment of ventricular tachycardia in patients with coronary artery disease. *Clin Cardiol*. 1992;15:181–188.

359. Krijne R. Rate acceleration of ventricular tachycardia after a precordial chest thump. *Am J Cardiol*. 1984;53:964–965.

360. Sclarovsky S, Kracoff OH, Agmon J. Acceleration of ventricular tachycardia induced by a chest thump. *Chest.* 1981;80:596–599.

361. Yakaitis RW, Redding JS. Precordial thumping during cardiac resuscitation. *Crit Care Med.* 1973;1:22–26.

362. 2005 American Heart Association Guidelines for Cardiopulmonary Resuscitation and Emergency Cardiovascular Care. *Circulation.* 2005; 112(24 suppl):IV1–IV203.

363. Smith I, Monk TG, White PF. Comparison of transesophageal atrial pacing with anticholinergic drugs for the treatment of intraoperative bradycardia. *Anesth Analg.* 1994;78:245–252.

364. Brady WJ, Swart G, DeBehnke DJ, Ma OJ, Aufderheide TP. The efficacy of atropine in the treatment of hemodynamically unstable bradycardia and atrioventricular block: prehospital and emergency department considerations. *Resuscitation.* 1999;41:47–55.

365. Swart G, Brady WJJ, DeBehnke DJ, John OM, Aufderheide TP. Acute myocardial infarction complicated by hemodynamically unstable bradyarrhythmia: prehospital and ED treatment with atropine. *Am J Emerg Med.* 1999;17:647–652.

366. Chadda KD, Lichstein E, Gupta PK, Choy R. Bradycardia-hypotension syndrome in acute myocardial infarction. Reappraisal of the overdrive effects of atropine. *Am J Med.* 1975;59:158–164.

367. Chadda KD, Lichstein E, Gupta PK, Kourtesis P. Effects of atropine in patients with bradyarrhythmia complicating myocardial infarction: usefulness of an optimum dose for overdrive. *Am J Med.* 1977;63:503–510.

368. Dauchot P, Gravenstein JS. Effects of atropine on the electrocardiogram in different age groups. *Clin Pharmacol Ther.* 1971;12:274–280.

369. Bernheim A, Fatio R, Kiowski W, Weilenmann D, Rickli H, Rocca HP. Atropine often results in complete atrioventricular block or sinus arrest after cardiac transplantation: an unpredictable and dose-independent phenomenon. *Transplantation.* 2004;77:1181–1185.

370. Morrison LJ, Long J, Vermeulen M, Schwartz B, Sawadsky B, Frank J, Cameron B, Burgess R, Shield J, Bagley P, Mausz V, Brewer JE, Dorian P. A randomized controlled feasibility trial comparing safety and effectiveness of prehospital pacing versus conventional treatment: 'PrePACE.' *Resuscitation.* 2008;76:341–349.

371. Lown B. Electrical reversion of cardiac arrhythmias. *Br Heart J.* 1967; 29:469–489.

372. Mittal S, Ayati S, Stein KM, Schwartzman D, Cavlovich D, Tchou PJ, Markowitz SM, Slotwiner DJ, Scheiner MA, Lerman BB. Transthoracic cardioversion of atrial fibrillation: comparison of rectilinear biphasic versus damped sine wave monophasic shocks. *Circulation.* 2000;101: 1282–1287.

373. Page RL, Kerber RE, Russell JK, Trouton T, Waktare J, Gallik D, Olgin JE, Ricard P, Dalzell GW, Reddy R, Lazzara R, Lee K, Carlson M, Halperin B, Bardy GH. Biphasic versus monophasic shock waveform for conversion of atrial fibrillation: the results of an international randomized, double-blind multicenter trial. *J Am Coll Cardiol.* 2002;39: 1956–1963.

374. Scholten M, Szili-Torok T, Klootwijk P, Jordaens L. Comparison of monophasic and biphasic shocks for transthoracic cardioversion of atrial fibrillation. *Heart.* 2003;89:1032–1034.

375. Glover BM, Walsh SJ, McCann CJ, Moore MJ, Manoharan G, Dalzell GW, McAllister A, McClements B, McEneaney DJ, Trouton TG, Mathew TP, Adgey AA. Biphasic energy selection for transthoracic cardioversion of atrial fibrillation. The BEST AF Trial. *Heart.* 2008;94: 884–887.

376. Reisinger J, Gstrein C, Winter T, Zeindlhofer E, Hollinger K, Mori M, Schiller A, Winter A, Geiger H, Siostrzonek P. Optimization of initial energy for cardioversion of atrial tachyarrhythmias with biphasic shocks. *Am J Emerg Med.* 2010;28:159–165.

377. Kerber RE, Martins JB, Kienzle MG, Constantin L, Olshansky B, Hopson R, Charbonnier F. Energy, current, and success in defibrillation and cardioversion: clinical studies using an automated impedance-based method of energy adjustment. *Circulation.* 1988;77:1038–1046.

378. Lim SH, Anantharaman V, Teo WS, Goh PP, Tan AT. Comparison of treatment of supraventricular tachycardia by Valsalva maneuver and carotid sinus massage. *Ann Emerg Med.* 1998;31:30–35.

379. Wen ZC, Chen SA, Tai CT, Chiang CE, Chiou CW, Chang MS. Electrophysiological mechanisms and determinants of vagal maneuvers for termination of paroxysmal supraventricular tachycardia. *Circulation.* 1998;98:2716–2723.

380. Ornato JP, Hallagan LF, Reese WA, Clark RF, Tayal VS, Garnett AR, Gonzalez ER. Treatment of paroxysmal supraventricular tachycardia in the emergency department by clinical decision analysis. *Am J Emerg Med.* 1988;6:555–560.

381. DiMarco JP, Miles W, Akhtar M, Milstein S, Sharma AD, Platia E, McGovern B, Scheinman MM, Govier WC. Adenosine for paroxysmal supraventricular tachycardia: dose ranging and comparison with verapamil: assessment in placebo-controlled, multicenter trials. The Adenosine for PSVT Study Group [published correction appears in *Ann Intern Med.* 1990;113:996]. *Ann Intern Med.* 1990;113:104–110.

382. Lim SH, Anantharaman V, Teo WS, Chan YH. Slow infusion of calcium channel blockers compared with intravenous adenosine in the emergency treatment of supraventricular tachycardia. *Resuscitation.* 2009;80:523–528.

383. Cheng KA. [A randomized, multicenter trial to compare the safety and efficacy of adenosine versus verapamil for termination of paroxysmal supraventricular tachycardia]. *Zhonghua Nei Ke Za Zhi.* 2003;42: 773–776.

384. Hood MA, Smith WM. Adenosine versus verapamil in the treatment of supraventricular tachycardia: a randomized double-crossover trial. *Am Heart J.* 1992;123:1543–1549.

385. Rankin AC, Oldroyd KG, Chong E, Dow JW, Rae AP, Cobbe SM. Adenosine or adenosine triphosphate for supraventricular tachycardias? Comparative double-blind randomized study in patients with spontaneous or inducible arrhythmias. *Am Heart J.* 1990;119:316–323.

386. Brady WJ Jr, DeBehnke DJ, Wickman LL, Lindbeck G. Treatment of out-of-hospital supraventricular tachycardia: adenosine vs verapamil. *Acad Emerg Med.* 1996;3:574–585.

387. Morrison LJ, Allan R, Vermeulen M, Dong SL, McCallum AL. Conversion rates for prehospital paroxysmal supraventricular tachycardia (PSVT) with the addition of adenosine: a before-and-after trial. *Prehosp Emerg Care.* 2001;5:353–359.

388. Glatter K, Cheng J, Dorostkar P, Modin G, Talwar S, Al-Nimri M, Lee R, Saxon L, Lesh M, Scheinman M. Electrophysiologic effects of adenosine in patients with supraventricular tachycardia. *Circulation.* 1999;99:1034–1040.

389. Cairns CB, Niemann JT. Intravenous adenosine in the emergency department management of paroxysmal supraventricular tachycardia. *Ann Emerg Med.* 1991;20:717–721.

390. Davis R, Spitalnic SJ, Jagminas L. Cost-effective adenosine dosing for the treatment of PSVT. *Am J Emerg Med.* 1999;17:633–634.

391. Gausche M, Persse DE, Sugarman T, Shea SR, Palmer GL, Lewis RJ, Brueske PJ, Mahadevan S, Melio FR, Kuwata JH, Niemann JT. Adenosine for the prehospital treatment of paroxysmal supraventricular tachycardia. *Ann Emerg Med.* 1994;24:183–189.

392. McIntosh-Yellin NL, Drew BJ, Scheinman MM. Safety and efficacy of central intravenous bolus administration of adenosine for termination of supraventricular tachycardia. *J Am Coll Cardiol.* 1993;22:741–745.

393. Riccardi A, Arboscello E, Ghinatti M, Minuto P, Lerza R. Adenosine in the treatment of supraventricular tachycardia: 5 years of experience (2002–2006). *Am J Emerg Med.* 2008;26:879–882.

394. Sellers TD, Kirchhoffer JB, Modesto TA. Adenosine: a clinical experience and comparison with verapamil for the termination of supraventricular tachycardias. *Prog Clin Biol Res.* 1987;230:283–299.

395. Marco CA, Cardinale JF. Adenosine for the treatment of supraventricular tachycardia in the ED. *Am J Emerg Med.* 1994;12:485–488.

396. Seet CM. Efficacy of intravenous adenosine in treatment of paroxysmal supraventricular tachycardia in the local population. *Singapore Med J.* 1997;38:525–528.

397. Tan H, Spekhorst H, Peters R, Wilde A. Adenosine induced ventricular arrhythmias in the emergency room. *Pacing Clin Electrophysiol.* 2001; 24:450–455.

398. Madsen CD, Pointer JE, Lynch TG. A comparison of adenosine and verapamil for the treatment of supraventricular tachycardia in the prehospital setting. *Ann Emerg Med.* 1995;25:649–655.

399. Cybulski J, Kulakowski P, Makowska E, Czepiel A, Sikora-Frac M, Ceremuzynski L. Intravenous amiodarone is safe and seems to be effective in termination of paroxysmal supraventricular tachyarrhythmias. *Clin Cardiol.* 1996;19:563–566.

400. Gowda RM, Khan IA, Mehta NJ, Vasavada BC, Sacchi TJ. Cardiac arrhythmias in pregnancy: clinical and therapeutic considerations. *Int J Cardiol.* 2003;88:129–133.

401. Camm AJ, Garratt CJ. Adenosine and supraventricular tachycardia. *N Engl J Med.* 1991;325:1621–1629.

402. Lim SH, Anantharaman V, Teo WS. Slow-infusion of calcium channel blockers in the emergency management of supraventricular tachycardia. *Resuscitation.* 2002;52:167–174.

403. Ferreira JF, Pamplona D, Cesar LA, Leite PF, Sosa EA, da Luz PL, Bellotti G. [Comparative study between verapamil and adenosine

triphosphate in the treatment of paroxysmal supraventricular tachycardia]. *Arq Bras Cardiol*. 1996;66:55–57.

404. Rankin AC, Rae AP, Oldroyd KG, Cobbe SM. Verapamil or adenosine for the immediate treatment of supraventricular tachycardia. *Q J Med*. 1990;74:203–208.

405. Joshi PP, Deshmukh PK, Salkar RG. Efficacy of intravenous magnesium sulphate in supraventricular tachyarrhythmias. *J Assoc Physicians India*. 1995;43:529–531.

406. Gupta A, Naik A, Vora A, Lokhandwala Y. Comparison of efficacy of intravenous diltiazem and esmolol in terminating supraventricular tachycardia. *J Assoc Physicians India*. 1999;47:969–972.

407. Boudonas G, Lefkos N, Efthymiadis AP, Styliadis IG, Tsapas G. Intravenous administration of diltiazem in the treatment of supraventricular tachyarrhythmias. *Acta Cardiol*. 1995;50:125–134.

408. Marill KA, Wolfram S, Desouza IS, Nishijima DK, Kay D, Setnik GS, Stair TO, Ellinor PT. Adenosine for wide-complex tachycardia: efficacy and safety. *Crit Care Med*. 2009;37:2512–2518.

409. Domanovits H, Laske H, Stark G, Sterz F, Schmidinger H, Schreiber W, Mullner M, Laggner AN. Adenosine for the management of patients with tachycardias—a new protocol. *Eur Heart J*. 1994;15:589–593.

410. Ilkhanipour K, Berrol R, Yealy DM. Therapeutic and diagnostic efficacy of adenosine in wide-complex tachycardia. *Ann Emerg Med*. 1993;22:1360–1364.

411. Rankin AC, Oldroyd KG, Chong E, Rae AP, Cobbe SM. Value and limitations of adenosine in the diagnosis and treatment of narrow and broad complex tachycardias. *Br Heart J*. 1989;62:195–203.

412. Wilber DJ, Baerman J, Olshansky B, Kall J, Kopp D. Adenosine-sensitive ventricular tachycardia. Clinical characteristics and response to catheter ablation. *Circulation*. 1993;87:126–134.

413. Armengol RE, Graff J, Baerman JM, Swiryn S. Lack of effectiveness of lidocaine for sustained, wide QRS complex tachycardia. *Ann Emerg Med*. 1989;18:254–257.

414. Exner DV, Muzyka T, Gillis AM. Proarrhythmia in patients with the Wolff-Parkinson-White syndrome after standard doses of intravenous adenosine. *Ann Intern Med*. 1995;122:351–352.

415. Gupta AK, Shah CP, Maheshwari A, Thakur RK, Hayes OW, Lokhandwala YY. Adenosine induced ventricular fibrillation in Wolff-Parkinson-White syndrome. *Pacing Clin Electrophysiol*. 2002;25:477–480.

416. Shah CP, Gupta AK, Thakur RK, Hayes OW, Mehrotra A, Lokhandwala YY. Adenosine-induced ventricular fibrillation. *Indian Heart J*. 2001;53:208–210.

417. Parham WA, Mehdirad AA, Biermann KM, Fredman CS. Case report: adenosine induced ventricular fibrillation in a patient with stable ventricular tachycardia. *J Interv Card Electrophysiol*. 2001;5:71–74.

418. Buxton AE, Marchlinski FE, Doherty JU, Flores B, Josephson ME. Hazards of intravenous verapamil for sustained ventricular tachycardia. *Am J Cardiol*. 1987;59:1107–1110.

419. Gorgels AP, van den Dool A, Hofs A, Mulleneers R, Smeets JL, Vos MA, Wellens HJ. Comparison of procainamide and lidocaine in terminating sustained monomorphic ventricular tachycardia. *Am J Cardiol*. 1996;78:43–46.

420. Ho DS, Zecchin RP, Richards DA, Uther JB, Ross DL. Double-blind trial of lignocaine versus sotalol for acute termination of spontaneous sustained ventricular tachycardia. *Lancet*. 1994;344:18–23.

421. Ho DSW, Zecchin RP, Cooper MJ, Richards DAB, Uther JB, Ross DL. Rapid intravenous infusion of d-1 sotalol: time to onset of effects on ventricular refractoriness, and safety. *Eur Heart J*. 1995;16:81–86.

422. Marill KA, deSouza IS, Nishijima DK, Stair TO, Setnik GS, Ruskin JN. Amiodarone is poorly effective for the acute termination of ventricular tachycardia. *Ann Emerg Med*. 2006;47:217–224.

423. Schutzenberger W, Leisch F, Kerschner K, Harringer W, Herbinger W. Clinical efficacy of intravenous amiodarone in the short term treatment of recurrent sustained ventricular tachycardia and ventricular fibrillation. *Br Heart J*. 1989;62:367–371.

424. Tomlinson DR, Cherian P, Betts TR, Bashir Y. Intravenous amiodarone for the pharmacological termination of haemodynamically-tolerated sustained ventricular tachycardia: is bolus dose amiodarone an appropriate first-line treatment? *Emerg Med J*. 2008;25:15–18.

425. Nasir N Jr, Taylor A, Doyle TK, Pacifico A. Evaluation of intravenous lidocaine for the termination of sustained monomorphic ventricular

426. Marill KA, Greenberg GM, Kay D, Nelson BK. Analysis of the treatment of spontaneous sustained stable ventricular tachycardia. *Acad Emerg Med*. 1997;4:1122–1128.

427. Koster RW, Dunning AJ. Intramuscular lidocaine for prevention of lethal arrhythmias in the prehospitalization phase of acute myocardial infarction. *N Engl J Med*. 1985;313:1105–1110.

428. Roth A, Malov N, Bloch Y, Schlesinger Z, Laniado S, Kaplinski E. Usefulness of self-administration of intramuscular lidocaine in the pre-hospital setting for ventricular tachyarrhythmias unassociated with acute myocardial infarction (The "SHAHAL" experience in Israel). *Am J Cardiol*. 1997;79:611–614.

429. Fuster V, Ryden LE, Cannom DS, Crijns HJ, Curtis AB, Ellenbogen KA, Halperin JL, Le Heuzey JY, Kay GN, Lowe JE, Olsson SB, Prystowsky EN, Tamargo JL, Wann S, Smith SC Jr, Jacobs AK, Adams CD, Anderson JL, Antman EM, Halperin JL, Hunt SA, Nishimura R, Ornato JP, Page RL, Riegel B, Priori SG, Blanc JJ, Budaj A, Camm AJ, Dean V, Deckers JW, Despres C, Dickstein K, Lekakis J, McGregor K, Metra M, Morais J, Osterspey A, Tamargo JL, Zamorano JL. ACC/AHA/ESC 2006 Guidelines for the Management of Patients with Atrial Fibrillation: a report of the American College of Cardiology/American Heart Association Task Force on Practice Guidelines and the European Society of Cardiology Committee for Practice Guidelines (Writing Committee to Revise the 2001 Guidelines for the Management of Patients With Atrial Fibrillation): developed in collaboration with the European Heart Rhythm Association and the Heart Rhythm Society. *Circulation*. 2006;114:e257–e354.

430. Sticherling C, Tada H, Hsu W, Bares AC, Oral H, Pelosi F, Knight BP, Strickberger SA, Morady F. Effects of diltiazem and esmolol on cycle length and spontaneous conversion of atrial fibrillation. *J Cardiovasc Pharmacol Ther*. 2002;7:81–88.

431. Chiladakis JA, Stathopoulos C, Davlouros P, Manolis AS. Intravenous magnesium sulfate versus diltiazem in paroxysmal atrial fibrillation. *Int J Cardiol*. 2001;79:287–291.

432. Schreck DM, Rivera AR, Tricarico VJ. Emergency management of atrial fibrillation and flutter: intravenous diltiazem versus intravenous digoxin. *Ann Emerg Med*. 1997;29:135–140.

433. Siu CW, Lau CP, Lee WL, Lam KF, Tse HF. Intravenous diltiazem is superior to intravenous amiodarone or digoxin for achieving ventricular rate control in patients with acute uncomplicated atrial fibrillation. *Crit Care Med*. 2009;37:2174–2179, quiz 2180.

434. Intravenous digoxin in acute atrial fibrillation. Results of a randomized, placebo-controlled multicentre trial in 239 patients. The Digitalis in Acute Atrial Fibrillation (DAAF) Trial Group. *Eur Heart J*. 1997;18:649–654.

435. Jordaens L, Trouerbach J, Calle P, Tavernier R, Derycke E, Vertongen P, Bergez B, Vandekerckhove Y. Conversion of atrial fibrillation to sinus rhythm and rate control by digoxin in comparison to placebo. *Eur Heart J*. 1997;18:643–648.

436. Wattanasuwan N, Khan IA, Mehta NJ, Arora P, Singh N, Vasavada BC, Sacchi TJ. Acute ventricular rate control in atrial fibrillation: IV combination of diltiazem and digoxin vs IV diltiazem alone. *Chest*. 2001;119:502–506.

437. Galve E, Rius T, Ballester R, Artaza MA, Arnau JM, Garcia-Dorado D, Soler-Soler J. Intravenous amiodarone in treatment of recent-onset atrial fibrillation: results of a randomized, controlled study. *J Am Coll Cardiol*. 1996;27:1079–1082.

438. Thomas SP, Guy D, Wallace E, Crampton R, Kijvanit P, Eipper V, Ross DL, Cooper MJ. Rapid loading of sotalol or amiodarone for management of recent onset symptomatic atrial fibrillation: a randomized, digoxin-controlled trial. *Am Heart J*. 2004;147:E3.

439. Keren A, Tzivoni D, Gavish D, Levi J, Gottlieb S, Benhorin J, Stern S. Etiology, warning signs and therapy of torsade de pointes: a study of 10 patients. *Circulation*. 1981;64:1167–1174.

440. Nguyen PT, Scheinman MM, Seger J. Polymorphous ventricular tachycardia: clinical characterization, therapy, and the QT interval. *Circulation*. 1986;74:340–349.

KEY WORDS: arrhythmia ■ cardiac arrest ■ drugs ■ ventricular arrhythmia ■ ventricular fibrillation

# Part 9: Post–Cardiac Arrest Care
## 2010 American Heart Association Guidelines for Cardiopulmonary Resuscitation and Emergency Cardiovascular Care

Mary Ann Peberdy, Co-Chair*; Clifton W. Callaway, Co-Chair*; Robert W. Neumar;
Romergryko G. Geocadin; Janice L. Zimmerman; Michael Donnino; Andrea Gabrielli;
Scott M. Silvers; Arno L. Zaritsky; Raina Merchant; Terry L. Vanden Hoek; Steven L. Kronick

There is increasing recognition that systematic post–cardiac arrest care after return of spontaneous circulation (ROSC) can improve the likelihood of patient survival with good quality of life. This is based in part on the publication of results of randomized controlled clinical trials as well as a description of the post–cardiac arrest syndrome.[1–3] Post–cardiac arrest care has significant potential to reduce early mortality caused by hemodynamic instability and later morbidity and mortality from multiorgan failure and brain injury.[3,4] This section summarizes our evolving understanding of the hemodynamic, neurological, and metabolic abnormalities encountered in patients who are initially resuscitated from cardiac arrest.

The initial objectives of post–cardiac arrest care are to

- Optimize cardiopulmonary function and vital organ perfusion.
- After out-of-hospital cardiac arrest, transport patient to an appropriate hospital with a comprehensive post–cardiac arrest treatment system of care that includes acute coronary interventions, neurological care, goal-directed critical care, and hypothermia.
- Transport the in-hospital post–cardiac arrest patient to an appropriate critical-care unit capable of providing comprehensive post–cardiac arrest care.
- Try to identify and treat the precipitating causes of the arrest and prevent recurrent arrest.

Subsequent objectives of post–cardiac arrest care are to

- Control body temperature to optimize survival and neurological recovery
- Identify and treat acute coronary syndromes (ACS)
- Optimize mechanical ventilation to minimize lung injury
- Reduce the risk of multiorgan injury and support organ function if required
- Objectively assess prognosis for recovery
- Assist survivors with rehabilitation services when required

## Systems of Care for Improving Post–Cardiac Arrest Outcomes

Post–cardiac arrest care is a critical component of advanced life support (Figure). Most deaths occur during the first 24 hours after cardiac arrest.[5,6] The best hospital care for patients with ROSC after cardiac arrest is not completely known, but there is increasing interest in identifying and optimizing practices that are likely to improve outcomes (Table 1).[7] Positive associations have been noted between the likelihood of survival and the number of cardiac arrest cases treated at any individual hospital.[8,9] Because multiple organ systems are affected after cardiac arrest, successful post–cardiac arrest care will benefit from the development of system-wide plans for proactive treatment of these patients. For example, restoration of blood pressure and gas exchange does not ensure survival and functional recovery. Significant cardiovascular dysfunction can develop, requiring support of blood flow and ventilation, including intravascular volume expansion, vasoactive and inotropic drugs, and invasive devices. Therapeutic hypothermia and treatment of the underlying cause of cardiac arrest impacts survival and neurological outcomes. Protocolized hemodynamic optimization and multidisciplinary early goal-directed therapy protocols have been introduced as part of a bundle of care to improve survival rather than single interventions.[10–12] The data suggests that proactive titration of post–cardiac arrest hemodynamics to levels intended to ensure organ perfusion and oxygenation may improve outcomes. There are multiple specific options for acheiving these goals, and it is difficult to distinguish between the benefit of protocols or any specific component of care that is most important.

A comprehensive, structured, multidisciplinary system of care should be implemented in a consistent manner for the treatment of post–cardiac arrest patients (Class I, LOE B). Programs should include as part of structured interventions therapeutic hypothermia; optimization of hemodynamics and gas exchange; immediate coronary reperfusion when indicated for restoration of coronary blood flow with percutaneous coronary intervention (PCI); glycemic control; and neurological diagnosis, management, and prognostication.

## Overview of Post–Cardiac Arrest Care
The provider of CPR should ensure an adequate airway and support breathing immediately after ROSC. Unconscious

---

The American Heart Association requests that this document be cited as follows: Peberdy MA, Callaway CW, Neumar RW, Geocadin RG, Zimmerman JL, Donnino M, Gabrielli A, Silvers SM, Zaritsky AL, Merchant R, Vanden Hoek TL, Kronick SL. Part 9: post–cardiac arrest care: 2010 American Heart Association Guidelines for Cardiopulmonary Resuscitation and Emergency Cardiovascular Care. *Circulation.* 2010;122(suppl 3):S768–S786.
*Co-chairs and equal first co-authors.
**(*Circulation.* 2010;122[suppl 3]:S768–S786.)**
© 2010 American Heart Association, Inc.

*Circulation* is available at http://circ.ahajournals.org          DOI: 10.1161/CIRCULATIONAHA.110.971002

### Adult Immediate Post–Cardiac Arrest Care

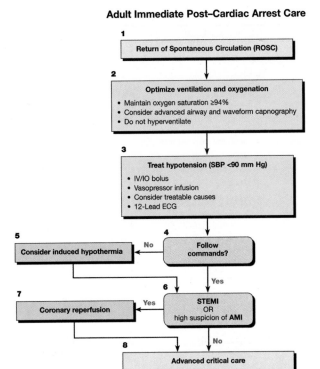

© 2010 American Heart Association

**Figure.** Post–cardiac arrest care algorithm.

patients usually require an advanced airway for mechanical support of breathing. It may be necessary to replace a supraglottic airway used for initial resuscitation with an endotracheal tube, although the timing of replacement may vary. Methods for securing an advanced airway are discussed in Part 8.1: "Airway Management," but several simple maneuvers deserve consideration. For example, rescuers and long-term hospital providers should avoid using ties that pass circumferentially around the patient's neck, potentially obstructing venous return from the brain. They should also elevate the head of the bed 30° if tolerated to reduce the incidence of cerebral edema, aspiration, and ventilatory-associated pneumonia. Correct placement of an advanced airway, particularly during patient transport, should be monitored using waveform capnography as described in other sections of the *2010 AHA Guidelines for CPR and ECC.* Oxygenation of the patient should be monitored continuously with pulse oximetry.

Although 100% oxygen may have been used during initial resuscitation, providers should titrate inspired oxygen to the lowest level required to achieve an arterial oxygen saturation of ≥94%, so as to avoid potential oxygen toxicity. It is recognized that titration of inspired oxygen may not be possible immediately after out-of-hospital cardiac arrest until the patient is transported to the emergency department or, in the case of in-hospital arrest, the intensive care unit (ICU). Hyperventilation or "overbagging" the patient is common after cardiac arrest and should be avoided because of potential adverse hemodynamic effects. Hyperventilation increases intrathoracic pressure and inversely lowers cardiac output. The decrease in $PaCO_2$ seen with hyperventilation can also potentially decrease cerebral blood flow directly. Ventilation may be started at 10 to 12 breaths per minute and titrated to achieve a $PETCO_2$ of 35 to 40 mm Hg or a $PaCO_2$ of 40 to 45 mm Hg.

The clinician should assess vital signs and monitor for recurrent cardiac arrhythmias. Continuous electrocardiographic (ECG) monitoring should continue after ROSC, during transport, and throughout ICU care until stability has been achieved. Intravenous (IV) access should be obtained if not already established and the position and function of any intravenous catheter verified. IV lines should be promptly established to replace emergent intraosseous access achieved during resuscitation. If the patient is hypotensive (systolic blood pressure <90 mm Hg), fluid boluses can be considered. Cold fluid may be used if therapeutic hypothermia is elected. Vasoactive drug infusions such as dopamine, norepinephrine, or epinephrine may be initiated if necessary and titrated to achieve a minimum systolic blood pressure of ≥90 mm Hg or a mean arterial pressure of ≥65 mm Hg.

Brain injury and cardiovascular instability are the major determinants of survival after cardiac arrest.[13] Because therapeutic hypothermia is the only intervention demonstrated to improve neurological recovery, it should be considered for any patient who is unable to follow verbal commands after ROSC. The patient should be transported to a facility that reliably provides this therapy in addition to coronary reperfusion (eg, PCI) and other goal-directed postarrest care therapies.

Overall the most common cause of cardiac arrest is cardiovascular disease and coronary ischemia.[14,15] Therefore, a 12-lead ECG should be obtained as soon as possible to detect ST elevation or new or presumably new left bundle-branch block. When there is high suspicion of acute myocardial infarction (AMI), local protocols for treatment of AMI and coronary reperfusion should be activated. Even in the absence of ST elevation, medical or interventional treatments may be considered for treatment of ACS[14,16,17] and should not be deferred in the presence of coma or in conjunction with

**Table 1.    Multiple System Approach to Post–Cardiac Arrest Care**

| Ventilation | Hemodynamics | Cardiovascular | Neurological | Metabolic |
|---|---|---|---|---|
| • Capnography | • Frequent Blood Pressure Monitoring/Arterial-line | • Continuous Cardiac Monitoring | • Serial Neurological Exam | • Serial Lactate |
| • Rationale: Confirm secure airway and titrate ventilation | • Rationale: Maintain perfusion and prevent recurrent hypotension | • Rationale: Detect recurrent arrhythmia | • Rationale: Serial examinations define coma, brain injury, and prognosis | • Rationale: Confirm adequate perfusion |
| • Endotracheal tube when possible for comatose patients | • Mean arterial pressure ≥65 mm Hg or systolic blood pressure ≥90 mm Hg | • No prophylactic antiarrhythmics | • Response to verbal commands or physical stimulation | |
| • $P_{ETCO_2} \sim$ 35–40 mm Hg | | • Treat arrhythmias as required | • Pupillary light and corneal reflex, spontaneous eye movement | |
| • $Paco_2 \sim$ 40–45 mm Hg | | • Remove reversible causes | • Gag, cough, spontaneous breaths | |
| • Chest X-ray | • Treat Hypotension | • 12-lead ECG/Troponin | • EEG Monitoring If Comatose | • Serum Potassium |
| • Rationale: Confirm secure airway and detect causes or complications of arrest: pneumonitis, pneumonia, pulmonary edema | • Rationale: Maintain perfusion | • Rationale: Detect Acute Coronary Syndrome/ST-Elevation Myocardial Infarction; Assess QT interval | • Rationale: Exclude seizures | • Rationale: Avoid hypokalemia which promotes arrhythmias |
| | • Fluid bolus if tolerated | | • Anticonvulsants if seizing | • Replace to maintain K >3.5 mEq/L |
| | • Dopamine 5–10 mcg/kg per min | | | |
| | • Norepinephrine 0.1–0.5 mcg/kg per min | | | |
| | • Epinephrine 0.1–0.5 mcg/kg per min | | | |
| • Pulse Oximetry/ABG | ... | • Treat Acute Coronary Syndrome | • Core Temperature Measurement If Comatose | • Urine Output, Serum Creatinine |
| • Rationale: Maintain adequate oxygenation and minimize $F_{IO_2}$ | ... | • Aspirin/heparin | • Rationale: Minimize brain injury and improve outcome | • Rationale: Detect acute kidney injury |
| • $Spo_2$ ≥94% | ... | • Transfer to acute coronary treatment center | • Prevent hyperpyrexia >37.7°C | • Maintain euvolemia |
| • $Pao_2 \sim$ 100 mm Hg | ... | • Consider emergent PCI or fibrinolysis | • Induce therapeutic hypothermia if no contraindications | • Renal replacement therapy if indicated |
| • Reduce $F_{IO_2}$ as tolerated | ... | | • Cold IV fluid bolus 30 mL/kg if no contraindication | |
| • $Pao_2/F_{IO_2}$ ratio to follow acute lung injury | ... | | • Surface or endovascular cooling for 32°C–34°C×24 hours | |
| | ... | | • After 24 hours, slow rewarming 0.25°C/hr | |
| • Mechanical Ventilation | ... | • Echocardiogram | • Consider Non-enhanced CT Scan | • Serum Glucose |
| • Rationale: Minimize acute lung injury, potential oxygen toxicity | ... | • Rationale: Detect global stunning, wall-motion abnormalities, structural problems or cardiomyopathy | • Rationale: Exclude primary intracranial process | • Rationale: Detect hyperglycemia and hypoglycemia |
| • Tidal Volume 6–8 mL/kg | ... | | | • Treat hypoglycemia (<80 mg/dL) with dextrose |
| • Titrate minute ventilation to $P_{ETCO_2} \sim$ 35–40 mm Hg $Paco_2 \sim$ 40–45 mm Hg | ... | | | • Treat hyperglycemia to target glucose 144–180 mg/dL |
| • Reduce $F_{IO_2}$ as tolerated to keep $Spo_2$ or $Sao_2$ ≥94% | ... | | | • Local insulin protocols |
| | ... | • Treat Myocardial Stunning | • Sedation/Muscle Relaxation | • Avoid Hypotonic Fluids |
| | ... | • Fluids to optimize volume status (requires clinical judgment) | • Rationale: To control shivering, agitation, or ventilator desynchrony as needed | • Rationale: May increase edema, including cerebral edema |
| | ... | • Dobutamine 5–10 mcg/kg per min | | |
| | ... | • Mechanical augmentation (IABP) | | |

hypothermia. Concurrent PCI and hypothermia are safe, with good outcomes reported for some comatose patients who undergo PCI.

Patients who are unconscious or unresponsive after cardiac arrest should be directed to an inpatient critical-care facility with a comprehensive care plan that includes acute cardiovascular interventions, use of therapeutic hypothermia, standardized medical goal-directed therapies, and advanced neu-

rological monitoring and care. Neurological prognosis may be difficult to determine during the first 72 hours, even for patients who are not undergoing therapeutic hypothermia. This time frame for prognostication is likely to be extended in patients being cooled.[18] Many initially comatose survivors of cardiac arrest have the potential for full recovery such that they are able to lead normal lives.[1,2,19] Between 20% and 50% or more of survivors of out-of-hospital cardiac arrest who are comatose on arrival at the hospital may have good one-year neurological outcome.[1,2,11] Therefore, it is important to place patients in a hospital critical-care unit where expert care and neurological evaluation can be performed and where appropriate testing to aid prognosis is available and performed in a timely manner.

Attention should be directed to treating the precipitating cause of cardiac arrest after ROSC. The provider should initiate or request studies that will further aid in evaluation of the patient. It is important to identify and treat any cardiac, electrolyte, toxicological, pulmonary, and neurological precipitants of arrest. The clinician may find it helpful to review the H's and T's mnemonic to recall factors that may contribute to cardiac arrest or complicate resuscitation or postresuscitation care: hypovolemia, hypoxia, hydrogen ion (acidosis of any etiology), hyper-/hypokalemia, moderate to severe hypothermia, toxins, tamponade (cardiac), tension pneumothorax, and thrombosis of the coronary or pulmonary vasculature. For further information on treating other causes of cardiac arrest, see Part 12: "Special Resuscitation Situations."

## Targeted Temperature Management

### Induced Hypothermia

For protection of the brain and other organs, hypothermia is a helpful therapeutic approach in patients who remain comatose (usually defined as a lack of meaningful response to verbal commands) after ROSC. Questions remain about specific indications and populations, timing and duration of therapy, and methods for induction, maintenance, and subsequent reversal of hypothermia. One good randomized trial[1] and a pseudorandomized trial[2] reported improved neurologically intact survival to hospital discharge when comatose patients with out-of-hospital ventricular fibrillation (VF) cardiac arrest were cooled to 32°C to 34°C for 12 or 24 hours beginning minutes to hours after ROSC. Additional studies with historical control groups show improved neurological outcome after therapeutic hypothermia for comatose survivors of VF cardiac arrest.[20,21]

No randomized controlled trials have compared outcome between hypothermia and normothermia for non-VF arrest. However, 6 studies with historical control groups reported a beneficial effect on outcome from use of therapeutic hypothermia in comatose survivors of out-of-hospital cardiac arrest associated with any arrest rhythm.[11,22–26] Only one study with historical controls reported better neurological outcome after VF cardiac arrest but no difference in outcome after cardiac arrest associated with other rhythms.[27] Two nonrandomized studies with concurrent controls[28,29] indicate a possible benefit of hypothermia after in- and out-of-hospital cardiac arrest associated with non-VF initial rhythms.

Case series have reported the feasibility of using therapeutic hypothermia after ROSC in the setting of cardiogenic shock[23,30,31] and therapeutic hypothermia in combination with emergent PCI.[32–36] Case series also report successful use of fibrinolytic therapy for AMI after ROSC,[37,38] but data are lacking about interactions between fibrinolytics and hypothermia in this population.

The impact of the timing of initiating hypothermia after cardiac arrest is not completely understood. Studies of animal models of cardiac arrest showed that short-duration hypothermia (≤1 hour) achieved <10 to 20 minutes after ROSC had a beneficial effect that was lost when hypothermia was delayed.[39–41] Beyond the initial minutes of ROSC and when hypothermia is prolonged (>12 hours), the relationship between the onset of hypothermia and the resulting neuroprotection is less clear.[42,43] Two prospective clinical trials in which hypothermia was achieved within 2 hours[2] or at a median of 8 hours (interquartile range [IQR] 4 to 16 hours)[1] after ROSC both demonstrated better outcomes in the hypothermia-treated than the normothermia-treated subjects. Subsequent to these studies, one registry-based case series of 986 comatose post–cardiac arrest patients[35] suggested that time to initiation of cooling (IQR 1 to 1.8 hours) and time to achieving target temperature (IQR 3 to 6.7 hours) were not associated with improved neurological outcome after discharge. A case series of 49 consecutive comatose post–cardiac arrest patients[44] cooled intravascularly after out-of-hospital cardiac arrest also documented that time to target temperature (median 6.8 hours [IQR 4.5 to 9.2 hours]) was not an independent predictor of neurological outcome.

The optimal duration of induced hypothermia is at least 12 hours and may be >24 hours. Hypothermia was maintained for 12[2] or 24 hours[1] in the studies of out-of-hospital patients presenting in VF. Most case series of adult patients have reported 24 hours of hypothermia. The effect of a longer duration of cooling on outcome has not been studied in adults, but hypothermia for up to 72 hours was used safely in newborns.[45,46]

Although there are multiple methods for inducing hypothermia, no single method has proved to be optimal. Feedback-controlled endovascular catheters and surface cooling devices are available.[47–49] Other techniques (eg, cooling blankets and frequent application of ice bags) are readily available and effective but may require more labor and closer monitoring. As an adjunct, iced isotonic fluid can be infused to initiate core cooling but must be combined with a follow-up method for maintenance of hypothermia.[50–52] Although a theoretical concern is that rapid fluid loading could have adverse cardiopulmonary effects such as pulmonary edema, 9 case series indicate that cooling can be initiated safely with IV ice-cold fluids (500 mL to 30 mL/kg of saline 0.9% or Ringer's lactate).[51–59] One human case series[56] showed that the deterioration in oxygenation that often occurs after ROSC was not significantly affected by the infusion of cold fluids (3427 mL ± 210 mL). Two randomized controlled trials,[60,61] one study with concurrent controls,[62] and 3 case series[63,64] indicate that cooling with IV cold saline can be initiated safely in the prehospital setting.

Clinicians should continuously monitor the patient's core temperature using an esophageal thermometer, bladder catheter in nonanuric patients, or pulmonary artery catheter if one is placed for other indications.[1,2] Axillary and oral temperatures are inadequate for measurement of core temperature changes, especially during active manipulation of temperature for therapeutic hypothermia,[65,66] and true tympanic temperature probes are rarely available and often unreliable.

Bladder temperatures in anuric patients and rectal temperatures may differ from brain or core temperature.[66,67] A secondary source of temperature measurement should be considered, especially if a closed feedback cooling system is used for temperature management.

A number of potential complications are associated with cooling, including coagulopathy, arrhythmias, and hyperglycemia, particularly with an unintended drop below target temperature.[35] The likelihood of pneumonia and sepsis may increase in patients treated with therapeutic hypothermia.[1,2] Although these complications were not significantly different between groups in the published clinical trials, infections are common in this population, and prolonged hypothermia is known to decrease immune function. Hypothermia also impairs coagulation, and any ongoing bleeding should be controlled before decreasing temperature.

In summary, we recommend that comatose (ie, lack of meaningful response to verbal commands) adult patients with ROSC after out-of-hospital VF cardiac arrest should be cooled to 32°C to 34°C (89.6°F to 93.2°F) for 12 to 24 hours (Class I, LOE B). Induced hypothermia also may be considered for comatose adult patients with ROSC after in-hospital cardiac arrest of any initial rhythm or after out-of-hospital cardiac arrest with an initial rhythm of pulseless electric activity or asystole (Class IIb, LOE B). Active rewarming should be avoided in comatose patients who spontaneously develop a mild degree of hypothermia (>32°C [89.6°F]) after resuscitation from cardiac arrest during the first 48 hours after ROSC. (Class III, LOE C).

### Hyperthermia

After resuscitation, temperature elevation above normal can impair brain recovery. The etiology of fever after cardiac arrest may be related to activation of inflammatory cytokines in a pattern similar to that observed in sepsis.[68,69] There are no randomized controlled trials evaluating the effect of treating pyrexia with either frequent use of antipyretics or "controlled normothermia" using cooling techniques compared to no temperature intervention in post–cardiac arrest patients. Case series[70–74] and studies[75–80] suggest that there is an association between poor survival outcomes and pyrexia $\geq 37.6°C$. In patients with a cerebrovascular event leading to brain ischemia, studies[75–80] demonstrate worsened short-term outcome and long-term mortality. By extrapolation this data may be relevant to the global ischemia and reperfusion of the brain that follows cardiac arrest. Patients can develop hyperthermia after rewarming posthypothermia treatment. This late hyperthermia should also be identified and treated. Providers should closely monitor patient core temperature after ROSC and actively intervene to avoid hyperthermia (Class I, LOE C).

## Organ-Specific Evaluation and Support

The remainder of Part 9 focuses on organ-specific measures that should be included in the immediate post–cardiac arrest period.

### Pulmonary System

Pulmonary dysfunction after cardiac arrest is common. Etiologies include hydrostatic pulmonary edema from left ventricular dysfunction; noncardiogenic edema from inflammatory, infective, or physical injuries; severe pulmonary atelectasis; or aspiration occurring during cardiac arrest or resuscitation. Patients often develop regional mismatch of ventilation and perfusion, contributing to decreased arterial oxygen content. The severity of pulmonary dysfunction often is measured in terms of the $PaO_2/FIO_2$ ratio. A $PaO_2/FIO_2$ ratio of $\leq 300$ mm Hg usually defines acute lung injury. The acute onset of bilateral infiltrates on chest x-ray and a pulmonary artery pressure $\leq 18$ mm Hg or no evidence of left atrial hypertension are common to both acute lung injury and acute respiratory distress syndrome (ARDS). A $PaO_2/FIO_2$ ratio $<300$ or $<200$ mm Hg separates acute lung injury from ARDS, respectively.[81] Positive end-expiratory pressure (PEEP), a lung-protective strategy for mechanical ventilation, and titrated $FIO_2$ are strategies that can improve pulmonary function and $PaO_2$ while the practitioner is determining the pathophysiology of the pulmonary dysfunction.

Essential diagnostic tests in intubated patients include a chest radiograph and arterial blood gas measurements. Other diagnostic tests may be added based on history, physical examination, and clinical circumstances. Evaluation of a chest radiograph should verify the correct position of the endotracheal tube and the distribution of pulmonary infiltrates or edema and identify complications from chest compressions (eg, rib fracture, pneumothorax, and pleural effusions) or pneumonia.

Providers should adjust mechanical ventilatory support based on the measured oxyhemoglobin saturation, blood gas values, minute ventilation (respiratory rate and tidal volume), and patient-ventilator synchrony. In addition, mechanical ventilatory support to reduce the work of breathing should be considered as long as the patient remains in shock. As spontaneous ventilation becomes more efficient and as concurrent medical conditions allow, the level of support may be gradually decreased.

The optimal $FIO_2$ during the immediate period after cardiac arrest is still debated. The beneficial effect of high $FIO_2$ on systemic oxygen delivery should be balanced with the deleterious effect of generating oxygen-derived free radicals during the reperfusion phase. Animal data suggests that ventilations with 100% oxygen (generating $PaO_2 >350$ mm Hg at 15 to 60 minutes after ROSC) increase brain lipid peroxidation, increase metabolic dysfunctions, increase neurological degeneration, and worsen short-term functional outcome when compared with ventilation with room air or an inspired oxygen fraction titrated to a pulse oximeter reading between 94% and 96%.[82–87] One randomized prospective clinical trial compared ventilation for the first 60 minutes after ROSC with 30% oxygen (resulting in $PaO_2=110\pm25$ mm Hg at 60 minutes) or 100% oxygen (resulting in $PaO_2=345\pm174$ mm Hg at 60 minutes).[88] This small trial detected no difference in serial markers of acute brain injury, survival to hospital discharge, or percentage of patients with good neurological outcome at hospital discharge but was inadequately powered to detect important differences in survival or neurological outcome.

Once the circulation is restored, monitor systemic arterial oxyhemoglobin saturation. It may be reasonable, when the appropriate equipment is available, to titrate oxygen administration to maintain the arterial oxyhemoglobin saturation ≥94%. Provided appropriate equipment is available, once ROSC is achieved, adjust the $FIO_2$ to the minimum concentration needed to achieve arterial oxyhemoglobin saturation ≥94%, with the goal of avoiding hyperoxia while ensuring adequate oxygen delivery. Since an arterial oxyhemoglobin saturation of 100% may correspond to a $PaO_2$ anywhere between ~80 and 500 mm Hg, in general it is appropriate to wean $FIO_2$ when saturation is 100%, provided the oxyhemoglobin saturation can be maintained ≥94% (Class I, LOE C).

Because patients may have significant metabolic acidosis after cardiac arrest, there is a temptation to institute hyperventilation to normalize blood pH. However, metabolic acidosis is likely to be reversed once adequate perfusion is restored, and there are several physiological reasons why hyperventilation may be detrimental. Minute ventilation alters the partial pressure of carbon dioxide ($PaCO_2$), which in turn can affect cerebral blood flow. In a normal brain a 1-mm Hg decrease in $PaCO_2$ results in a decrease in cerebral blood flow of approximately 2.5% to 4%; cerebral blood flow remains $CO_2$-reactive after cardiac arrest,[89,90] although the magnitude of the $CO_2$ reactivity (magnitude of change in cerebral blood flow per millimeters of mercury [mm Hg] change in $PCO_2$) may be diminished or suppressed for 1 to 3 hours after reperfusion,[91,92] especially after prolonged ischemia (≥15 minutes).[93,94] After ROSC there is an initial hyperemic blood flow response that lasts 10 to 30 minutes, followed by a more prolonged period of low blood flow.[95,96] During this latter period of late hypoperfusion, a mismatch between blood flow (as a component of oxygen delivery) and oxygen requirement may occur. Hyperventilation at this stage may lower $PaCO_2$, cause cerebral vasoconstriction, and exacerbate cerebral ischemic injury.

Physiological data in humans suggests that hyperventilation could cause additional cerebral ischemia in the post–cardiac arrest patient because sustained hypocapnia (low $PCO_2$) may reduce cerebral blood flow.[97,98] Transcranial Doppler measurements of the middle cerebral artery and jugular bulb oxygen saturation measurements in 10 comatose subjects after cardiac arrest revealed that hyperventilation with hypocapnia did not affect median flow velocity but did decrease jugular bulb oxygen saturation below the ischemic threshold (55%). Conversely, hypoventilation with hypercapnia produced the opposite effect.[99] In one study, controlled ventilation with specific goals to keep $PaCO_2$ 37.6 to 45.1 mm Hg (5 to 6 kPa) and $SaO_2$ 95% to 98% as part of a bundle with multiple other goals (including hypothermia and blood pressure goals) increased survival from 26% to 56%.[11] In that study it was impossible to ascertain an independent effect of controlled ventilation separate from all other components of the bundle.

Hyperventilation also may compromise systemic blood flow because of occult or auto-PEEP and is deleterious in all low-flow states, including cardiopulmonary resuscitation (CPR)[100,101] and hypovolemia.[102,103] Auto-PEEP, also known as *intrinsic PEEP* or *gas trapping*, occurs preferentially in patients with obstructive lung disease and is aggravated by hyperventilation that does not allow sufficient time for complete exhalation. A gradual increase in end-expiratory volume and pressure in the lung (hyperinflation) is transmitted to the great veins in the thorax and depresses both venous return and cardiac output.[104,105] Similar effects may occur after cardiac arrest, suggesting that hyperventilation should be avoided, especially in hypotensive patients.

Other ventilatory parameters may affect the outcome of patients on mechanical ventilation after cardiac arrest, particularly when acute lung injury or ARDS develops. Over the last decade attention has focused on low-volume/high-rate ventilation. In a comparison of high- and low-tidal-volume ventilation, the death rate of patients with ARDS was reduced from 40% to 31% in the group with reduced tidal volume ($V_T$).[106] This and subsequent studies recommend ventilating patients to maintain $V_T$ of 6 to 8 mL/kg predicted body weight and inspiratory plateau pressure ≤30 cm $H_2O$ to reduce ventilator-associated lung injury.[107] Because low $V_T$ ventilation (6 mL/kg) is associated with an increased incidence of atelectasis, PEEP and other lung "recruitment maneuver" procedures may be warranted.[108] However, one study reported no difference in the rate of discharge or survival between ARDS patients receiving high- or low-PEEP regimens.[109] Furthermore, a recent historical comparison of ventilation practice after cardiac arrest reported no differences in pneumonia, oxygenation, lung compliance, and ventilator days when a low $V_T$ strategy versus a more liberal "old practice" $V_T$ was applied.[110]

In conclusion, post–cardiac arrest patients are at risk of acute lung injury and ARDS, but refractory hypoxemia is not a frequent mode of death after cardiac arrest. There is no reason to recommend hyperventilation and "permissive hypercapnia" (hypoventilation) for these patients, and normocapnia should be considered the standard. There is also no data to recommend unique ventilation strategies in this population different from usual care of other mechanically ventilated patients at risk for acute lung injury and ARDS.

Routine hyperventilation with hypocapnia should be avoided after ROSC because it may worsen global brain ischemia by excessive cerebral vasoconstriction (Class III, LOE C). Hyperventilation or excessive tidal volumes resulting in increased intrathoracic pressure may also contribute to hemodynamic instability in certain patients. Ventilation rate and volume may be titrated to maintain high-normal $PaCO_2$ (40 to 45 mm Hg) or $PETCO_2$ (35 to 40 mm Hg) while avoiding hemodynamic compromise (Class IIb, LOE C).

### Treatment of Pulmonary Embolism After CPR

Fibrinolytic use may benefit patients with massive pulmonary emboli who have not had CPR,[111] and use of fibrinolytics to treat pulmonary embolism after CPR has been reported.[112] The use of fibrinolytics during CPR has been studied, and CPR itself does not appear to pose an unacceptable risk of bleeding.[113–121] Alternatively, surgical embolectomy has also been used successfully in some patients after PE-induced cardiac arrest.[117,122–125] Mechanical thrombectomy was employed in a small case series and only one of seven patients died and pulmonary perfusion was restored in the majority (85.7%).[115] In post–cardiac arrest patients with arrest due to presumed or known pulmonary embolism, fibrinolytics may be considered (Class IIb, LOE C).

## Sedation After Cardiac Arrest

Patients with coma or respiratory dysfunction after ROSC are routinely intubated and maintained on mechanical ventilation for a period of time, which results in discomfort, pain, and anxiety. Intermittent or continuous sedation and/or analgesia can be used to achieve specific goals. Patients with post–cardiac arrest cognitive dysfunction may display agitation or frank delirium with purposeless movement and are at risk of self-injury. Opioids, anxiolytics, and sedative-hypnotic agents can be used in various combinations to improve patient-ventilator interaction and blunt the stress-related surge of endogenous catecholamines. Other agents with sedative and antipsychotic-tranquilizer properties, such as $\alpha_2$-adrenergic agonists,[126] and butyrophenones[127] are also used based on individual clinical circumstances.

If patient agitation is life-threatening, neuromuscular blocking agents can be used for short intervals with adequate sedation. Caution should be used in patients at high risk of seizures unless continuous electroencephalographic (EEG) monitoring is available. In general sedative agents should be administered cautiously with daily interruptions and titrated to the desired effect. A number of sedation scales[128–133] and motor activity scales[134] were developed to titrate these pharmacological interventions to a clinical goal.

Shorter-acting medications that can be used as a single bolus or continuous infusion are usually preferred. There is little evidence to guide sedation/analgesia therapy immediately after ROSC. One observational study[135] found an association between use of sedation and development of pneumonia in intubated patients during the first 48 hours of therapy. However, the study was not designed to investigate sedation as a risk factor for either pneumonia or death in patients with cardiac arrest.

Although minimizing sedation allows a better clinical estimate of neurological status, sedation, analgesia, and occasionally neuromuscular relaxation are routinely used to facilitate induced hypothermia and to control shivering. The duration of neuromuscular blocker use should be minimized and the depth of neuromuscular blockade should be monitored with a nerve twitch stimulator.

It is reasonable to consider the titrated use of sedation and analgesia in critically ill patients who require mechanical ventilation or shivering suppression during induced hypothermia after cardiac arrest (Class IIb, LOE C). Duration of neuromuscular blocking agents should be kept to a minimum or avoided altogether.

## Cardiovascular System

ACS is a common cause of cardiac arrest.[14,16,34,35,134–147] The clinician should evaluate the patient's 12-lead ECG and cardiac markers after ROSC. A 12-lead ECG should be obtained as soon as possible after ROSC to determine whether acute ST elevation is present (Class I, LOE B). Because it is impossible to determine the final neurological status of comatose patients in the first hours after ROSC, aggressive treatment of ST-elevation myocardial infarction

(STEMI) should begin as in non–cardiac arrest patients, regardless of coma or induced hypothermia. Because of the high incidence of acute coronary ischemia, consideration of emergent coronary angiography may be reasonable even in the absence of STEMI.[14,16] Notably, PCI, alone or as part of a bundle of care, is associated with improved myocardial function[14] and neurological outcomes.[11,16] Therapeutic hypothermia can be safely combined with primary PCI after cardiac arrest caused by AMI.[11,31,33–35] Other details of ACS treatment are discussed in Part 10.

Patients with cardiac arrest may receive antiarrhythmic drugs such as lidocaine or amiodarone during initial resuscitation. There is no evidence to support or refute continued or prophylactic administration of these medications.[7,148–152]

## Vasoactive Drugs for Use in Post–Cardiac Arrest Patients

### Vasopressors

Vasoactive drugs may be administered after ROSC to support cardiac output, especially blood flow to the heart and brain. Drugs may be selected to improve heart rate (chronotropic effects), myocardial contractility (inotropic effects), or arterial pressure (vasoconstrictive effects), or to reduce afterload (vasodilator effects). Unfortunately many adrenergic drugs are not selective and may increase or decrease heart rate and afterload, increase cardiac arrhythmias, and increase myocardial ischemia by creating a mismatch between myocardial oxygen demand and delivery. Myocardial ischemia, in turn, may further decrease heart function. Some agents may also have metabolic effects that increase blood glucose, lactate, and metabolic rate. There is a paucity of data about which vasoactive drug to select first, although providers should become familiar with the differing adverse effects associated with these drugs, which might make a particular agent more or less appropriate for a specific patient.[153]

Specific drug infusion rates cannot be recommended because of variations in pharmacokinetics (relation between drug dose and concentration) and pharmacodynamics (relation between drug concentration and effect) in critically ill patients,[154,155] so commonly used initial dose ranges are listed in Table 2. Vasoactive drugs must be titrated at the bedside to secure the intended effect while limiting side effects. Providers must also be aware of the concentrations delivered and compatibilities with previously and concurrently administered drugs.

In general, adrenergic drugs should not be mixed with sodium bicarbonate or other alkaline solutions in the IV line because there is evidence that adrenergic agents are inactivated in alkaline solutions.[156,157] Norepinephrine (levarterenol) and other catecholamines that activate $\beta$-adrenergic receptors may produce tissue necrosis if extravasation occurs. Therefore, administration through a central line is preferred whenever possible. If extravasation develops, infiltrate 5 to 10 mg of phentolamine diluted in 10 to 15 mL of saline into the site of extravasation as soon as possible to prevent tissue death and sloughing.

**Table 2.    Common Vasoactive Drugs**

| Drug | Typical Starting Dose (Then Titrate to Effect) |
|---|---|
| Epinephrine | 0.1–0.5 mcg/kg/min (In 70-kg adult, 7–35 mcg/min) |
| | • Useful for symptomatic bradycardia if atropine and transcutaneous pacing fail or if pacing is not available |
| | • Used to treat severe hypotension (eg, systolic blood pressure <70 mm Hg) |
| | • Useful for anaphylaxis associated with hemodynamic instability or respiratory distress[158] |
| Norepinephrine | 0.1–0.5 mcg/kg/min (In 70-kg adult, 7–35 mcg/min) |
| | • Used to treat severe hypotension (eg, systolic blood pressure <70 mm Hg) and a low total peripheral resistance |
| | • Relatively contraindicated in patients with hypovolemia. It may increase myocardial oxygen requirements, mandating cautious use in patients with ischemic heart disease |
| | • Usually induces renal and mesenteric vasoconstriction; in sepsis, however, norepinephrine improves renal blood flow and urine output[159,160] |
| Phenylephrine | 0.5–2.0 mcg/kg/min (In 70-kg adult, 35–140 mcg/min) |
| | • Used to treat severe hypotension (eg, systolic blood pressure <70 mm Hg) and a low total peripheral resistance |
| Dopamine | 5–10 mcg/kg/min |
| | • Used to treat hypotension, especially if it is associated with symptomatic bradycardia |
| | • Although low-dose dopamine infusion has frequently been recommended to maintain renal blood flow or improve renal function, more recent data have failed to show a beneficial effect from such therapy[161,162] |
| Dobutamine | 5–10 mcg/kg/min |
| | • The (+) isomer is a potent beta-adrenergic agonist, whereas the (–) isomer is a potent alpha-1-agonist[163] |
| | • The vasodilating beta$_2$-adrenergic effects of the (+) isomer counterbalance the vasoconstricting alpha-adrenergic effects, often leading to little change or a reduction in systemic vascular resistance |
| Milrinone | Load 50 mcg/kg over 10 minutes then infuse at 0.375 mcg/kg/min |
| | • Used to treat low cardiac output |
| | • May cause less tachycardia than dobutamine |

## Use of Vasoactive Drugs After Cardiac Arrest

Hemodynamic instability is common after cardiac arrest.[6] Death due to multiorgan failure is associated with a persistently low cardiac index during the first 24 hours after resuscitation.[6,164] Vasodilation may occur from loss of sympathetic tone and from metabolic acidosis. In addition, the ischemia/reperfusion of cardiac arrest and electric defibrillation both can cause transient myocardial stunning and dysfunction[165] that can last many hours but may improve with use of vasoactive drugs.[158] Echocardiographic evaluation within the first 24 hours after arrest is a useful way to assess myocardial function in order to guide ongoing management.[14,17]

There is no proven benefit or harm associated with administration of routine IV fluids or vasoactive drugs (pressor and inotropic agents) to patients experiencing myocardial dysfunction after ROSC. Although some studies found improved outcome associated with these therapies, the outcome could not be solely ascribed to these specific interventions because they were only one component of standardized treatment protocols (eg, PCI and therapeutic hypothermia).[6,11,12,166] Invasive monitoring may be necessary to measure hemodynamic parameters accurately and to determine the most appropriate combination of medications to optimize perfusion.

Fluid administration as well as vasoactive (eg, norepinephrine), inotropic (eg, dobutamine), and inodilator (eg, milrinone) agents should be titrated as needed to optimize blood pressure, cardiac output, and systemic perfusion (Class I , LOE B). Although human studies have not established ideal targets for blood pressure or blood oxygenation,[11,12] a mean arterial pressure ≥65 mm Hg and an ScvO$_2$ ≥70% are generally considered reasonable goals.

Although mechanical circulatory support improves hemodynamics in patients not experiencing cardiac arrest,[167–171] it has not been associated with improved clinical outcome and routine use of mechanical circulatory support after cardiac arrest is not recommended.

## Modifying Outcomes From Critical Illness

Cardiac arrest is thought to involve multiorgan ischemic injury and microcirculatory dysfunction.[68,69,172] Implementing a protocol for goal-directed therapy using fluid and vasoactive drug administration along with monitoring of central venous oxygen saturation may improve survival from sepsis,[173] suggesting that a similar approach may benefit post–cardiac arrest patients. By analogy, studies have explored several other interventions believed to be beneficial in sepsis or other critical illness.

### Glucose Control

The post–cardiac arrest patient is likely to develop metabolic abnormalities such as hyperglycemia that may be detrimental. Evidence from several retrospective studies[7,73,174–176] suggests an association of higher glucose levels with increased mortality or worse neurological outcomes. Variable ranges for optimum glucose values were suggested, and the studies do not provide evidence that an interventional strategy to manage glucose levels will alter outcomes. Only one study examined patients with induced hypothermia.[175]

The optimum blood glucose concentration and interventional strategy to manage blood glucose in the post–cardiac arrest period is unknown. A consistent finding in clinical trials of glucose control[177–185] is that intensive therapy leads to more frequent episodes of severe hypoglycemia (usually defined as blood glucose level ≤40 mg/dL [2.2 mmol/L]). Hypoglycemia may be associated with worse outcomes in critically ill patients.[186,187]

Strategies to target moderate glycemic control (144 to 180 mg/dL [8 to 10 mmol/L]) may be considered in adult patients with ROSC after cardiac arrest (Class IIb, LOE B). Attempts to control glucose concentration within a lower range (80 to 110 mg/dL [4.4 to 6.1 mmol/L]) should not be implemented after cardiac arrest due to the increased risk of hypoglycemia (Class III, LOE B).

## Steroids

Corticosteroids have an essential role in the physiological response to severe stress, including maintenance of vascular tone and capillary permeability. In the post–cardiac arrest phase, several authors report a relative adrenal insufficiency compared with the metabolic demands of the body.[188,189] Relative adrenal insufficiency in the post–cardiac arrest phase was associated with higher rates of mortality.[188–190]

At present there are no human randomized trials investigating corticosteroid use after ROSC. One investigation combined steroid therapy with use of vasopressin, which made interpretation of results specific to steroids impossible.[191] The post–cardiac arrest syndrome has similarities to septic shock, but the efficacy of corticosteroids remains controversial in patients with sepsis as well.[68,192–194] Whether the provision of corticosteroids in the post–cardiac arrest phase improves outcome remains unknown and the value of the routine use of corticosteroids for patients with ROSC following cardiac arrest is uncertain.

## Hemofiltration

Hemofiltration has been proposed as a method to modify the humoral response to the ischemic-reperfusion injury that occurs after cardiac arrest. In a single randomized controlled trial there was no difference in 6-month survival among the groups.[195] Future investigations are required to determine whether hemofiltration will improve outcome in post–cardiac arrest patients.

## Central Nervous System

Brain injury is a common cause of morbidity and mortality in post–cardiac arrest patients. Brain injury is the cause of death in 68% of patients after out-of-hospital cardiac arrest and in 23% after in-hospital cardiac arrest.[13] The pathophysiology of post–cardiac arrest brain injury involves a complex cascade of molecular events that are triggered by ischemia and reperfusion and then executed over hours to days after ROSC. Events and conditions in the post–cardiac arrest period have the potential to exacerbate or attenuate these injury pathways and impact ultimate outcomes. Clinical manifestations of post–cardiac arrest brain injury include coma, seizures, myoclonus, various degrees of neurocognitive dysfunction (ranging from memory deficits to persistent vegetative state), and brain death.[3]

### Seizure Management

Whether there is any disease-specific management of seizures after cardiac arrest remains unknown and the true incidence of post–cardiac arrest electrographic seizures may be higher as the clinical diagnosis of seizures may not be readily apparent. It is accepted in other settings that prolonged, untreated seizures are detrimental to the brain, and seizures are common after ROSC, occurring in 5% to 20% of comatose cardiac arrest survivors with or without therapeutic hypothermia.[11,196,197]

An EEG for the diagnosis of seizure should be performed with prompt interpretation as soon as possible and should be monitored frequently or continuously in comatose patients after ROSC (Class I , LOE C). More clinical data are needed to define the diagnosis and management of seizures after cardiac arrest. Neuroprotective agents with anticonvulsant properties such as thiopental[196] and single-dose diazepam or magnesium or both[198] given after ROSC have not improved neurological outcome in survivors. No studies have addressed whether anticonvulsant therapy improves outcome after cardiac arrest, and several studies demonstrated that post–cardiac arrest seizures were refractory to traditional anticonvulsant agents.[199–201] The same anticonvulsant regimens for the treatment of seizures used for status epilepticus caused by other etiologies may be considered after cardiac arrest. (Class IIb, LOE C).

## Neuroprotective Drugs

The molecular events that cause neurodegeneration after cardiac arrest occur over hours to days after ROSC. This time course suggests a potentially broad therapeutic window for neuroprotective drug therapy. However, the number of clinical trials performed to date is limited and has failed to demonstrate improved neurological outcome with potential neuroprotective drugs given after cardiac arrest.

Few neuroprotective drugs have been tested in clinical trials, and only one published randomized trial[202] was performed in which a neuroprotective drug was combined with therapeutic hypothermia. No neuroprotection benefit was observed when patients (without hypothermia) were treated with thiopental, glucocorticoids, nimodipine, lidoflazine, diazepam, and magnesium sulfate. One trial using coenzyme Q10 in patients receiving hypothermia failed to show improved survival with good neurological outcome.[202] The routine use of coenzyme Q10 in patients treated with hypothermia is uncertain (Class IIb, LOE B).

## Prognostication of Neurological Outcome in Comatose Cardiac Arrest Survivors

The goal of post–cardiac arrest management is to return patients to their prearrest functional level. However, many patients will die, remain permanently unresponsive, or remain permanently unable to perform independent activities. Early prognostication of neurological outcome is an essential component of post–cardiac arrest care. Most importantly, when decisions to limit or withdraw life-sustaining care are being considered, tools used to prognosticate poor outcome must be accurate and reliable with a false-positive rate (FPR) approaching 0%. Poor outcome is defined as death, persistent unresponsiveness, or the inability to undertake independent activities after 6 months.[203] No prearrest or intra-arrest parameters (including arrest duration, bystander CPR, or presenting rhythm) alone or in combination accurately predict outcome in individual patients who achieve ROSC.

A thorough neurological evaluation is needed to obtain accurate prognostic findings. No postarrest physical examination finding or diagnostic study has as yet predicted poor outcome of comatose cardiac arrest survivors during the first 24 hours after ROSC. After 24 hours somatosensory evoked potentials (SSEPs) and select physical examination findings at specific time points after ROSC in the absence of confounders (such as hypotension, seizures, sedatives, or neuromuscular blockers) are the most reliable early predictors of poor outcome in patients not undergoing therapeutic hypothermia. However, the decision to limit care should never be made on the basis of a single prognostic parameter, and expert consultation may be needed.

## Neurological Assessment

The neurological examination is the most widely studied parameter to predict outcome in comatose post–cardiac arrest patients. Prognostication of functional outcome has not been established in noncomatose patients. Neurological examination for this purpose can be reliably undertaken only in the absence of confounding factors (hypotension, seizures, sedatives, or neuromuscular blockers). On the basis of existing studies, no clinical neurological signs reliably predict poor outcome <24 hours after cardiac arrest.[204,205] Among adult patients who are comatose and have *not* been treated with hypothermia, the absence of both pupillary light and corneal reflexes at ≥72 hours after cardiac arrest predicted poor outcome with high reliability.[204] The absence of vestibulo-ocular reflexes at ≥24 hours (FPR 0%, 95% CI 0% to 14%)[205,206] or Glasgow Coma Scale (GCS) score <5 at ≥72 hours (FPR 0%, 95% CI 0% to 6%)[204,207,208] are less reliable for predicting poor outcome or were studied only in limited numbers of patients. Other clinical signs, including myoclonus,[209–213] are not recommended for predicting poor outcome (Class III, LOE C).

## EEG

No electrophysiological study reliably predicts outcome in comatose patients during the first 24 hours after ROSC. In *normothermic* patients without significant confounders (sedatives, hypotension, hypothermia, neuromuscular blockade, or hypoxemia), an EEG pattern showing generalized suppression to <20 $\mu$V, burst-suppression pattern associated with generalized epileptic activity, or diffuse periodic complexes on a flat background is associated with a poor outcome (FPR 3%, 95% CI 0.9% to 11%).[203] One week after the initial arrest event, specific EEG findings may be useful for predicting poor outcomes in comatose cardiac arrest survivors.[161,203,204,206,214–221] The prognostic accuracy of malignant EEG patterns appears to be less reliable in patients treated with hypothermia. Status epilepticus in post-ROSC patients treated with hypothermia has an FPR of 7% (95% CI 1% to 25%) to 11.5% (95% CI 3% to 31%) for predicting poor outcome.[218,222]

In the absence of confounding factors such as sedatives, hypotension, hypothermia, neuromuscular blockade, seizures, or hypoxemia, it may be helpful to use an unprocessed EEG interpretation observed ≥24 hours after ROSC to assist with the prediction of a poor outcome in comatose survivors of cardiac arrest not treated with hypothermia (Class IIb, LOE B).

## Evoked Potentials

Abnormalities in evoked potentials are associated with poor outcomes. Bilateral absence of the N20 cortical response to median nerve SSEPs predicts poor outcome (FPR 0%, 95% CI 0% to 3%).[161,203] Although other evoked potential measurements

(for example, Brain stem Auditory Evoked Potentials) have been associated with poor outcomes in comatose cardiac arrest survivors, they are either less reliable predictors of poor outcome than SSEPs or have not been studied in enough patients to establish their reliability. Bilateral absence of the N20 cortical response to median nerve stimulation after 24 hours predicts poor outcome in comatose cardiac arrest survivors not treated with therapeutic hypothermia (Class IIa, LOE A).

The impact of therapeutic hypothermia on the prognostic accuracy of SSEPs has not been adequately studied.

## Neuroimaging

The most studied neuroimaging modalities are magnetic resonance imaging (MRI) and computed tomography (CT) of the brain. Extensive cortical and subcortical lesions on MRI are associated with poor neurological outcome.[223–253] These studies varied widely in the MRI parameters used, sample size, and interval after arrest when testing occurred.

CT imaging to detect brain injury and predict functional outcome is supported by several studies.[233,244,245,247,248,254–267] The timing of CT in these studies varied widely. CT parameters associated with poor outcome were varied and included quantitative measure of gray matter:white matter Hounsfield unit ratio and qualitative description of brain structures. A nonenhanced CT scan can also provide information about structural lesions, stroke, or intracranial hemorrhage that may have contributed to cardiac arrest.[268,269]

Other less utilized and investigated neuroimaging modalities have included single-photon emission computed tomography,[253,267,270] cerebral angiography[244] and transcranial Doppler[240] A nuclear imaging study observed that abnormal tracer uptake in the cerebral cortices was associated with poor outcome in one case report.[248]

Despite tremendous potential, neuroimaging has yet to be proved as an independently accurate modality for prediction of outcome in individual comatose survivors of cardiac arrest and specific neuroimaging modalities cannot be recommended for predicting poor outcome after cardiac arrest.

## Blood and Cerebrospinal Fluid Biomarkers

There has been extensive clinical research exploring biomarkers in the blood (plasma or serum) and cerebrospinal fluid (CSF) as early predictors of poor outcome in comatose cardiac arrest survivors. Biomarkers that are predictive of neurological outcome are typically released from dying neurons or glial cells in the brain (eg, neuron-specific enolase [NSE], S100B, GFAP, CK-BB) and can be measured in the blood or CSF. The primary advantage of biomarkers is that levels are unlikely to be confounded by sedation or neuromuscular blockade, which are commonly used in the first few days after cardiac arrest. However, for most biomarkers, only an association with outcome has been reported. When using a cutoff value that results in an FPR of 0% for predicting poor outcome, the 95% CI is unacceptably high due to the small number of patients studied.

The most promising and extensively studied biomarker is serum NSE, which has been reported to have a 0% FPR (95% CI 0% to 3%) for predicting poor outcome when measured between 24 and 72 hours after cardiac arrest.[203,204] Other guidelines have recommended the use of serum NSE to predict poor outcome in patients after ROSC.[203] However, the primary limitation of serum NSE is the variability among studies in both the assays used and the cutoff value that results in an FPR of 0% for predicting poor outcome.[271–282] Furthermore, interventions such as therapeutic hypothermia appear to variably alter the NSE cutoff value that is predictive of poor outcome.[283–285] Finally a number of clinical disorders, such as abdominal organ injury, have been associated with elevated NSE levels independent of cardiac arrest.[286]

The routine use of any serum or CSF biomarker as a sole predictor of poor outcome in comatose patients after cardiac arrest is not recommended (Class III, LOE B).

## Changes in Prognostication With Hypothermia

There is a paucity of data about the utility of physical examination, EEG, and evoked potentials in patients who have been treated with induced hypothermia. Physical examination (motor response, pupillary light and corneal reflexes), EEG, SSEP, and imaging studies are less reliable for predicting poor outcome in patients treated with hypothermia. Durations of observation greater than 72 hours after ROSC should be considered before predicting poor outcome in patients treated with hypothermia (Class I, Level C).

## Organ Donation After Cardiac Arrest

Despite maximal support and adequate observation, some patients will be brain-dead after cardiac arrest. Studies sug-gest that there is no difference in functional outcomes of organs transplanted from patients who are brain-dead as a consequence of cardiac arrest when compared with donors who are brain-dead due to other causes.[287–290] Adult patients who progress to brain death after resuscitation from cardiac arrest should be considered for organ donation (Class I, LOE B).

## Summary

The goal of immediate post–cardiac arrest care is to optimize systemic perfusion, restore metabolic homeostasis, and support organ system function to increase the likelihood of intact neurological survival. The post–cardiac arrest period is often marked by hemodynamic instability as well as metabolic abnormalities. Support and treatment of acute myocardial dysfunction and acute myocardial ischemia can increase the probability of survival. Interventions to reduce secondary brain injury, such as therapeutic hypothermia, can improve survival and neurological recovery. Every organ system is at risk during this period, and patients are at risk of developing multiorgan dysfunction.

The comprehensive treatment of diverse problems after cardiac arrest involves multidisciplinary aspects of critical care, cardiology, and neurology. For this reason, it is important to admit patients to appropriate critical-care units with a prospective plan of care to anticipate, monitor, and treat each of these diverse problems. It is also important to appreciate the relative strengths and weaknesses of different tools for estimating the prognosis of patients after cardiac arrest.

## Disclosures

### Guidelines Part 9: Post–Cardiac Arrest Care: Writing Group Disclosures

| Writing Group Member | Employment | Research Grant | Other Research Support | Speakers' Bureau/Honoraria | Ownership Interest | Consultant/Advisory Board | Other |
|---|---|---|---|---|---|---|---|
| Mary Ann Peberdy | Virginia Commonwealth University–Professor of Medicine & Emergency Medicine | None | None | None | None | None | None |
| Clifton W. Callaway | University of Pittsburgh School of Medicine–Associate Professor; UPMC Health System–Physician | †Grants to University of Pittsburgh: NHLBI-Resuscitation Outcomes Consortium HRSA-Development and Dissemination of Program Tools for Uncontrolled Donation After Cardiac Death (UDCD) | *Loan of an Arctic Sun cooling device (without disposables) to human physiology laboratory for experiments on hypothermia by Medivance, Inc. | None | †Co-inventor on patent about ventricular fibrillation waveform analysis, licensed by University of Pittsburgh to Medtronic ERS, Inc. | None | None |
| Robert W. Neumar | University of Pennsylvania–Associate Professor of Emergency Medicine | †Funding Source: NIH/NINDS Grant Number: R21 NS054654 Funding Period 06/01/07 to 06/31/2010 Role on Project: Principal Investigator Title: Optimizing Therapeutic Hypothermia After Cardiac Arrest Description: The goal of this project is to evaluate how the onset and duration of therapeutic hypothermia after cardiac arrest impacts survival and neuroprotection | None | None | None | None | None |
| Romergryko G. Geocadin | Johns Hopkins University School of Medicine–Associate Professor of Neurology, Anesthesiology-Critical Care Medicine and Neurosurgery | †NIH RO1 Grant: "Consequence of Cardiac Arrest: Brain Injury" *NIH R44 Grant: "Cortical Injury Monitor Phase IIB" | None | *Academic Grand Rounds American Academy of Neurology | None | None | *Guest Editor: Neurology Clinics, Emergency Medicine Clinics, and Seminars in Neurology |
| Janice L. Zimmerman | The Methodist Hospital Physician Organization–Head, Critical Care Division and Director, MICU | None | None | *Society of Critical Care Medicine American College of Chest Physicians Center for Biomedical Communications | None | None | *Callaway and Associates Andrews and Kurth |
| Michael Donnino | Harvard Medical Faculty Physicians–Physician | †Corticosteroids in Post-cardiac Arrest Patients [Scientist Development Grant, American Heart Association] Thiamine as a Metabolic Resuscitator in Septic Shock [Pending] *Thiamine Deficiency in Septic Shock [completed, NIH through Harvard Medical School] Statin Therapy in Sepsis [Eleanor Shores Grant-nonindustry] | None | None | None | None | None |

(Continued)

**Guidelines Part 9: Post–Cardiac Arrest Care: Writing Group Disclosures, *Continued***

| Writing Group Member | Employment | Research Grant | Other Research Support | Speakers' Bureau/Honoraria | Ownership Interest | Consultant/Advisory Board | Other |
|---|---|---|---|---|---|---|---|
| Andrea Gabrielli | University of Florida–Professor of Anesthesiology and Surgery | †NIH-Biomarkers and Traumatic Brain Injury | None | None | None | None | None |
| Scott M. Silvers | Mayo Clinic Florida–Chair, Department of Emergency Medicine | None | None | None | None | None | None |
| Arno L. Zaritsky | Children's Hospital of the King's Daughters–Sr. VP for Clinical Services | None | None | None | None | *Data Safety Monitoring Board for NIH-sponsored clinical trial of therapeutic hypothermia after pediatric cardiac arrest | None |
| Raina Merchant | University of Pennsylvania–Research fellow | None | None | None | None | None | None |
| Terry L. Vanden Hoek | University of Chicago–Associate Professor | *Principal Investigator 09/06/04–04/30/10 DOD/Office of Naval Research $885,639 Proteomic Development of Molecular Vital Signs: Mapping a Mitochondrial Injury Severity Score to Triage and Guide Resuscitation of Hemorrhagic Shock. This research grant is awarded to the University of Chicago | None | None | *Hypothermia Induction Patents (3 approved, 3 pending) no income | None | None |
| Steven L. Kronick | University of Michigan Health System Healthcare institution Assistant Professor | None | None | None | None | None | *Expert Witness: Reviewed a single case for an attorney. Less than 4 hours work total |

This table represents the relationships of writing group members that may be perceived as actual or reasonably perceived conflicts of interest as reported on the Disclosure Questionnaire, which all members of the writing group are required to complete and submit. A relationship is considered to be "significant" if (a) the person receives $10 000 or more during any 12-month period, or 5% or more of the person's gross income; or (b) the person owns 5% or more of the voting stock or share of the entity, or owns $10 000 or more of the fair market value of the entity. A relationship is considered to be "modest" if it is less than "significant" under the preceding definition.

*Modest.
†Significant.

# References

1. HACA. Hypothermia After Cardiac Arrest Study Group. Mild therapeutic hypothermia to improve the neurologic outcome after cardiac arrest. *N Engl J Med.* 2002;346:549–556.

2. Bernard SA, Gray TW, Buist MD, Jones BM, Silvester W, Gutteridge G, Smith K. Treatment of comatose survivors of out-of-hospital cardiac arrest with induced hypothermia. *N Engl J Med.* 2002;346:557–563.

3. Neumar RW, Nolan JP, Adrie C, Aibiki M, Berg RA, Bottiger BW, Callaway C, Clark RS, Geocadin RG, Jauch EC, Kern KB, Laurent I, Longstreth WT, Jr., Merchant RM, Morley P, Morrison LJ, Nadkarni V, Peberdy MA, Rivers EP, Rodriguez-Nunez A, Sellke FW, Spaulding C, Sunde K, Vanden Hoek T. Post-cardiac arrest syndrome: epidemiology, pathophysiology, treatment, and prognostication. A consensus statement from the International Liaison Committee on Resuscitation (American Heart Association, Australian and New Zealand Council on Resuscitation, European Resuscitation Council, Heart and Stroke Foundation of Canada, InterAmerican Heart Foundation, Resuscitation Council of Asia, and the Resuscitation Council of Southern Africa); the American Heart Association Emergency Cardiovascular Care Committee; the Council on Cardiovascular Surgery and Anesthesia; the Council on Cardiopulmonary, Perioperative, and Critical Care; the Council on Clinical Cardiology; and the Stroke Council. *Circulation.* 2008;118:2452–2483.

4. Safar P. Resuscitation from clinical death: Pathophysiologic limits and therapeutic potentials. *Crit Care Med.* 1988;16:923–941.

5. Negovsky VA. The second step in resuscitation–the treatment of the 'post-resuscitation disease.' *Resuscitation.* 1972;1:1–7.

6. Laurent I, Monchi M, Chiche JD, Joly LM, Spaulding C, Bourgeois B, Cariou A, Rozenberg A, Carli P, Weber S, Dhainaut JF. Reversible myocardial dysfunction in survivors of out-of-hospital cardiac arrest. *J Am Coll Cardiol.* 2002;40:2110–2116.

7. Skrifvars MB, Pettila V, Rosenberg PH, Castren M. A multiple logistic regression analysis of in-hospital factors related to survival at six months in patients resuscitated from out-of-hospital ventricular fibrillation. *Resuscitation.* 2003;59:319–328.

8. Carr BG, Kahn JM, Merchant RM, Kramer AA, Neumar RW. Inter-hospital variability in post-cardiac arrest mortality. *Resuscitation.* 2009;80:30–34.

9. Callaway CW, Schmicker R, Kampmeyer M, Powell J, Rea TD, Daya MR, Aufderheide TP, Davis DP, Rittenberger JC, Idris AH, Nichol G Receiving hospital characteristics associated with survival after out-of-hospital cardiac arrest. *Resuscitation*; 2010;81:524–529.

10. Kirves H, Skrifvars MB, Vahakuopus M, Ekstrom K, Martikainen M, Castren M. Adherence to resuscitation guidelines during prehospital care of cardiac arrest patients. *Eur J Emerg Med.* 2007;14:75–81.

11. Sunde K, Pytte M, Jacobsen D, Mangschau A, Jensen LP, Smedsrud C, Draegni T, Steen PA. Implementation of a standardised treatment protocol for post resuscitation care after out-of-hospital cardiac arrest. *Resuscitation.* 2007;73:29–39.

12. Gaieski DF, Band RA, Abella BS, Neumar RW, Fuchs BD, Kolansky DM, Merchant RM, Carr BG, Becker LB, Maguire C, Klair A, Hylton J, Goyal M. Early goal-directed hemodynamic optimization combined with therapeutic hypothermia in comatose survivors of out-of-hospital cardiac arrest. *Resuscitation.* 2009;80:418–424.

13. Laver S, Farrow C, Turner D, Nolan J. Mode of death after admission to an intensive care unit following cardiac arrest. *Intensive Care Med.* 2004;30:2126–2128.

14. Spaulding CM, Joly LM, Rosenberg A, Monchi M, Weber SN, Dhainaut JF, Carli P. Immediate coronary angiography in survivors of out-of-hospital cardiac arrest. *N Engl J Med.* 1997;336:1629–1633.

15. Anyfantakis ZA, Baron G, Aubry P, Himbert D, Feldman LJ, Juliard JM, Ricard-Hibon A, Burnod A, Cokkinos DV, Steg PG. Acute coronary angiographic findings in survivors of out-of-hospital cardiac arrest. *Am Heart J.* 2009;157:312–318.

16. Reynolds JC, Callaway CW, El Khoudary SR, Moore CG, Alvarez RJ, Rittenberger JC. Coronary angiography predicts improved outcome following cardiac arrest: propensity-adjusted analysis. *J Intensive Care Med.* 2009;24:179–186.

17. Dumas F, Cariou A, Manzo-Silberman S, Grimaldi D, Vivien B, Rosencher J, Empana J-P, Carli P, Mira J-P, Jouven X, Spaulding C. Immediate percutaneous coronary intervention is associated with better survival after out-of-hospital cardiac arrest: insights from the PROCAT (Parisian Region Out of Hospital Cardiac Arrest) Registry. *Circ Cardiovasc Interv.* 2010;3:200–207.

18. Booth CM, Boone RH, Tomlinson G, Detsky AS. Is this patient dead, vegetative, or severely neurologically impaired? Assessing outcome for comatose survivors of cardiac arrest. *JAMA.* 2004;291:870–879.

19. Bunch TJ, White RD, Gersh BJ, Meverden RA, Hodge DO, Ballman KV, Hammill SC, Shen WK, Packer DL. Long-term outcomes of out-of-hospital cardiac arrest after successful early defibrillation. *N Engl J Med.* 2003;348:2626–2633.

20. Belliard G, Catez E, Charron C, Caille V, Aegerter P, Dubourg O, Jardin F, Vieillard-Baron A. Efficacy of therapeutic hypothermia after out-of-hospital cardiac arrest due to ventricular fibrillation. *Resuscitation.* 2007;75:252–259.

21. Castrejon S, Cortes M, Salto ML, Benittez LC, Rubio R, Juarez M, Lopez de Sa E, Bueno H, Sanchez PL, Fernandez Aviles F. Improved prognosis after using mild hypothermia to treat cardiorespiratory arrest due to a cardiac cause: comparison with a control group. *Rev Esp Cardiol.* 2009;62:733–741.

22. Bernard SA, Jones BM, Horne MK. Clinical trial of induced hypothermia in comatose survivors of out-of-hospital cardiac arrest. *Ann Emerg Med.* 1997;30:146–153.

23. Oddo M, Schaller MD, Feihl F, Ribordy V, Liaudet L. From evidence to clinical practice: effective implementation of therapeutic hypothermia to improve patient outcome after cardiac arrest. *Crit Care Med.* 2006;34: 1865–1873.

24. Busch M, Soreide E, Lossius HM, Lexow K, Dickstein K. Rapid implementation of therapeutic hypothermia in comatose out-of-hospital cardiac arrest survivors. *Acta Anaesthesiol Scand.* 2006;50:1277–1283.

25. Storm C, Steffen I, Schefold JC, Krueger A, Oppert M, Jorres A, Hasper D. Mild therapeutic hypothermia shortens intensive care unit stay of survivors after out-of-hospital cardiac arrest compared to historical controls. *Crit Care.* 2008;12:R78.

26. Don CW, Longstreth WT, Jr., Maynard C, Olsufka M, Nichol G, Ray T, Kupchik N, Deem S, Copass MK, Cobb LA, Kim F. Active surface cooling protocol to induce mild therapeutic hypothermia after out-of-hospital cardiac arrest: a retrospective before-and-after comparison in a single hospital. *Crit Care Med.* 2009;37:3062–3069.

27. Bro-Jeppesen J, Kjaergaard J, Horsted TI, Wanscher MC, Nielsen SL, Rasmussen LS, Hassager C. The impact of therapeutic hypothermia on neurological function and quality of life after cardiac arrest. *Resuscitation.* 2009;80:171–176.

28. Arrich J. Clinical application of mild therapeutic hypothermia after cardiac arrest. *Crit Care Med.* 2007;35:1041–1047.

29. Holzer M, Mullner M, Sterz F, Robak O, Kliegel A, Losert H, Sodeck G, Uray T, Zeiner A, Laggner AN. Efficacy and safety of endovascular cooling after cardiac arrest: cohort study and Bayesian approach. *Stroke.* 2006;37:1792–1797.

30. Skulec R, Kovarnik T, Dostalova G, Kolar J, Linhart A. Induction of mild hypothermia in cardiac arrest survivors presenting with cardiogenic shock syndrome. *Acta Anaesthesiol Scand.* 2008;52:188–194.

31. Hovdenes J, Laake JH, Aaberge L, Haugaa H, Bugge JF. Therapeutic hypothermia after out-of-hospital cardiac arrest: experiences with patients treated with percutaneous coronary intervention and cardiogenic shock. *Acta Anaesthesiol Scand.* 2007;51:137–142.

32. Batista LM, Lima FO, Januzzi JL, Jr., Donahue V, Snydeman C, Greer DM. Feasibility and safety of combined percutaneous coronary intervention and therapeutic hypothermia following cardiac arrest. *Resuscitation.* 2010;81: 398–403.

33. Wolfrum S, Pierau C, Radke PW, Schunkert H, Kurowski V. Mild therapeutic hypothermia in patients after out-of-hospital cardiac arrest due to acute ST-segment elevation myocardial infarction undergoing immediate percutaneous coronary intervention. *Crit Care Med.* 2008; 36:1780–1786.

34. Knafelj R, Radsel P, Ploj T, Noc M. Primary percutaneous coronary intervention and mild induced hypothermia in comatose survivors of ventricular fibrillation with ST-elevation acute myocardial infarction. *Resuscitation.* 2007;74:227–234.

35. Nielsen N, Hovdenes J, Nilsson F, Rubertsson S, Stammet P, Sunde K, Valsson F, Wanscher M, Friberg H. Outcome, timing and adverse events in therapeutic hypothermia after out-of-hospital cardiac arrest. *Acta Anaesthesiol Scand.* 2009;53:926–934.

36. Sunde K, Pytte M, Jacobsen D, Mangschau A, Jensen LP, Smedsrud C, Draegni T, Steen PA. Implementation of a standardised treatment protocol for post resuscitation care after out-of-hospital cardiac arrest. *Resuscitation.* 2007;73:29–39.

37. Voipio V, Kuisma M, Alaspaa A, Manttari M, Rosenberg P. Thrombolytic treatment of acute myocardial infarction after out-of-hospital cardiac arrest. *Resuscitation.* 2001;49:251–258.

38. Weston CF, Avery P. Thrombolysis following pre-hospital cardiopulmonary resuscitation. *Int J Cardiol.* 1992;37:195–198.

39. Kuboyama K, Safar P, Radovsky A, Tisherman SA, Stezoski SW, Alexander H. Delay in cooling negates the beneficial effect of mild resuscitative cerebral hypothermia after cardiac arrest in dogs: a prospective, randomized study. *Crit Care Med.* 1993;21:1348–1358.

40. Abella BS, Zhao D, Alvarado J, Hamann K, Vanden Hoek TL, Becker LB. Intra-arrest cooling improves outcomes in a murine cardiac arrest model. *Circulation.* 2004;109:2786–2791.

41. Takata K, Takeda Y, Sato T, Nakatsuka H, Yokoyama M, Morita K. Effects of hypothermia for a short period on histologic outcome and extracellular glutamate concentration during and after cardiac arrest in rats. *Crit Care Med.* 2005;33:1340–1345.

42. Hicks SD, DeFranco DB, Callaway CW. Hypothermia during reperfusion after asphyxial cardiac arrest improves functional recovery and selectively alters stress-induced protein expression. *J Cereb Blood Flow Metab.* 2000;20:520–530.

43. Colbourne F, Li H, Buchan AM. Indefatigable CA1 sector neuroprotection with mild hypothermia induced 6 hours after severe forebrain ischemia in rats. *J Cereb Blood Flow Metab.* 1999;19:742–749.

44. Wolff B, Machill K, Schumacher D, Schulzki I, Werner D. Early achievement of mild therapeutic hypothermia and the neurologic outcome after cardiac arrest. *Int J Cardiol.* 2009;133:223–228.

45. Gluckman PD, Wyatt JS, Azzopardi D, Ballard R, Edwards AD, Ferriero DM, Polin RA, Robertson CM, Thoresen M, Whitelaw A, Gunn AJ. Selective head cooling with mild systemic hypothermia after neonatal encephalopathy: multicentre randomised trial. *Lancet.* 2005;365(9460): 663–670.

46. Shankaran S, Laptook AR, Ehrenkranz RA, Tyson JE, McDonald SA, Donovan EF, Fanaroff AA, Poole WK, Wright LL, Higgins RD, Finer NN, Carlo WA, Duara S, Oh W, Cotten CM, Stevenson DK, Stoll BJ, Lemons JA, Guillet R, Jobe AH. Whole-body hypothermia for neonates with hypoxic-ischemic encephalopathy. *N Engl J Med.* 2005;353: 1574–1584.

47. Heard KJ, Peberdy MA, Sayre MR, Sanders A, Geocadin RG, Dixon SR, Larabee TM, Hiller K, Fiorello A, Paradis NA, O'Neil BJ. A randomized controlled trial comparing the Arctic Sun to standard cooling for induction of hypothermia after cardiac arrest. *Resuscitation.* 81:9–14.

48. Flint AC, Hemphill JC, Bonovich DC. Therapeutic hypothermia after cardiac arrest: performance characteristics and safety of surface cooling with or without endovascular cooling. *Neurocrit Care.* 2007;7:109–118.

49. Pichon N, Amiel JB, Francois B, Dugard A, Etchecopar C, Vignon P. Efficacy of and tolerance to mild induced hypothermia after out-of-hospital cardiac arrest using an endovascular cooling system. *Crit Care.* 2007;11:R71.

50. Kliegel A, Losert H, Sterz F, Kliegel M, Holzer M, Uray T, Domanovits H. Cold simple intravenous infusions preceding special endovascular cooling for faster induction of mild hypothermia after cardiac arrest–a feasibility study. *Resuscitation.* 2005;64:347–351.

51. Kliegel A, Janata A, Wandaller C, Uray T, Spiel A, Losert H, Kliegel M, Holzer M, Haugk M, Sterz F, Laggner AN. Cold infusions alone are effective for induction of therapeutic hypothermia but do not keep patients cool after cardiac arrest. *Resuscitation.* 2007;73:46–53.

52. Kim F, Olsufka M, Carlbom D, Deem S, Longstreth WT, Jr., Hanrahan M, Maynard C, Copass MK, Cobb LA. Pilot study of rapid infusion of 2 L of 4 degrees C normal saline for induction of mild hypothermia in hospitalized, comatose survivors of out-of-hospital cardiac arrest. *Circulation.* 2005;112:715–719.

53. Kliegel A, Losert H, Sterz F, Kliegel M, Holzer M, Uray T, Domanovits H. Cold simple intravenous infusions preceding special endovascular cooling for faster induction of mild hypothermia after cardiac arrest–a feasibility study. *Resuscitation.* 2005;64:347–351.

54. Bernard S, Buist M, Monteiro O, Smith K. Induced hypothermia using large volume, ice-cold intravenous fluid in comatose survivors of out-of-hospital cardiac arrest: a preliminary report. *Resuscitation.* 2003; 56:9–13.

55. Virkkunen I, Yli-Hankala A, Silfvast T. Induction of therapeutic hypothermia after cardiac arrest in prehospital patients using ice-cold Ringer's solution: a pilot study. *Resuscitation.* 2004;62:299–302.

56. Jacobshagen C, Pax A, Unsold BW, Seidler T, Schmidt-Schweda S, Hasenfuss G, Maier LS. Effects of large volume, ice-cold intravenous fluid infusion on respiratory function in cardiac arrest survivors. *Resuscitation.* 2009;80:1223–1228.

57. Kilgannon JH, Roberts BW, Stauss M, Cimino MJ, Ferchau L, Chansky ME, Dellinger RP, Parrillo JE, Trzeciak S. Use of a standardized order set for achieving target temperature in the implementation of therapeutic hypothermia after cardiac arrest: a feasibility study. *Acad Emerg Med.* 2008;15:499–505.

58. Spiel AO, Kliegel A, Janata A, Uray T, Mayr FB, Laggner AN, Jilma B, Sterz F. Hemostasis in cardiac arrest patients treated with mild hypothermia initiated by cold fluids. *Resuscitation.* 2009;80:762–765.

59. Larsson IM, Wallin E, Rubertsson S. Cold saline infusion and ice packs alone are effective in inducing and maintaining therapeutic hypothermia after cardiac arrest. *Resuscitation.* 2010;81:15–19.

60. Kim F, Olsufka M, Longstreth WT, Jr., Maynard C, Carlbom D, Deem S, Kudenchuk P, Copass MK, Cobb LA. Pilot randomized clinical trial of prehospital induction of mild hypothermia in out-of-hospital cardiac arrest patients with a rapid infusion of 4 degrees C normal saline. *Circulation.* 2007;115:3064–3070.

61. Kamarainen A, Virkkunen I, Tenhunen J, Yli-Hankala A, Silfvast T. Prehospital therapeutic hypothermia for comatose survivors of cardiac arrest: a randomized controlled trial. *Acta Anaesthesiol Scand.* 2009;53: 900–907.

62. Hammer L, Vitrat F, Savary D, Debaty G, Santre C, Durand M, Dessertaine G, Timsit JF. Immediate prehospital hypothermia protocol in comatose survivors of out-of-hospital cardiac arrest. *Am J Emerg Med.* 2009;27:570–573.

63. Kamarainen A, Virkkunen I, Tenhunen J, Yli-Hankala A, Silfvast T. Prehospital induction of therapeutic hypothermia during CPR: a pilot study. *Resuscitation.* 2008;76:360–363.

64. Kamarainen A, Virkkunen I, Tenhunen J, Yli-Hankala A, Silfvast T. Induction of therapeutic hypothermia during prehospital CPR using ice-cold intravenous fluid. *Resuscitation.* 2008;79:205–211.

65. Imamura M, Matsukawa T, Ozaki M, Sessler DI, Nishiyama T, Kumazawa T. The accuracy and precision of four infrared aural canal thermometers during cardiac surgery. *Acta Anaesthesiol Scand.* 1998; 42:1222–1226.

66. Pujol A, Fusciardi J, Ingrand P, Baudouin D, Le Guen AF, Menu P. Afterdrop after hypothermic cardiopulmonary bypass: the value of tympanic membrane temperature monitoring. *J Cardiothorac Vasc Anesth.* 1996;10:336–341.

67. Akata T, Setoguchi H, Shirozu K, Yoshino J. Reliability of temperatures measured at standard monitoring sites as an index of brain temperature during deep hypothermic cardiopulmonary bypass conducted for thoracic aortic reconstruction. *J Thorac Cardiovasc Surg.* 2007;133: 1559–1565.

68. Adrie C, Adib-Conquy M, Laurent I, Monchi M, Vinsonneau C, Fitting C, Fraisse F, Dinh-Xuan AT, Carli P, Spaulding C, Dhainaut JF, Cavaillon JM. Successful cardiopulmonary resuscitation after cardiac arrest as a "sepsis-like" syndrome. *Circulation.* 2002;106:562–568.

69. Adrie C, Laurent I, Monchi M, Cariou A, Dhainaou JF, Spaulding C. Postresuscitation disease after cardiac arrest: a sepsis-like syndrome? *Curr Opin Crit Care.* 2004;10:208–212.

70. Takino M, Okada Y. Hyperthermia following cardiopulmonary resuscitation. *Intensive Care Med.* 1991;17:419–420.

71. Zeiner A, Holzer M, Sterz F, Schorkhuber W, Eisenburger P, Havel C, Kliegel A, Laggner AN. Hyperthermia after cardiac arrest is associated with an unfavorable neurologic outcome. *Arch Intern Med.* 2001;161: 2007–2012.

72. Hickey RW, Kochanek PM, Ferimer H, Graham SH, Safar P. Hypothermia and hyperthermia in children after resuscitation from cardiac arrest. *Pediatrics.* 2000;106(pt 1):118–122.

73. Langhelle A, Tyvold SS, Lexow K, Hapnes SA, Sunde K, Steen PA. In-hospital factors associated with improved outcome after out-of-hospital cardiac arrest. A comparison between four regions in Norway. *Resuscitation.* 2003;56:247–263.

74. Takasu A, Saitoh D, Kaneko N, Sakamoto T, Okada Y. Hyperthermia: is it an ominous sign after cardiac arrest? *Resuscitation.* 2001;49: 273–277.

75. Wang Y, Lim LL, Levi C, Heller RF, Fisher J. Influence of admission body temperature on stroke mortality. *Stroke.* 2000;31:404–409.

76. Diringer MN. Treatment of fever in the neurologic intensive care unit with a catheter-based heat exchange system. *Crit Care Med.* 2004;32: 559–564.

77. Diringer MN, Reaven NL, Funk SE, Uman GC. Elevated body temperature independently contributes to increased length of stay in neurologic intensive care unit patients. *Crit Care Med.* 2004;32:1489–1495.

78. Reith J, Jorgensen HS, Pedersen PM, Nakayama H, Raaschou HO, Jeppesen LL, Olsen TS. Body temperature in acute stroke: relation to stroke severity, infarct size, mortality, and outcome. *Lancet.* 1996; 347(8999):422–425.

79. Hanchaiphiboolkul S. Body temperature and mortality in acute cerebral infarction. *J Med Assoc Thai.* 2005;88:26–31.

80. Kammersgaard LP, Jorgensen HS, Rungby JA, Reith J, Nakayama H, Weber UJ, Houth J, Olsen TS. Admission body temperature predicts long-term mortality after acute stroke: the Copenhagen Stroke Study. *Stroke.* 2002;33:1759–1762.

81. Bernard GR, Artigas A, Brigham KL, Carlet J, Falke K, Hudson L, Lamy M, Legall JR, Morris A, Spragg R. The Am-European Consensus Conference on ARDS. Definitions, mechanisms, relevant outcomes, and clinical trial coordination. *Am J Respir Crit Care Med.* 1994;149(3 Pt 1): 818–824.

82. Marsala J, Marsala M, Vanicky I, Galik J, Orendacova J. Post cardiac arrest hyperoxic resuscitation enhances neuronal vulnerability of the respiratory rhythm generator and some brainstem and spinal cord neuronal pools in the dog. *Neurosci Lett.* 1992;146:121–124.

83. Zwemer CF, Whitesall SE, D'Alecy LG. Cardiopulmonary-cerebral resuscitation with 100% oxygen exacerbates neurological dysfunction following nine minutes of normothermic cardiac arrest in dogs. *Resuscitation.* 1994;27:159–170.

84. Liu Y, Rosenthal RE, Haywood Y, Miljkovic-Lolic M, Vanderhoek JY, Fiskum G. Normoxic ventilation after cardiac arrest reduces oxidation of brain lipids and improves neurological outcome. *Stroke.* 1998;29: 1679–1686.

85. Vereczki V, Martin E, Rosenthal RE, Hof PR, Hoffman GE, Fiskum G. Normoxic resuscitation after cardiac arrest protects against hippocampal oxidative stress, metabolic dysfunction, and neuronal death. *J Cereb Blood Flow Metab.* 2006;26:821–835.

86. Richards EM, Fiskum G, Rosenthal RE, Hopkins I, McKenna MC. Hyperoxic reperfusion after global ischemia decreases hippocampal energy metabolism. *Stroke.* 2007;38:1578–1584.

87. Richards EM, Rosenthal RE, Kristian T, Fiskum G. Postischemic hyperoxia reduces hippocampal pyruvate dehydrogenase activity. *Free Radic Biol Med.* 2006;40:1960–1970.

88. Kuisma M, Boyd J, Voipio V, Alaspaa A, Roine RO, Rosenberg P. Comparison of 30 and the 100% inspired oxygen concentrations during early post-resuscitation period: a randomised controlled pilot study. *Resuscitation.* 2006;69:199–206.

89. Safar P, Xiao F, Radovsky A, Tanigawa K, Ebmeyer U, Bircher N, Alexander H, Stezoski SW. Improved cerebral resuscitation from cardiac arrest in dogs with mild hypothermia plus blood flow promotion. *Stroke.* 1996;27:105–113.

90. Kagstrom E, Smith ML, Siesjo BK. Cerebral circulatory responses to hypercapnia and hypoxia in the recovery period following complete and incomplete cerebral ischemia in the rat. *Acta Physiol Scand.* 1983;118: 281–291.

91. Krep H, Brinker G, Pillekamp F, Hossmann KA. Treatment with an endothelin type A receptor-antagonist after cardiac arrest and resuscitation improves cerebral hemodynamic and functional recovery in rats. *Crit Care Med.* 2000;28:2866–2872.

92. Krep H, Brinker G, Schwindt W, Hossmann KA. Endothelin type A-antagonist improves long-term neurological recovery after cardiac arrest in rats. *Crit Care Med.* 2000;28:2873–2880.

93. Nemoto EM, Snyder JV, Carroll RG, Morita H. Global ischemia in dogs: cerebrovascular CO2 reactivity and autoregulation. *Stroke.* 1975; 6:425–431.

94. Vanicky I, Marsala M, Murar J, Marsala J. Prolonged postischemic hyperventilation reduces acute neuronal damage after 15 min of cardiac arrest in the dog. *Neurosci Lett.* 1992;135:167–170.

95. Wolfson SK, Jr., Safar P, Reich H, Clark JM, Gur D, Stezoski W, Cook EE, Krupper MA. Dynamic heterogeneity of cerebral hypoperfusion after prolonged cardiac arrest in dogs measured by the stable xenon/CT technique: a preliminary study. *Resuscitation.* 1992;23:1–20.

96. Fischer M, Hossmann KA. No-reflow after cardiac arrest. *Intensive Care Med.* 1995;21:132–141.

97. Ausina A, Baguena M, Nadal M, Manrique S, Ferrer A, Sahuquillo J, Garnacho A. Cerebral hemodynamic changes during sustained hypocapnia in severe head injury: can hyperventilation cause cerebral ischemia? *Acta Neurochir Suppl.* 1998;71:1–4.

98. Yundt KD, Diringer MN. The use of hyperventilation and its impact on cerebral ischemia in the treatment of traumatic brain injury. *Crit Care Clin.* 1997;13:163–184.

99. Buunk G, van der Hoeven JG, Meinders AE. Cerebrovascular reactivity in comatose patients resuscitated from a cardiac arrest. *Stroke.* 1997;28: 1569–1573.

100. Yannopoulos D, Aufderheide TP, Gabrielli A, Beiser DG, McKnite SH, Pirrallo RG, Wigginton J, Becker L, Vanden Hoek T, Tang W, Nadkarni VM, Klein JP, Idris AH, Lurie KG. Clinical and hemodynamic comparison of 15:2 and 30:2 compression-to-ventilation ratios for cardiopulmonary resuscitation. *Crit Care Med.* 2006;34:1444–1449.

101. Yannopoulos D, Tang W, Roussos C, Aufderheide TP, Idris AH, Lurie KG. Reducing ventilation frequency during cardiopulmonary resuscitation in a porcine model of cardiac arrest. *Respir Care.* 2005;50: 628–635.

102. Herff H, Paal P, von Goedecke A, Lindner KH, Severing AC, Wenzel V. Influence of ventilation strategies on survival in severe controlled hemorrhagic shock. *Crit Care Med.* 2008;36:2613–2620.

103. Pepe PE, Raedler C, Lurie KG, Wigginton JG. Emergency ventilatory management in hemorrhagic states: elemental or detrimental? *J Trauma.* 2003;54:1048–1055.

104. Pepe PE, Marini JJ. Occult positive end-expiratory pressure in mechanically ventilated patients with airflow obstruction: the auto-PEEP effect. *Am Rev Respir Dis.* 1982;126:166–170.

105. Franklin C, Samuel J, Hu TC. Life-threatening hypotension associated with emergency intubation and the initiation of mechanical ventilation. *Am J Emerg Med.* 1994;12:425–428.

106. The Acute Respiratory Distress Syndrome Network. Ventilation with lower tidal volumes as compared with traditional tidal volumes for acute lung injury and the acute respiratory distress syndrome. *N Engl J Med.* 2000;342:1301–1308.

107. Tremblay LN, Slutsky AS. Ventilator-induced lung injury: from the bench to the bedside. *Intensive Care Med.* 2006;32:24–33.

108. Borges JB, Okamoto VN, Matos GF, Caramez MP, Arantes PR, Barros F, Souza CE, Victorino JA, Kacmarek RM, Barbas CS, Carvalho CR, Amato MB. Reversibility of lung collapse and hypoxemia in early acute respiratory distress syndrome. *Am J Respir Crit Care Med.* 2006;174: 268–278.

109. Brower RG, Lanken PN, MacIntyre N, Matthay MA, Morris A, Ancukiewicz M, Schoenfeld D, Thompson BT. Higher versus lower positive end-expiratory pressures in patients with the acute respiratory distress syndrome. *N Engl J Med.* 2004;351:327–336.

110. Wongsurakiat P, Pierson DJ, Rubenfeld GD. Changing pattern of ventilator settings in patients without acute lung injury: changes over 11 years in a single institution. *Chest.* 2004;126:1281–1291.

111. Wan S, Quinlan DJ, Agnelli G, Eikelboom JW. Thrombolysis compared with heparin for the initial treatment of pulmonary embolism: a meta-analysis of the randomized controlled trials. *Circulation.* 2004;110: 744–749.

112. Scholz KH, Hilmer T, Schuster S, Wojcik J, Kreuzer H, Tebbe U. Thrombolysis in resuscitated patients with pulmonary embolism. *Dtsch Med Wochenschr.* 1990;115:930–935.

113. Bottiger BW, Bode C, Kern S, Gries A, Gust R, Glatzer R, Bauer H, Motsch J, Martin E. Efficacy and safety of thrombolytic therapy after initially unsuccessful cardiopulmonary resuscitation: a prospective clinical trial. *Lancet.* 2001;357(9268):1583–1585.

114. Fatovich DM, Dobb GJ, Clugston RA. A pilot randomised trial of thrombolysis in cardiac arrest (The TICA trial). *Resuscitation.* 2004;61: 309–313.

115. Fava M, Loyola S, Bertoni H, Dougnac A. Massive pulmonary embolism: percutaneous mechanical thrombectomy during cardiopulmonary resuscitation. *J Vasc Interv Radiol.* 2005;16:119–123.

116. Janata K, Holzer M, Kurkciyan I, Losert H, Riedmuller E, Pikula B, Laggner AN, Laczika K. Major bleeding complications in cardiopulmonary resuscitation: the place of thrombolytic therapy in cardiac arrest due to massive pulmonary embolism. *Resuscitation.* 2003;57:49–55.

117. Konstantinov IE, Saxena P, Koniuszko MD, Alvarez J, Newman MA. Acute massive pulmonary embolism with cardiopulmonary resuscitation: management and results. *Tex Heart Inst J.* 2007;34:41–45; discussion 45–46.

118. Lederer W, Lichtenberger C, Pechlaner C, Kroesen G, Baubin M. Recombinant tissue plasminogen activator during cardiopulmonary resuscitation in 108 patients with out-of-hospital cardiac arrest. *Resuscitation.* 2001;50:71–76.

119. Lederer W, Lichtenberger C, Pechlaner C, Kinzl J, Kroesen G, Baubin M. Long-term survival and neurological outcome of patients who received recombinant tissue plasminogen activator during out-of-hospital cardiac arrest. *Resuscitation.* 2004;61:123–129.

120. Zahorec R. Rescue systemic thrombolysis during cardiopulmonary resuscitation. *Bratisl Lek Listy.* 2002;103(7–8):266–269.

121. Spohr F, Bottiger BW. Thrombolytic therapy during or after cardiopulmonary resuscitation: efficacy and safety of a new therapeutic approach. *Minerva Anestesiol.* 2003;69:357–364.

122. Schmid C, Zietlow S, Wagner TO, Laas J, Borst HG. Fulminant pulmonary embolism: symptoms, diagnostics, operative technique, and results. *Ann Thorac Surg.* 1991;52:1102–1105.

123. Dauphine C, Omari B. Pulmonary embolectomy for acute massive pulmonary embolism. *Ann Thorac Surg.* 2005;79:1240–1244.

124. Doerge HC, Schoendube FA, Loeser H, Walter M, Messmer BJ. Pulmonary embolectomy: review of a 15-year experience and role in the age of thrombolytic therapy. *Eur J Cardiothorac Surg.* 1996;10: 952–957.

125. Ullmann M, Hemmer W, Hannekum A. The urgent pulmonary embolectomy: mechanical resuscitation in the operating theatre determines the outcome. *Thorac Cardiovasc Surg.* 1999;47:5–8.

126. Hall JE, Uhrich TD, Barney JA, Arain SR, Ebert TJ. Sedative, amnestic, and analgesic properties of small-dose dexmedetomidine infusions. *Anesth Analg.* 2000;90:699–705.

127. Milbrandt EB, Kersten A, Kong L, Weissfeld LA, Clermont G, Fink MP, Angus DC. Haloperidol use is associated with lower hospital mortality in mechanically ventilated patients. *Crit Care Med.* 2005;33: 226–229, discussion 263–225.

128. De Jonghe B, Cook D, Griffith L, Appere-de-Vecchi C, Guyatt G, Theron V, Vagnerre A, Outin H. Adaptation to the Intensive Care Environment (ATICE): development and validation of a new sedation assessment instrument. *Crit Care Med.* 2003;31:2344–2354.

129. Weinert C, McFarland L. The state of intubated ICU patients: development of a two-dimensional sedation rating scale for critically ill adults. *Chest.* 2004;126:1883–1890.

130. Ramsay MA, Savege TM, Simpson BR, Goodwin R. Controlled sedation with alphaxalone-alphadolone. *Br Med J.* 1974;2(5920): 656–659.

131. Sessler CN, Gosnell MS, Grap MJ, Brophy GM, O'Neal PV, Keane KA, Tesoro EP, Elswick RK. The Richmond Agitation-Sedation Scale: validity and reliability in adult intensive care unit patients. *Am J Respir Crit Care Med.* 2002;166:1338–1344.

132. Riker RR, Fraser GL, Cox PM. Continuous infusion of haloperidol controls agitation in critically ill patients. *Crit Care Med.* 1994;22: 433–440.

133. de Lemos J, Tweeddale M, Chittock D. Measuring quality of sedation in adult mechanically ventilated critically ill patients: the Vancouver Interaction and Calmness Scale. Sedation Focus Group. *J Clin Epidemiol.* 2000;53:908–919.

134. Devlin JW, Boleski G, Mlynarek M, Nerenz DR, Peterson E, Jankowski M, Horst HM, Zarowitz BJ. Motor Activity Assessment Scale: a valid and reliable sedation scale for use with mechanically ventilated patients in an adult surgical intensive care unit. *Crit Care Med.* 1999;27: 1271–1275.

135. Rello J, Diaz E, Roque M, Valles J. Risk factors for developing pneumonia within 48 hours of intubation. *Am J Respir Crit Care Med.* 1999;159:1742–1746.

136. Bendz B, Eritsland J, Nakstad AR, Brekke M, Klow NE, Steen PA, Mangschau A. Long-term prognosis after out-of-hospital cardiac arrest and primary percutaneous coronary intervention. *Resuscitation.* 2004; 63:49–53.

137. Engdahl J, Abrahamsson P, Bang A, Lindqvist J, Karlsson T, Herlitz J. Is hospital care of major importance for outcome after out-of-hospital cardiac arrest? Experience acquired from patients with out-of-hospital cardiac arrest resuscitated by the same Emergency Medical Service and admitted to one of two hospitals over a 16-year period in the municipality of Goteborg. *Resuscitation.* 2000;43:201–211.

138. Gorjup V, Radsel P, Kocjancic ST, Erzen D, Noc M. Acute ST-elevation myocardial infarction after successful cardiopulmonary resuscitation. *Resuscitation.* 2007;72:379–385.

139. Garot P, Lefevre T, Eltchaninoff H, Morice MC, Tamion F, Abry B, Lesault PF, Le Tarnec JY, Pouges C, Margenet A, Monchi M, Laurent I, Dumas P, Garot J, Louvard Y. Six-month outcome of emergency percutaneous coronary intervention in resuscitated patients after cardiac arrest complicating ST-elevation myocardial infarction. *Circulation.* 2007;115:1354–1362.

140. Lettieri C, Savonitto S, De Servi S, Guagliumi G, Belli G, Repetto A, Piccaluga E, Politi A, Ettori F, Castiglioni B, Fabbiocchi F, De Cesare N, Sangiorgi G, Musumeci G, Onofri M, D'Urbano M, Pirelli S, Zanini R, Klugmann S. Emergency percutaneous coronary intervention in patients with ST-elevation myocardial infarction complicated by out-of-hospital cardiac arrest: early and medium-term outcome. *Am Heart J.* 2009;157:569–575.

141. Kahn JK, Glazier S, Swor R, Savas V, O'Neill WW. Primary coronary angioplasty for acute myocardial infarction complicated by out-of-hospital cardiac arrest. *Am J Cardiol.* 1995;75:1069–1070.

142. Marcusohn E, Roguin A, Sebbag A, Aronson D, Dragu R, Amikam S, Boulus M, Grenadier E, Kerner A, Nikolsky E, Markiewicz W, Hammerman H, Kapeliovich M. Primary percutaneous coronary intervention after out-of-hospital cardiac arrest: patients and outcomes. *Isr Med Assoc J*. 2007;9:257–259.

143. McCullough PA, Prakash R, Tobin KJ, O'Neill WW, Thompson RJ. Application of a cardiac arrest score in patients with sudden death and ST segment elevation for triage to angiography and intervention. *J Interv Cardiol*. 2002;15:257–261.

144. Nagao K, Hayashi N, Kanmatsuse K, Arima K, Ohtsuki J, Kikushima K, Watanabe I. Cardiopulmonary cerebral resuscitation using emergency cardiopulmonary bypass, coronary reperfusion therapy and mild hypothermia in patients with cardiac arrest outside the hospital. *J Am Coll Cardiol*. 2000;36:776–783.

145. Peels HO, Jessurun GA, van der Horst IC, Arnold AE, Piers LH, Zijlstra F. Outcome in transferred and nontransferred patients after primary percutaneous coronary intervention for ischaemic out-of-hospital cardiac arrest. *Catheter Cardiovasc Interv*. 2008;71:147–151.

146. Pleskot M, Babu A, Hazukova R, Stritecky J, Bis J, Matejka J, Cermakova E. Out-of-hospital cardiac arrests in patients with acute ST elevation myocardial infarctions in the East Bohemian region over the period 2002–2004. *Cardiology*. 2008;109:41–51.

147. Quintero-Moran B, Moreno R, Villarreal S, Perez-Vizcayno MJ, Hernandez R, Conde C, Vazquez P, Alfonso F, Banuelos C, Escaned J, Fernandez-Ortiz A, Azcona L, Macaya C. Percutaneous coronary intervention for cardiac arrest secondary to ST-elevation acute myocardial infarction. Influence of immediate paramedical/medical assistance on clinical outcome. *J Invasive Cardiol*. 2006;18:269–272.

148. Investigators A. A comparison of antiarrhythmic-drug therapy with implantable defibrillators in patients resuscitated from near-fatal ventricular arrhythmias. The Antiarrhythmics versus Implantable Defibrillators (AVID) Investigators. *N Engl J Med*. 1997;337:1576–1583.

149. Buxton AE, Lee KL, Fisher JD, Josephson ME, Prystowsky EN, Hafley G. A randomized study of the prevention of sudden death in patients with coronary artery disease. Multicenter Unsustained Tachycardia Trial Investigators. *N Engl J Med*. 1999;341:1882–1890.

150. Connolly SJ, Gent M, Roberts RS, Dorian P, Roy D, Sheldon RS, Mitchell LB, Green MS, Klein GJ, O'Brien B. Canadian implantable defibrillator study (CIDS): a randomized trial of the implantable cardioverter defibrillator against amiodarone. *Circulation*. 2000;101: 1297–1302.

151. Kuck KH, Cappato R, Siebels J, Ruppel R. Randomized comparison of antiarrhythmic drug therapy with implantable defibrillators in patients resuscitated from cardiac arrest: the Cardiac Arrest Study Hamburg (CASH). *Circulation*. 2000;102:748–754.

152. Wever EFD, Hauer RNW, Van Capelle FJL, Tijssen JGP, Crijns HJGM, Algra A, Wiesfeld ACP, Bakker PFA, Robles de Medina EO. Randomized study of implantable defibrillator as first-choice therapy versus conventional strategy in postinfarct sudden death survivors. *Circulation*. 1995;91:2195–2203.

153. De Backer D, Biston P, Devriendt J, Madl C, Chochrad D, Aldecoa C, Brasseur A, Defrance P, Gottignies P, Vincent JL. Comparison of dopamine and norepinephrine in the treatment of shock. *N Engl J Med*. 2010;362:779–789.

154. Kellum JA, Pinsky MR. Use of vasopressor agents in critically ill patients. *Curr Opin Crit Care*. 2002;8:236–241.

155. Zaritsky AL. Catecholamines, inotropic medications, and vasopressor agents. In: Chernow B, ed. *The Pharmacologic Approach to the Critically Ill Patient*. III ed. Baltimore, MD: Williams & Wilkins;1994: 387–404.

156. Grillo JA, Gonzalez ER, Ramaiya A, Karnes HT, Wells B. Chemical compatibility of inotropic and vasoactive agents delivered via a multiple line infusion system. *Crit Care Med*. 1995;23:1061–1066.

157. Bonhomme L, Benhamou D, Comoy E, Preaux N. Stability of epinephrine in alkalinized solutions. *Ann Emerg Med*. 1990;19:1242–1244.

158. Vasquez A, Kern KB, Hilwig RW, Heidenreich J, Berg RA, Ewy GA. Optimal dosing of dobutamine for treating post-resuscitation left ventricular dysfunction. *Resuscitation*. 2004;61:199–207.

159. Gisvold SE, Sterz F, Abramson NS, Bar-Joseph G, Ebmeyer U, Gervais H, Ginsberg M, Katz LM, Kochanek PM, Kuboyama K, Miller B, Obrist W, Roine RO, Safar P, Sim KM, Vandevelde K, White RJ, Xiao F. Cerebral resuscitation from cardiac arrest: treatment potentials. *Crit Care Med*. 1996;24(2 Suppl):S69–80.

160. del Zoppo GJ, Mabuchi T. Cerebral microvessel responses to focal ischemia. *J Cereb Blood Flow Metab*. 2003;23:879–894.

161. Zandbergen EG, de Haan RJ, Stoutenbeek CP, Koelman JH, Hijdra A. Systematic review of early prediction of poor outcome in anoxic-ischaemic coma. *Lancet*. 1998;352(9143):1808–1812.

162. Rothstein TL. Recovery from near death following cerebral anoxia: A case report demonstrating superiority of median somatosensory evoked potentials over EEG in predicting a favorable outcome after cardiopulmonary resuscitation. *Resuscitation*. 2004;60:335–341.

163. Kaplan PW, Genoud D, Ho TW, Jallon P. Etiology, neurologic correlations, and prognosis in alpha coma. *Clin Neurophysiol*. 1999;110: 205–213.

164. Mullner M, Domanovits H, Sterz F, Herkner H, Gamper G, Kurkciyan I, Laggner AN. Measurement of myocardial contractility following successful resuscitation: quantitated left ventricular systolic function utilising non-invasive wall stress analysis. *Resuscitation*. 1998;39: 51–59.

165. Weaver WD, Cobb LA, Copass MK, Hallstrom AP. Ventricular defibrillation: a comparative trial using 175-J and 320-J shocks. *N Engl J Med*. 1982;307:1101–1106.

166. Mayr V, Luckner G, Jochberger S, Wenzel V, Ulmer H, Pajk W, Knotzer H, Friesenecker B, Lindner K, Hasibeder W, Dunser M. Arginine vasopressin in advanced cardiovascular failure during the postresuscitation phase after cardiac arrest. *Resuscitation*. 2007;72:35–44.

167. Stevenson LW, Miller LW, Desvigne-Nickens P, Ascheim DD, Parides MK, Renlund DG, Oren RM, Krueger SK, Costanzo MR, Wann LS, Levitan RG, Mancini D. Left ventricular assist device as destination for patients undergoing intravenous inotropic therapy: a subset analysis from REMATCH (Randomized Evaluation of Mechanical Assistance in Treatment of Chronic Heart Failure). *Circulation*. 2004;110:975–981.

168. Thiele H, Sick P, Boudriot E, Diederich KW, Hambrecht R, Niebauer J, Schuler G. Randomized comparison of intra-aortic balloon support with a percutaneous left ventricular assist device in patients with revascularized acute myocardial infarction complicated by cardiogenic shock. *Eur Heart J*. 2005;26:1276–1283.

169. Burkhoff D, Cohen H, Brunckhorst C, O'Neill WW. A randomized multicenter clinical study to evaluate the safety and efficacy of the TandemHeart percutaneous ventricular assist device versus conventional therapy with intraaortic balloon pumping for treatment of cardiogenic shock. *Am Heart J*. 2006;152:469 e461–e468.

170. Greenberg SB, Deshur M, Khavkin Y, Karaikovic E, Vender J. Successful resuscitation of a patient who developed cardiac arrest from pulsed saline bacitracin lavage during thoracic laminectomy and fusion. *J Clin Anesth*. 2008;20:294–296.

171. Seyfarth M, Sibbing D, Bauer I, Frohlich G, Bott-Flugel L, Byrne R, Dirschinger J, Kastrati A, Schomig A. A randomized clinical trial to evaluate the safety and efficacy of a percutaneous left ventricular assist device versus intra-aortic balloon pumping for treatment of cardiogenic shock caused by myocardial infarction. *J Am Coll Cardiol*. 2008;52: 1584–1588.

172. Dellinger RP, Carlet JM, Masur H, Gerlach H, Calandra T, Cohen J, Gea-Banacloche J, Keh D, Marshall JC, Parker MM, Ramsay G, Zimmerman JL, Vincent JL, Levy MM. Surviving Sepsis Campaign guidelines for management of severe sepsis and septic shock. *Crit Care Med*. 2004;32:858–873.

173. Rivers E, Nguyen B, Havstad S, Ressler J, Muzzin A, Knoblich B, Peterson E, Tomlanovich M. Early goal-directed therapy in the treatment of severe sepsis and septic shock. *N Engl J Med*. 2001;345: 1368–1377.

174. Nolan JP, Laver SR, Welch CA, Harrison DA, Gupta V, Rowan K. Outcome following admission to UK intensive care units after cardiac arrest: a secondary analysis of the ICNARC Case Mix Programme Database. *Anaesthesia*. 2007;62:1207–1216.

175. Losert H, Sterz F, Roine RO, Holzer M, Martens P, Cerchiari E, Tiainen M, Mullner M, Laggner AN, Herkner H, Bischof MG. Strict normoglycaemic blood glucose levels in the therapeutic management of patients within 12h after cardiac arrest might not be necessary. *Resuscitation*. 2008;76:214–220.

176. Mullner M, Sterz F, Binder M, Schreiber W, Deimel A, Laggner AN. Blood glucose concentration after cardiopulmonary resuscitation influences functional neurological recovery in human cardiac arrest survivors. *J Cereb Blood Flow Metab*. 1997;17:430–436.

177. Oksanen T, Skrifvars MB, Varpula T, Kuitunen A, Pettila V, Nurmi J, Castren M. Strict versus moderate glucose control after resuscitation from ventricular fibrillation. *Intensive Care Med*. 2007;33:2093–2100.

178. van den Berghe G, Wouters P, Weekers F, Verwaest C, Bruyninckx F, Schetz M, Vlasselaers D, Ferdinande P, Lauwers P, Bouillon R.

Intensive insulin therapy in the critically ill patients. *N Engl J Med.* 2001;345:1359–1367.

179. Van den Berghe G, Wilmer A, Hermans G, Meersseman W, Wouters PJ, Milants I, Van Wijngaerden E, Bobbaers H, Bouillon R. Intensive insulin therapy in the medical ICU. *N Engl J Med.* 2006;354:449–461.

180. Arabi YM, Dabbagh OC, Tamim HM, Al-Shimemeri AA, Memish ZA, Haddad SH, Syed SJ, Giridhar HR, Rishu AH, Al-Daker MO, Kahoul SH, Britts RJ, Sakkijha MH. Intensive versus conventional insulin therapy: a randomized controlled trial in medical and surgical critically ill patients. *Crit Care Med.* 2008;36:3190–3197.

181. Brunkhorst FM, Engel C, Bloos F, Meier-Hellmann A, Ragaller M, Weiler N, Moerer O, Gruendling M, Oppert M, Grond S, Olthoff D, Jaschinski U, John S, Rossaint R, Welte T, Schaefer M, Kern P, Kuhnt E, Kiehntopf M, Hartog C, Natanson C, Loeffler M, Reinhart K. Intensive insulin therapy and pentastarch resuscitation in severe sepsis. *N Engl J Med.* 2008;358:125–139.

182. Finfer S, Chittock DR, Su SY, Blair D, Foster D, Dhingra V, Bellomo R, Cook D, Dodek P, Henderson WR, Hebert PC, Heritier S, Heyland DK, McArthur C, McDonald E, Mitchell I, Myburgh JA, Norton R, Potter J, Robinson BG, Ronco JJ. Intensive versus conventional glucose control in critically ill patients. *N Engl J Med.* 2009;360:1283–1297.

183. Preiser JC, Devos P, Ruiz-Santana S, Melot C, Annane D, Groeneveld J, Iapichino G, Leverve X, Nitenberg G, Singer P, Wernerman J, Joannidis M, Stecher A, Chiolero R. A prospective randomised multicentre controlled trial on tight glucose control by intensive insulin therapy in adult intensive care units: the Glucontrol study. *Intensive Care Med.* 2009;35:1738–1748.

184. Griesdale DE, de Souza RJ, van Dam RM, Heyland DK, Cook DJ, Malhotra A, Dhaliwal R, Henderson WR, Chittock DR, Finfer S, Talmor D. Intensive insulin therapy and mortality among critically ill patients: a meta-analysis including NICE-SUGAR study data. *CMAJ.* 2009;180: 821–827.

185. Wiener RS, Wiener DC, Larson RJ. Benefits and risks of tight glucose control in critically ill adults: a meta-analysis. *JAMA.* 2008;300: 933–944.

186. Krinsley JS, Grover A. Severe hypoglycemia in critically ill patients: risk factors and outcomes. *Crit Care Med.* 2007;35:2262–2267.

187. Arabi YM, Tamim HM, Rishu AH. Hypoglycemia with intensive insulin therapy in critically ill patients: predisposing factors and association with mortality. *Crit Care Med.* 2009;37:2536–2544.

188. Schultz CH, Rivers EP, Feldkamp CS, Goad EG, Smithline HA, Martin GB, Fath JJ, Wortsman J, Nowak RM. A characterization of hypothalamic-pituitary-adrenal axis function during and after human cardiac arrest. *Crit Care Med.* 1993;21:1339–1347.

189. Kim JJ, Lim YS, Shin JH, Yang HJ, Kim JK, Hyun SY, Rhoo I, Hwang SY, Lee G. Relative adrenal insufficiency after cardiac arrest: impact on postresuscitation disease outcome. *Am J Emerg Med.* 2006;24:684–688.

190. Pene F, Hyvernat H, Mallet V, Cariou A, Carli P, Spaulding C, Dugue MA, Mira JP. Prognostic value of relative adrenal insufficiency after out-of-hospital cardiac arrest. *Intensive Care Med.* 2005;31:627–633.

191. Mentzelopoulos SD, Zakynthinos SG, Tzoufi M, Katsios N, Papastylianou A, Gkisioti S, Stathopoulos A, Kollintza A, Stamataki E, Roussos C. Vasopressin, epinephrine, and corticosteroids for in-hospital cardiac arrest. *Arch Intern Med.* 2009;169:15–24.

192. Minneci PC, Deans KJ, Banks SM, Eichacker PQ, Natanson C. Corticosteroids for septic shock. *Ann Intern Med.* 2004;141:742–743.

193. Sprung CL, Annane D, Keh D, Moreno R, Singer M, Freivogel K, Weiss YG, Benbenishty J, Kalenka A, Forst H, Laterre PF, Reinhart K, Cuthbertson BH, Payen D, Briegel J. Hydrocortisone therapy for patients with septic shock. *N Engl J Med.* 2008;358:111–124.

194. Annane D, Sebille V, Charpentier C, Bollaert PE, Francois B, Korach JM, Capellier G, Cohen Y, Azoulay E, Troche G, Chaumet-Riffaud P, Bellissant E. Effect of treatment with low doses of hydrocortisone and fludrocortisone on mortality in patients with septic shock. *JAMA.* 2002; 288:862–871.

195. Laurent I, Adrie C, Vinsonneau C, Cariou A, Chiche JD, Ohanessian A, Spaulding C, Carli P, Dhainaut JF, Monchi M. High-volume hemofiltration after out-of-hospital cardiac arrest: a randomized study. *J Am Coll Cardiol.* 2005;46:432–437.

196. Brain Resuscitation Clinical Trial I Study Group. Randomized clinical study of thiopental loading in comatose survivors of cardiac arrest. *N Engl J Med.* 1986;314:397–403.

197. Holzer M, Sterz F, Behringer W, Oschatz E, Kofler J, Eisenburger P, Kittler H, Konschitzky R, Laggner AN. Endothelin-1 elevates regional cerebral perfusion during prolonged ventricular fibrillation cardiac arrest in pigs. *Resuscitation.* 2002;55:317–327.

198. Longstreth WT, Jr., Fahrenbruch CE, Olsufka M, Walsh TR, Copass MK, Cobb LA. Randomized clinical trial of magnesium, diazepam, or both after out-of-hospital cardiac arrest. *Neurology.* 2002;59:506–514.

199. Krumholz A, Stern BJ, Weiss HD. Outcome from coma after cardiopulmonary resuscitation: relation to seizures and myoclonus. *Neurology.* 1988;38:401–405.

200. Wijdicks EF, Parisi JE, Sharbrough FW. Prognostic value of myoclonus status in comatose survivors of cardiac arrest. *Ann Neurol.* 1994;35: 239–243.

201. Hui AC, Cheng C, Lam A, Mok V, Joynt GM. Prognosis following Postanoxic Myoclonus Status epilepticus. *Eur Neurol.* 2005;54:10–13.

202. Damian MS, Ellenberg D, Gildemeister R, Lauermann J, Simonis G, Sauter W, Georgi C. Coenzyme Q10 combined with mild hypothermia after cardiac arrest: a preliminary study. *Circulation.* 2004;110: 3011–3016.

203. Wijdicks EF, Hijdra A, Young GB, Bassetti CL, Wiebe S. Practice parameter: prediction of outcome in comatose survivors after cardiopulmonary resuscitation (an evidence-based review): report of the Quality Standards Subcommittee of the American Academy of Neurology. *Neurology.* 2006;67:203–210.

204. Zandbergen EG, Hijdra A, Koelman JH, Hart AA, Vos PE, Verbeek MM, de Haan RJ. Prediction of poor outcome within the first 3 days of postanoxic coma. *Neurology.* 2006;66:62–68.

205. Edgren E, Hedstrand U, Nordin M, Rydin E, Ronquist G. Prediction of outcome after cardiac arrest. *Crit Care Med.* 1987;15:820–825.

206. Young GB, Doig G, Ragazzoni A. Anoxic-ischemic encephalopathy: clinical and electrophysiological associations with outcome. *Neurocrit Care.* 2005;2:159–164.

207. Bassetti C, Bomio F, Mathis J, Hess CW. Early prognosis in coma after cardiac arrest: a prospective clinical, electrophysiological, and biochemical study of 60 patients. *J Neurol Neurosurg Psychiatry.* 1996;61: 610–615.

208. Edgren E, Hedstrand U, Kelsey S, Sutton-Tyrrell K, Safar P. Assessment of neurological prognosis in comatose survivors of cardiac arrest. BRCT I Study Group. *Lancet.* 1994;343(8905):1055–1059.

209. Arnoldus EP, Lammers GJ. Postanoxic coma: good recovery despite myoclonus status. *Ann Neurol.* 1995;38:697–698.

210. Celesia GG, Grigg MM, Ross E. Generalized status myoclonicus in acute anoxic and toxic-metabolic encephalopathies. *Arch Neurol.* 1988; 45:781–784.

211. Datta S, Hart GK, Opdam H, Gutteridge G, Archer J. Post-hypoxic myoclonic status: the prognosis is not always hopeless. *Crit Care Resusc.* 2009;11:39–41.

212. English WA, Giffin NJ, Nolan JP. Myoclonus after cardiac arrest: pitfalls in diagnosis and prognosis. *Anaesthesia.* 2009;64:908–911.

213. Morris HR, Howard RS, Brown P. Early myoclonic status and outcome after cardiorespiratory arrest. *J Neurol Neurosurg Psychiatry.* 1998;64: 267–268.

214. Rundgren M, Rosen I, Friberg H. Amplitude-integrated EEG (aEEG) predicts outcome after cardiac arrest and induced hypothermia. *Intensive Care Med.* 2006;32:836–842.

215. Shibata S, Imota T, Shigeomi S, Sato W, Enzan K. Use of the bispectral index during the early postresuscitative phase after out-of-hospital cardiac arrest. *J Anesth.* 2005;19:243–246.

216. Stammet P, Werer C, Mertens L, Lorang C, Hemmer M. Bispectral index (BIS) helps predicting bad neurological outcome in comatose survivors after cardiac arrest and induced therapeutic hypothermia. *Resuscitation.* 2009;80:437–442.

217. Ajisaka H. Early electroencephalographic findings in patients with anoxic encephalopathy after cardiopulmonary arrest and successful resuscitation. *J Clin Neurosci.* 2004;11:616–618.

218. Rossetti AO, Logroscino G, Liaudet L, Ruffieux C, Ribordy V, Schaller MD, Despland PA, Oddo M. Status epilepticus: an independent outcome predictor after cerebral anoxia. *Neurology.* 2007;69:255–260.

219. Berkhoff M, Donati F, Bassetti C. Postanoxic alpha (theta) coma: a reappraisal of its prognostic significance. *Clin Neurophysiol.* 2000;111: 297–304.

220. Thomke F, Brand A, Weilemann SL. The temporal dynamics of postanoxic burst-suppression EEG. *J Clin Neurophysiol.* 2002;19:24–31.

221. Fatovich DM, Jacobs IG, Celenza A, Paech MJ. An observational study of bispectral index monitoring for out of hospital cardiac arrest. *Resuscitation.* 2006;69:207–212.

222. Rossetti AO, Oddo M, Liaudet L, Kaplan PW. Predictors of awakening from postanoxic status epilepticus after therapeutic hypothermia. *Neurology.* 2009;72:744–749.

223. Allen JS, Tranel D, Bruss J, Damasio H. Correlations between regional brain volumes and memory performance in anoxia. *J Clin Exp Neuropsychol.* 2006;28:457–476.

224. De Volder AG, Michel C, Guerit JM, Bol A, Georges B, de Barsy T, Laterre C. Brain glucose metabolism in postanoxic syndrome due to cardiac arrest. *Acta Neurol Belg.* 1994;94:183–189.

225. Fujioka M, Nishio K, Miyamoto S, Hiramatsu KI, Sakaki T, Okuchi K, Taoka T, Fujioka S. Hippocampal damage in the human brain after cardiac arrest. *Cerebrovasc Dis.* 2000;10:2–7.

226. Tommasino C, Grana C, Lucignani G, Torri G, Fazio F. Regional cerebral metabolism of glucose in comatose and vegetative state patients. *J Neurosurg Anesthesiol.* 1995;7:109–116.

227. Lovblad K, Senn P, Walpoth BH, Walpoth BN, Mattle HP, Radanov BP, Ozdoba C, Schroth G. Increased brain tolerance for ischemia in accidental deep hypothermia and circulatory arrest. *Riv Neuroradiol* 1998;11(SUPPL 2):224–226.

228. Edgren E, Enblad P, Grenvik A, Lilja A, Valind S, Wiklund L, Hedstrand U, Stjernstrom H, Persson L, Ponten U, Langstrom B. Cerebral blood flow and metabolism after cardiopulmonary resuscitation. A pathophysiologic and prognostic positron emission tomography pilot study. *Resuscitation.* 2003;57:161–170.

229. Grubb NR, Fox KA, Smith K, Best J, Blane A, Ebmeier KP, Glabus MF, O'Carroll RE. Memory impairment in out-of-hospital cardiac arrest survivors is associated with global reduction in brain volume, not focal hippocampal injury. *Stroke.* 2000;31:1509–1514.

230. Gut E, Fritz R, Leyhe T, et al. MRT after cerebral hypoxia. Correlation of imaging findings with clinical outcome and functional rehabilitation. *Klin Neuroradiol.* 1999;9:147–152.

231. Els T, Kassubek J, Kubalek R, Klisch J. Diffusion-weighted MRI during early global cerebral hypoxia: a predictor for clinical outcome? *Acta Neurol Scand.* 2004;110:361–367.

232. Kano H, Houkin K, Harada K, Koyanagi I, Nara S, Itou Y, Imaizumi H, Asai Y, Saitou M. Neuronal cell injury in patients after cardiopulmonary resuscitation: evaluation by diffusion-weighted imaging and magnetic resonance spectroscopy. *Neurosurg Rev.* 2006;29:88–92.

233. Nogami K, Fujii M, Kato S, Nishizaki T, Suzuki M, Yamashita S, Oda Y, Sadamitsu D, Maekawa T. Analysis of magnetic resonance imaging (MRI) morphometry and cerebral blood flow in patients with hypoxic-ischemic encephalopathy. *J Clin Neurosci.* 2004;11:376–380.

234. Wijdicks EF, Campeau NG, Miller GM. MR imaging in comatose survivors of cardiac resuscitation. *AJNR Am J Neuroradiol.* 2001;22:1561–1565.

235. Wijman CA, Mlynash M, Caulfield AF, Hsia AW, Eyngorn I, Bammer R, Fischbein N, Albers GW, Moseley M. Prognostic value of brain diffusion-weighted imaging after cardiac arrest. *Ann Neurol.* 2009;65:394–402.

236. Wu O, Sorensen AG, Benner T, Singhal AB, Furie KL, Greer DM. Comatose patients with cardiac arrest: predicting clinical outcome with diffusion-weighted MR imaging. *Radiology.* 2009;252:173–181.

237. Arbelaez A, Castillo M, Mukherji SK. Diffusion-weighted MR imaging of global cerebral anoxia. *AJNR Am J Neuroradiol.* 1999;20:999–1007.

238. Barrett KM, Freeman WD, Weindling SM, Brott TG, Broderick DF, Heckman MG, Crook JE, Divertie GD, Meschia JF. Brain injury after cardiopulmonary arrest and its assessment with diffusion-weighted magnetic resonance imaging. *Mayo Clin Proc.* 2007;82:828–835.

239. Berek K, Lechleitner P, Luef G, Felber S, Saltuari L, Schinnerl A, Traweger C, Dienstl F, Aichner F. Early determination of neurological outcome after prehospital cardiopulmonary resuscitation. *Stroke.* 1995;26:543–549.

240. Iida K, Satoh H, Arita K, Nakahara T, Kurisu K, Ohtani M. Delayed hyperemia causing intracranial hypertension after cardiopulmonary resuscitation. *Crit Care Med.* 1997;25:971–976.

241. Ettl A, Felber S, Birbamer G, Daxer A. Corticol blindness following cerebral hypoxia. Proton nuclear magnetic resonance imaging and spectroscopy observations. *Neuroophthalmology.* 1994;14:259–263.

242. Greer DM. MRI in anoxic brain injury. *Neurocrit Care.* 2004;1:213–215.

243. Kuoppamaki M, Bhatia KP, Quinn N. Progressive delayed-onset dystonia after cerebral anoxic insult in adults. *Mov Disord.* 2002;17:1345–1349.

244. Arishima H, Ishii H, Kubota T, Maeda H, Shigemori K. [Angiographic features of anoxic encephalopathy in the acute phase: a case report]. *No To Shinkei.* 2003;55:977–982.

245. Verslegers W, Crols R, van den Kerchove M, de Potter W, Appel B, Lowenthal A. Parkinsonian syndrome after cardiac arrest: radiological and neurochemical changes. *Clin Neurol Neurosurg.* 1988;90:177–179.

246. Bolouri MR, Small GA. Neuroimaging of hypoxia and cocaine-induced hippocampal stroke. *J Neuroimaging.* 2004;14:290–291.

247. Fujioka M, Okuchi K, Sakaki T, Hiramatsu K, Miyamoto S, Iwasaki S. Specific changes in human brain following reperfusion after cardiac arrest. *Stroke.* 1994;25:2091–2095.

248. Hung GU, Lee JD, Lee JK. Bilateral cranial Tc-99m MDP uptake due to hypoxic-ischemic encephalopathy. *Clin Nucl Med.* 2007;32:328–329.

249. Johkura K, Naito M. Wernicke's encephalopathy-like lesions in global cerebral hypoxia. *J Clin Neurosci.* 2008;15:318–319.

250. Konaka K, Miyashita K, Naritomi H. Changes in diffusion-weighted magnetic resonance imaging findings in the acute and subacute phases of anoxic encephalopathy. *J Stroke Cerebrovasc Dis.* 2007;16:82–83.

251. Singhal AB, Topcuoglu MA, Koroshetz WJ. Diffusion MRI in three types of anoxic encephalopathy. *J Neurol Sci.* 2002;196(1–2):37–40.

252. Wartenberg KE, Patsalides A, Yepes MS. Is magnetic resonance spectroscopy superior to conventional diagnostic tools in hypoxic-ischemic encephalopathy? *J Neuroimaging.* 2004;14:180–186.

253. Zhang YX, Liu JR, Jiang B, Liu HQ, Ding MP, Song SJ, Zhang BR, Zhang H, Xu B, Chen HH, Wang ZJ, Huang JZ. Lance-Adams syndrome: a report of two cases. *J Zhejiang Univ Sci.* 2007;8:715–720.

254. Choi SP, Park HK, Park KN, Kim YM, Ahn KJ, Choi KH, Lee WJ, Jeong SK. The density ratio of grey to white matter on computed tomography as an early predictor of vegetative state or death after cardiac arrest. *Emerg Med J.* 2008;25:666–669.

255. De Reuck J, Decoo D, Vienne J, Strijckmans K, Lemahieu I. Significance of white matter lucencies in posthypoxic-ischemic encephalopathy: comparison of clinical status and of computed and positron emission tomographic findings. *Eur Neurol.* 1992;32:334–339.

256. Inoue Y, Shiozaki T, Irisawa T, Mohri T, Yoshiya K, Ikegawa H, Tasaki O, Tanaka H, Shimazu T, Sugimoto H. Acute cerebral blood flow variations after human cardiac arrest assessed by stable xenon enhanced computed tomography. *Curr Neurovasc Res.* 2007;4:49–54.

257. Nunes B, Pais J, Garcia R, Magalhaes Z, Granja C, Silva MC. Cardiac arrest: long-term cognitive and imaging analysis. *Resuscitation.* 2003;57:287–297.

258. Yanagawa Y, Un-no Y, Sakamoto T, Okada Y. Cerebral density on CT immediately after a successful resuscitation of cardiopulmonary arrest correlates with outcome. *Resuscitation.* 2005;64:97–101.

259. Della Corte F, Barelli A, Giordano A, Iacobucci T, Valente MR, Pennisi MA. CBF determination in post-ischemic-anoxic comatose patients. *Minerva Anestesiol.* 1993;59:637–641.

260. Kjos BO, Brant-Zawadzki M, Young RG. Early CT findings of global central nervous system hypoperfusion. *AJR.* 1983;141:1227–1232.

261. Morimoto Y, Kemmotsu O, Kitami K, Matsubara I, Tedo I. Acute brain swelling after out-of-hospital cardiac arrest: pathogenesis and outcome. *Crit Care Med.* 1993;21:104–110.

262. Torbey MT, Geocadin R, Bhardwaj A. Brain arrest neurological outcome scale (BrANOS): predicting mortality and severe disability following cardiac arrest. *Resuscitation.* 2004;63:55–63.

263. Torbey MT, Selim M, Knorr J, Bigelow C, Recht L. Quantitative analysis of the loss of distinction between gray and white matter in comatose patients after cardiac arrest. *Stroke.* 2000;31:2163–2167.

264. Imaizumi H, Tsuruoka K, Ujike Y, Kaneko M, Namiki A. [Hypoxic brain damage after prolonged cardiac arrest during anesthesia–changes in CT and serum NSE concentration]. *Masui.* 1994;43:1256–1260.

265. Kelsen J, Obel A. Images in clinical medicine. Fatal cerebral hypoxemia after cardiac arrest. *N Engl J Med.* 2003;348:817.

266. Schwab SA, Richter G, Bautz WA, Uder M, Alibek S. [Hypoxic injury of all deep nuclei of the brain–a case report from computed tomography]. *Rontgenpraxis.* 2008;56:245–248.

267. Tanaka H, Masugata H, Fukunaga R, Mandai K, Sueyoshi K, Abe H. Sequential change of heterogeneous cerebral blood blow patterns after diffuse brain ischemia. *Resuscitation.* 1992;24:273–281.

268. Inamasu J, Miyatake S, Tomioka H, Suzuki M, Nakatsukasa M, Maeda N, Ito T, Arai K, Komura M, Kase K, Kobayashi K. Subarachnoid haemorrhage as a cause of out-of-hospital cardiac arrest: a prospective computed tomography study. *Resuscitation.* 2009;80:977–980.

269. Naples R, Ellison E, Brady WJ. Cranial computed tomography in the resuscitated patient with cardiac arrest. *Am J Emerg Med.* 2009;27: 63–67.

270. Heckmann JG, Lang CJ, Pfau M, Neundorfer B. Electrocerebral silence with preserved but reduced cortical brain perfusion. *Eur J Emerg Med.* 2003;10:241–243.

271. Grubb NR, Simpson C, Sherwood RA, Abraha HD, Cobbe SM, O'Carroll RE, Deary I, Fox KA. Prediction of cognitive dysfunction after resuscitation from out-of-hospital cardiac arrest using serum neuron-specific enolase and protein S-100. *Heart.* 2007;93:1268–1273.

272. Reisinger J, Hollinger K, Lang W, Steiner C, Winter T, Zeindlhofer E, Mori M, Schiller A, Lindorfer A, Wiesinger K, Siostrzonek P. Prediction of neurological outcome after cardiopulmonary resuscitation by serial determination of serum neuron-specific enolase. *Eur Heart J.* 2007;28: 52–58.

273. Prohl J, Rother J, Kluge S, de Heer G, Liepert J, Bodenburg S, Pawlik K, Kreymann G. Prediction of short-term and long-term outcomes after cardiac arrest: a prospective multivariate approach combining biochemical, clinical, electrophysiological, and neuropsychological investigations. *Crit Care Med.* 2007;35:1230–1237.

274. Rech TH, Vieira SR, Nagel F, Brauner JS, Scalco R. Serum neuron-specific enolase as early predictor of outcome after in-hospital cardiac arrest: a cohort study. *Crit Care.* 2006;10:R133.

275. Pfeifer R, Borner A, Krack A, Sigusch HH, Surber R, Figulla HR. Outcome after cardiac arrest: predictive values and limitations of the neuroproteins neuron-specific enolase and protein S-100 and the Glasgow Coma Scale. *Resuscitation.* 2005;65:49–55.

276. Meynaar IA, Straaten HM, van der Wetering J, Verlooy P, Slaats EH, Bosman RJ, van der Spoel JI, Zandstra DF. Serum neuron-specific enolase predicts outcome in post-anoxic coma: a prospective cohort study. *Intensive Care Med.* 2003;29:189–195.

277. Zingler VC, Krumm B, Bertsch T, Fassbender K, Pohlmann-Eden B. Early prediction of neurological outcome after cardiopulmonary resuscitation: a multimodal approach combining neurobiochemical and electrophysiological investigations may provide high prognostic certainty in patients after cardiac arrest. *Eur Neurol.* 2003;49:79–84.

278. Rosen H, Sunnerhagen KS, Herlitz J, Blomstrand C, Rosengren L. Serum levels of the brain-derived proteins S-100 and NSE predict long-term outcome after cardiac arrest. *Resuscitation.* 2001;49:183–191.

279. Schoerkhuber W, Kittler H, Sterz F, Behringer W, Holzer M, Frossard M, Spitzauer S, Laggner AN. Time course of serum neuron-specific enolase. A predictor of neurological outcome in patients resuscitated from cardiac arrest. *Stroke.* 1999;30:1598–1603.

280. Fogel W, Krieger D, Veith M, Adams HP, Hund E, Storch-Hagenlocher B, Buggle F, Mathias D, Hacke W. Serum neuron-specific enolase as early predictor of outcome after cardiac arrest. *Crit Care Med.* 1997; 25:1133–1138.

281. Martens P, Raabe A, Johnsson P. Serum S-100 and neuron-specific enolase for prediction of regaining consciousness after global cerebral ischemia. *Stroke.* 1998;29:2363–2366.

282. Dauberschmidt R, Zinsmeyer J, Mrochen H, Meyer M. Changes of neuron-specific enolase concentration in plasma after cardiac arrest and resuscitation. *Mol Chem Neuropathol.* 1991;14:237–245.

283. Tiainen M, Roine RO, Pettila V, Takkunen O. Serum neuron-specific enolase and S-100B protein in cardiac arrest patients treated with hypothermia. *Stroke.* 2003;34:2881–2886.

284. Oksanen T, Tiainen M, Skrifvars MB, Varpula T, Kuitunen A, Castren M, Pettila V. Predictive power of serum NSE and OHCA score regarding 6-month neurologic outcome after out-of-hospital ventricular fibrillation and therapeutic hypothermia. *Resuscitation.* 2009;80: 165–170.

285. Rundgren M, Karlsson T, Nielsen N, Cronberg T, Johnsson P, Friberg H. Neuron specific enolase and S-100B as predictors of outcome after cardiac arrest and induced hypothermia. *Resuscitation.* 2009;80: 784–789.

286. Pelinka LE, Hertz H, Mauritz W, Harada N, Jafarmadar M, Albrecht M, Redl H, Bahrami S. Nonspecific increase of systemic neuron-specific enolase after trauma: clinical and experimental findings. *Shock (Augusta, Ga.)* 2005;24:119–123.

287. Adrie C, Haouache H, Saleh M, Memain N, Laurent I, Thuong M, Darques L, Guerrini P, Monchi M. An underrecognized source of organ donors: patients with brain death after successfully resuscitated cardiac arrest. *Intensive Care Med.* 2008;34:132–137.

288. Ali AA, Lim E, Thanikachalam M, Sudarshan C, White P, Parameshwar J, Dhital K, Large SR. Cardiac arrest in the organ donor does not negatively influence recipient survival after heart transplantation. *Eur J Cardiothorac Surg.* 2007;31:929–933.

289. Matsumoto CS, Kaufman SS, Girlanda R, Little CM, Rekhtman Y, Raofi V, Laurin JM, Shetty K, Fennelly EM, Johnson LB, Fishbein TM. Utilization of donors who have suffered cardiopulmonary arrest and resuscitation in intestinal transplantation. *Transplantation.* 2008;86: 941–946.

290. Mercatello A, Roy P, Ng-Sing K, Choux C, Baude C, Garnier JL, Colpart JJ, Finaz J, Petit P, Moskovtchenko JF, et al. Organ transplants from out-of-hospital cardiac arrest patients. *Transplant Proc.* 1988;20: 749–750.

---

KEY WORDS: cardiac arrest ■ drug ■ imaging ■ moderate hypothermia

# Part 10: Acute Coronary Syndromes
## 2010 American Heart Association Guidelines for Cardiopulmonary Resuscitation and Emergency Cardiovascular Care

Robert E. O'Connor, Chair; William Brady; Steven C. Brooks; Deborah Diercks; Jonathan Egan;
Chris Ghaemmaghami; Venu Menon; Brian J. O'Neil; Andrew H. Travers; Demetris Yannopoulos

The *2010 AHA Guidelines for CPR and ECC* for the evaluation and management of acute coronary syndromes (ACS) are intended to define the scope of training for healthcare providers who treat patients with suspected or definite ACS within the first hours after onset of symptoms. These guidelines summarize key out-of-hospital, emergency department (ED), and related initial critical-care topics that are relevant to diagnosis and initial stabilization and are not intended to guide treatment beyond the ED. Emergency providers should use these contents to supplement other recommendations from the ACC/AHA Guidelines, which are used throughout the United States and Canada.[1–3] As with any guidelines, these general recommendations must be considered within the context of local resources and their application to individual patients by knowledgeable healthcare providers. The healthcare providers managing the individual patients are best suited to determine the most appropriate treatment strategy.

The primary goals of therapy for patients with ACS are to

- Reduce the amount of myocardial necrosis that occurs in patients with acute myocardial infarction (AMI), thus preserving left ventricular (LV) function, preventing heart failure, and limiting other cardiovascular complications
- Prevent major adverse cardiac events (MACE): death, nonfatal MI, and need for urgent revascularization
- Treat acute, life-threatening complications of ACS, such as ventricular fibrillation (VF), pulseless ventricular tachycardia (VT), unstable tachycardias, symptomatic bradycardias (See Part 8: "Advanced Cardiovascular Life Support"), pulmonary edema, cardiogenic shock and mechanical complications of AMI
- An overview of recommended care for the ACS patient is illustrated in Figure 1, the Acute Coronary Syndromes Algorithm. Part 10 provides details of the care highlighted in the numbered algorithm boxes; box numbers in the text correspond to the numbered boxes in the algorithm. In this part, the abbreviation "AMI" refers to acute myocardial infarction, whether associated with ST-elevation myocardial infarction (STEMI) or non-ST-elevation myocardial

infarction (NSTEMI). The diagnosis and treatment of AMI, however, will often differ for patients with STEMI versus NSTEMI. Please note carefully which AMI type is being discussed.

## Prehospital Management

### Patient and Healthcare Provider Recognition of ACS (Figure 1, Box 1)

Prompt diagnosis and treatment offers the greatest potential benefit for myocardial salvage in the first hours of STEMI; and early, focused management of unstable angina and NSTEMI reduces adverse events and improves outcome.[4] Thus, it is imperative that healthcare providers recognize patients with potential ACS in order to initiate the evaluation, appropriate triage, and management as expeditiously as possible; in the case of STEMI, this recognition also allows for prompt notification of the receiving hospital and preparation for emergent reperfusion therapy. Potential delays to therapy occur during 3 intervals: from onset of symptoms to patient recognition, during prehospital transport, and during emergency department (ED) evaluation.

Patient-based delay in recognition of ACS and activation of the emergency medical services (EMS) system often constitutes the longest period of delay to treatment.[5] With respect to the prehospital recognition of ACS, numerous issues have been identified as independent factors for prehospital treatment delay (ie, symptom-to-door time), including older age,[6] racial and ethnic minorities,[7,8] female gender,[9] lower socioeconomic status,[10,11] and solitary living arrangements.[7,12]

Hospital-based delays in ACS recognition range from nonclassical patient presentations and other confounding diagnostic issues to provider misinterpretation of patient data and inefficient in-hospital system of care.[9,13–16]

Symptoms of ACS may be used in combination with other important information (biomarkers, risk factors, ECG, and other diagnostic tests) in making triage and some treatment decisions in the out-of-hospital and ED settings. The symptoms of AMI may be more intense than angina and most often

The American Heart Association requests that this document be cited as follows: O'Connor RE, Brady W, Brooks SC, Diercks D, Egan J, Ghaemmaghami C, Menon V, O'Neil BJ, Travers AH, Yannopoulos D. Part 10: acute coronary syndromes: 2010 American Heart Association Guidelines for Cardiopulmonary Resuscitation and Emergency Cardiovascular Care. *Circulation.* 2010;122(suppl 3):S787–S817.

(*Circulation.* 2010;122[suppl 3]:S787–S817.)

*Circulation* is available at http://circ.ahajournals.org

DOI: 10.1161/CIRCULATIONAHA.110.971028

## Acute Coronary Syndromes

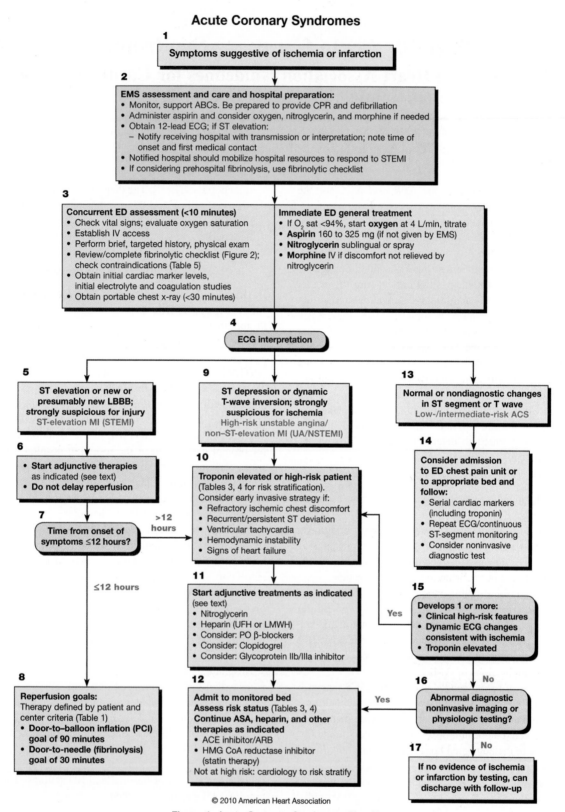

**Figure 1.** Acute Coronary Syndromes Algorithm.

persist for longer periods of time (eg, longer than 15–20 minutes). The classic symptom associated with ACS is chest discomfort, but symptoms may also include discomfort in other areas of the upper body, shortness of breath, sweating, nausea, vomiting, and dizziness. Most often the patient will note chest or upper body discomfort and dyspnea as the predominant presenting symptoms accompanied by diaphoresis, nausea, vomiting, and dizziness.[17–19] Isolated diaphoresis, nausea, vomiting, or dizziness are unusual predominant presenting symptoms.[20] Atypical or unusual symptoms are

## Prehospital Fibrinolytic Checklist

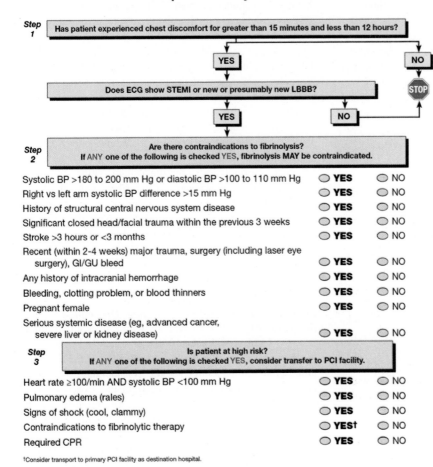

**Figure 2.** Prehospital fibrinolytic checklist. Adapted from Antman EM, et al. ACC/AHA guidelines for the management of patients with ST-elevation myocardial infarction: a report of the American College of Cardiology/American Heart Association Task Force on Practice Guidelines (Committee to Revise the 1999 Guidelines for the Management of Patients with Acute Myocardial Infarction). *Circulation.* 2004;110:e82-e292, with permission from Lippincott Williams & Wilkins. Copyright 2004, American Heart Association.

more common in women, the elderly, and diabetic patients.[21–23] The physical examination of the patient with ACS is often normal.

Public education campaigns increase patient awareness and knowledge of the symptoms of ACS, yet have only transient effects on time to presentation.[24,25] For patients at risk for ACS (and for their families), primary care physicians and other healthcare providers should consider discussing the appropriate use of aspirin and activation of EMS system. Furthermore, an awareness of the location of the nearest hospital that offers 24-hour emergency cardiovascular care can also be included in this discussion. Previous guidelines have recommended that the patient, family member, or companion activate the EMS system rather than call their physician or drive to the hospital if chest discomfort is unimproved or worsening 5 minutes after taking 1 nitroglycerin treatment.[2]

### Initial EMS Care (Figure 1, Box 2)

Half the patients who die of ACS do so before reaching the hospital. VF or pulseless VT is the precipitating cardiac arrest rhythm in most of these deaths,[26,27] and it is most likely to develop in the early phase of ACS evolution.[28] Communities should develop programs to respond to cardiac emergencies that include the prompt recognition of ACS symptoms by

patients and their companions as well as by healthcare and public safety providers and early activation of the EMS system. Additional features of such a program include high-quality CPR for patients in cardiac arrest (see Part 5: "Adult Basic Life Support") and rapid access to and use of an automated external defibrillator (AED) through community AED programs (see Part 6: "Electrical Therapies").[29] Emergency dispatch center personnel should be educated in the provision of CPR instructions for lay rescuers before the arrival of EMS. EMS providers should be trained to respond to cardiovascular emergencies, including ACS and its acute complications.

Emergency dispatch center personnel can provide instructions to the patient or caller before EMS arrival. Because aspirin should be administered as soon as possible after symptom onset to patients with suspected ACS, it is reasonable for EMS dispatchers to instruct patients with no history of aspirin allergy and without signs of active or recent gastrointestinal bleeding to chew an aspirin (160 to 325 mg) while awaiting the arrival of EMS providers (Class IIa, LOE C).[30–35]

EMS providers should be familiar with the presentation of ACS and trained to determine the time of symptom onset. EMS providers should monitor vital signs and cardiac rhythm and be prepared to provide CPR and defibrillation if needed.

EMS providers administer oxygen during the initial assessment of patients with suspected ACS. However, there is insufficient evidence to support its routine use in uncomplicated ACS. If the patient is dyspneic, hypoxemic, or has obvious signs of heart failure, providers should titrate therapy, based on monitoring of oxyhemoglobin saturation, to ≥94% (Class I, LOE C).[36]

EMS providers should administer nonenteric aspirin (160 [Class I, LOE B] to 325 mg [Class I, LOE C]). The patient should chew the aspirin tablet to hasten absorption.[30,37–39] EMS providers should administer up to 3 nitroglycerin doses (tablets or spray) at intervals of 3 to 5 minutes. Nitrates in all forms are contraindicated in patients with initial systoloic blood pressure <90 mm Hg or ≥30 mm Hg below baseline and in patients with right ventricular infarction.[40–42] Caution is advised in patients with known inferior wall STEMI, and a right-sided ECG should be performed to evaluate RV infarction. Administer nitrates with extreme caution, if at all, to patients with inferior STEMI and suspected right ventricular (RV) involvement because these patients require adequate RV preload. Nitrates are contraindicated when patients have taken a phosphodiesterase-5 (PDE-5) inhibitor within 24 hours (48 hours for tadalafil).[43] Morphine is indicated in STEMI when chest discomfort is unresponsive to nitrates (Class I, LOE C); morphine should be used with caution in unstable angina (UA)/NSTEMI due to an association with increased mortality in a large registry (Class IIa, LOE C).[44] The efficacy of other analgesics is unknown.

## Prehospital ECGs (Figure 1, Box 2)

Prehospital 12-lead ECGs speed the diagnosis, shorten the time to reperfusion (fibrinolytics[45–52] or primary percutaneous coronary intervention [PPCI][53–60]). EMS personnel should routinely acquire a 12-lead electrocardiogram (ECG) as soon as possible for all patients exhibiting signs and symptoms of ACS. The ECG may be transmitted for remote interpretation by a physician or screened for STEMI by properly trained paramedics, with or without the assistance of computer-interpretation. Advance notification should be provided to the receiving hospital for patients identified as having STEMI (Class I, LOE B).

Implementation of 12-lead ECG diagnostic programs with concurrent medically-directed quality assurance is recommended (Class I, LOE B). Prehospital personnel can accurately identify ST-segment elevation from the 12-lead ECG.[47,50,61–74] If providers are not trained to interperet the 12-lead ECG, field transmission of the ECG or a computer report to the receiving hospital is recommended (Class I, LOE B).

## Prehospital Fibrinolysis

Clinical trials have shown the benefit of initiating fibrinolysis as soon as possible after onset of ischemic-type chest discomfort in patients with confirmed STEMI or new or presumably new left bundle branch block (LBBB).[75,76] Several prospective studies[77–79] have documented reduced time to administration of fibrinolytics and decreased mortality rates when out-of-hospital fibrinolytics were administered to patients with STEMI. Physicians in the Grampian Region Early

Anistreplase Trial (GREAT) trial administered fibrinolytic therapy to patients at home 130 minutes earlier than to patients at the hospital with both a 50% reduction in hospital mortality and greater 1-year and 5-year survival in those treated earlier.[79–81] Meta-analyses have demonstrated reduced mortality and improved outcomes with prehospital fibrinolysis regardless of the training and experience of the prehospital provider.[75,77]

When fibrinolysis is the chosen reperfusion strategy the fibrinolytic agent should be initiated as soon as possible, preferably within 30 minutes of first medical contact (Class I, LOE A). It is strongly recommended that systems which administer fibrinolytics in the prehospital setting include the following features: protocols using fibrinolytic checklists, 12-lead ECG acquisition and interpretation, experience in advanced life support, communication with the receiving institution, medical director with training and experience in STEMI management, and continuous quality improvement (Class I, LOE C).

## Triage and Transfer

### Prehospital Triage and EMS Hospital Destination

In approximately 40% of patients with a myocardial infarction, the EMS provider establishes first medical contact.[82,83] In these patients, the ability to identify STEMI in the prehospital setting allows for the consideration of specific hospital destination. Direct triage from the scene to a PCI-capable hospital may reduce the time to definitive therapy and improve outcome. In a large historically controlled clinical trial, the mortality rate was significantly reduced (8.9% versus 1.9%) when transport time was *less than 30 minutes*.[84] Increased out-of-hospital times with longer EMS-initiated diversion to a PCI-capable hospital may worsen outcomes. If PCI is the chosen method of reperfusion for the prehospital STEMI patient, it is reasonable to transport patients directly to the nearest PCI facility, bypassing closer EDs as necessary, in systems where time intervals between first medical contact and balloon times are <90 minutes and transport times are relatively short (ie, <30 minutes) (Class IIa, LOE B).

In patients presenting within 2 hours of symptom onset or when delays to PCI are anticipated, fibrinolytic therapy is recommended. In these circumstances fibrinolytic therapy has equivalent or improved outcomes compared to PCI, especially when the benefit to bleeding risk is favorable (eg, young age, anterior location of MI) (Class 1, LOE B).[85,86]

### Interfacility Transfer

Hospital and ED protocols should clearly identify criteria for expeditious transfer of patients to PCI facilities. These include patients who are ineligible for fibrinolytic therapy or who are in cardiogenic shock (Class I, LOE C).[1] A door-to-departure time <30 minutes is recommended by ACC/AHA Guidelines.[2] Transfer of high-risk patients who have received primary reperfusion with fibrinolytic therapy is reasonable (Class IIa, LOE B).[87,88]

## Systems of Care

A well-organized approach to STEMI care requires integration of community, EMS, physician, and hospital resources.

The most appropriate STEMI system of care starts "on the phone" with activation of EMS. Hospital-based issues include ED protocols, activation of the cardiac catheterization laboratory, and admission to the coronary intensive care unit.

In PCI-capable hospitals an established "STEMI Alert" activation plan is critical. Components include prehospital ECGs and notification of the receiving facility,[45–60] and activation of the cardiac catherization team to shorten reperfusion time[54,59,82,89–92] and other hospital personnel important for treatment and resource allocation.

Continuous review and quality improvement involving EMS and prehospital care providers are important to achieve ongoing optimal reperfusion time. Quality assurance, real-time feedback, and healthcare provider education can also reduce the time to therapy in STEMI.[89,93–97] Involvement of hospital leadership in the process and commitment to support rapid access to STEMI reperfusion therapy are critical factors associated with successful programs.

If the emergency physician activates the STEMI reperfusion protocol, including the cardiac catheterization team, significant reductions in time to reperfusion are seen, and the rate of "false-positive" activations are infrequent, ranging from 0% to 14%.[89,93,95,96,98–107]

## ED Evaluation and Risk Stratification (Figure 1, Boxes 3 and 4)

### Focused Assessment and ECG Risk Stratification

ED providers should quickly assess patients with possible ACS. Ideally within 10 minutes of ED arrival providers should obtain a targeted history while a monitor is attached to the patient and a 12-lead ECG is obtained (if not done in the prehospital setting).[108] The evaluation should focus on chest discomfort, associated signs and symptoms, prior cardiac history, risk factors for ACS, and historical features that may preclude the use of fibrinolytics or other therapies. This initial evaluation must be efficient because if the patient has STEMI, the goals of reperfusion are to administer fibrinolytics within 30 minutes of arrival (30-minute interval "door-to-drug") or to provide PCI within 90 minutes of arrival (90-minute interval "door-to-balloon") (Class I, LOE A).

Potential delay during the in-hospital evaluation period may occur from door to data, from data (ECG) to decision, and from decision to drug (or PCI). These 4 major points of in-hospital therapy are commonly referred to as the "4 D's."[109] All providers must focus on minimizing delays at each of these points. Prehospital transport time constitutes only 5% of delay to treatment time; ED evaluation constitutes 25% to 33% of this delay.[3,109–111]

The physical examination is performed to aid diagnosis, rule out other causes of the patient's symptoms, and evaluate the patient for complications related to ACS. Although the presence of clinical signs and symptoms may increase suspicion of ACS, evidence does not support the use of any single sign or combination of clinical signs and symptoms alone to confirm the diagnosis.[17–19,112]

When the patient presents with symptoms and signs of potential ACS, the clinician uses ECG findings (Figure 1, Box 4) to classify the patient into 1 of 3 groups:

1. ST-segment elevation or presumed new LBBB (Box 5) is characterized by ST-segment elevation in 2 or more contiguous leads and is classified as *ST-segment elevation MI (STEMI)*. Threshold values for ST-segment elevation consistent with STEMI are J-point elevation 0.2 mV (2 mm) in leads V2 and V3 and 0.1 mV (1 mm) in all other leads (men ≥40 years old); J-point elevation 0.25 mV (2.5 mm) in leads V2 and V3 and 0.1 mV (1 mm) in all other leads (men <40 years old); J-point elevation 0.15 mV (2.5 mm) in leads V2 and V3 and 0.1 mV (1 mm) in all other leads (women).[113]

2. Ischemic ST-segment depression >0.5 mm (0.05 mV) or dynamic T-wave inversion with pain or discomfort (Box 9) is classified as UA/NSTEMI. Nonpersistent or transient ST-segment elevation ≥0.5 mm for <20 minutes is also included in this category. Threshold values for ST-segment depression consistent with ischemia are J-point depression 0.05 mV (-.5 mm) in leads V2 and V3 and -0.1 mV (-1 mm) in all other leads (men and women).[113]

3. The nondiagnostic ECG with either normal or minimally abnormal (ie, nonspecific ST-segment or T-wave changes, Box 13). This ECG is nondiagnostic and inconclusive for ischemia, requiring further risk stratification. This classification includes patients with normal ECGs and those with ST-segment deviation of <0.5 mm (0.05 mV) or T-wave inversion of ≤0.2 mV. This category of ECG is termed *nondiagnostic*.

The interpretation of the 12-lead ECG is a key step in this process, allowing not only for this classification but also the selection of the most appropriate diagnostic and management strategies. Not all providers are skilled in the interpretation of the ECG; as a consequence, the use of computer-aided ECG interpretation has been studied. While expert ECG intepretation is ideal, computer-aided ECG interpretation may have a role, particularly in assisting inexperienced clinicians in achieving a diagnosis (Class IIa, LOE B).

### *Cardiac Biomarkers*

Serial cardiac biomarkers are often obtained during evaluation of patients suspected of ACS. Cardiac troponin is the preferred biomarker and is more sensitive than creatine kinase isoenzyme (CK-MB). Cardiac troponins are useful in diagnosis, risk stratification, and determination of prognosis. An elevated level of *troponin* correlates with an increased risk of death, and greater elevations predict greater risk of adverse outcome.[114]

In the patients with STEMI reperfusion therapy should not be delayed pending results of biomarkers. Important limitations to these tests exist because they are insensitive during the first 4 to 6 hours of presentation unless continuous persistent pain has been present for 6 to 8 hours. For this reason cardiac biomarkers are not useful in the prehospital setting.[115–120]

Clinicians should take into account the timing of symptom onset and the sensitivity, precision, and institutional norms of the assay, as well as the release kinetics and clearance of the measured biomarker. If biomarkers are initially negative within 6 hours of symptom onset, it is recommended that biomarkers should be remeasured between 6 to 12 hours after symptom onset (Class I, LOE A). A diagnosis of myocardial infarction can be made when clinical symptoms or new ECG abnormalities are consistent with ischemia and one biomarker is elevated above the 99th percentile of the upper reference limit (URL) using a test with optimal precision defined as a CV ≤10%.

There is insufficient evidence to support the use of troponin point-of-care testing (POCT) either in or out of hospital. There is also insufficient evidence to support the use of myoglobin, β-natriuretic peptide (BNP), NT-proBNP, D-dimer, C-reactive protein, ischemia-modified albumin pregnancy-associated plasma protein A (PAPP-A) or interleukin-6 in isolation.

## STEMI (Figure 1, Boxes 5 Through 8)

Patients with STEMI usually have complete occlusion of an epicardial coronary artery. The primary goal of initial treatment is early reperfusion therapy through administration of fibrinolytics (pharmacological reperfusion) or PPCI (mechanical reperfusion). Providers should rapidly identify patients with STEMI and quickly screen them for indications and contraindications to fibrinolytic therapy and PCI. Patients who are ineligible for fibrinolytic therapy should be considered for transfer to a PCI facility regardless of delay.

Within a STEMI system of care, the first physician who encounters a patient with STEMI determines the need and strategy (fibrinolytic or PPCI) for reperfusion therapy (see Table 1). If the patient meets the criteria for fibrinolytic therapy, a door-to-needle time (initiation of fibrinolytic agent) <30 minutes is recommended—the earlier the better (Class I, LOE A). Routine consultation with a cardiologist or another physician is not recommended except in equivocal or uncertain cases.[89,121] Consultation delays therapy and is associated with increased hospital mortality rates (Class III, LOE B).

## UA and NSTEMI (Figure 1, Boxes 9 Through 12)

Unstable angina (UA) and NSTEMI are difficult to distinguish initially. These patients usually have a partially or intermittently occluding thrombus. Both ACS syndromes may present with similar symptoms and ECG. Clinical features can correlate with the dynamic nature of clot formation and degradation (eg, waxing and waning clinical symptoms). The ECG will demonstrate a range of findings short of diagnostic ST-segment deviation; these ECG presentations include normal, minimal nonspecific ST-segment/T-wave changes, and significant ST-segment depression and T-wave inversions.

An elevated biomarker separates NSTEMI from UA and has incremental value in addition to the ECG. Elevation of cardiac troponin indicates increased risk for major adverse cardiac events and benefit from an invasive strategy. Cardiac troponins indicate myocardial necrosis, although numerous conditions other than ACS may cause elevated biomarkers (eg, myocarditis, heart failure, and pulmonary embolism).

Management strategies for UA/NSTEMI include antiplatelet, antithrombin, and antianginal therapy and are based on risk stratification. Fibrinolysis is contraindicated in this het-

**Table 1.    ST-Segment Elevation or New or Presumably New LBBB: Evaluation for Reperfusion**

**Step 1: Assess time and risk**

Time since onset of symptoms

Risk of STEMI

Risk of fibrinolysis

Time required to transport to skilled PCI catheterization suite

**Step 2: Select reperfusion (fibrinolysis or invasive) strategy**

*Note:* If presentation <3 hours and no delay for PCI, then no preference for either strategy.

| Fibrinolysis is generally preferred if: | An invasive strategy is generally preferred if: |
|---|---|
| • Early presentation (≤3 hours from symptom onset) | • Late presentation (symptom onset >3 hours ago) |
| • Invasive strategy is not an option (eg, lack of access to skilled PCI facility or difficult vascular access) or would be delayed | • Skilled PCI facility available with surgical backup |
| – Medical contact-to-balloon or door-balloon >90 minutes | • Medical contact-to-balloon or door-to-balloon <90 minutes |
| – (Door-to-balloon) minus (door-to-needle) is >1 hour | • (Door-to-balloon) minus (door-to-needle) is <1 hour |
| • No contraindications to fibrinolysis | • Contraindications to fibrinolysis, including increased risk of bleeding and ICH |
| | • High risk from STEMI (CHF, Killip class is ≥3) |
| | • Diagnosis of STEMI is in doubt |

Modified from ACC/AHA 2004 Update Recommendations.[2]

erogenous group of patients and may be harmful; an invasive strategy is indicated in patients with positive biomarkers or unstable clinical features.

### The Process of Risk Stratification

Diagnosis of ACS and risk stratification become an integrated process in patients presenting to an acute care setting with possible ACS and an initially nondiagostic evaluation. This nondiagnostic evaluation includes a normal or nondiagnostic 12-lead ECG and normal serum cardiac biomarker concentrations. The majority of these patients will not be experiencing an ACS, but many may have underlying CAD or other clinical features putting them at subsequent risk for major adverse cardiac events over the course of a few days to several months.

A major goal of the risk stratification process is to identify those patients who do not appear to have high-risk features on initial assessment but are found, through the course of the diagnostic process, to have ACS and clinically significant CAD. This strategy allows physicians to target patients who would benefit from guidelines-based ACS therapies while avoiding unnecessary procedural and pharmacological risks (eg, anticoagulation therapy and invasive cardiac catheterization) in patients with low risk for major adverse cardiac events.

Although the diagnosis of ACS is important and will help to guide immediate therapy, the estimation of risk for major adverse cardiac events in the immediate, short-term, and long-term time frames helps the physician determine the urgency in completing the diagnostic workup not just for ACS but also for CAD. Many patients can be managed in the outpatient setting once it is determined that they are at very low risk for short-term (30 days) major adverse cardiac events.

### Braunwald Risk Stratification

ACC/AHA Guidelines recommend that all patients be risk stratified for the selection of an initial management strategy and site of care.[3] A well-recognized approach is the one initially proposed and later refined by Braunwald and colleagues and published in ACC/AHA Guidelines on the Management of Patients With Unstable Angina and Non-ST Segment Elevation MI.[122–126] This approach is based on a combination of historical, clinical, laboratory, and ECG variables and answers two questions: what is the likelihood that signs and symptoms represent ACS secondary to obstructive CAD, and what is the likelihood of an adverse clinical outcome?

Table 2[127] is a modified version of Braunwald and colleagues' approach updated over several publications.[124,126,128] Patients are initially risk-stratified according to the likelihood that symptoms are due to unstable CAD. Patients at intermediate or high risk for CAD are further classified by their risk of major adverse cardiac events. This second classification is useful for prospectively identifying patients at intermediate or high risk who can benefit from an invasive strategy and more aggressive pharmacology with antiplatelet and antithrombin agents. Other risk stratification schemes include the TIMI, GRACE, and PURSUIT risk scores developed for short- and longer-term risk assessment.[129–133] Stratification tools cannot be used to determine discharge from the ED.

### TIMI Risk Score

The risk of major adverse cardiac events has been further studied and refined. Researchers who derived the important Thrombolysis in Myocardial Ischemia (TIMI) risk score used data from the TIMI-11B and ESSENCE (Efficacy and Safety of Subcutaneous Enoxaparin in Non–Q-Wave Coronary Events) trials for UA/NSTEMI[134,135] and from the In-TIME trial for STEMI.[136]

The TIMI risk score comprises 7 independent prognostic variables (Table 3). These 7 variables were significantly associated with the occurrence within 14 days of at least one of the primary end points: death, new or recurrent MI, or need for urgent revascularization. The score is derived from complex multivariate logistic regression. It is useful to note that traditional cardiac risk factors are only weakly associated with major adverse cardiac events. Aspirin use was found to be one of the most powerful predictors.[134] It is possible that aspirin use identified a subgroup of patients at higher risk or on active but failed therapy for CAD.

The TIMI risk score was validated with 3 groups of patients, and 4 clinical trials showed a significant interaction between the TIMI risk score and outcome (Table 3).[136–139]

These findings confirm the value of the TIMI risk score as a guide to therapeutic decisions (Class IIa, LOE B).

### Indicators for Early Invasive Strategies

Risk stratification (Figure 1, Boxes 9, 13, 14, 15) helps the clinician identify patients with non–ST-elevation ACS who should be managed with an early invasive strategy versus a selectively invasive one. Early coronary angiography may allow the clinician to determine whether patients are appropriate candidates for revascularization with PCI or coronary artery bypass grafting (CABG).

The 2007 Focused Update of the ACC/AHA/SCAI 2005 Guideline Update for Percutaneous Coronary Intervention contains the following recommendations related to the selection of early invasive PCI versus conservative strategies.

1. An early invasive PCI strategy is indicated for patients with non–ST-elevation ACS who have no serious co-morbidity and who have coronary lesions amenable to PCI and an elevated risk for clinical events (Class I, LOE A). (See Table 4 and Section 3.3 of the ACC/AHA 2007 UA/NSTEMI Guidelines).
2. An early invasive strategy (ie, diagnostic angiography with intent to perform revascularization) is indicated in non–ST-elevation ACS patients who have refractory angina or hemodynamic or electric instability (without serious comorbidities or contraindications to such procedures) (Class I, LOE B).
3. In initially stabilized patients, an initially conservative (ie, a selectively invasive) strategy may be considered as a treatment strategy for non–ST-elevation ACS patients (without serious comorbidities or contraindications to such procedures) who have an elevated risk for clinical events including those with abnormal troponin elevations (Class IIb, LOE B).
4. The decision to implement an initial conservative (versus initial invasive) strategy in these patients may be made by considering physician and patient preference (Class IIb, LOE C).

### Normal or Nondiagnostic ECG Changes (Figure 1, Boxes 13 Through 17)

The majority of patients with normal or nondiagnostic ECGs do not have ACS. Patients in this category with ACS are most often at low or intermediate risk. The physician's goal involves risk stratification (see above) to provide appropriate diagnostic or treatment strategies for an individual patient. These strategies then target patients at increased risk for benefit while avoiding risk (eg, anticoagulation therapy and invasive cardiac catheterization) in patients with low or minimal risk.

### The Chest Pain Unit Model

Chest pain observation protocols may be employed in a dedicated space (ie, a physical chest pain unit [CPU]) or throughout an ED/hospital (ie, virtual CPU). These chest pain observation protocols are a rapid system of patient assessment that should generally include a history and physical examination, a period of observation, serial electrocardiography, and serial measurement of serum cardiac markers. In selected patients, an evaluation for inducible myocardial ischemia or anatomic coronary disease after AMI is excluded

**Table 2. Likelihood That Signs and Symptoms Represent ACS Secondary to CAD**

| Feature | High Likelihood *Any of the following:* | Intermediate Likelihood *Absence of high-likelihood features and presence of any of the following:* | Low Likelihood *Absence of high- or intermediate-likelihood features but may have the following:* |
|---|---|---|---|
| History | Chest or left arm pain or discomfort as chief symptom reproducing prior documented angina; known history of CAD including MI | Chest or left arm pain or discomfort as chief symptom; age >70 years; male sex; diabetes mellitus | Probable ischemic symptoms in absence of any intermediate-likelihood characteristics; recent cocaine use |
| Examination | Transient MR murmur, hypotension, diaphoresis, pulmonary edema, or rales | Extracardiac vascular disease | Chest discomfort reproduced by palpation |
| ECG | New or presumably new transient ST-segment deviation (≥1 mm) or T-wave inversion in multiple precordial leads | Fixed Q waves ST depression 0.5 to 1 mm or T-wave inversion >1 mm | T-wave flattening or inversion <1 mm in leads with dominant R waves Normal ECG |
| Cardiac markers | Elevated cardiac TnI, TnT, or CK-MB | Normal | Normal |

CAD indicates coronary artery disease; CK-MB, MB fraction of creatine kinase; ECG, electrocardiogram; MI, myocardial infarction; MR, mitral regurgitation; TnI, troponin I; and TnT, troponin T.

Modified from Braunwald E, et al. *Unstable Angina: Diagnosis and Management.* 1994;3-1-AHCPR Publication No 94-0602:1-154. In the public domain.[127]

when indicated. Eleven randomized trials[140–150] suggest that these protocols may be used to improve accuracy in identifying patients requiring inpatient admission or further diagnostic testing and, thereby, reduce length of stay, rate of hospital admission, and health care costs while improving quality of life measures.

In patients with suspicion for ACS, normal initial biomarkers, and nonischemic ECG, chest pain observation protocols may be recommended as a safe and effective strategy for evaluating patients in the ED (Class I, LOE A). There is no direct evidence demonstrating that CPUs/observation protocols reduce adverse cardiovascular outcomes, including mortality for patients presenting with possible ACS, normal serum cardiac biomarkers, and a nondiagnostic ECG.

### Advanced Testing to Detect Coronary Ischemia and CAD

For ED/CPU patients who are suspected of having ACS, have nonischemic ECG's and negative biomarkers, a noninvasive test for inducible myocardial ischemia or anatomic evaluation of the coronary arteries (eg, computed tomography [CT] angiography, cardiac magnetic resonance, myocardial perfusion imaging, stress echocardiography) can be useful in identifying patients suitable for discharge from the ED (Class IIa, LOE B). This strategy may be considered to increase diagnostic accuracy for ACS thereby decreasing costs, length of stay, time to diagnosis, and can provide valuable short-term and long-term prognostic information of future major cardiac events.

Myocardial perfusion scintigraphy (MPS) has a high negative predictive value (NPV) for ruling out ACS; 99% in patients presenting to the ED with acute chest pain, nondiagnostic ECG, and negative cardiac markers. MPS can also be used for risk stratification, especially in low- to intermediate-likelihood of cardiac events according to traditional cardiac markers (Class IIa, LOE B).[151–154] MPS is best utilized in patients with an intermediate probability or LOE of risk stratification.

The use of multidetector computed tomography (MDCT) angiography (64-slice scanner) after presentation to the ED with chest discomfort, a nondiagnostic ECG, and negative cardiac biomarkers has also been demonstrated to have high sensitivity and specificity for CAD and ACS.[155,156] The use of MDCT angiography for selected low-risk patients can be useful to allow for safe early discharge from the ED (Class IIa, LOE B).[157–159]

It is reasonable to consider both the exposure to radiation and iodinated contrast agents when using MDCT angiography and myocardial perfusion imaging. Little evidence is available to support the use of MRI in this patient population.

### Safety of Discharge and Risk of Major Adverse Cardiac Events After Discharge From the ED/CPU

The final step in the CPU risk-stratification process is the decision to discharge or admit the patient. No simple clinical decision rule is adequate and appropriate to identify ED chest discomfort patients with suspected ACS who can be safely discharged from the ED.[160] The use of inpatient-derived risk scoring systems are useful for prognosis (Class I, LOE A) but are not recommended to identify patients who may be safely discharged from the ED (Class III, LOE C).

The Bayesian process of serial assignment of pretest risk, diagnostic testing, and reclassification into post-test risk levels based on the test results is the most reliable method to identify patients at the lowest risk for short term major adverse cardiac events and those patients in need of further evaluation for underlying CAD.

Patients at low and intermediate clinical risk for ACS who have remained stable in the CPU and have negative serial ECGs, serial cardiac biomarker measurements, and noninvasive physiological or anatomic testing for ACS have very low rates of major adverse cardiac events at 30 days from ED discharge.[161–165] Patients younger than 40 years-of-age with nonclassical presentations and no significant past medical history have very low short-term rates of major adverse cardiac events when serial biomarkers and 12-lead ECGs are

**Table 3. TIMI Risk Score for Patients With Unstable Angina and Non–ST-Segment Elevation MI: Predictor Variables**

| Predictor Variable | Point Value of Variable | Definition |
|---|---|---|
| Age ≥65 years | 1 | |
| ≥3 risk factors for CAD | 1 | Risk factors |
| | | • Family history of CAD |
| | | • Hypertension |
| | | • Hypercholesterolemia |
| | | • Diabetes |
| | | • Current smoker |
| Aspirin use in last 7 days | 1 | |
| Recent, severe symptoms of angina | 1 | ≥2 anginal events in last 24 hours |
| Elevated cardiac markers | 1 | CK-MB or cardiac-specific troponin level |
| ST deviation ≥0.5 mm | 1 | ST depression >0.5 mm is significant; transient ST elevation ≥0.5 mm for <20 minutes is treated as ST-segment depression and is high risk; ST elevation ≥1 mm for more than 20 minutes places these patients in the STEMI treatment category |
| Prior coronary artery stenosis ≥50% | 1 | Risk predictor remains valid even if this information is unknown |

| Calculated TIMI Risk Score | Risk of ≥1 Primary End Point* in ≤14 Days | Risk Status |
|---|---|---|
| 0 or 1 | 5% | Low |
| 2 | 8% | Low |
| 3 | 13% | Intermediate |
| 4 | 20% | Intermediate |
| 5 | 26% | High |

*Primary end points: death, new or recurrent MI, or need for urgent revascularization.

**Table 4. Selection of Initial Treatment Strategy for Patients With Non-ST-Elevation ACS: Invasive Versus Conservative Strategy***

| Preferred Strategy | Patient Characteristics |
|---|---|
| Invasive | • Recurrent angina or ischemia at rest or with low-level activities despite intensive medical therapy |
| | • Elevated cardiac biomarkers (TnT or TnI) |
| | • New or presumably new ST-segment depression |
| | • Signs or symptoms of HF or new or worsening mitral regurgitation |
| | • High-risk findings from noninvasive testing |
| | • Hemodynamic instability |
| | • Sustained ventricular tachycardia |
| | • PCI within 6 months |
| | • Prior CABG |
| | • High-risk score (eg, TIMI, GRACE) |
| | • Reduced LV function (LVEF less than 40%) |
| Conservative | • Low-risk score (eg, TIMI, GRACE) |
| | • Patient or physician preference in absence of high-risk features |

CABG indicates coronary artery bypass graft surgery; GRACE, Global Registry of Acute Coronary Events; HF, heart failure; LV, left ventricular; LVEF, left ventricular ejection fraction; PCI, percutaneous coronary intervention; TIMI, Thrombolysis in Myocardial Infarction; TnI, troponin I; and TnT, troponin T.
*Adapted from the ACC/AHA 2007 UA/NSTEMI Guidelines.

normal. These patients may be discharged directly from the ED/CPU if appropriate outpatient testing can be arranged within 72 hours.[3,161–163,165–167] Any system that attempts to facilitate outpatient testing should include mechanisms to ensure patient access to outpatient clinics and testing facilities and should consider nonmedical barriers to discharge from the ED that may require inpatient admission.

## Initial General Therapy for ACS

Several initial therapeutic measures are appropriate for all patients with suspected ACS in the ED setting. These include continuous cardiac monitoring, establishment of intravenous (IV) access, and consideration of several medications discussed below.

## Oxygen

Oxygen should be administered to patients with breathlessness, signs of heart failure, shock, or an arterial oxyhemoglobin saturation <94% (Class I, LOE C). Noninvasive monitoring of blood oxygen saturation can be useful to decide on the need for oxygen administration.

In the absence of compelling evidence for established benefit in uncomplicated cases, ACC/AHA Guidelines have noted that there appeared to be little justification for continuing routine oxygen use beyond 6 hours.[2] There is insufficient evidence to recommend the routine usage of oxygen therapy in patients suffering from an uncomplicated AMI or an ACS without signs of hypoxemia or heart failure. Supplementary oxygen has been shown to limit ischemic myocardial injury in animals,[168–171] but evidence of benefit from supplementary oxygen from human trials is limited.[168] A case study found improvement in ST changes with the use of oxygen in humans.[172] Others suggested harm with *high*-flow oxygen administration.[173,174]

## Aspirin and Nonsteriodal Anti-Inflammatory Drugs

Early administration of aspirin (acetylsalicylic acid [ASA]), has been associated with decreased mortality rates in several clinical trials.[30,32,175,176] Multiple studies support the safety of aspirin administration. Therefore, unless the patient has a known aspirin allergy or active gastrointestinal hemorrhage, nonenteric aspirin should be given as soon as possible to all patients with suspected ACS (Class I, LOE A).

Aspirin produces a rapid clinical antiplatelet effect with near-total inhibition of thromboxane A2 production. It reduces coronary reocclusion and recurrent ischemic events after fibrinolytic therapy. Aspirin alone reduced death from AMI in the Second International Study of Infarct Survival (ISIS-2), and its effect was additive to that of streptokinase.[32] Aspirin was found to substantially reduce vascular events in all patients with AMI, and in high-risk patients it reduced nonfatal AMI and vascular death.[177] Aspirin is also effective in patients with NSTEMI. The recommended dose is 160 to 325 mg. Chewable or soluble aspirin is absorbed more quickly than swallowed tablets.[178,179]

Aspirin suppositories (300 mg) are safe and can be considered for patients with severe nausea, vomiting, or disorders of the upper gastrointestinal tract.

Other nonsteroidal anti-inflammatory medications (NSAIDS) are contraindicated and should be discontinued in patients who are taking these medications. NSAIDs (except for aspirin), both nonselective as well as COX-2 selective agents, should not be administered during hospitalization for STEMI because of the increased risk of mortality, reinfarction, hypertension, heart failure, and myocardial rupture associated with their use (Class III, LOE C).[180–182]

## Nitroglycerin (or Glyceryl Trinitrate)

Nitroglycerin has beneficial hemodynamic effects, including dilation of the coronary arteries (particularly in the region of plaque disruption), the peripheral arterial bed, and venous capacitance vessels. The treatment benefits of nitroglycerin are limited, however, and no conclusive evidence has been shown to support the routine use of IV, oral, or topical nitrate therapy in patients with AMI.[183] With this in mind, these agents should be carefully considered, especially in the patient with low blood pressure and when their use would preclude the use of other agents known to be beneficial, such as angiotensin-converting enzyme (ACE) inhibitors.

Patients with ischemic discomfort should receive up to 3 doses of sublingual or aerosol nitroglycerin at 3- to 5-minute intervals until pain is relieved or low blood pressure limits its use (Class I, LOE B). Topical nitrates are acceptable alternatives for patients who require anti-anginal therapy but who are hemodynamically stable and do not have ongoing refractory ischemic symptoms. Parenteral formulations, rather than long acting oral preparations, can be used acutely to enable titration in patients with obvious ACS, objective test abnormality, and ongoing discomfort. In patients with recurrent ischemia, nitrates are indicated in the first 24 to 48 hours.

The use of nitrates in patients with hypotension (SBP <90 mm Hg or ≥30 mm Hg below baseline), extreme bradycardia (<50 bpm), or tachycardia in the absence of heart failure (>100 bpm) and in patients with right ventricular infarction is contraindicated (Class III, LOE C). Caution is advised in patients with known inferior wall STEMI, and a right-sided ECG should be performed to evaluate RV infarction. Administer nitrates with extreme caution, if at all, to patients with inferior-wall MI and suspected right ventricular (RV) involvement because these patients require adequate RV preload. Nitroglycerin should not be administered to patients who had taken a phosphodiesterase inhibitor (eg, sildenafil) for erectile dysfunction within 24 hours (48 hours if tadalafil use).

Relief of chest discomfort with nitroglycerin is neither sensitive nor specific for ACS; gastrointestinal etiologies as well as other causes of chest discomfort can "respond" to nitroglycerin administration.[18,184–186]

## Analgesia

Providers should administer analgesics, such as intravenous morphine, for chest discomfort unresponsive to nitrates. Morphine is the preferred analgesic for patients with STEMI (Class I, LOE C). However, analysis of retrospective registry data raised a question about the potentially adverse effects of morphine in patients with UA/NSTEMI.[44] As a result, the ACC AHA UA/NSTEMI writing group reduced morphine use to a Class IIa recommendation for that patient population.[3]

## Reperfusion Therapies (Figure 1, Box 7, 8)

Acute reperfusion therapy using PPCI or fibrinolytic therapy in patients with STEMI restores flow in the infarct-related artery, limits infarct size, and translates into early mortality benefit that is sustained over the next decade.[187,188] While optimal fibrinolysis restores normal coronary flow (TIMI 3) in 50% to 60% of subjects, PPCI is able to achieve restored flow in >90% of subjects. The patency rates achieved with PPCI translates into reduced mortality and reinfarction rates as compared to fibrinolytic therapy.[189] This benefit is even greater in patients presenting with cardiogenic shock. PPCI also results in a decreased risk of intracranial hemorrhage and stroke, making it the reperfusion strategy of choice in the elderly and those at risk for bleeding complications.

## Fibrinolytics

Early fibrinolytic therapy is a well-established treatment modality for patients with STEMI who present within 12 hours of the onset of symptoms and who lack contraindications to its use.[188,190–193] Early reperfusion results in reduced mortality, and the shorter the time to reperfusion, the greater the benefit. A 47% reduction in mortality was noted when fibrinolytic therapy was provided within the first hour after onset of symptoms.[188,193]

The major determinants of myocardial salvage and long-term prognosis are short time to reperfusion,[190,193] complete and sustained patency of the infarct-related artery with normal (TIMI grade 3) flow,[194,195] and normal microvascular perfusion.[22,196–198]

In the absence of contraindications, fibrinolytic therapy is recommended for STEMI if symptom onset has been within 12 hours of presentation and PCI is not available within 90 minutes of first medical contact (Class I, LOE A). Patients are evaluated for risk and benefit; for absolute and relative contraindications to therapy (see Table 5).

If fibrinolysis is chosen for reperfusion, the ED physician should administer fibrinolytics to eligible patients as early as possible according to a predetermined process of care developed by the ED and cardiology staff (Class I, LOE A). The goal is a door-to-needle time of less than 30 minutes with effort focused on shortening the time to therapy. Patients treated within the first 70 minutes of onset of symptoms have >50% reduction in infarct size and 75% reduction in mortality rates.[199] For fibrinolytic therapy, it is estimated that 65 lives will be saved per 1000 patients treated if fibrinolytics are provided in the first hour, with a pooled total of 131 lives saved per 1000 patients treated if fibrinolytics are provided within the first 3 hours of onset of symptoms.[200] Although fibrinolytics may be beneficial if given within 12 hours after

**Table 5.    Fibrinolytic Therapy**

Contraindications and cautions for fibrinolytic use in STEMI from ACC/AHA 2004 Guideline Update*

Absolute Contraindications

- Any prior intracranial hemorrhage
- Known structural cerebral vascular lesion (eg, AVM)
- Known malignant intracranial neoplasm (primary or metastatic)
- Ischemic stroke within 3 months EXCEPT acute ischemic stroke within 3 hours
- Suspected aortic dissection
- Active bleeding or bleeding diathesis (excluding menses)
- Significant closed head trauma or facial trauma within 3 months

Relative Contraindications

- History of chronic, severe, poorly controlled hypertension
- Severe uncontrolled hypertension on presentation (SBP >180 mm Hg or DBP >110 mm Hg)†
- History of prior ischemic stroke >3 months, dementia, or known intracranial pathology not covered in contraindications
- Traumatic or prolonged (>10 minutes) CPR or major surgery (<3 weeks)
- Recent (within 2 to 4 weeks) internal bleeding
- Noncompressible vascular punctures
- For streptokinase/anistreplase: prior exposure (>5 days ago) or prior allergic reaction to these agents
- Pregnancy
- Active peptic ulcer
- Current use of anticoagulants: the higher the INR, the higher the risk of bleeding

CPR, cardiopulmonary resuscitation; AVM indicates arteriovenous malformation; SBP, systolic blood pressure; DBP, diastolic blood pressure; INR, International Normalized Ratio.

*Viewed as advisory for clinical decision making and may not be all-inclusive or definitive.

†Could be an absolute contraindication in low-risk patients with myocardial infarction.

onset of symptoms, the mortality benefit is time sensitive, with shorter intervals to administration being associated with better outcomes.[201,202]

Patients with STEMI presenting at later times in the myocardial infarction evolution are much less likely to benefit from fibrinolysis. In fact, fibrinolytic therapy is generally not recommended for patients presenting between 12 and 24 hours after onset of symptoms based on the results of the LATE and EMERAS trials,[201,204] unless continuing ischemic pain is present with continuing ST-segment elevation (Class IIb, LOE B). Fibrinolytic therapy should not be administered (Class III, LOE B) to patients who present greater than 24 hours after the onset of symptoms.

### Risks of Fibrinolytic Therapy

Physicians who administer fibrinolytic agents must be aware of the indications, contraindications, benefits, and major risks of administration so that they are able to weigh the net clinical benefit for each patient (see Table 5).[203,204] This net clinical benefit requires integration of relative and absolute contraindications versus overall potential clinical gain.

Patients who present early after symptom onset with extensive ECG changes (consistent with a large AMI) and a low risk of intracranial bleeding receive the greatest benefit from fibrinolytic therapy.[190] Patients who have symptoms highly suggestive of ACS and ECG findings consistent with LBBB are also appropriate candidates for intervention because they have the highest mortality rate when LBBB is due to extensive AMI. Inferior wall STEMI also benefits from fibrinolysis, yet the magnitude of this outcome improvement is markedly less robust. More extensive inferior STEMI presentations, of course, demonstrate more robust benefit when undergoing fibrinolysis; inferior wall STEMI with RV involement is such an example. Fibrinolytics have been shown to be beneficial across a spectrum of patient subgroups with comorbidities such as previous MI, diabetes, tachycardia, and hypotension.[190] Although superior to placebo, the lack of efficacy in the setting of cardiogenic shock makes referral for PPCI an optimal strategy in this setting.

Although older patients (>75 years) have a higher risk of death, their absolute benefit appears to be similar to that of younger patients. The incidence of stroke does increase with advancing age,[205,206] reducing the relative benefit of fibrinolytic therapy. Older age is the most important baseline variable predicting nonhemorrhagic stroke.[206] Although 1 large trial reported lower early and 1-year mortality rates with accelerated administration of tissue plasminogen activator (rtPA) in patients <85 years of age,[207] a retrospective analysis found no specific survival advantage and possible risk for patients >75 years of age.[208]

### Intracranial Hemorrhage

Fibrinolytic therapy is associated with a small but definite increase in the risk of hemorrhagic stroke, which contributes to increased mortality.[190] More intensive fibrinolytic regimens using rtPA (alteplase) and heparin pose a greater risk than streptokinase and aspirin.[200,209] Clinical factors that may help risk-stratify patients at the time of presentation are age (≥65 years), low body weight (<70 kg), hypertension on presentation (>180/110 mm Hg), and use of rtPA. The number of risk factors can be used to estimate the frequency of stroke, which ranges from 0.25% with no risk factors to 2.5% with 3 risk factors.[204] Several risk factor estimates are available for use by clinicians, including Simoons,[204] the Co-Operative Cardiovascular Project,[210] and the In-Time 2 trial.[211]

### Percutaneous Coronary Intervention (PCI)

Coronary angioplasty with or without stent placement is the treatment of choice for the management of STEMI when it can be performed effectively with a door-to-balloon time <90 minutes by a skilled provider (performing >75 PCIs per year) at a skilled PCI facility (performing >200 PCIs annually, of which at least 36 are primary PCI for STEMI) (Class I, LOE A).[2,212,213] PPCI may also be offered to patients presenting to non-PCI centers when prompt transfer can result in an effective ballon time of <90 minutes from first medical contact as a systems goal.[214] The TRANSFER AMI trial supports the transfer of high-risk patients who receive fibrinolysis in a non-PCI center to a PCI center within 6 hours of presentation to receive routine early PCI.[87]

### PCI Following ROSC After Cardiac Arrest

Each year in the United States, 236 000 to 325 000 patients experience out-of-hospital cardiac arrest, and the prognosis is generally grim with a median survival to discharge rate of only 8.4%.[215] Large variations in outcome have been observed across EMS systems, and this has resulted in a call for regionalization of care with a goal to optimize the utilization of proven beneficial therapies and interventions.[216] Despite the lack of data from RCTs in this situation, the performance of PCI has been associated with favorable outcomes in this setting and is supported by the observation that following early angiography, half of the studied population is noted to have an acute coronary occlusion.[217] The data are strongest for patients with out-of-hospital cardiac arrest due to VF in the setting of STEMI (or new or presumably new LBBB), and emergent angiography with prompt recanalization of the infarct-related artery is recommended (Class I, LOE B). PPCI also appears applicable in the setting of NSTEMI subjects in whom emergent revascularization may result in hemodynamic and electric stability. PPCI after ROSC in subjects with arrest of presumed ischemic cardiac etiology may be reasonable, even in the absence of a clearly defined STEMI (Class IIb, LOE B).

There is concern that the poor prognosis for out-of-hospital cardiac arrest will prove detrimental to the public perception and reputation of interventional programs dedicated to treating patients following ROSC because of poorer outcome that could adversely affect mortality data for PCI programs. As a result, the AHA policy statement strongly supports a mechanism to report PCI outcomes for out-of-hospital cardiac arrest separate from PCI outcomes following STEMI, as this will remove potential barriers for interventional cardiologists to actively participate in the care of this population.[216] In contrast to PCI, randomized control trials of acute reperfusion therapy using fibrinolytic agents have been performed in subjects with out-of-hospital cardiac arrest without a favorable outcome.[218,219]

A 12-lead ECG should be performed as soon as possible after ROSC. Clinical findings of coma in patients prior to PCI are commonly present in patients with out-of-hospital cardiac arrest, and should not be a contraindication to consider immediate angiography and PCI. It is reasonable to include cardiac catheterization and coronary angiography in standardized post–cardiac arrest protocols as part of an overall strategy to improve neurologically intact survival in this patient group (Class IIa, LOE B) and appropriate treatment of ACS or STEMI, including PCI or fibrinolysis, should be initiated regardless of coma (Class I, LOE B). Angiography and/or PCI need not preclude or delay other therapeutic strategies including therapeutic hypothermia (Class IIa, LOE B).

Cardiac angiography and PCI, when used as part of a standardized advanced post–cardiac arrest protocol, may result in improved survival to hospital discharge.[220] Acute coronary artery occlusion is frequent in survivors of out-of-hospital cardiac arrest. PCI is feasible following ROSC, and almost 50% of cardiac arrest survivors have an acute thrombotic occlusion, or culprit lesion, that is amenable to reperfusion.[217,221–235] In addition, successful PCI can result in improved cardiac ejection fraction and survival.[217] Cardiac catheterization alone (without PCI) has been associated with improved neurologically intact survival.[235] Although coronary artery occlusion after cardiac arrest is associated with ST elevation or LBBB, specific ECG findings may also be conspicuously absent.[217,235]

Outcomes after angiography and PCI vary considerably depending on patient subsets. Survival in post–cardiac arrest patients with STEMI is as high as 70% to almost 100% with shorter durations of witnessed arrest due to VF.[221,223] A significant number of eventual survivors may initially be comatose before PCI.[221]

A 12-lead ECG should be performed as soon as possible after ROSC (Class I, LOE A). Appropriate treatment of ACS or STEMI, including PCI or fibrinolysis, should be initiated regardless of coma (Class I, LOE B). Coma and the use of induced hypothermia are not contraindications or reasons to delay PCI or fibrinolysis.

### PCI Versus Fibrinolytic Therapy

For patients admitted to hospitals with PCI facilities, PPCI confers clinical benefit as compared to fibrinolysis (both in terms of death and reinfarction or stroke) for the majority of patients.[189,236] There is scant evidence for incremental benefit of PCI over fibrinolysis for specific subgroups such as post-CABG patients[235] or patients with renal failure.[238]

PCI is the preferred reperfusion strategy in the STEMI patient who can arrive in the catheterization laboratory with ballon inflation within 90 minutes of initial hospital arrival. As a system goal, PCI should ideally be performed within 90 minutes of first medical contact. PCI should be performed by an experienced provider (an individual who performs >75 PCI procedures per year) in a high-volume center (a laboratory that performs more than 200 PCI procedures per year, of which at least 36 are PCI for STEMI). High-risk STEMI patients, "late presenters" (ie, >3 hours since the onset of STEMI symptoms), and individuals with contraindication to fibrinolysis are all candidates for PCI as well. And, of course, if the diagnosis of STEMI is in doubt, regardless of the reason, initial coronary angiography followed by PCI is the most appropriate diagnostic and therapeutic strategy.

Although PCI may offer an improved outcome over fibrinolysis, catheter-based techniques must be applied early without prolonged delay. If applied without delay by experienced providers, PCI provides improved outcome in the STEMI patient. As noted in the DANAMI-2 study,[239] PCI initiated within 3 hours of initial hospital arrival was superior to fibrinolysis. For patients admitted in hospital without PCI capabilities, there may be some benefit associated with transferring patients for PPCI versus on-site fibrinolytics in terms of reinfarction, stroke and a trend to a lower mortality in the PPCI group.[214,240] For patients with cardiogenic shock, early revascularization was associated with improved survival at six months, especially in patients younger than 75 years-of-age.[241] Transfer for PCI instead of more immediate fibrinolysis has shown the combined rate of death, nonfatal MI, and stroke to be reduced by 42% if the mean transfer to PCI time could be less than 80 to 122 minutes.

If the time required to mobilize staff and arrange for PCI is prolonged or delays in transfer are anticipated, the treating physician must consider fibrinolysis, assuming that the patient is an appropriate candidate. Time delays to PCI range from 45 to 120 minutes and are associated with age, symptom duration, and location of infarction. These delays may negate the benefit of PCI over fibrinolytics.[86,242] In addition, the benefit of PCI over fibrinolytics is offset when PCI is carried out in low-volume PCI centers.[212] PCI has been shown to be superior to fibrinolysis on the combined end points of short-term death, nonfatal myocardial infarction, and stroke.

Pinto and colleagues[86] have performed a very important analysis of the "PCI versus fibrinolysis" consideration in the STEMI patient. Their analysis asked the following questions for the patient with STEMI: How long should the practitioner wait for PCI in a patient who is fibrinolytic eligible? And, in this waiting period for PCI, when is the benefit of the catheter-based therapy lost and fibrinolysis becomes the preferred option? Time recommendations—essentially the answer to the above questions—are provided with respect to patient age, infarct duration, and MI anatomic location. This paper provides the emergency physician with the total elapsed time that he or she should wait for PCI, at which point the survival benefit of the invasive strategy is lost and the patient should receive a fibrinolytic agent. These times include the following:

- For patients presenting within 2 hours of symptom onset: 94 minutes
- For patients presenting beyond 2 hours of symptom onset: 190 minutes
- For patients less than 65 years of age: 71 minutes
- For patients greater than 65 years of age: 155 minutes
- Anterior STEMI: 115 minutes
- Nonanterior STEMI: 112 minutes

Further analysis combined commonly encountered clinical variables in typical STEMI presentations:

- Patient presentation within 2 hours of symptom onset and

    —anterior STEMI with age <65 years: 40 minutes
    —anterior STEMI with age >65 years: 107 minutes
    —non-anterior STEMI with age <65 years: 58 minutes
    —non-anterior STEMI with age >65 years: 168 minutes

- Patient presentation beyond 2 hours of symptom onset and

    —anterior STEMI with age <65 years: 43 minutes
    —anterior STEMI with age >65 years: 148 minutes
    —nonanterior STEMI with age <65 years: 103 minutes
    —nonanterior STEMI with age >65 years: 179 minutes

Post hoc analysis and theoretical constructs have addressed the time delay that mitigates the benefit of PPCI as compared to fibrinolytic therapy in the absence of randomized trials. The time delay has been analyzed to be between 60 and 120 minutes.[86,243–243b] Taking these into consideration, the recent European Society of Cardiology recommendation extended the time delay indicating that PPCI should be performed within 2 hours from first medical contact except in those

patients with a large amount of myocardium is at risk (maximum delay of 90 minutes).[242c] The ACC AHA 2009 Focused STEMI Writing Group noted, "There has been discussion about whether the recommended door-to-balloon time (or first medical contact to balloon time) should be greater than 90 minutes. However, the writing group continues to believe that the focus should be on developing systems of care to increase the number of patients with timely access to PCI rather than extending the acceptable window for door-to-balloon time."[1]

Delays to reperfusion therapy are not without negative consequence as noted in a subset of patients in the GRACE (Global Registry of Acute Coronary Events) database. The authors of this registry examined the outcome impact of treatment delays on STEMI patients receiving reperfusion therapy. This study involved 3959 patients from 106 hospitals in 14 countries who presented within 6 hours of chest pain onset and underwent either PCI (55%) or fibrinolysis (45%). Delays in reperfusion were associated with increased mortality for both treatment strategies, yet were more pronounced in those patients receiving fibrinolysis.[243d]

A cooperative and interdisciplinary effort between emergency medicine and cardiology, as well as among the EMS agencies, the catheterization laboratory, and the CCU, has the potential to reduce markedly the door-to-therapy time in STEMI patients and therefore limit delays in providing this time-sensitive treatment. Prior agreement between the ED and cardiovascular physicians at institutions with invasive capability must be obtained so that consideration of PCI does not introduce further delays in fibrinolytic drug administration; such cooperation can limit additional delays in the administration of fibrinolytic agents in patients who are considered for PCI in AMI.

A systems of care approach involving a reperfusion team or "STEMI alert" system mobilizes hospital-based resources, optimizing the approach to the patient. This system, whether activated by data gathered in the ED or prehospital-based information, has the potential to offer time-sensitive therapies in a rapid fashion to these ill patients.

In summary, for patients presenting within 12 hours of symptom onset and electrocardiographic findings consistent with STEMI, reperfusion should be initiated as soon as possible – independent of the method chosen (Class I, LOE A). Primary PCI performed at a high-volume center within 90 minutes of first medical contact by an experienced operator that maintains an appropriate expert status is reasonable, as it improves morbidity and mortality as compared with immediate fibrinolysis (<30 minutes door-to-needle) (Class I, LOE A). If PCI cannot be accomplished within 90 minutes of first medical contact, independent of the need for emergent transfer, then fibrinolysis is recommended, assuming the patient lacks contraindications to such therapy (Class I, LOE B). For those patients with a contraindication to fibrinolysis, PCI is recommended despite the delay, rather than foregoing reperfusion therapy (Class I, LOE A). For those STEMI patients presenting in shock, PCI (or CABG) is the preferred reperfusion treatment. Fibrinolysis should only be considered in consultation with the cardiologist if there is a substantial delay to PCI.

## Complicated AMI

### Cardiogenic Shock, LV Failure, and Congestive Heart Failure

Infarction of ≥40% of the LV myocardium usually results in cardiogenic shock and carries a high mortality rate. Of those who developed shock,[244] patients with ST-segment elevation developed shock significantly earlier than patients without ST-segment elevation. Cardiogenic shock and congestive heart failure are not contraindications to fibrinolysis, but PCI is preferred if the patient is at a facility with PCI capabilities. Based on the results of the SHOCK trial ACC/AHA guidelines note that PPCI is reasonable in those who develop shock within 36 hours of symptom onset and who are suitable candidates for revascularization that can be performed within 18 hours of the onset of shock.[3] Although the benefits in the SHOCK trial were observed only in patients ≤75 years of age, selected elderly patients also appear to benefit from this strategy. The guidelines also support the use of hemodynamic support with intra-aortic balloon counterpulsation (IABP) in this setting as part of aggressive medical treatment. The IABP works synergistically with fibrinolytic agents in this setting, and the benefits observed with early revascularization strategy in the SHOCK trial were also obtained in the setting of IABP support. The use of PPCI for patients with cardiogenic shock has increased over time and contributes to the observed decrease in hospital mortality.[245,246] The majority of survivors following cardiogenic shock experience a good quality of life, and the early mortality benefit with revascularization is sustained over time.[247–249] In hospitals without PCI facilities, fibrinolytic administration needs to be considered with prompt transfer to a tertiary care facility where adjunct PCI can be performed if cardiogenic shock or ongoing ischemia ensues.[250] The ACC/AHA STEMI guidelines recommend a door-to-departure time of ≤30 minutes for transfer to a PCI-capable center.[3]

### RV Infarction

RV infarction or ischemia may occur in up to 50% of patients with inferior wall MI. The clinician should suspect RV infarction in patients with inferior wall infarction, hypotension, and clear lung fields. In patients with inferior wall infarction, obtain an ECG with right-sided leads. ST-segment elevation (>1 mm) in lead V4R is sensitive (sensitivity, 88%; specificity, 78%; diagnostic accuracy, 83%) for RV infarction and is a strong predictor of increased in-hospital complications and mortality.[251]

The in-hospital mortality rate of patients with RV dysfunction is 25% to 30%, and these patients should be routinely considered for reperfusion therapy. Fibrinolytic therapy reduces the incidence of RV dysfunction.[252] Similarly PCI is an alternative for patients with RV infarction and is preferred for patients in shock. Patients with shock caused by RV failure have a mortality rate similar to that for patients with shock due to LV failure.

Patients with RV dysfunction and acute infarction are dependent on maintenance of RV "filling" pressure (RV end-diastolic pressure) to maintain cardiac output.[253] Thus, nitrates, diuretics, and other vasodilators (ACE inhibitors) should be avoided because severe hypotension may result. Hypotension is initially treated with an IV fluid bolus.

## Adjunctive Therapies for ACS and AMI

### Thienopyridines

#### Clopidogrel

Clopidogrel is an oral thienopyridine prodrug that irreversibly inhibits the adenosine diphosphate receptor on the platelet, resulting in a reduction in platelet aggregation through a different mechanism than aspirin. Since the publication of the *2005 AHA Guidelines,* several important clopidogrel studies have been published that document its efficacy for patients with both NSTEMI and STEMI.

There is a reduction in combined event rate (cardiovascular mortality, nonfatal infarction, and nonfatal stroke) and/or mortality; with a resultant small increase in major bleeding when clopidogrel is administered by providers in the ED or in hospital to patients with NSTEMI ACS.[254–256] Patients with ACS and a rise in cardiac biomarkers or ECG changes consistent with ischemia had reduced stroke and major adverse cardiac events if clopidogrel was added to aspirin and heparin within 4 hours of hospital presentation.[257] Clopidogrel given 6 hours or more before elective PCI for patients with ACS without ST elevation reduces adverse ischemic events at 28 days.[258]

The Clopidogrel in Unstable angina to prevent Recurrent ischemic Events (CURE) trial documented an increased rate of bleeding (but not intracranial hemorrhage) in the 2072 patients undergoing CABG within 5 to 7 days of administration.[259] Although a posthoc analysis of this trial reported a trend toward life-threatening bleeding[257]and a prospective study failed to show increased bleeding in 1366 patients undergoing CABG,[260] a subsequent risk-to-benefit ratio analysis concluded that the bleeding risk with clopidogrel in patients undergoing CABG was modest. The use of clopidogrel in ACS patients with a high likelihood of needing CABG requires weighing the risk of bleeding if given against the potential for perioperative ACS events if withheld. The current ACC/AHA guidelines recommend withholding clopidogrel for 5 to 7 days in patients for whom CABG is anticipated.

In patients up to 75 years of age with STEMI managed by fibrinolysis, a consistent improvement in combined event rate (cardiovascular mortality, nonfatal infarction, and nonfatal stroke) and/or mortality, with a resultant small increase in major bleeding, is observed when clopidogrel, in a 300-mg loading dose, was administered in addition to aspirin and heparin (low-molecular-weight heparin [LMWH] or unfractionated heparin [UFH]), at the time of initial management (followed by a 75 mg daily dose for up to 8 days in hospital).[260–265]

In patients with STEMI managed with PPCI, there is a reduction in combined event rate (cardiovascular mortality, nonfatal infarction, and nonfatal stroke) and/or mortality with a resultant small increase in major bleeding when clopidogrel is administered by ED, hospital, or prehospital providers.[261,264–267]

On the basis of these findings, providers should administer a loading dose of clopidogrel in addition to standard care (aspirin, anticoagulants, and reperfusion) for patients determined to have moderate- to high-risk non-ST-segment elevation ACS and STEMI (Class I, LOE A).[257] In patients <75 years of age a loading dose of clopidogrel 300 to 600 mg with non-STE ACS and STEMI, regardless of approach to management, is recommended. It is reasonable to administer a 300-mg oral dose of clopidogrel to ED patients with suspected ACS (without ECG or cardiac marker changes) who are unable to take aspirin because of hypersensitivity or major gastrointestinal intolerance (Class IIa, LOE B). Providers should administer a 300-mg oral dose of clopidogrel to ED patients up to 75 years of age with STEMI who receive aspirin, heparin, and fibrinolysis (Class I, LOE B). There is little evidence on the use of a loading dose of clopidogrel in patients aged ≥75 years of age with NSTEMI and STEMI treated by PPCI, and patients >75 years of age were excluded in the studies on STEMI treated by fibrinolysis, therefore the ideal dose of clopidogrel in patients over 75 years of age has yet to be delineated. In the ED the choice of immediate antiplatelet therapy (as well as protocols for STEMI and NSTEMI) should be guided by local interdisciplinary review of ongoing clinical trials, guidelines, and recommendations.

### Prasugrel

Prasugrel is an oral thienopyridine prodrug that irreversibly binds to the ADP receptor to inhibit platelet aggregation. Prasugrel may be associated with a reduction in combined event rate (cardiovascular mortality, nonfatal infarction, and nonfatal stroke) with no benefit in mortality compared to clopidogrel but with an overall resultant increase in major bleeding (as compared to clopidogrel) when administered after angiography to patients with NSTEMI undergoing PCI.[268–272] Risk factors associated with a higher rate of bleeding with prasugrel use are age ≥75 years, previous stroke or TIA, and body weight less than 60 kg.

Small improvements in combined event rate (cardiovascular mortality, nonfatal infarction, and nonfatal stroke) and/or mortality are observed when prasugrel (compared to clopidogrel) is administered before or after angiography to patients with NSTEMI and STEMI managed with PCI.[268–271,273,274]

Prasugrel (60 mg oral loading dose) may be substituted for clopidogrel after angiography in patients determined to have non-ST-segment elevation ACS or STEMI who are more than 12 hours after symptom onset prior to planned PCI (Class IIa, LOE B). There is no direct evidence for the use of prasugrel in the ED or prehospital settings. In patients who are not at high risk for bleeding, administration of prasugrel (60-mg oral loading dose) prior to angiography in patients determined to have STEMI ≤12 hours after the initial symptoms may be substituted for administration of clopidogrel (Class IIa, LOE B). Prasugrel is not recommended in STEMI patients managed with fibrinolysis or NSTEMI patients before angiography.

### Glycoprotein IIb/IIIa Inhibitors

The use and efficacy of glycoprotein IIb/IIIa receptor inhibitors for treatment of patients with UA/NSTEMI has been well established.[274–279] These trials were conducted prior to contemporary conservative and invasive strategies, and ongoing questions have been investigated concerning their timing (eg, upsteam initiation) and use combined with other contemporary agents (eg, clopidogrel).

Two recent studies do not support the *routine* use of upstream GP IIb/IIIa inhibitors.[280,281] Other studies have documented benefit largely in patients who have elevated cardiac troponin and a planned invasive strategy or specific subsets such as those patients with diabetes or significant ST-segment depression on the presenting ECG.[282–286] The current evidence supports a selective strategy for the use of GP IIb/IIIa inhibitors in the use of dual platelet inhibitor treatment of patients with planned invasive strategy taking into consideration the ACS risk of the patient and weighing this against the potential bleeding risk. There is no current evidence supporting the routine use of GP IIb/ IIIa inhibitor therapy prior to angiography in patients with STEMI and use of these agents upstream is uncertain. Use of GP IIb/ IIIa inhibitors should be guided by local interdisciplinary review of ongoing clinical trials, guidelines, and recommendations.

### β-Adrenergic Receptor Blockers

Controversy surrounds the administration of β-adrenergic receptor blockers in the setting of ACS. Several studies have shown reduced mortality[287,288] and decreased infarct size[289–291] with early IV β-blocker use. Early β-blocker administration may help prevent dangerous arrhythmias[288,290,292,293] and reduce reinfarction, but there is an increased incidence of cardiogenic shock.

Recent evidence shows no particular benefit to the IV administration of β-blockers on either mortality, infarct size, prevention of arrhythmias, or reinfarction[294–301] There may be, however, a statistically significant short-term benefit to 6-week mortality when IV β-blockers were given to low-risk (ie, Killip Class I) patients. [296] IV β-blockers may also be beneficial for NSTEMI. One study[302] suggested that the earlier the IV β-blockers were administered, the greater the effect seen on infarct size and mortality. Of note, none of the papers reviewed showed that β-blockers caused irreversible harm when given early in the development of suspected ACS. Balancing the evidence overall for non-ST-segment elevation ACS patients, current ACC/AHA Guidelines recommend β-blockers be initiated orally within the first 24 hours after hospitalization.[3]

Contraindications to β-blockers are moderate to severe LV failure and pulmonary edema, bradycardia (<60 bpm), hypotension (SBP <100 mm Hg), signs of poor peripheral perfusion, second-degree or third-degree heart block, or reactive airway disease. Studies of β-blockers varied significantly in the treatment times used, with no high quality papers studying the administration of β-blockers in the prehospital setting or in the very early ED setting (ie, within the first hour of a suspected ACS).

For patients with ACS, there is no evidence to support the routine administration of IV β-blockers in the prehospital setting or during initial assessment in the ED. IV β-blocker therapy may be considered as reasonable in specific situations such as severe hypertension or tachyarrhythmias in patients without contraindications (Class IIa, LOE B). In the absence of contraindications, PO β-blockers should be administered within the first 24 hours to patients with suspected ACS (Class 1, LOE A). Patients with initial contraindications should be re-evaluated periodically. It is reasonable to start oral β-blockers with low doses after the patient is stabilized prior to discharge (Class IIa, LOE B).

## Heparins

Heparin is an indirect inhibitor of thrombin that has been widely used in ACS as adjunctive therapy for fibrinolysis and in combination with aspirin and other platelet inhibitors for the treatment of non-ST-segment elevation ACS. UFH has several disadvantages, including (1) the need for IV administration; (2) the requirement for frequent monitoring of the activated partial thromboplastin time (aPTT); (3) an unpredictable anticoagulant response in individual patients; and (4) heparin can also stimulate platelet activation, causing thrombocytopenia. Because of the limitations of heparin, newer preparations of LMWH have been developed.

### Unfractionated Heparin Versus Low-Molecular-Weight Heparin in UA/NSTEMI

#### Enoxaparin
Eleven in-hospital randomized clinical trials,[303–313] and additional studies (including 7 meta-analyses)[314–320] document similar or improved composite outcomes (death, MI, and/or recurrent angina or recurrent ischemia or revascularization) when enoxaparin was administered instead of UFH to patients with non-ST-segment elevation ACS with an increase in the proportion of patients with minor bleeding complications.

#### Fondaparinux
There was similar[321–323] or improved[324,325] outcomes of combined end points (death, MI, urgent revascularization) without increased bleeding when fondaparinux was administered in-hospital rather than UFH in patients with non-ST-segment elevation ACS. Fondaparinux was associated with increased risk of catheter thrombosis in PCI.[324]

#### Bivalirudin
No benefit in combined outcome was observed when bivalirudin was administered in hospital compared to UFH in patients with non-ST-segment elevation ACS, however less bleeding was observed with bivalirudin and no renal dosing is required.[326–329]

### Treatment Recommendations for UA/NSTEMI
For in-hospital patients with NSTEMI managed with a planned initial conservative approach, either fondaparinux (Class IIa, LOE B) or enoxaparin (Class IIa, LOE A) are reasonable alternatives to UFH or placebo. For in-hospital patients with NSTEMI managed with a planned invasive approach, either enoxaparin or UFH are reasonable choices (Class IIa, LOE A). Fondaparinux may be used in the setting of PCI, but requires co-administration of UFH and does not appear to offer an advantage over UFH alone (Class IIb, LOE A). For in-hospital patients with NSTEMI and renal insufficiency, bivalirudin or UFH may be considered (Class IIb, LOE A). For in-hospital patients with NSTEMI and increased bleeding risk, where anticoagulant therapy is not contraindicated, fondaparinux (Class IIa, LOE B) or bivalirudin (Class IIa, LOE A) are reasonable and UFH may be considered (Class IIb, LOE C) There is no specific evidence for or against anticoagulant use in NSTEMI in the prehospital setting.

### Unfractionated Heparin Versus Low-Molecular-Weight Heparin With Fibrinolysis in STEMI
Nine randomized clinical trials[320,331–338] and additional studies (including one meta-analyses)[339] document similar or improved composite outcomes (death, MI, and/or recurrent angina or recurrent ischemia or revascularization) when enoxaparin was administered instead of UFH to patients with STEMI undergoing fibrinolysis. This must be balanced against an increase in intracranial hemorrhage in patients >75 years of age who received enoxaparin documented in one of these randomized controlled trials.[338]

One randomized clinical trial[340] demonstrated superiority in clinical outcomes when fondaparinux was compared to UFH in patients treated with fibrinolysis.

There is insufficient evidence to provide a recommendation on bivalirudin, nadroparin, reviparin, or parnaparin for use in STEMI patients undergoing fibrinolysis.

#### Enoxaparin
For patients with STEMI managed with fibrinolysis in the hospital, it is reasonable to administer enoxaparin instead of UFH (Class IIa, LOE A). In addition, for prehospital patients with STEMI managed with fibrinolysis, adjunctive enoxaparin instead of UFH may be considered (Class IIb, LOE A). Patients initially treated with enoxaparin should not be switched to UFH and vice versa because of increased risk of bleeding (Class III, LOE C).[341] In younger patients <75 years the initial dose of enoxaparin is 30 mg IV bolus followed by 1 mg/kg SC every 12 hours (first SC dose shortly after the IV bolus) (Class IIb, LOE A). Patients ≥75 years may be treated with 0.75 mg/kg SC enoxaparin every 12 hours without an initial IV bolus (Class IIb, LOE B). Patients with impaired renal function (creatinine clearance <30 mL/min) may be given 1 mg/kg enoxaparin SC once daily (Class IIb, LOE B). Patients with known impaired renal function may alternatively be managed with UFH (Class IIb, LOE B).

#### Fondaparinux
Fondaparinux (initially 2.5 mg IV followed by 2.5 mg SC once daily) may be considered in the hospital for patients treated specifically with non-fibrin-specific thrombolytics (ie, streptokinase), provided the creatinine is <3 mg/dL (Class IIb, LOE B).

There are insufficient data to recommend other LMWH or bivalirudin over UFH in patients treated with fibrinolysis in STEMI.

### Unfractionated Heparin Versus Low-Molecular-Weight Heparin With PPCI in STEMI

Two registry studies[342,343] and other studies demonstrated similar or improved outcomes when enoxaparin was compared to UFH in patients undergoing PPCI combined with a GP IIb/IIIa antagonist and thienopyridine inhibitor.

One large clinical trial[340] demonstrated better outcomes in terms of acute cardiac events and bleeding using fondaparinux and PPCI. Thrombus formation on catheter material in patients on fondaparinux, however, required the addition of UFH during PCI.[324]

Two large randomized clinical trials resulted in less bleeding and a short- and long-term reduction in cardiac events and overall mortality with bivalirudin compared to UFH plus a glycoprotein inhibitor in patients with STEMI and PPCI.[344,345]

For patients with STEMI undergoing contemporary PCI (ie, additional broad use of glycoprotein IIb/IIIa inhibitors and a thienopyridine) enoxaparin may be considered a safe and effective alternative to UFH (Class IIb, LOE B). Patients initially treated with enoxaparin should not be switched to UFH and vice versa to avoid increased risk of bleeding. Fondaparinux may be considered as an alternative to UFH, however, there is an increased risk of catheter thrombi with fondaparinux alone. Additional UFH (50 to 100 U/kg bolus) may help to avoid this complication (Class IIb, LOE B), but using these two agents is not recommended over UFH alone. For fondaparinux and enoxaparin it is necessary to adjust the dose in patients with renal impairment. Bivalirudin may be considered as an alternative to UFH and GP IIb/IIIa inhibitors (Class IIb, LOE A).

## Calcium Channel Blockers

There is little evidence that calcium channel blocking agents can be safely used as an alternative or additional therapy to β-blockers when the later are contraindicated or their maximum dose has been achieved.

Calcium channel blocking agents have not been shown to reduce mortality after acute MI, and in certain patients with cardiovascular disease there are data to suggest that they are harmful. β-blockers have been used much more boadly, have a much safer profile, and appear to be a more appropriate choice for patients presenting with myocardial infarction compared to calcium channel blockers.

## ACE Inhibitor Therapy

### ACE Inhibitors and ARBs in the Hospital

ACE inhibitor therapy has improved survival rates in patients with AMI, particularly when started early after the initial hospitalization.[183,346–349] Evidence from 7 large clinical trials,[183,346–351] 2 meta-analyses,[352,353] and 10 minor trials[348,351,354–362] documents consistent improvement in mortality when oral ACE inhibitors are administered in the hospital setting to patients with AMI with or without early reperfusion therapy. In these studies ACE inhibitors were not administered in the presence of hypotension (SBP <100 mm Hg or ≥30 mm Hg below baseline). *The beneficial effects are most pronounced in patients with anterior infarction, pulmonary congestion, or LV ejection fraction <40%.*

Administration of an oral ACE inhibitor is recommended within the first 24 hours after onset of symptoms in STEMI patients with pulmonary congestion or LV ejection fraction <40%, in the absence of hypotension (SBP <100 mm Hg or ≥30 mm Hg below baseline) (Class I, LOE A). Oral ACE inhibitor therapy can also be useful for all other patients with AMI with or without early reperfusion therapy (Class IIa, LOE B). IV administration of ACE inhibitors is contraindicated in the first 24 hours because of risk of hypotension (Class III, LOE C).

### ACE Inhibitors in the Prehospital Setting

Despite multiple studies that have shown a benefit of ACE inhibitors and ARBs in patients with a myocardial infarction when therapy is started during the first 24 hours of the index hospitalization, no trial specifically evaluates patients in the ED or prehospital settings. An older randomized trial showed a reduction in mortality with an increased risk of hypotension in patients treated soon after presentation in the inpatient setting.[183] Several trials showed a reduction in the rate of heart failure and mortality in patients treated soon after fibrinolysis,[363–365] and several others showed no benefit with the early or prehospital use of angiotensin converting enzyme.[364,366,367]

In conclusion, although ACE inhibitors and ARBs have been shown to reduce long-term risk of mortality in patients suffering an AMI, there is insufficient evidence to support the routine initiation of ACE inhibitors and ARBs in the prehospital or ED setting (Class IIb, LOE C).

## HMG Coenzyme A Reductase Inhibitors (Statins)

A variety of studies documented consistent reduction in indicators of inflammation and complications such as reinfarction, recurrent angina, and arrhythmias when statin treatment is administered within a few days after onset of an ACS.[368–371] There is little data to suggest that this therapy should be initiated within the ED; however, early initiation (within 24 hours of presentation) of statin therapy is recommended in patients with an ACS or AMI (Class I, LOE C). If patients are already on statin therapy, continue the therapy (Class IIb, LOE C).

An increase in short-term mortality and incidence of major adverse cardiac events have been reported with discontinuation of statin treatment in ACS patients at hospital admission. Statins should not be discontinued during the index hospitalization unless contraindicated (Class III, LOE C).[372–381]

Pretreatment with statins in patients undergoing elective percutaneous angioplasty for stable angina or hemodynamicaly stable ACS has been shown to significantly reduce biomarkers of myocardial necrosis or inflammation compared to placebo when given between 3 and 7 days prior to the procedure.[382,383]

Furthermore, pretreatment with atorvastatin 80 mg 12 hours before and an additional 40 mg immediately before PCI for NSTEMI or documented ischemia has been shown to significanty decrease the 30 day composite of death, MI, and unplanned revascularization compared to placebo in a prospective randomized trial. There were no deaths in any of the two groups and the primary end point was driven by periprocedural myocardial infarction in concordance to the previously published studies.[384]

In conclusion, intensive (target LDL values optimally <70 mg/dL) statin treatment should be initiated within the first 24 hours after onset of an ACS event (eg, immediately after hospital admission) in all patients presenting with any form of ACS unless strictly contraindicated (eg, by proven intolerance) (Class I, LOE A).

It is reasonable to use statin pretreatment for patients who will be undergoing elective or urgent angioplasty in order to decrease perioperative myocardial infarction. There are no reports on risk or safety considerations of early initiation of statin treatment in ACS.

### Glucose-Insulin-Potassium

Although glucose-insulin-potassium (GIK) therapy was formerly thought to reduce the chance of mortality during AMI by several mechanisms, recent clinical trials found that GIK did not show any benefit in STEMI.[385,386] At this time there is little evidence to suggest that this intervention is helpful (Class IIb, LOE C).

## Management of Arrhythmias

This section discusses management of arrhythmias during acute ischemia and infarction.

### Ventricular Rhythm Disturbances

Treatment of ventricular arrhythmias during and after AMI has been a controversial topic for three decades. Primary VF accounts for the majority of early deaths during AMI.[387–389] The incidence of primary VF is highest during the first 4 hours after onset of symptoms[28,390–392] but remains an important contributor to mortality during the first 24 hours. Secondary VF occurring in the setting of CHF or cardiogenic shock can also contribute to death from AMI. VF is a less common cause of death in the hospital setting with the use of fibrinolytics and percutaneous revascularization as early reperfusion strategies. Broad use of $\beta$-blockers also contributes significantly in the reduction of VF incidence in the after AMI.

Although prophylaxis with lidocaine reduces the incidence of VF, an analysis of data from ISIS-3 and a meta-analysis suggest that lidocaine increased all-cause mortality rates.[393] Thus, the practice of prophylactic administration of lidocaine is not recommended (Class III, LOE A).

Sotalol has not been adequately studied (Class IIb, LOE C).

Amiodarone in a single RCT did not appear to improve survival in low doses and may increase mortality in high doses when used early in patients with suspected myocardial infarction (Class IIb, LOE C).[394]

Twenty published studies including 14 RCTs and 4 meta-analyses/reviews provide no good evidence that prophylactic antiarrhythmics improve outcomes (survival to discharge, 30/60 day mortality) and despite a documented decrease in the incidence of malignant ventricular arrhythmias, they may cause harm. Therefore prophylactic antiarrhythmics are not recommended for patients with suspected ACS or myocardial infarction in the prehospital or ED (Class III, LOE A).

Routine IV administration of $\beta$-blockers to patients without hemodynamic or electric contraindications is associated with a reduced incidence of primary VF (Class IIb, LOE C).

Low serum potassium, but not magnesium, has been associated with ventricular arrhythmias. It is prudent clinical practice to maintain serum potassium >4 mEq/L and magnesium >2 mEq/L (Class IIB, LOE A).

Routine administration of magnesium to patients with MI has no significant clinical mortality benefit, particularly in patients receiving fibrinolytic therapy.[183] ISIS-4 enrolled >58 000 patients and showed a trend toward increased mortality rates when magnesium was given in-hospital for primary prophylaxis to patients within the first 4 hours of known or suspected AMI.

Following an episode of VF, there is no conclusive data to support the use of lidocaine or any particular strategy for preventing VF recurrence. Further management of ventricular rhythm disturbances is discussed in Part 8.2: "Management of Cardiac Arrest" and Part 8.3: "Management of Symptomatic Bradycardia and Tachycardia."

## Summary

There has been tremendous progress in reducing disability and death from ACS. But many patients still die before reaching the hospital because patients and family members fail to recognize the signs of ACS and fail to activate the EMS system. Once the patient with ACS contacts the healthcare system, providers must focus on support of cardiorespiratory function, rapid transport, and early classification of the patient based on ECG characteristics. Patients with STEMI require prompt reperfusion; the shorter the interval from symptom onset to reperfusion, the greater the benefit. In the STEMI population, mechanical reperfusion with percutaneous coronary intervention improves survival and decreases major cardiovascular events compared to fibrinolysis. Patients with UA/NSTEMI (non-STEMI ACS) or nonspecific or normal ECGs require risk stratification and appropriate monitoring and therapy. Healthcare providers can improve survival rates and myocardial function of patients with ACS by providing skilled, efficient, and coordinated out-of-hospital and in-hospital care.

# Disclosures

## Guidelines Part 10: ACS Writing Group Disclosures

| Writing Group Member | Employment | Research Grant | Other Research Support | Speakers' Bureau/Honoraria | Ownership Interest | Consultant/Advisory Board | Other |
|---|---|---|---|---|---|---|---|
| Robert E. O'Connor | University of Virginia Health System–Professor and Chair of Emergency Medicine | None | None | None | None | None | None |
| William Brady | University of Virginia | None | None | None | None | None | *Expert Witness: If contacted by attorneys, I will consider reviewing cases under litigation/potentially under litigation. I am not affiliated with any agency or business entity in this regard. When paid, the money is paid to my department at the University of Virginia–I can then use the money for professional issues and/or receive a certain amount in my personal pay check from the University. |
| Steven C. Brooks | University of Toronto–Clinician-Scientist | None | None | None | None | None | None |
| Deborah Diercks | University of California, Davis Medical Center–Professor of Emergency Medicine | *Collaborator on Research Grant Nanosphere and Heartscape with money going to the University | None | *Speakers Bureau for Sanofi-Aventis and Bristol Myer Squibb *Sanofi Aventis, Heartscape, Bristol Myers Squibb, and Schering Plough | None | *Scheuring Plough, Heartscape, Sanofi-Aventis | None |
| Jonathan Egan | Children's hopital at Westmead, Sydney–Paediatric Intensivist | None | None | None | None | None | None |
| Chris Ghaemmaghami | University of Virginia School of medicine Faculty Department of Emergency Medicine Associate Professor and Vice Chair | None | None | *Speaker and program chair for the 2010 national meeting of the Society of Chest Pain Centers | None | None | None |
| Venu Menon | Cleveland Clinic–Director CCU | None | None | None | None | None | None |
| Brian J. O'Neil | Wayne State, Associate Chair | †Medivance Corporation, Zoll Circulation, Heartscape Technologies | *Somanetics Corp | Speakers bureau †Sanofi- Aventis, Bristol Meyer Squibb *Glaxo-Smith Kline; Medivance Corp; Heartscape Technologies Honoraria* Heartscape Technologies | None | Advisory board- *Heartscape Technologies; *Zoll Circulation | Expert witness- *Seimien Huckabay law offices |
| Andrew H. Travers | Emergency Health Services–Provincial Medical Director; Dalhousie University–Associate Professor; QE-II Hospital–Attending Physician | None | None | None | None | None | None |
| Demetris Yannopoulos | University of Minnesota–Interventional cardiologist | None | None | None | None | None | None |

This table represents the relationships of writing group members that may be perceived as actual or reasonably perceived conflicts of interest as reported on the Disclosure Questionnaire, which all members of the writing group are required to complete and submit. A relationship is considered to be "significant" if (a) the person receives $10 000 or more during any 12-month period, or 5% or more of the person's gross income; or (b) the person owns 5% or more of the voting stock or share of the entity, or owns $10 000 or more of the fair market value of the entity. A relationship is considered to be "modest" if it is less than "significant" under the preceding definition

*Modest.

†Significant.

# References

1. Kushner FG, Hand M, Smith SC Jr, King SB III, Anderson JL, Antman EM, Bailey SR, Bates ER, Blankenship JC, Casey DE Jr, Green LA, Hochman JS, Jacobs AK, Krumholz HM, Morrison DA, Ornato JP, Pearle DL, Peterson ED, Sloan MA, Whitlow PL, Williams DO. 2009 Focused Updates: ACC/AHA Guidelines for the Management of Patients With ST-Elevation Myocardial Infarction (updating the 2004 Guideline and 2007 Focused Update) and ACC/AHA/SCAI Guidelines on Percutaneous Coronary Intervention (updating the 2005 Guideline and 2007 Focused Update): a report of the Am College of Cardiology Foundation/Am Heart Association Task Force on Practice Guidelines. *Circulation.* 2009;120:2271–2306.

2. Antman EM, Anbe DT, Armstrong PW, Bates ER, Green LA, Hand M, Hochman JS, Krumholz HM, Kushner FG, Lamas GA, Mullany CJ, Ornato JP, Pearle DL, Sloan MA, Smith SC Jr, Alpert JS, Anderson JL, Faxon DP, Fuster V, Gibbons RJ, Gregoratos G, Halperin JL, Hiratzka LF, Hunt SA, Jacobs AK. ACC/AHA guidelines for the management of patients with ST-elevation myocardial infarction–executive summary: a report of the Am College of Cardiology/Am Heart Association Task Force on Practice Guidelines (Writing Committee to Revise the 1999 Guidelines for the Management of Patients With Acute Myocardial Infarction). *Circulation.* 2004;110:588–636.

3. Anderson JL, Adams CD, Antman EM, Bridges CR, Califf RM, Casey DE Jr, Chavey WE II, Fesmire FM, Hochman JS, Levin TN, Lincoff AM, Peterson ED, Theroux P, Wenger NK, Wright RS, Smith SC Jr, Jacobs AK, Halperin JL, Hunt SA, Krumholz HM, Kushner FG, Lytle BW, Nishimura R, Ornato JP, Page RL, Riegel B. ACC/AHA 2007 guidelines for the management of patients with unstable angina/non ST-elevation myocardial infarction: a report of the Am College of Cardiology/Am Heart Association Task Force on Practice Guidelines

(Writing Committee to Revise the 2002 Guidelines for the Management of Patients With Unstable Angina/Non ST-Elevation Myocardial Infarction): developed in collaboration with the Am College of Emergency Physicians, the Society for Cardiovascular Angiography and Interventions, and the Society of Thoracic Surgeons: endorsed by the Am Association of Cardiovascular and Pulmonary Rehabilitation and the Society for Academic Emergency Medicine. *Circulation.* 2007;116: e148–e304.

4. Steg PG, Bonnefoy E, Chabaud S, Lapostolle F, Dubien PY, Cristofini P, Leizorovicz A, Touboul P. Impact of time to treatment on mortality after prehospital fibrinolysis or primary angioplasty: data from the CAPTIM randomized clinical trial. *Circulation.* 2003;108:2851–2856.

5. Nallamothu BK, Bates ER, Herrin J, Wang Y, Bradley EH, Krumholz HM. Times to treatment in transfer patients undergoing primary percutaneous coronary intervention in the United States: National Registry of Myocardial Infarction (NRMI)-3/4 analysis. *Circulation.* 2005;111: 761–767.

6. Saczynski JS, Yarzebski J, Lessard D, Spencer FA, Gurwitz JH, Gore JM, Goldberg RJ. Trends in prehospital delay in patients with acute myocardial infarction (from the Worcester Heart Attack Study). *Am J Cardiol .* 2008;102:1589–1594.

7. Lefler LL, Bondy KN. Women's delay in seeking treatment with myocardial infarction: a meta-synthesis. *J Cardiovasc Nurs.* 2004;19: 251–268.

8. McGinn AP, Rosamond WD, Goff DC Jr, Taylor HA, Miles JS, Chambless L. Trends in prehospital delay time and use of emergency medical services for acute myocardial infarction: experience in 4 US communities from 1987–2000. *Am Heart J.* 2005;150:392–400.

9. Jneid H, Fonarow GC, Cannon CP, Hernandez AF, Palacios IF, Maree AO, Wells Q, Bozkurt B, Labresh KA, Liang L, Hong Y, Newby LK, Fletcher G, Peterson E, Wexler L. Sex differences in medical care and early death after acute myocardial infarction. *Circulation.* 2008;118: 2803–2810.

10. Foraker RE, Rose KM, McGinn AP, Suchindran CM, Goff DC Jr, Whitsel EA, Wood JL, Rosamond WD. Neighborhood income, health insurance, and prehospital delay for myocardial infarction: the atherosclerosis risk in communities study. *Arch Intern Med.* 2008;168: 1874–1879.

11. Sari I, Acar Z, Ozer O, Erer B, Tekbas E, Ucer E, Genc A, Davutoglu V, Aksoy M. Factors associated with prolonged prehospital delay in patients with acute myocardial infarction. *Turk Kardiyol Dern Ars.* 2008;36:156–162.

12. Gibler WB, Armstrong PW, Ohman EM, Weaver WD, Stebbins AL, Gore JM, Newby LK, Califf RM, Topol EJ. Persistence of delays in presentation and treatment for patients with acute myocardial infarction: The GUSTO-I and GUSTO-III experience. *Ann Emerg Med.* 2002;39: 123–130.

13. Mehta RH, Bufalino VJ, Pan W, Hernandez AF, Cannon CP, Fonarow GC, Peterson ED. Achieving rapid reperfusion with primary percutaneous coronary intervention remains a challenge: insights from Am Heart Association's Get With the Guidelines program. *Am Heart J.* 2008;155: 1059–1067.

14. Rathore SS, Curtis JP, Chen J, Wang Y, Nallamothu BK, Epstein AJ, Krumholz HM. Association of door-to-balloon time and mortality in patients admitted to hospital with ST elevation myocardial infarction: national cohort study. *BMJ.* 2009;338:b1807.

15. Song YB, Hahn JY, Gwon HC, Kim JH, Lee SH, Jeong MH. The impact of initial treatment delay using primary angioplasty on mortality among patients with acute myocardial infarction: from the Korea acute myocardial infarction registry. *J Korean Med Sci.* 2008;23:357–364.

16. Moser DK, Kimble LP, Alberts MJ, Alonzo A, Croft JB, Dracup K, Evenson KR, Go AS, Hand MM, Kothari RU, Mensah GA, Morris DL, Pancioli AM, Riegel B, Zerwic JJ. Reducing delay in seeking treatment by patients with acute coronary syndrome and stroke: a scientific statement from the Am Heart Association Council on cardiovascular nursing and stroke council. *Circulation.* 2006;114:168–182.

17. Goodacre SW, Angelini K, Arnold J, Revill S, Morris F. Clinical predictors of acute coronary syndromes in patients with undifferentiated chest pain. *QJM.* 2003;96:893–898.

18. Goodacre S, Locker T, Morris F, Campbell S. How useful are clinical features in the diagnosis of acute, undifferentiated chest pain? *Acad Emerg Med.* 2002;9:203–208.

19. Everts B, Karlson BW, Wahrborg P, Hedner T, Herlitz J. Localization of pain in suspected acute myocardial infarction in relation to final diagnosis, age and sex, and site and type of infarction. *Heart Lung .* 1996;25:430–437.

20. Panju AA, B.R. Hemmelgarn, G.G. Guyatt, and DLSimel. Is this patient having a myocardial infarction? *JAMA.* 1998;280:1256–1263.

21. Douglas PS, Ginsburg GS. The evaluation of chest pain in women. N *Engl J Med.* 1996;334:1311–1315.

22. Solomon CG, Lee TH, Cook EF, Weisberg MC, Brand DA, Rouan GW, Goldman L. Comparison of clinical presentation of acute myocardial infarction in patients older than 65 years of age to younger patients: the Multicenter Chest Pain Study experience. *Am J Cardiol.* 1989;63: 772–776.

23. Peberdy MA, Ornato JP. Coronary artery disease in women. Heart *Dis Stroke.* 1992;1:315–319.

24. Blohm M, Herlitz J, Schroder U, Hartford M, Karlson BW, Risenfors M, Larsson E, Luepker R, Wennerblom B, Holmberg S. Reaction to a media campaign focusing on delay in acute myocardial infarction. *Heart Lung.* 1991;20:661–666.

25. Hedges JR, Feldman HA, Bittner V, Goldberg RJ, Zapka J, Osganian SK, Murray DM, Simons-Morton DG, Linares A, Williams J, Luepker RV, Eisenberg MS. Impact of community intervention to reduce patient delay time on use of reperfusion therapy for acute myocardial infarction: rapid early action for coronary treatment (REACT) trial. REACT Study Group. *Acad Emerg Med.* 2000;7:862–872.

26. Antman EM, Berlin JA. Declining incidence of ventricular fibrillation in myocardial infarction: implications for the prophylactic use of lidocaine. *Circulation.* 1992;86:764–773.

27. Wyman MG, Wyman RM, Cannom DS, Criley JM. Prevention of primary ventricular fibrillation in acute myocardial infarction with prophylactic lidocaine. *Am J Cardiol.* 2004;94:545–551.

28. Chiriboga D, Yarzebski J, Goldberg RJ, Gore JM, Alpert JS. Temporal trends (1975 through 1990) in the incidence and case-fatality rates of primary ventricular fibrillation complicating acute myocardial infarction: a communitywide perspective. *Circulation.* 1994;89: 998–1003.

29. The Public Access Defibrillation Trial Investigators. Public-access defibrillation and survival after out-of-hospital cardiac arrest. *N Engl J Med.* 2004;351:637–646.

30. Freimark D, Matetzky S, Leor J, Boyko V, Barbash IM, Behar S, Hod H. Timing of aspirin administration as a determinant of survival of patients with acute myocardial infarction treated with thrombolysis. *Am J Cardiol.* 2002;89:381–385.

31. Barbash IM, Freimark D, Gottlieb S, Hod H, Hasin Y, Battler A, Crystal E, Matetzky S, Boyko V, Mandelzweig L, Behar S, Leor J. Outcome of myocardial infarction in patients treated with aspirin is enhanced by pre-hospital administration. *Cardiology.* 2002;98:141–147.

32. Randomised trial of intravenous streptokinase, oral aspirin, both, or neither among 17,187 cases of suspected acute myocardial infarction: ISIS-2. ISIS-2 (Second International Study of Infarct Survival) Collaborative Group. *Lancet.* 1988;2(8607):349–360.

33. Casaccia M, Bertello F, De Bernardi A, Sicuro M, Scacciatella P. Prehospital management of acute myocardial infarct in an experimental metropolitan system of medical emergencies [in Italian]. *G Ital Cardiol.* 1996;26:657–672.

34. Quan D, LoVecchio F, Clark B, Gallagher JV, III. Prehospital use of aspirin rarely is associated with adverse events. *Prehosp Disaster Med.* 2004;19:362–365.

35. Eisenberg MJ, Topol EJ. Prehospital administration of aspirin in patients with unstable angina and acute myocardial infarction. *Arch Intern Med.* 1996;156:1506–1510.

36. Wijesinghe M, Perrin K, Ranchord A, Simmonds M, Weatherall M, Beasley R. Routine use of oxygen in the treatment of myocardial infarction: systematic review. *Heart.* 2009;95:198–202.

37. Haynes BE, Pritting J. A rural emergency medical technician with selected advanced skills. *Prehosp Emerg Care.* 1999;3:343–346.

38. Funk D, Groat C, Verdile VP. Education of paramedics regarding aspirin use. *Prehosp Emerg Care.* 2000;4:62–64.

39. Verheugt FW, van der Laarse A, Funke-Kupper AJ, Sterkman LG, Galema TW, Roos JP. Effects of early intervention with low-dose aspirin (100 mg) on infarct size, reinfarction and mortality in anterior wall acute myocardial infarction. *Am J Cardiol.* 1990;66:267–270.

40. Bussmann WD, Passek D, Seidel W, Kaltenbach M. Reduction of CK and CK-MB indexes of infarct size by intravenous nitroglycerin. *Circulation.* 1981;63:615–622.

41. Charvat J, Kuruvilla T, al Amad H. Beneficial effect of intravenous nitroglycerin in patients with non-Q myocardial infarction. *Cardiologia.* 1990;35:49–54.

42. Jugdutt BI, Warnica JW. Intravenous nitroglycerin therapy to limit myocardial infarct size, expansion, and complications. Effect of timing, dosage, and infarct location. *Circulation.* 1988;78:906–919.

43. Madsen JK, Chevalier B, Darius H, Rutsch W, Wojcik J, Schneider S, Allikmets K. Ischaemic events and bleeding in patients undergoing percutaneous coronary intervention with concomitant bivalirudin treatment. *EuroIntervention.* 2008;3:610–616.

44. Meine TJ, Roe MT, Chen AY, Patel MR, Washam JB, Ohman EM, Peacock WF, Pollack CV Jr, Gibler WB, Peterson ED. Association of intravenous morphine use and outcomes in acute coronary syndromes: results from the CRUSADE Quality Improvement Initiative. *Am Heart J.* 2005;149:1043–1049.

45. Karagounis L, Ipsen SK, Jessop MR, Gilmore KM, Valenti DA, Clawson JJ, Teichman S, Anderson JL. Impact of field-transmitted electrocardiography on time to in-hospital thrombolytic therapy in acute myocardial infarction. *Am J Cardiol.* 1990;66:786–791.

46. Kereiakes DJ, Gibler WB, Martin LH, Pieper KS, Anderson LC. Relative importance of emergency medical system transport and the prehospital electrocardiogram on reducing hospital time delay to therapy for acute myocardial infarction: a preliminary report from the Cincinnati Heart Project. *Am Heart J.* 1992;123(4 Pt 1):835–840.

47. Foster DB, Dufendach JH, Barkdoll CM, Mitchell BK. Prehospital recognition of AMI using independent nurse/paramedic 12-lead ECG evaluation: impact on in-hospital times to thrombolysis in a rural community hospital. *The Am journal of emergency medicine.* 1994;12:25–31.

48. Banerjee S, Rhoden WE. Fast-tracking of myocardial infarction by paramedics. *J R Coll Physicians Lond.* 1998;32:36–38.

49. Melville MR, Gray D, al. e. The potential impact of prehospital electrocardiography and telemetry on time to thrombolysis in a United Kingdom center. *Ann Noninvasive Electrocardiol.* 1998;3:327–333.

50. Millar-Craig MW, Joy AV, Adamowicz M, Furber R, Thomas B. Reduction in treatment delay by paramedic ECG diagnosis of myocardial infarction with direct CCU admission. *Heart .* 1997;78:456–461.

51. Brainard AH, Raynovich W, Tandberg D, Bedrick EJ. The prehospital 12-lead electrocardiogram's effect on time to initiation of reperfusion therapy: a systematic review and meta-analysis of existing literature. *Am J Emerg Med.* 2005;23:351–356.

52. Morrison LJ, Brooks S, Sawadsky B, McDonald A, Verbeek PR. Prehospital 12-lead electrocardiography impact on acute myocardial infarction treatment times and mortality: a systematic review. *Acad Emerg Med.* 2006;13:84–89.

53. Adams GL, Campbell PT, Adams JM, Strauss DG, Wall K, Patterson J, Shuping KB, Maynard C, Young D, Corey C, Thompson A, Lee BA, Wagner GS. Effectiveness of prehospital wireless transmission of electrocardiograms to a cardiologist via hand-held device for patients with acute myocardial infarction (from the Timely Intervention in Myocardial Emergency, NorthEast Experience [TIME-NE]). *Am J Cardiol.* 2006;98:1160–1164.

54. Afolabi BA, Novaro GM, Pinski SL, Fromkin KR, Bush HS. Use of the prehospital ECG improves door-to-balloon times in ST segment elevation myocardial infarction irrespective of time of day or day of week. *Emerg Med J.* 2007;24:588–591.

55. Terkelsen CJ, Lassen JF, Norgaard BL, Gerdes JC, Poulsen SH, Bendix K, Ankersen JP, Gotzsche LB, Romer FK, Nielsen TT, Andersen HR. Reduction of treatment delay in patients with ST-elevation myocardial infarction: impact of pre-hospital diagnosis and direct referral to primary percutanous coronary intervention. *Eur Heart J.* 2005;26:770–777.

56. Wall T, Albright J, Livingston B, Isley L, Young D, Nanny M, Jacobowitz S, Maynard C, Mayer N, Pierce K, Rathbone C, Stuckey T, Savona M, Leibrandt P, Brodie B, Wagner G. Prehospital ECG transmission speeds reperfusion for patients with acute myocardial infarction. *North Carolina Medical Journal.* 2000;61:104–108.

57. Dhruva VN, Abdelhadi SI, Anis A, Gluckman W, Hom D, Dougan W, Kaluski E, Haider B, Klapholz M. ST-Segment Analysis Using Wireless Technology in Acute Myocardial Infarction (STAT-MI) trial. *J Am Coll Cardiol.* 2007;50:509–513.

58. Sekulic M, Hassunizadeh B, McGraw S, David S. Feasibility of early emergency room notification to improve door-to-balloon times for patients with acute ST segment elevation myocardial infarction. *Catheter Cardiovasc Interv.* 2005;66:316–319.

59. Swor R, Hegerberg S, McHugh-McNally A, Goldstein M, McEachin CC. Prehospital 12-lead ECG: efficacy or effectiveness? *Prehosp Emerg Care.* 2006;10:374–377.

60. Campbell PT, Patterson J, Cromer D, Wall K, Adams GL, Albano A, Corey C, Fox P, Gardner J, Hawthorne B, Lipton J, Sejersten M, Thompson A, Wilfong S, Maynard C, Wagner G. Prehospital triage of acute myocardial infarction: wireless transmission of electrocardiograms to the on-call cardiologist via a handheld computer. *J Electrocardiol.* 2005;38(4):300–309.

61. Feldman JA, Brinsfield K, Bernard S, White D, Maciejko T. Real-time paramedic compared with blinded physician identification of ST-segment elevation myocardial infarction: results of an observational study. *Am J Emerg Med.* 2005;23:443–448.

62. Le May MR, Dionne R, Maloney J, Trickett J, Watpool I, Ruest M, Stiell I, Ryan S, Davies RF. Diagnostic performance and potential clinical impact of advanced care paramedic interpretation of ST-segment elevation myocardial infarction in the field. *CJEM.* 2006;8:401–407.

63. van't Hof AW, Rasoul S, van de Wetering H, Ernst N, Suryapranata H, Hoorntje JC, Dambrink JH, Gosselink M, Zijlstra F, Ottervanger JP, de Boer MJ Feasibility and benefit of prehospital diagnosis, triage, and therapy by paramedics only in patients who are candidates for primary angioplasty for acute myocardial infarction. *Am heart journal.* 2006; 151:1255 e1251–1255.

64. Pitt K. Prehospital selection of patients for thrombolysis by paramedics. *Emerg Med J .* 2002;19:260–263.

65. Trivedi K, Schuur JD, Cone DC. Can paramedics read ST-segment elevation myocardial infarction on prehospital 12-lead electrocardiograms? *Prehosp Emerg Care.* 2009;13:207–214.

66. Whitbread M, Leah V, Bell T, Coats TJ. Recognition of ST elevation by paramedics. *Emerg Med J.* 2002;19:66–67.

67. Lloyd G, Roberts A, Bashir I, Mumby M, Kamalvand K, Cooke R. An audit of clinical nurse practitioner led thrombolysis to improve the treatment of acute myocardial infarction. *J Public Health Med.* 2000; 22:462–465.

68. Qasim A, Malpass K, O'Gorman DJ, Heber ME. Safety and efficacy of nurse initiated thrombolysis in patients with acute myocardial infarction. *BMJ.* 2002;324(7349):1328–1331.

69. Heath SM, Bain RJ, Andrews A, Chida S, Kitchen SI, Walters MI. Nurse initiated thrombolysis in the accident and emergency department: safe, accurate, and faster than fast track. *Emerg Med J.* 2003;20: 418–420.

70. Bouten MJ, Simoons ML, Hartman JA, van Miltenburg AJ, van der Does E, Pool J. Prehospital thrombolysis with alteplase (rt-PA) in acute myocardial infarction. *Eur Heart J.* 1992;13:925–931.

71. Kremser AK, Lyneham J. Can Australian nurses safely assess for thrombolysis on EKG criteria? *J Emerg Nurs.* 2007;33:102–109.

72. Wilmshurst P, Purchase A, Webb C, Jowett C, Quinn T. Improving door to needle times with nurse initiated thrombolysis. *Heart.* 2000;84: 262–266.

73. Quinn T. Can nurses safely assess suitability for thrombolytic therapy? A pilot study. *Intensive Crit Care Nurs.* 1995;11:126–129.

74. Ioannidis JP, Salem D, Chew PW, Lau J. Accuracy and clinical effect of out-of-hospital electrocardiography in the diagnosis of acute cardiac ischemia: a meta-analysis. *Ann Emerg Med.* 2001;37:461–470.

75. Prehospital thrombolytic therapy in patients with suspected acute myocardial infarction. The European Myocardial Infarction Project Group. *N Engl J Med.* 1993;329:383–389.

76. Weaver WD, Cerqueira M, Hallstrom AP, Litwin PE, Martin JS, Kudenchuk PJ, Eisenberg M. Prehospital-initiated vs hospital-initiated thrombolytic therapy. The Myocardial Infarction Triage and Intervention Trial. *JAMA.* 1993;270:1211–1216.

77. Morrison LJ, Verbeek PR, McDonald AC, Sawadsky BV, Cook DJ. Mortality and prehospital thrombolysis for acute myocardial infarction: A meta-analysis. *JAMA .* 2000;283:2686–2692.

78. Dussoix P, Reuille O, Verin V, Gaspoz JM, Unger PF. Time savings with prehospital thrombolysis in an urban area. *Eur J Emerg Med.* 2003;10:2–5.

79. Feasibility, safety, and efficacy of domiciliary thrombolysis by general practitioners: Grampian region early anistreplase trial. GREAT Group. *BMJ.* 1992;305(6853):548–553.

80. Rawles JM. Quantification of the benefit of earlier thrombolytic therapy: five- year results of the Grampian Region Early Anistreplase Trial (GREAT). *J Am Coll Cardiol.* 1997;30:1181–1186.

81. Rawles J. Halving of mortality at 1 year by domiciliary thrombolysis in the Grampian Region Early Anistreplase Trial (GREAT). *J Am Coll Cardiol.* 1994;23:1–5.

82. Le May MR, So DY, Dionne R, Glover CA, Froeschl MP, Wells GA, Davies RF, Sherrard HL, Maloney J, Marquis JF, O'Brien ER, Trickett J, Poirier P, Ryan SC, Ha A, Joseph PG, Labinaz M. A citywide protocol for primary PCI in ST-segment elevation myocardial infarction. *N Engl J Med.* 2008;358:231–240.

83. Stenestrand U, Lindback J, Wallentin L. Long-term outcome of primary percutaneous coronary intervention vs prehospital and in-hospital thrombolysis for patients with ST-elevation myocardial infarction. *Jama.* 2006;296:1749–1756.

84. Le May MR, Davies RF, Dionne R, Maloney J, Trickett J, So D, Ha A, Sherrard H, Glover C, Marquis JF, O'Brien ER, Stiell IG, Poirier P, Labinaz M. Comparison of early mortality of paramedic-diagnosed ST-segment elevation myocardial infarction with immediate transport to a designated primary percutaneous coronary intervention center to that of similar patients transported to the nearest hospital. *Am J Cardiol.* 2006;98:1329–1333.

85. Bonnefoy E, Steg PG, Boutitie F, Dubien PY, Lapostolle F, Roncalli J, Dissait F, Vanzetto G, Leizorowicz A, Kirkorian G, Mercier C, McFadden EP, Touboul P. Comparison of primary angioplasty and pre-hospital fibrinolysis in acute myocardial infarction (CAPTIM) trial: a 5-year follow-up. *Eur Heart J.* 2009;30:1598–1606.

86. Pinto DS, Kirtane AJ, Nallamothu BK, Murphy SA, Cohen DJ, Laham RJ, Cutlip DE, Bates ER, Frederick PD, Miller DP, Carrozza JP Jr, Antman EM, Cannon CP, Gibson CM. Hospital delays in reperfusion for ST-elevation myocardial infarction: implications when selecting a reperfusion strategy. *Circulation.* 2006;114:2019–2025.

87. Cantor WJ, Fitchett D, Borgundvaag B, Ducas J, Heffernan M, Cohen EA, Morrison LJ, Langer A, Dzavik V, Mehta SR, Lazzam C, Schwartz B, Casanova A, Goodman SG. Routine early angioplasty after fibrinolysis for acute myocardial infarction. *N Engl J Med.* 2009;360: 2705–2718.

88. Di Mario C, Dudek D, Piscione F, Mielecki W, Savonitto S, Murena E, Dimopoulos K, Manari A, Gaspardone A, Ochala A, Zmudka K, Bolognese L, Steg PG, Flather M. Immediate angioplasty versus standard therapy with rescue angioplasty after thrombolysis in the Combined Abciximab REteplase Stent Study in Acute Myocardial Infarction (CARESS-in-AMI): an open, prospective, randomised, multicentre trial. *Lancet.* 2008;371(9612):559–568.

89. Bradley EH, Herrin J, Wang Y, Barton BA, Webster TR, Mattera JA, Roumanis SA, Curtis JP, Nallamothu BK, Magid DJ, McNamara RL, Parkosewich J, Loeb JM, Krumholz HM. Strategies for reducing the door-to-balloon time in acute myocardial infarction. *N Engl J Med.* 2006;355:2308–2320.

90. Brown JP, Mahmud E, Dunford JV, Ben-Yehuda O. Effect of pre-hospital 12-lead electrocardiogram on activation of the cardiac catheterization laboratory and door-to-balloon time in ST-segment elevation acute myocardial infarction. *Am J Cardiol.* 2008;101:158–161.

91. Gross BW, Dauterman KW, Moran MG, Kotler TS, Schnugg SJ, Rostykus PS, Ross AM, Weaver WD. An approach to shorten time to infarct artery patency in patients with ST-segment elevation myocardial infarction. *Am J Cardiol.* 2007;99:1360–1363.

92. van de Loo A, Saurbier B, Kalbhenn J, Koberne F, Zehender M. Primary percutaneous coronary intervention in acute myocardial infarction: direct transportation to catheterization laboratory by emergency teams reduces door-to-balloon time. *Clin Cardiol.* 2006;29:112–116.

93. Bradley EH, Curry LA, Webster TR, Mattera JA, Roumanis SA, Radford MJ, McNamara RL, Barton BA, Berg DN, Krumholz HM. Achieving rapid door-to-balloon times: how top hospitals improve complex clinical systems. *Circulation .* 2006;113:1079–1085.

94. Holmboe ES, Bradley EH, Mattera JA, Roumanis SA, Radford MJ, Krumholz HM. Characteristics of physician leaders working to improve the quality of care in acute myocardial infarction. *Jt Comm J Qual Saf.* 2003;29:289–296.

95. Huang RL, Donelli A, Byrd J, Mickiewicz MA, Slovis C, Roumie C, Elasy TA, Dittus RS, Speroff T, Disalvo T, Zhao D. Using quality improvement methods to improve door-to-balloon time at an academic medical center. *J Invasive Cardiol.* 2008;20:46–52.

96. Lipton JA, Broce M, Lucas D, Mimnagh K, Matthews A, Reyes B, Burdette J, Wagner GS, Warren SG. Comprehensive hospital care improvement strategies reduce time to treatment in ST-elevation acute myocardial infarction. *Crit Pathw Cardiol.* 2006;5:29–33.

97. Ward MR, Lo ST, Herity NA, Lee DP, Yeung AC Effect of audit on door-to-inflation times in primary angioplasty/stenting for acute myocardial infarction. *Am J Cardiol.* 2001;87:336–338, A339.

98. Krumholz HM, Bradley EH, Nallamothu BK, Ting HH, Batchelor WB, Kline-Rogers E, Stern AF, Byrd JR, Brush JE Jr. A campaign to improve the timeliness of primary percutaneous coronary intervention: Door-to-Balloon: An Alliance for Quality. *J Am Coll Cardiol Cardiovasc Interv.* 2008;1:97–104.

99. Bradley EH, Roumanis SA, Radford MJ, Webster TR, McNamara RL, Mattera JA, Barton BA, Berg DN, Portnay EL, Moscovitz H, Parkosewich J, Holmboe ES, Blaney M, Krumholz HM. Achieving door-to-balloon times that meet quality guidelines: how do successful hospitals do it? *J Am Coll Cardiol.* 2005;46:1236–1241.

100. Jacoby J, Axelband J, Patterson J, Belletti D, Heller M. Cardiac cath lab activation by the emergency physician without prior consultation decreases door-to-balloon time. *J Invasive Cardiol.* 2005;17:154–155.

101. Khot UN, Johnson ML, Ramsey C, Khot MB, Todd R, Shaikh SR, Berg WJ. Emergency department physician activation of the catheterization laboratory and immediate transfer to an immediately available catheterization laboratory reduce door-to-balloon time in ST-elevation myocardial infarction. *Circulation.* 2007;116:67–76.

102. Kraft PL, Newman S, Hanson D, Anderson W, Bastani A. Emergency physician discretion to activate the cardiac catheterization team decreases door-to-balloon time for acute ST-elevation myocardial infarction. *Ann Emerg Med.* 2007;50:520–526.

103. Kurz MC, Babcock C, Sinha S, Tupesis JP, Allegretti J. The impact of emergency physician-initiated primary percutaneous coronary intervention on mean door-to-balloon time in patients with ST-segment-elevation myocardial infarction. *Ann Emerg Med.* 2007;50:527–534.

104. Lee CH, Ooi SB, Tay EL, Low AF, Teo SG, Lau C, Tai BC, Lim I, Lam S, Lim IH, Chai P, Tan HC. Shortening of median door-to-balloon time in primary percutaneous coronary intervention in Singapore by simple and inexpensive operational measures: clinical practice improvement program. *J Interv Cardiol.* 2008;21:414–423.

105. Singer AJ, Shembekar A, Visram F, Schiller J, Russo V, Lawson W, Gomes CA, Santora C, Maliszewski M, Wilbert L, Dowdy E, Viccellio P, Henry MC. Emergency department activation of an interventional cardiology team reduces door-to-balloon times in ST-segment-elevation myocardial infarction. *Ann Emerg Med.* 2007;50:538–544.

106. Thatcher JL, Gilseth TA, Adlis S. Improved efficiency in acute myocardial infarction care through commitment to emergency department-initiated primary PCI. *J Invasive Cardiol.* 2003;15:693–698.

107. Zarich SW, Sachdeva R, Fishman R, Werdmann MJ, Parniawski M, Bernstein L, Dilella M. Effectiveness of a multidisciplinary quality improvement initiative in reducing door-to-balloon times in primary angioplasty. *J Interv Cardiol.* 2004;17:191–195.

108. Emergency department: rapid identification and treatment of patients with acute myocardial infarction. National Heart Attack Alert Program Coordinating Committee, 60 Minutes to Treatment Working Group. *Ann Emerg Med.* 1994;23:311–329.

109. Lambrew CT, Bowlby LJ, Rogers WJ, Chandra NC, Weaver WD. Factors influencing the time to thrombolysis in acute myocardial infarction. Time to Thrombolysis Substudy of the National Registry of Myocardial Infarction-1. *Arch Intern Med.* 1997;157:2577–2582.

110. Bleeker JK, Simoons ML, Erdman RA, Leenders CM, Kruyssen HA, Lamers LM, van der Does E. Patient and doctor delay in acute myocardial infarction: a study in Rotterdam, The Netherlands. *Br J Gen Pract.* 1995;45(393):181–184.

111. Goldberg RJ, McGovern PG, Guggina T, Savageau J, Rosamond WD, Luepker RV. Prehospital delay in patients with acute coronary heart disease: concordance between patient interviews and medical records. *Am Heart J.* 135(pt 1):293–299, 1998.

112. McSweeney JC, Cody M, O'Sullivan P, Elberson K, Moser DK, Garvin BJ. Women's early warning symptoms of acute myocardial infarction. *Circulation.* 2003;108:2619–2623.

113. Wagner GS, Macfarlane P, Wellens H, Josephson M, Gorgels A, Mirvis DM, Pahlm O, Surawicz B, Kligfield P, Childers R, Gettes LS, Bailey JJ, Deal BJ, Gorgels A, Hancock EW, Kors JA, Mason JW, Okin P, Rautaharju PM, van Herpen G. AHA/ACCF/HRS recommendations for the standardization and interpretation of the electrocardiogram: part VI: acute ischemia/infarction: a scientific statement from the Am Heart Association Electrocardiography and Arrhythmias Committee, Council on Clinical Cardiology; the Am College of Cardiology Foundation; and the Heart Rhythm Society. Endorsed by the International Society for

Computerized Electrocardiology. *Journal of the Am College of Cardiology.* 2009;53:1003–1011.

114. Antman EM, Tanasijevic MJ, Thompson B, Schactman M, McCabe CH, Cannon CP, Fischer GA, Fung AY, Thompson C, Wybenga D, Braunwald E. Cardiac-specific troponin I levels to predict the risk of mortality in patients with acute coronary syndromes. *N Engl J Med.* 1996;335:1342–1349.

115. Svensson L, Axelsson C, Nordlander R, Herlitz J. Elevation of biochemical markers for myocardial damage prior to hospital admission in patients with acute chest pain or other symptoms raising suspicion of acute coronary syndrome. *J Intern Med.* 2003;253:311–319.

116. Gust R, Gust A, Bottiger BW, Bohrer H, Martin E. Bedside troponin T testing is not useful for early out-of-hospital diagnosis of myocardial infarction. *Acta Anaesthesiol Scand.* 1998;42:414–417.

117. Newman J, Aulick N, Cheng T, Faynor S, Curtis R, Mercer D, Williams J, Hobbs G. Prehospital identification of acute coronary ischemia using a troponin T rapid assay. *Prehosp Emerg Care.* 1999;3:97–101.

118. Svensson L, Axelsson C, Nordlander R, Herlitz J. Prognostic value of biochemical markers, 12-lead ECG and patient characteristics amongst patients calling for an ambulance due to a suspected acute coronary syndrome. *J Intern Med.* 2004;255:469–477.

119. Schuchert A, Hamm C, Scholz J, Klimmeck S, Goldmann B, Meinertz T. Prehospital testing for troponin T in patients with suspected acute myocardial infarction. *Am Heart J.* 1999;138(1 Pt 1):45–48.

120. Tanaka K, Seino Y, Ohbayashi K, Takano T. Cardiac emergency triage and therapeutic decisions using whole blood rapid troponin T test for patients with suspicious acute coronary syndrome. *Jpn Circ J.* 2001;65:424–428.

121. Al-Mubarak N, Rogers WJ, Lambrew CT, Bowlby LJ, French WJ Consultation before thrombolytic therapy in acute myocardial infarction. Second National Registry of Myocardial Infarction (NRMI 2) Investigators. *The Am journal of cardiology.* 1999;83:89–93, A88.

122. Braunwald E, Antman EM, Beasley JW, Califf RM, Cheitlin MD, Hochman JS, Jones RH, Kereiakes D, Kupersmith J, Levin TN, Pepine CJ, Schaeffer JW, Smith EE, III, Steward DE, Theroux P, Gibbons RJ, Alpert JS, Faxon DP, Fuster V, Gregoratos G, Hiratzka LF, Jacobs AK, Smith SC Jr. ACC/AHA 2002 guideline update for the management of patients with unstable angina and non-ST-segment elevation myocardial infarction–summary article: a report of the Am College of Cardiology/Am Heart Association task force on practice guidelines (Committee on the Management of Patients With Unstable Angina). *J Am Coll Cardiol.* 2002;40:1366–1374.

123. Braunwald E, Antman EM, Beasley JW, Califf RM, Cheitlin MD, Hochman JS, Jones RH, Kereiakes D, Kupersmith J, Levin TN, Pepine CJ, Schaeffer JW, Smith EE, III, Steward DE, Theroux P, Gibbons RJ, Alpert JS, Faxon DP, Fuster V, Gregoratos G, Hiratzka LF, Jacobs AK, Smith SC Jr. ACC/AHA guideline update for the management of patients with unstable angina and non-ST-segment elevation myocardial infarction–2002: summary article: a report of the Am College of Cardiology/Am Heart Association Task Force on Practice Guidelines (Committee on the Management of Patients With Unstable Angina). *Circulation.* 2002;106:1893–1900.

124. Braunwald E, Antman EM, Beasley JW, Califf RM, Cheitlin MD, Hochman JS, Jones RH, Kereiakes D, Kupersmith J, Levin TN, Pepine CJ, Schaeffer JW, Smith EE III, Steward DE, Theroux P, Alpert JS, Eagle KA, Faxon DP, Fuster V, Gardner TJ, Gregoratos G, Russell RO, Smith SC Jr. ACC/AHA guidelines for the management of patients with unstable angina and non-ST-segment elevation myocardial infarction. A report of the Am College of Cardiology/Am Heart Association Task Force on Practice Guidelines (Committee on the Management of Patients With Unstable Angina). *J Am Coll Cardiol.* 2000;36:970–1062.

125. Effects of tissue plasminogen activator and a comparison of early invasive and conservative strategies in unstable angina and non-Q-wave myocardial infarction. Results of the TIMI IIIB Trial. Thrombolysis in Myocardial Ischemia. *Circulation.* 1994;89:1545–1556.

126. Scanlon PJ, Faxon DP, Audet AM, Carabello B, Dehmer GJ, Eagle KA, Legako RD, Leon DF, Murray JA, Nissen SE, Pepine CJ, Watson RM, Ritchie JL, Gibbons RJ, Cheitlin MD, Gardner TJ, Garson A Jr, Russell RO Jr, Ryan TJ, Smith SC Jr. ACC/AHA guidelines for coronary angiography: executive summary and recommendations. A report of the Am College of Cardiology/Am Heart Association Task Force on Practice Guidelines (Committee on Coronary Angiography) developed in collaboration with the Society for Cardiac Angiography and Interventions. *Circulation.* 1999;99:2345–2357.

127. King SB, III, Smith SC Jr, Hirshfeld JW Jr, Jacobs AK, Morrison DA, Williams DO, Feldman TE, Kern MJ, O'Neill WW, Schaff HV, Whitlow PL, Adams CD, Anderson JL, Buller CE, Creager MA, Ettinger SM, Halperin JL, Hunt SA, Krumholz HM, Kushner FG, Lytle BW, Nishimura R, Page RL, Riegel B, Tarkington LG, Yancy CW. 2007 Focused Update of the ACC/AHA/SCAI 2005 Guideline Update for Percutaneous Coronary Intervention: a report of the Am College of Cardiology/Am Heart Association Task Force on Practice Guidelines: 2007 Writing Group to Review New Evidence and Update the ACC/AHA/SCAI 2005 Guideline Update for Percutaneous Coronary Intervention, Writing on Behalf of the 2005 Writing Committee. *Circulation.* 2008;117:261–295.

128. Alpert JS, Thygesen K, Antman E, Bassand JP. Myocardial infarction redefined–a consensus document of The Joint European Society of Cardiology/Am College of Cardiology Committee for the redefinition of myocardial infarction. *Journal of the Am College of Cardiology.* 2000;36:959–969.

129. Pollack CV Jr, Sites FD, Shofer FS, Sease KL, Hollander JE. Application of the TIMI risk score for unstable angina and non-ST elevation acute coronary syndrome to an unselected emergency department chest pain population. *Acad Emerg Med.* 2006;13:13–18.

130. Antman EM, Cohen M, Bernink PJ, McCabe CH, Horacek T, Papuchis G, Mautner B, Corbalan R, Radley D, Braunwald E. The TIMI risk score for unstable angina/non-ST elevation MI: A method for prognostication and therapeutic decision making. *JAMA.* 2000;284:835–842.

131. Boersma E, Pieper KS, Steyerberg EW, Wilcox RG, Chang WC, Lee KL, Akkerhuis KM, Harrington RA, Deckers JW, Armstrong PW, Lincoff AM, Califf RM, Topol EJ, Simoons ML. Predictors of outcome in patients with acute coronary syndromes without persistent ST-segment elevation. Results from an international trial of 9461 patients. The PURSUIT Investigators. *Circulation.* 2000;101:2557–2567.

132. Granger CB, Goldberg RJ, Dabbous O, Pieper KS, Eagle KA, Cannon CP, Van De Werf F, Avezum A, Goodman SG, Flather MD, Fox KA. Predictors of hospital mortality in the global registry of acute coronary events. *Archives of internal medicine.* 2003;163:2345–2353.

133. Eagle KA, Lim MJ, Dabbous OH, Pieper KS, Goldberg RJ, Van de Werf F, Goodman SG, Granger CB, Steg PG, Gore JM, Budaj A, Avezum A, Flather MD, Fox KAA, for the GRACE Investigators. A validated prediction model for all forms of acute coronary syndrome: estimating the risk of 6-month postdischarge death in an international registry. *JAMA.* 2004;291:2727–2733.

134. Guideline for the management of patients with acute coronary syndromes without persistent ECG ST segment elevation. British Cardiac Society Guidelines and Medical Practice Committee and Royal College of Physicians Clinical Effectiveness and Evaluation Unit. *Heart.* 2001;85:133–142.

135. Clinical policy: critical issues in the evaluation and management of adult patients presenting with suspected acute myocardial infarction or unstable angina. Am College of Emergency Physicians. *Ann Emerg Med.* 2000;35:521–525.

136. Doukky R, Calvin JE. Risk stratification in patients with unstable angina and non-ST segment elevation myocardial infarction: evidence-based review. *J Invasive Cardiol.* 2002;14:215–220.

137. Doukky R, Calvin JE. Part II: risk stratification in patients with unstable angina and non-ST segment elevation myocardial infarction: evidence-based review. *The Journal of Invasive Cardiology.* 2002;14:254–262.

138. Braunwald E, Jones RH, Mark DB, Brown J, Brown L, Cheitlin MD, Concannon CA, Cowan M, Edwards C, Fuster V, et al. Diagnosing and managing unstable angina. Agency for Health Care Policy and Research. *Circulation.* 1994;90:613–622.

139. Smith SC Jr, Dove JT, Jacobs AK, Kennedy JW, Kereiakes D, Kern MJ, Kuntz RE, Popma JJ, Schaff HV, Williams DO, Gibbons RJ, Alpert JP, Eagle KA, Faxon DP, Fuster V, Gardner TJ, Gregoratos G, Russell RO, Smith SC Jr. ACC/AHA guidelines for percutaneous coronary intervention (revision of the 1993 PTCA guidelines)-executive summary: a report of the Am College of Cardiology/Am Heart Association task force on practice guidelines (Committee to revise the 1993 guidelines for percutaneous transluminal coronary angioplasty) endorsed by the Society for Cardiac Angiography and Interventions. *Circulation.* 2001;103:3019–3041.

140. Farkouh ME, Smars PA, Reeder GS, Zinsmeister AR, Evans RW, Meloy TD, Kopecky SL, Allen M, Allison TG, Gibbons RJ, Gabriel SE. A clinical trial of a chest-pain observation unit for patients with unstable

angina. Chest Pain Evaluation in the Emergency Room (CHEER) Investigators. *N Engl J Med.* 1998;339:1882–1888.

141. Udelson JE, Beshansky JR, Ballin DS, Feldman JA, Griffith JL, Handler J, Heller GV, Hendel RC, Pope JH, Ruthazer R, Spiegler EJ, Woolard RH, Selker HP. Myocardial perfusion imaging for evaluation and triage of patients with suspected acute cardiac ischemia: a randomized controlled trial. *JAMA.* 2002;288:2693–2700.

142. Bedetti G, Pasanisi EM, Tintori G, Fonseca L, Tresoldi S, Minneci C, Jambrik Z, Ghelarducci B, Orlandini A, Picano E. Stress echo in chest pain unit: the SPEED trial. *International journal of cardiology.* 2005; 102:461–467.

143. Caragher TE, Fernandez BB, Barr LA. Long-term experience with an accelerated protocol for diagnosis of chest pain. *Archives of pathology & laboratory medicine.* 2000;124:1434–1439.

144. deFilippi CR, Rosanio S, Tocchi M, Parmar RJ, Potter MA, Uretsky BF, Runge MS. Randomized comparison of a strategy of predischarge coronary angiography versus exercise testing in low-risk patients in a chest pain unit: in-hospital and long-term outcomes. *Journal of the Am College of Cardiology.* 2001;37:2042–2049.

145. Gomez MA, Anderson JL, Karagounis LA, Muhlestein JB, Mooers FB. An emergency department-based protocol for rapidly ruling out myocardial ischemia reduces hospital time and expense: results of a randomized study (ROMIO). *J Am Coll Cardiol.* 1996;28:25–33.

146. Lee TH, Juarez G, Cook EF, Weisberg MC, Rouan GW, Brand DA, Goldman L. Ruling out acute myocardial infarction. A prospective multicenter validation of a 12-hour strategy for patients at low risk. *N Engl J Med.* 1991;324:1239–1246.

147. Nucifora G, Badano LP, Sarraf-Zadegan N, Karavidas A, Trocino G, Scaffidi G, Pettinati G, Astarita C, Vysniauskas V, Gregori D, Ilerigelen B, Fioretti PM. Effect on quality of life of different accelerated diagnostic protocols for management of patients presenting to the emergency department with acute chest pain. *The Am journal of cardiology.* 2009; 103:592–597.

148. Ramakrishna G, Milavetz JJ, Zinsmeister AR, Farkouh ME, Evans RW, Allison TG, Smars PA, Gibbons RJ. Effect of exercise treadmill testing and stress imaging on the triage of patients with chest pain: CHEER substudy. *Mayo Clinic proceedings.* 2005;80:322–329.

149. Roberts RR, Zalenski RJ, Mensah EK, Rydman RJ, Ciavarella G, Gussow L, Das K, Kampe LM, Dickover B, McDermott MF, Hart A, Straus HE, Murphy DG, Rao R. Costs of an emergency department-based accelerated diagnostic protocol vs hospitalization in patients with chest pain: a randomized controlled trial. *JAMA.* 1997; 278:1670–1676.

150. Zalenski RJ, McCarren M, Roberts R, Rydman RJ, Jovanovic B, Das K, Mendez J, el-Khadra M, Fraker L, McDermott M. An evaluation of a chest pain diagnostic protocol to exclude acute cardiac ischemia in the emergency department. *Archives of internal medicine.* 1997;157: 1085–1091.

151. Paventi S, Parafati MA, Luzio ED, Pellegrino CA. Usefulness of two-dimensional echocardiography and myocardial perfusion imaging for immediate evaluation of chest pain in the emergency department. *Resuscitation.* 2001;49:47–51.

152. Conti A, Sammicheli L, Gallini C, Costanzo EN, Antoniucci D, Barletta G. Assessment of patients with low-risk chest pain in the emergency department: Head-to-head comparison of exercise stress echocardiography and exercise myocardial SPECT. *Am Heart J.* 2005;149:894–901.

153. Gallagher MJ, Ross MA, Raff GL, Goldstein JA, O'Neill WW, O'Neil B. The diagnostic accuracy of 64-slice computed tomography coronary angiography compared with stress nuclear imaging in emergency department low-risk chest pain patients. *Ann Emerg Med.* 2007;49: 125–136.

154. Forberg JL, Hilmersson CE, Carlsson M, Arheden H, Bjork J, Hjalte K, Ekelund U. Negative predictive value and potential cost savings of acute nuclear myocardial perfusion imaging in low risk patients with suspected acute coronary syndrome: a prospective single blinded study. *BMC Emerg Med.* 2009;9:12.

155. Athappan G, Habib M, Ponniah T, Jeyaseelan L Multi-detector computerized tomography angiography for evaluation of acute chest pain - A meta analysis and systematic review of literature. *Int J Cardiol.* 2009.

156. Vanhoenacker PK, Decramer I, Bladt O, Sarno G, Bevernage C, Wijns W. Detection of non-ST-elevation myocardial infarction and unstable angina in the acute setting: meta-analysis of diagnostic performance of multi-detector computed tomographic angiography. *BMC Cardiovasc Disord.* 2007;7:39.

157. Hoffmann U, Bamberg F, Chae CU, Nichols JH, Rogers IS, Seneviratne SK, Truong QA, Cury RC, Abbara S, Shapiro MD, Moloo J, Butler J, Ferencik M, Lee H, Jang IK, Parry BA, Brown DF, Udelson JE, Achenbach S, Brady TJ, Nagurney JT. Coronary computed tomography angiography for early triage of patients with acute chest pain: the ROMICAT (Rule Out Myocardial Infarction using Computer Assisted Tomography) trial. *J Am Coll Cardiol.* 2009;53:1642–1650.

158. Hollander JE, Litt HI, Chase M, Brown AM, Kim W, Baxt WG. Computed tomography coronary angiography for rapid disposition of low-risk emergency department patients with chest pain syndromes. *Acad Emerg Med.* 2007;14:112–116.

159. Goldstein JA, Gallagher MJ, O'Neill WW, Ross MA, O'Neil BJ, Raff GL. A randomized controlled trial of multi-slice coronary computed tomography for evaluation of acute chest pain. *J Am Coll Cardiol.* 2007;49:863–871.

160. Hess EP, Thiruganasambandamoorthy V, Wells GA, Erwin P, Jaffe AS, Hollander JE, Montori VM, Stiell IG. Diagnostic accuracy of clinical prediction rules to exclude acute coronary syndrome in the emergency department setting: a systematic review. *Cjem.* 2008;10:373–382.

161. Hamm CW, Goldmann BU, Heeschen C, Kreymann G, Berger J, Meinertz T. Emergency room triage of patients with acute chest pain by means of rapid testing for cardiac troponin T or troponin I. *N Engl J Med.* 1997;337:1648–1653.

162. Lai C, Noeller TP, Schmidt K, King P, Emerman CL. Short-term risk after initial observation for chest pain. *J Emerg Med.* 2003;25:357–362.

163. Marsan RJ Jr, Shaver KJ, Sease KL, Shofer FS, Sites FD, Hollander JE. Evaluation of a clinical decision rule for young adult patients with chest pain. *Acad Emerg Med.* 2005;12:26–31.

164. Christenson J, Innes G, McKnight D, Thompson CR, Wong H, Yu E, Boychuk B, Grafstein E, Rosenberg F, Gin K, Anis A, Singer J. A clinical prediction rule for early discharge of patients with chest pain. *Ann Emerg Med.* 2006;47:1–10.

165. Challa PK, Smith KM, Conti CR. Initial presenting electrocardiogram as determinant for hospital admission in patients presenting to the emergency department with chest pain: a pilot investigation. *Clin Cardiol.* 2007;30:558–561.

166. Schillinger M, Sodeck G, Meron G, Janata K, Nikfardjam M, Rauscha F, Laggner AN, Domanovits H. Acute chest pain–identification of patients at low risk for coronary events. The impact of symptoms, medical history and risk factors. *Wien Klin Wochenschr.* 2004;116: 83–89.

167. Bassan R, Pimenta L, Scofano M, Gamarski R, Volschan A. Probability stratification and systematic diagnostic approach for chest pain patients in the emergency department. *Crit Pathw Cardiol.* 2004;3:1–7.

168. Maroko PR, Radvany P, Braunwald E, Hale SL. Reduction of infarct size by oxygen inhalation following acute coronary occlusion. *Circulation.* 1975;52:360–368.

169. Ribeiro LG, Louie EK, Davis MA, Maroko PR. Augmentation of collateral blood flow to the ischaemic myocardium by oxygen inhalation following experimental coronary artery occlusion. *Cardiovasc Res.* 1979;13:160–166.

170. Kelly RF, Hursey TL, Parrillo JE, Schaer GL. Effect of 100% oxygen administration on infarct size and left ventricular function in a canine model of myocardial infarction and reperfusion. *Am Heart J.* 1995;130: 957–965.

171. Ishikawa K, Kanamasa K, Yamakado T, Katori R. The beneficial effects of 40% and 100% O2 inhalations on acutely-induced myocardial ischemia in dogs. *The Tohoku journal of experimental medicine.* 1986;149: 107–117.

172. Madias JE, Hood WB Jr. Reduction of precordial ST-segment elevation in patients with anterior myocardial infarction by oxygen breathing. *Circulation.* 1976;53(3 Suppl):I198–I200.

173. Rawles JM, Kenmure AC. Controlled trial of oxygen in uncomplicated myocardial infarction. *BMJ.* 1976;1(6018):1121–1123.

174. Wilson AT, Channer KS. Hypoxaemia and supplemental oxygen therapy in the first 24 hours after myocardial infarction: the role of pulse oximetry. *J R Coll Physicians Lond.* 1997;31:657–661.

175. Gurfinkel EP, Manos EJ, Mejail RI, Cerda MA, Duronto EA, Garcia CN, Daroca AM, Mautner B. Low molecular weight heparin versus regular heparin or aspirin in the treatment of unstable angina and silent ischemia. *J Am Coll Cardiol.* 1995;26:313–318.

176. Collaborative meta-analysis of randomised trials of antiplatelet therapy for prevention of death, myocardial infarction, and stroke in high risk patients. *BMJ.* 2002;324(7329):71–86.

177. Collaborative overview of randomised trials of antiplatelet therapy–I: Prevention of death, myocardial infarction, and stroke by prolonged antiplatelet therapy in various categories of patients. Antiplatelet Trialists' Collaboration. *BMJ*. 1994;308(6921):81–106.

178. Feldman M, Cryer B. Aspirin absorption rates and platelet inhibition times with 325-mg buffered aspirin tablets (chewed or swallowed intact) and with buffered aspirin solution. *Am J Cardiol*. 1999;84:404–409.

179. Sagar KA, Smyth MR. A comparative bioavailability study of different aspirin formulations using on-line multidimensional chromatography. *J Pharm Biomed Anal*. 1999;21:383–392.

180. McGettigan P, Henry D. Cardiovascular risk and inhibition of cyclooxygenase: a systematic review of the observational studies of selective and nonselective inhibitors of cyclooxygenase 2. *Jama*. 2006;296: 1633–1644.

181. Kearney PM, Baigent C, Godwin J, Halls H, Emberson JR, Patrono C. Do selective cyclo-oxygenase-2 inhibitors and traditional non-steroidal anti-inflammatory drugs increase the risk of atherothrombosis? Meta-analysis of randomised trials. *BMJ (Clinical research ed.* 2006; 332(7553):1302–1308.

182. Gibson IR, Bonfield W. Novel synthesis and characterization of an AB-type carbonate-substituted hydroxyapatite. *J Biomed Mater Res*. 2002;59:697–708.

183. ISIS-4: a randomised factorial trial assessing early oral captopril, oral mononitrate, and intravenous magnesium sulphate in 58,050 patients with suspected acute myocardial infarction. ISIS-4 (Fourth International Study of Infarct Survival) Collaborative Group. *Lancet*. 1995; 345(8951):669–685.

184. Diercks DB, Boghos E, Guzman H, Amsterdam EA, Kirk JD. Changes in the numeric descriptive scale for pain after sublingual nitroglycerin do not predict cardiac etiology of chest pain. *Annals of emergency medicine*. 2005;45:581–585.

185. Henrikson CA, Howell EE, Bush DE, Miles JS, Meininger GR, Friedlander T, Bushnell AC, Chandra-Strobos N. Chest pain relief by nitroglycerin does not predict active coronary artery disease. *Ann Intern Med*. 2003;139:979–986.

186. Steele R, McNaughton T, McConahy M, Lam J. Chest pain in emergency department patients: if the pain is relieved by nitroglycerin, is it more likely to be cardiac chest pain? *CJEM*. 2006;8:164–169.

187. Baigent C, Collins R, Appleby P, Parish S, Sleight P, Peto R. ISIS-2: 10 year survival among patients with suspected acute myocardial infarction in randomised comparison of intravenous streptokinase, oral aspirin, both, or neither. The ISIS-2 (Second International Study of Infarct Survival) Collaborative Group. *Bmj*. 1998;316(7141):1337–1343.

188. Franzosi MG, Santoro E, De Vita C, Geraci E, Lotto A, Maggioni AP, Mauri F, Rovelli F, Santoro L, Tavazzi L, Tognoni G. Ten-year follow-up of the first megatrial testing thrombolytic therapy in patients with acute myocardial infarction: results of the Gruppo Italiano per lo Studio della Sopravvivenza nell'Infarto-1 study. The GISSI Investigators. *Circulation*. 1998;98:2659–2665.

189. Keeley EC, Boura JA, Grines CL. Primary angioplasty versus intravenous thrombolytic therapy for acute myocardial infarction: a quantitative review of 23 randomised trials. *Lancet*. 2003;361(9351):13–20.

190. Indications for fibrinolytic therapy in suspected acute myocardial infarction: collaborative overview of early mortality and major morbidity results from all randomised trials of more than 1000 patients. Fibrinolytic Therapy Trialists' (FTT) Collaborative Group. *Lancet*. 1994;343(8893):311–322.

191. A comparison of reteplase with alteplase for acute myocardial infarction. The Global Use of Strategies to Open Occluded Coronary Arteries (GUSTO III) Investigators. *N Engl J Med*. 1997;337:1118–1123.

192. Single-bolus tenecteplase compared with front-loaded alteplase in acute myocardial infarction: the ASSENT-2 double-blind randomised trial. Assessment of the Safety and Efficacy of a New Thrombolytic Investigators. *Lancet*. 1999;354(9180):716–722.

193. Effectiveness of intravenous thrombolytic treatment in acute myocardial infarction. Gruppo Italiano per lo Studio della Streptochinasi nell'Infarto Miocardico (GISSI). *Lancet*. 1986;1(8478):397–402.

194. Brodie BR, Stuckey TD, Kissling G, Hansen CJ, Weintraub RA, Kelly TA. Importance of infarct-related artery patency for recovery of left ventricular function and late survival after primary angioplasty for acute myocardial infarction. *J Am Coll Cardiol*. 1996;28:319–325.

195. Puma JA, Sketch MHJ, Thompson TD, Simes RJ, Morris DC, White HD, Topol EJ, Califf RM. Support for the open-artery hypothesis in survivors of acute myocardial infarction: analysis of 11,228 patients treated with thrombolytic therapy. *Am J Cardiol*. 1999;83:482–487.

196. de Lemos JA, Antman EM, Gibson CM, McCabe CH, Giugliano RP, Murphy SA, Coulter SA, Anderson K, Scherer J, Frey MJ, Van Der Wieken R, Van De Werf F, Braunwald E. Abciximab improves both epicardial flow and myocardial reperfusion in ST-elevation myocardial infarction: observations from the TIMI 14 trial. *Circulation*. 2000;101: 239–243.

197. Claeys MJ, Bosmans J, Veenstra L, Jorens P, De R, Vrints CJ. Determinants and prognostic implications of persistent ST-segment elevation after primary angioplasty for acute myocardial infarction: importance of microvascular reperfusion injury on clinical outcome. *Circulation*. 1999; 99:1972–1977.

198. Gibson CM, Murphy SA, Rizzo MJ, Ryan KA, Marble SJ, McCabe CH, Cannon CP, Van de Werf F, Braunwald E. Relationship between TIMI frame count and clinical outcomes after thrombolytic administration. Thrombolysis In Myocardial Infarction (TIMI) Study Group. *Circulation*. 1999;99:1945–1950.

199. Brouwer MA, Martin JS, Maynard C, Wirkus M, Litwin PE, Verheugt FW, Weaver WD. Influence of early prehospital thrombolysis on mortality and event-free survival (the Myocardial Infarction Triage and Intervention [MITI] Randomized Trial). MITI Project Investigators. *Am J Cardiol*. 1996;78:497–502.

200. An international randomized trial comparing four thrombolytic strategies for acute myocardial infarction. The GUSTO investigators. *N Engl J Med*. 1993;329:673–682.

201. Randomised trial of late thrombolysis in patients with suspected acute myocardial infarction. EMERAS (Estudio Multicentrico Estreptoquinasa Republicas de America del Sur) Collaborative Group. *Lancet*. 1993;342(8874):767–772.

202. Late Assessment of Thrombolytic Efficacy (LATE) study with alteplase 6–24 hours after onset of acute myocardial infarction. *Lancet*. 1993; 342(8874):759–766.

203. Hillis LD, Forman S, Braunwald E. Risk stratification before thrombolytic therapy in patients with acute myocardial infarction. The Thrombolysis in Myocardial Infarction (TIMI) Phase II Co-Investigators. *J Am Coll Cardiol*. 1990;16:313–315.

204. Simoons ML, Maggioni AP, Knatterud G, Leimberger JD, de Jaegere P, van Domburg R, Boersma E, Franzosi MG, Califf R, Schroder R, al. e. Individual risk assessment for intracranial haemorrhage during thrombolytic therapy. *Lancet*. 1993;342(8886–8887):1523–1528.

205. Mahaffey KW, Granger CB, Sloan MA, Thompson TD, Gore JM, Weaver WD, White HD, Simoons ML, Barbash GI, Topol EJ, Califf RM. Risk factors for in-hospital nonhemorrhagic stroke in patients with acute myocardial infarction treated with thrombolysis: results from GUSTO-I. *Circulation*. 1998;97:757–764.

206. Gore JM, Granger CB, Simoons ML, Sloan MA, Weaver WD, White HD, Barbash GI, Van de Werf F, Aylward PE, Topol EJ, et al. Stroke after thrombolysis. Mortality and functional outcomes in the GUSTO-I trial. Global Use of Strategies to Open Occluded Coronary Arteries. *Circulation*. 1995;92:2811–2818.

207. White HD, Barbash GI, Califf RM, Simes RJ, Granger CB, Weaver WD, Kleiman NS, Aylward PE, Gore JM, Vahanian A, Lee KL, Ross AM, Topol EJ. Age and outcome with contemporary thrombolytic therapy. Results from the GUSTO-I trial. Global Utilization of Streptokinase and TPA for Occluded coronary arteries trial. *Circulation*. 1996;94: 1826–1833.

208. Thiemann DR, Coresh J, Schulman SP, Gerstenblith G, Oetgen WJ, Powe NR. Lack of benefit for intravenous thrombolysis in patients with myocardial infarction who are older than 75 years. *Circulation*. 2000; 101:2239–2246.

209. Collins R, Peto R, Parish S, Sleight P. ISIS-3 and GISSI-2: no survival advantage with tissue plasminogen activator over streptokinase, but a significant excess of strokes with tissue plasminogen activator in both trials. *Am J Cardiol*. 1993;71:1127–1130.

210. Randomised placebo-controlled and balloon-angioplasty-controlled trial to assess safety of coronary stenting with use of platelet glycoprotein-IIb/IIIa blockade. The EPISTENT Investigators. Evaluation of Platelet IIb/IIIa Inhibitor for Stenting. *Lancet*. 1998;352(9122):87–92.

211. Selker HP, Griffith JL, D'Agostino RB. A tool for judging coronary care unit admission appropriateness, valid for both real-time and retrospective use. A time-insensitive predictive instrument (TIPI) for acute cardiac ischemia: a multicenter study. *Med Care*. 1991;29:610–627.

212. Magid DJ, Calonge BN, Rumsfeld JS, Canto JG, Frederick PD, Every NR, Barron HV. Relation between hospital primary angioplasty volume and mortality for patients with acute MI treated with primary angioplasty vs thrombolytic therapy. *JAMA*. 2000;284:3131–3138.

213. Canto JG, Every NR, Magid DJ, Rogers WJ, Malmgren JA, Frederick PD, French WJ, Tiefenbrunn AJ, Misra VK, Kiefe CI, Barron HV. The volume of primary angioplasty procedures and survival after acute myocardial infarction. National Registry of Myocardial Infarction 2 Investigators. *N Engl J Med*. 2000;342:1573–1580.

214. Dalby M, Bouzamondo A, Lechat P, Montalescot G. Transfer for primary angioplasty versus immediate thrombolysis in acute myocardial infarction: a meta-analysis. *Circulation*. 2003;108:1809–1814.

215. Nichol G, Thomas E, Callaway CW, Hedges J, Powell JL, Aufderheide TP, Rea T, Lowe R, Brown T, Dreyer J, Davis D, Idris A, Stiell I. Regional variation in out-of-hospital cardiac arrest incidence and outcome. *JAMA*. 2008;300:1423–1431.

216. Nichol G, Aufderheide TP, Eigel B, Neumar RW, Lurie KG, Bufalino VJ, Callaway CW, Menon V, Bass RR, Abella BS, Sayre M, Dougherty CM, Racht EM, Kleinman ME, O'Connor RE, Reilly JP, Ossmann EW, Peterson E. Regional systems of care for out-of-hospital cardiac arrest: A policy statement from the Am Heart Association. *Circulation*. 2010; 121:709–729.

217. Spaulding CM, Joly LM, Rosenberg A, Monchi M, Weber SN, Dhainaut JF, Carli P. Immediate coronary angiography in survivors of out-of-hospital cardiac arrest. *N Engl J Med*. 1997;336:1629–1633.

218. Abu-Laban RB, Christenson JM, Innes GD, van Beek CA, Wanger KP, McKnight RD, MacPhail IA, Puskaric J, Sadowski RP, Singer J, Schechter MT, Wood VM. Tissue plasminogen activator in cardiac arrest with pulseless electrical activity. *N Engl J Med*. 2002;346: 1522–1528.

219. Bottiger BW, Arntz HR, Chamberlain DA, Bluhmki E, Belmans A, Danays T, Carli PA, Adgey JA, Bode C, Wenzel V. Thrombolysis during resuscitation for out-of-hospital cardiac arrest. *N Engl J Med*. 2008;359:2651–2662.

220. Sunde K, Pytte M, Jacobsen D, Mangschau A, Jensen LP, Smedsrud C, Draegni T, Steen PA. Implementation of a standardised treatment protocol for post resuscitation care after out-of-hospital cardiac arrest. *Resuscitation*. 2007;73:29–39.

221. Bendz B, Eritsland J, Nakstad AR, Brekke M, Klow NE, Steen PA, Mangschau A. Long-term prognosis after out-of-hospital cardiac arrest and primary percutaneous coronary intervention. *Resuscitation*. 2004; 63:49–53.

222. Engdahl J, Abrahamsson P, Bang A, Lindqvist J, Karlsson T, Herlitz J. Is hospital care of major importance for outcome after out-of-hospital cardiac arrest? Experience acquired from patients with out-of-hospital cardiac arrest resuscitated by the same Emergency Medical Service and admitted to one of two hospitals over a 16-year period in the municipality of Goteborg. *Resuscitation*. 2000;43:201–211.

223. Gorjup V, Radsel P, Kocjancic ST, Erzen D, Noc M. Acute ST-elevation myocardial infarction after successful cardiopulmonary resuscitation. *Resuscitation*. 2007;72:379–385.

224. Garot P, Lefevre T, Eltchaninoff H, Morice MC, Tamion F, Abry B, Lesault PF, Le Tarnec JY, Pouges C, Margenet A, Monchi M, Laurent I, Dumas P, Garot J, Louvard Y. Six-month outcome of emergency percutaneous coronary intervention in resuscitated patients after cardiac arrest complicating ST-elevation myocardial infarction. *Circulation*. 2007;115:1354–1362.

225. Lettieri C, Savonitto S, De Servi S, Guagliumi G, Belli G, Repetto A, Piccaluga E, Politi A, Ettori F, Castiglioni B, Fabbiocchi F, De Cesare N, Sangiorgi G, Musumeci G, Onofri M, D'Urbano M, Pirelli S, Zanini R, Klugmann S Emergency percutaneous coronary intervention in patients with ST-elevation myocardial infarction complicated by out-of-hospital cardiac arrest: early and medium-term outcome. *Am Heart J*. 2009;157:569–575 e561.

226. Kahn JK, Glazier S, Swor R, Savas V, O'Neill WW. Primary coronary angioplasty for acute myocardial infarction complicated by out-of-hospital cardiac arrest. *The Am journal of cardiology*. 1995;75: 1069–1070.

227. Knafelj R, Radsel P, Ploj T, Noc M. Primary percutaneous coronary intervention and mild induced hypothermia in comatose survivors of ventricular fibrillation with ST-elevation acute myocardial infarction. *Resuscitation*. 2007;74:227–234.

228. Marcusohn E, Roguin A, Sebbag A, Aronson D, Dragu R, Amikam S, Boulus M, Grenadier E, Kerner A, Nikolsky E, Markiewicz W, Hammerman H, Kapeliovich M. Primary percutaneous coronary intervention after out-of-hospital cardiac arrest: patients and outcomes. *Isr Med Assoc J*. 2007;9:257–259.

229. McCullough PA, Prakash R, Tobin KJ, O'Neill WW, Thompson RJ. Application of a cardiac arrest score in patients with sudden death and ST segment elevation for triage to angiography and intervention. *J Interv Cardiol*. 2002;15:257–261.

230. Nagao K, Hayashi N, Kanmatsuse K, Arima K, Ohtsuki J, Kikushima K, Watanabe I. Cardiopulmonary cerebral resuscitation using emergency cardiopulmonary bypass, coronary reperfusion therapy and mild hypothermia in patients with cardiac arrest outside the hospital. *J Am Coll Cardiol*. 2000;36:776–783.

231. Nielsen N, Hovdenes J, Nilsson F, Rubertsson S, Stammet P, Sunde K, Valsson F, Wanscher M, Friberg H. Outcome, timing and adverse events in therapeutic hypothermia after out-of-hospital cardiac arrest. *Acta Anaesthesiol Scand*. 2009;53:926–934.

232. Peels HO, Jessurun GA, van der Horst IC, Arnold AE, Piers LH, Zijlstra F. Outcome in transferred and nontransferred patients after primary percutaneous coronary intervention for ischaemic out-of-hospital cardiac arrest. *Catheter Cardiovasc Interv*. 2008;71:147–151.

233. Pleskot M, Babu A, Hazukova R, Stritecky J, Bis J, Matejka J, Cermakova E. Out-of-hospital cardiac arrests in patients with acute ST elevation myocardial infarctions in the East Bohemian region over the period 2002–2004. *Cardiology*. 2008;109:41–51.

234. Quintero-Moran B, Moreno R, Villarreal S, Perez-Vizcayno MJ, Hernandez R, Conde C, Vazquez P, Alfonso F, Banuelos C, Escaned J, Fernandez-Ortiz A, Azcona L, Macaya C. Percutaneous coronary intervention for cardiac arrest secondary to ST-elevation acute myocardial infarction. Influence of immediate paramedical/medical assistance on clinical outcome. *J Invasive Cardiol*. 2006;18:269–272.

235. Reynolds JC, Callaway CW, El Khoudary SR, Moore CG, Alvarez RJ, Rittenberger JC. Coronary angiography predicts improved outcome following cardiac arrest: propensity-adjusted analysis. *J Intensive Care Med*. 2009;24:179–186.

236. Hartwell D, Colquitt J, Loveman E, Clegg AJ, Brodin H, Waugh N, Royle P, Davidson P, Vale L, MacKenzie L Clinical effectiveness and cost-effectiveness of immediate angioplasty for acute myocardial infarction: systematic review and economic evaluation. *Health Technol Assess*. 2005;9:1–99, iii–iv.

237. Peterson LR, Chandra NC, French WJ, Rogers WJ, Weaver WD, Tiefenbrunn AJ. Reperfusion therapy in patients with acute myocardial infarction and prior coronary artery bypass graft surgery (National Registry of Myocardial Infarction-2). *Am J Cardiol*. 1999;84: 1287–1291.

238. Dragu R, Behar S, Sandach A, Boyko V, Kapeliovich M, Rispler S, Hammerman H. Should primary percutaneous coronary intervention be the preferred method of reperfusion therapy for patients with renal failure and ST-elevation acute myocardial infarction? *Am J Cardiol*. 2006;97:1142–1145.

239. Andersen HR, Nielsen TT, Rasmussen K, Thuesen L, Kelbaek H, Thayssen P, Abildgaard U, Pedersen F, Madsen JK, Grande P, Villadsen AB, Krusell LR, Haghfelt T, Lomholt P, Husted SE, Vigholt E, Kjaergard HK, Mortensen LS. A comparison of coronary angioplasty with fibrinolytic therapy in acute myocardial infarction. *N Engl J Med*. 2003;349:733–742.

240. Scott I, Chan J, Aroney C, Carroll G. Local thrombolysis or rapid transfer for primary angioplasty for patients presenting with ST segment elevation myocardial infarction to hospitals without angioplasty facilities. *Internal medicine journal*. 2004;34:373–377.

241. Hochman JS, Sleeper LA, Webb JG, Sanborn TA, White HD, Talley JD, Buller CE, Jacobs AK, Slater JN, Col J, McKinlay SM, LeJemtel TH. Early revascularization in acute myocardial infarction complicated by cardiogenic shock. SHOCK Investigators. Should We Emergently Revascularize Occluded Coronaries for Cardiogenic Shock. *N Engl J Med*. 1999;341:625–634.

242. Kent DM, Ruthazer R, Griffith JL, Beshansky JR, Grines CL, Aversano T, Concannon TW, Zalenski RJ, Selker HP. Comparison of mortality benefit of immediate thrombolytic therapy versus delayed primary angioplasty for acute myocardial infarction. *Am J Cardiol*. 2007;99: 1384–1388.

243. Nallamothu BK, Bates ER. Percutaneous coronary intervention versus fibrinolytic therapy in acute myocardial infarction: is timing (almost) everything? *Am J Cardiol*. 2003;92:824–826.

243a.Betriu A, Masotti M. Comparison of mortality rates in acute myocardial infarction treated by percutaneous coronary intervention versus fibrinolysis. *Am J Cardiol*. 2005;95:100–101.

243b.Boersma E. Does time matter? A pooled analysis of randomized clinical trials comparing primary percutaneous coronary intervention and in-hospital fibrinolysis in acute myocardial infarction patients. *Eur Heart J*. 2006;27:779–788.

243c. Van de Werf F, Bax J, Betriu A, Blomstrom-Lundqvist C, Crea F, Falk V, Filippatos G, Fox K, Huber K, Kastrati A, Rosengren A, Steg PG, Tubaro M, Verheugt F, Weidinger F, Weis M, Vahanian A, Camm J, De Caterina R, Dean V, Dickstein K, Filippatos G, Funck-Brentano C, Hellemans I, Kristensen SD, McGregor K, Sechtem U, Silber S, Tendera M, Widimsky P, Zamorano JL, Silber S, Aguirre FV, Al-Attar N, Alegria E, Andreotti F, Benzer W, Breithardt O, Danchin N, Di Mario C, Dudek D, Gulba D, Halvorsen S, Kaufmann P, Kornowski R, Lip GY, Rutten F. Management of acute myocardial infarction in patients presenting with persistent ST-segment elevation: the Task Force on the Management of ST-Segment Elevation Acute Myocardial Infarction of the European Society of Cardiology. *Eur Heart J*. 2008;29:2909-2945.

243d. Nallamothu B, Fox KA, Kennelly BM, Van de Werf F, Gore JM, Steg PG, Granger CB, Dabbous OH, Kline-Rogers E, Eagle KA. Relationship of treatment delays and mortality in patients undergoing fibrinolysis and primary percutaneous coronary intervention. The Global Registry of Acute Coronary Events. *Heart (British Cardiac Society)*. 2007;93: 1552–1555.

244. Holmes DR Jr, Bates ER, Kleiman NS, Sadowski Z, Horgan JH, Morris DC, Califf RM, Berger PB, Topol EJ. Contemporary reperfusion therapy for cardiogenic shock: the GUSTO-I trial experience. The GUSTO-I Investigators. Global Utilization of Streptokinase and Tissue Plasminogen Activator for Occluded Coronary Arteries. *J Am Coll Cardiol*. 1995;26:668–674.

245. Babaev A, Frederick PD, Pasta DJ, Every N, Sichrovsky T, Hochman JS. Trends in management and outcomes of patients with acute myocardial infarction complicated by cardiogenic shock. *Jama*. 2005;294: 448–454.

246. Goldberg RJ, Spencer FA, Gore JM, Lessard D, Yarzebski J. Thirty-year trends (1975 to 2005) in the magnitude of, management of, and hospital death rates associated with cardiogenic shock in patients with acute myocardial infarction: a population-based perspective. *Circulation*. 2009;119:1211–1219.

247. Hochman JS, Sleeper LA, Webb JG, Dzavik V, Buller CE, Aylward P, Col J, White HD. Early revascularization and long-term survival in cardiogenic shock complicating acute myocardial infarction. *Jama*. 2006;295:2511–2515.

248. Singh M, White J, Hasdai D, Hodgson PK, Berger PB, Topol EJ, Califf RM, Holmes DR Jr. Long-term outcome and its predictors among patients with ST-segment elevation myocardial infarction complicated by shock: insights from the GUSTO-I trial. *J Am Coll Cardiol*. 2007; 50:1752–1758.

249. Sleeper LA, Ramanathan K, Picard MH, Lejemtel TH, White HD, Dzavik V, Tormey D, Avis NE, Hochman JS. Functional status and quality of life after emergency revascularization for cardiogenic shock complicating acute myocardial infarction. *J Am Coll Cardiol*. 2005;46: 266–273.

250. Califf RM, Bengtson JR. Cardiogenic shock. N Engl J Med. 1994;330: 1724–1730.

251. Zehender M, Kasper W, Kauder E, Schonthaler M, Geibel A, Olschewski M, Just H. Right ventricular infarction as an independent predictor of prognosis after acute inferior myocardial infarction. *N Engl J Med*. 1993;328:981–988.

252. Berger PB, Ruocco NA Jr, Ryan TJ, Jacobs AK, Zaret BL, Wackers FJ, Frederick MM, Faxon DP. Frequency and significance of right ventricular dysfunction during inferior wall left ventricular myocardial infarction treated with thrombolytic therapy (results from the thrombolysis in myocardial infarction [TIMI] II trial). The TIMI Research Group. *Am J Cardiol*. 1993;71:1148–1152.

253. Goldstein JA, Barzilai B, Rosamond TL, Eisenberg PR, Jaffe AS. Determinants of hemodynamic compromise with severe right ventricular infarction. *Circulation*. 1990;82:359–368.

254. Alexander D, Ou FS, Roe MT, Pollack CV Jr, Ohman EM, Cannon CP, Gibler WB, Fintel DJ, Peterson ED, Brown DL. Use of and inhospital outcomes after early clopidogrel therapy in patients not undergoing an early invasive strategy for treatment of non-ST-segment elevation myocardial infarction: results from Can Rapid risk stratification of Unstable angina patients Suppress ADverse outcomes with Early implementation of the Am College of Cardiology/Am Heart Association guidelines (CRUSADE). *Am Heart J*. 2008;156:606–612.

255. Chan AW, Moliterno DJ, Berger PB, Stone GW, DiBattiste PM, Yakubov SL, Sapp SK, Wolski K, Bhatt DL, Topol EJ. Triple antiplatelet therapy during percutaneous coronary intervention is associated with improved outcomes including one-year survival: results from the Do

Tirofiban and ReoProGive Similar Efficacy Outcome Trial (TARGET). *J Am Coll Cardiol*. 2003;42:1188–1195.

256. Zeymer U, Gitt AK, Zahn R, Junger C, Bauer T, Koth O, Heer T, Wienbergen H, Gottwik M, Senges J. Clopidogrel in addition to aspirin reduces one-year major adverse cardiac and cerebrovascular events in unselected patients with non-ST segment elevation myocardial infarction. *Acute Card Care*. 2008;10:43–48.

257. Fox KA, Mehta SR, Peters R, Zhao F, Lakkis N, Gersh BJ, Yusuf S. Benefits and risks of the combination of clopidogrel and aspirin in patients undergoing surgical revascularization for non-ST-elevation acute coronary syndrome: the Clopidogrel in Unstable angina to prevent Recurrent ischemic Events (CURE) Trial. *Circulation*. 2004;110: 1202–1208.

258. Steinhubl SR, Berger PB, Mann JT III, Fry ET, DeLago A, Wilmer C, Topol EJ. Early and sustained dual oral antiplatelet therapy following percutaneous coronary intervention: a randomized controlled trial. *JAMA*. 2002;288:2411–2420.

259. Yusuf S, Zhao F, Mehta SR, Chrolavicius S, Tognoni G, Fox KK. Effects of clopidogrel in addition to aspirin in patients with acute coronary syndromes without ST-segment elevation. *N Engl J Med*. 2001;345:494–502.

260. Sabatine MS, Cannon CP, Gibson CM, Lopez-Sendon JL, Montalescot G, Theroux P, Claeys MJ, Cools F, Hill KA, Skene AM, McCabe CH, Braunwald E. Addition of clopidogrel to aspirin and fibrinolytic therapy for myocardial infarction with ST-segment elevation. *N Engl J Med*. 2005;352:1179–1189.

261. Sabatine MS, Cannon CP, Gibson CM, Lopez-Sendon JL, Montalescot G, Theroux P, Lewis BS, Murphy SA, McCabe CH, Braunwald E. Effect of clopidogrel pretreatment before percutaneous coronary intervention in patients with ST-elevation myocardial infarction treated with fibrinolytics: the PCI-CLARITY study. *JAMA*. 2005;294:1224–1232.

262. Verheugt FW, Montalescot G, Sabatine MS, Soulat L, Lambert Y, Lapostolle F, Adgey J, Cannon CP. Prehospital fibrinolysis with dual antiplatelet therapy in ST-elevation acute myocardial infarction: a substudy of the randomized double blind CLARITY-TIMI 28 trial. *J Thromb Thrombolysis*. 2007;23:173–179.

263. Chen ZM, Jiang LX, Chen YP, Xie JX, Pan HC, Peto R, Collins R, Liu LS. Addition of clopidogrel to aspirin in 45,852 patients with acute myocardial infarction: randomised placebo-controlled trial. *Lancet*. 2005;366(9497):1607–1621.

264. Zeymer U, Gitt A, Junger C, Bauer T, Heer T, Koeth O, Mark B, Zahn R, Senges J, Gottwik M. Clopidogrel in addition to aspirin reduces in-hospital major cardiac and cerebrovascular events in unselected patients with acute ST segment elevation myocardial. *Thromb Haemost*. 2008;99:155–160.

265. Zeymer U, Gitt AK, Junger C, Heer T, Wienbergen H, Koeth O, Bauer T, Mark B, Zahn R, Gottwik M, Senges J. Effect of clopidogrel on 1-year mortality in hospital survivors of acute ST-segment elevation myocardial infarction in clinical practice. *Eur Heart J*. 2006;27: 2661–2666.

266. Lev EI, Kornowski R, Vaknin-Assa H, Brosh D, Fuchs S, Battler A, Assali A. Effect of clopidogrel pretreatment on angiographic and clinical outcomes in patients undergoing primary percutaneous coronary intervention for ST-elevation acute myocardial infarction. *Am J Cardiol*. 2008;101:435–439.

267. Vlaar PJ, Svilaas T, Damman K, de Smet BJ, Tijssen JG, Hillege HL, Zijlstra F. Impact of pretreatment with clopidogrel on initial patency and outcome in patients treated with primary percutaneous coronary intervention for ST-segment elevation myocardial infarction: a systematic review. *Circulation*. 2008;118:1828–1836.

268. Wiviott SD, Braunwald E, McCabe CH, Montalescot G, Ruzyllo W, Gottlieb S, Neumann FJ, Ardissino D, De Servi S, Murphy SA, Riesmeyer J, Weerakkody G, Gibson CM, Antman EM. Prasugrel versus clopidogrel in patients with acute coronary syndromes. *N Engl J Med*. 2007;357:2001–2015.

269. Antman EM, Wiviott SD, Murphy SA, Voitk J, Hasin Y, Widimsky P, Chandna H, Macias W, McCabe CH, Braunwald E. Early and late benefits of prasugrel in patients with acute coronary syndromes undergoing percutaneous coronary intervention: a TRITON-TIMI 38 (TRial to Assess Improvement in Therapeutic Outcomes by Optimizing Platelet InhibitioN with Prasugrel-Thrombolysis In Myocardial Infarction) analysis. *J Am Coll Cardiol*. 2008;51:2028–2033.

270. Murphy SA, Antman EM, Wiviott SD, Weerakkody G, Morocutti G, Huber K, Lopez-Sendon J, McCabe CH, Braunwald E. Reduction in recurrent cardiovascular events with prasugrel compared with clopi-

dogrel in patients with acute coronary syndromes from the TRITON-TIMI 38 trial. *Eur Heart J.* 2008;29:2473–2479.

271. Wiviott SD, Braunwald E, Angiolillo DJ, Meisel S, Dalby AJ, Verheugt FW, Goodman SG, Corbalan R, Purdy DA, Murphy SA, McCabe CH, Antman EM. Greater clinical benefit of more intensive oral antiplatelet therapy with prasugrel in patients with diabetes mellitus in the trial to assess improvement in therapeutic outcomes by optimizing platelet inhibition with prasugrel-Thrombolysis in Myocardial Infarction 38. *Circulation.* 2008;118:1626–1636.

272. Wiviott SD, Antman EM, Winters KJ, Weerakkody G, Murphy SA, Behounek BD, Carney RJ, Lazzam C, McKay RG, McCabe CH, Braunwald E. Randomized comparison of prasugrel (CS-747, LY640315), a novel thienopyridine P2Y12 antagonist, with clopidogrel in percutaneous coronary intervention: results of the Joint Utilization of Medications to Block Platelets Optimally (JUMBO)-TIMI 26 trial. *Circulation.* 2005;111:3366–3373.

273. Montalescot G, Wiviott SD, Braunwald E, Murphy SA, Gibson CM, McCabe CH, Antman EM. Prasugrel compared with clopidogrel in patients undergoing percutaneous coronary intervention for ST-elevation myocardial infarction (TRITON-TIMI 38): double-blind, randomised controlled trial. *Lancet.* 2009;373(9665):723–731.

274. Wiviott SD, Braunwald E, McCabe CH, Horvath I, Keltai M, Herrman JP, Van de Werf F, Downey WE, Scirica BM, Murphy SA, Antman EM. Intensive oral antiplatelet therapy for reduction of ischaemic events including stent thrombosis in patients with acute coronary syndromes treated with percutaneous coronary intervention and stenting in the TRITON-TIMI 38 trial: a subanalysis of a randomised trial. *Lancet.* 2008;371(9621):1353–1363.

275. Boersma E, Harrington RA, Moliterno DJ, White H, Theroux P, Van de Werf F, de Torbal A, Armstrong PW, Wallentin LC, Wilcox RG, Simes J, Califf RM, Topol EJ, Simoons ML. Platelet glycoprotein IIb/IIIa inhibitors in acute coronary syndromes: a meta-analysis of all major randomised clinical trials. *Lancet.* 2002;359:189–198.

276. Inhibition of the platelet glycoprotein IIb/IIIa receptor with tirofiban in unstable angina and non-Q-wave myocardial infarction. Platelet Receptor Inhibition in Ischemic Syndrome Management in Patients Limited by Unstable Signs and Symptoms (PRISM-PLUS) Study Investigators. *N Eng J Med.* 1998;338:1488–1497.

277. Inhibition of platelet glycoprotein IIb/IIIa with eptifibatide in patients with acute coronary syndromes. The PURSUIT Trial Investigators. Platelet Glycoprotein IIb/IIIa in Unstable Angina: Receptor Suppression Using Integrilin Therapy. *N Eng J Med.* 1998;339:436–443.

278. Randomised placebo-controlled trial of abciximab before and during coronary intervention in refractory unstable angina: the CAPTURE Study. *Lancet.* May 17 1997;349:1429–1435.

279. Cannon CP, Weintraub WS, Demopoulos LA, Vicari R, Frey MJ, Lakkis N, Neumann FJ, Robertson DH, DeLucca PT, DiBattiste PM, Gibson CM, Braunwald E. Comparison of early invasive and conservative strategies in patients with unstable coronary syndromes treated with the glycoprotein IIb/IIIa inhibitor tirofiban. *N Engl J Med.* 2001;344: 1879–1887.

280. Stone GW, Ware JH, Bertrand ME, Lincoff AM, Moses JW, Ohman EM, White HD, Feit F, Colombo A, McLaurin BT, Cox DA, Manoukian SV, Fahy M, Clayton TC, Mehran R, Pocock SJ. Antithrombotic strategies in patients with acute coronary syndromes undergoing early invasive management: one-year results from the ACUITY trial. *JAMA.* 2007;298:2497–2506.

281. Giugliano RP, White JA, Bode C, Armstrong PW, Montalescot G, Lewis BS, van't Hof A, Berdan LG, Lee KL, Strony JT, Hildemann S, Veltri E, Van de Werf F, Braunwald E, Harrington RA, Califf RM, Newby LK. Early versus delayed, provisional eptifibatide in acute coronary syndromes. *N Engl J Med.* 2009;360:2176–2190.

282. A comparison of aspirin plus tirofiban with aspirin plus heparin for unstable angina. Platelet Receptor Inhibition in Ischemic Syndrome Management (PRISM) Study Investigators. *N Engl J Med.* 1998;338: 1498–1505.

283. Hamm CW, Heeschen C, Goldmann B, Vahanian A, Adgey J, Miguel CM, Rutsch W, Berger J, Kootstra J, Simoons ML. Benefit of abciximab in patients with refractory unstable angina in relation to serum troponin T levels. c7E3 Fab Antiplatelet Therapy in Unstable Refractory Angina (CAPTURE) Study Investigators. *N Engl J Med.* 1999;340:1623–1629.

284. Heeschen C, Hamm CW, Goldmann B, Deu A, Langenbrink L, White HD. Troponin concentrations for stratification of patients with acute coronary syndromes in relation to therapeutic efficacy of tirofiban. PRISM Study Investigators. Platelet Receptor Inhibition in Ischemic Syndrome Management. *Lancet.* 1999;354:1757–1762.

285. Cannon CP, Weintraub WS, Demopoulos LA, Vicari R, Frey MJ, Lakkis N, Neumann FJ, Robertson DH, DeLucca PT, DiBattiste PM, Gibson CM, Braunwald E. Comparison of early invasive and conservative strategies in patients with unstable coronary syndromes treated with the glycoprotein IIb/IIIa inhibitor tirofiban. *N Engl J Med.* 2001;344: 1879–1887.

286. Roffi M, Chew DP, Mukherjee D, Bhatt DL, White JA, Heeschen C, Hamm CW, Moliterno DJ, Califf RM, White HD, Kleiman NS, Theroux P, Topol EJ. Platelet glycoprotein IIb/IIIa inhibitors reduce mortality in diabetic patients with non-ST-segment-elevation acute coronary syndromes. *Circulation.* 2001;104:2767–2771.

287. Randomised trial of intravenous atenolol among 16 027 cases of suspected acute myocardial infarction: ISIS-1. First International Study of Infarct Survival Collaborative Group. *Lancet.* 1986;2:57–66.

288. Hjalmarson A, Herlitz J, Holmberg S, Ryden L, Swedberg K, Vedin A, Waagstein F, Waldenstrom A, Waldenstrom J, Wedel H, Wilhelmsen L, Wilhelmsson C. The Goteborg metoprolol trial. Effects on mortality and morbidity in acute myocardial infarction: Limitation of infarct size by beta blockers and its potential role for prognosis. *Circulation.* 1983;67(6 Pt 2):I26–I32.

289. Reduction of infarct size by the early use of intravenous timolol in acute myocardial infarction. International Collaborative Study Group. *Am J Cardiol.* 1984;54:14E–15E.

290. Jurgensen HJ, Andersen MP, Bechsgaard P, Frederiksen J, Hansen DA, Nielsen PB, Pedersen F, Pedersen-Bjergaard O, Rasmussen SL. Effect of acute and long-term beta-adrenergic blockade with alprenolol in definite or suspected myocardial infarction. Study design, patient characteristics and conduct of the study. *Acta medica Scandinavica.* 1984; 680:8–17.

291. Galcera-Tomas J, Castillo-Soria FJ, Villegas-Garcia MM, Florenciano-Sanchez R, Sanchez-Villanueva JG, de La Rosa JA, Martinez-Caballero A, Valenti-Aldeguer JA, Jara-Perez P, Parraga-Ramirez M, Lopez-Martinez I, Inigo-Garcia L, Pico-Aracil F. Effects of early use of atenolol or captopril on infarct size and ventricular volume: A double-blind comparison in patients with anterior acute myocardial infarction. *Circulation.* 2001;103:813–819.

292. Chen ZM, Pan HC, Chen YP, Peto R, Collins R, Jiang LX, Xie JX, Liu LS. Early intravenous then oral metoprolol in 45,852 patients with acute myocardial infarction: randomised placebo-controlled trial. *Lancet.* 2005;366(9497):1622–1632.

293. Herlitz J, Edvardsson N, Holmberg S, Ryden L, Waagstein F, Waldenstrom A, Swedberg K, Hjalmarson A Goteborg Metoprolol Trial: effects on arrhythmias. *Am J Cardiol.* 1984;53:27D–31D.

294. Metoprolol in acute myocardial infarction (MIAMI). A randomised placebo-controlled international trial. The MIAMI Trial Research Group. *Eur Heart J.* 1985;6:199–226.

295. Roberts R, Rogers WJ, Mueller HS, Lambrew CT, Diver DJ, Smith HC, Willerson JT, Knatterud GL, Forman S, Passamani E, et al. Immediate versus deferred beta-blockade following thrombolytic therapy in patients with acute myocardial infarction. Results of the Thrombolysis in Myocardial Infarction (TIMI) II-B Study. *Circulation.* 1991;83: 422–437.

296. Al-Reesi A, Al-Zadjali N, Perry J, Fergusson D, Al-Shamsi M, Al-Thagafi M, Stiell I. Do beta-blockers reduce short-term mortality following acute myocardial infarction? A systematic review and meta-analysis. *CJEM.* 2008;10:215–223.

297. Yusuf S, Peto R, Lewis J, Collins R, Sleight P. Beta blockade during and after myocardial infarction: an overview of the randomized trials. *Prog Cardiovasc Dis.* 1985;27:335–371.

298. Basu S, Senior R, Raval U, van der Does R, Bruckner T, Lahiri A. Beneficial effects of intravenous and oral carvedilol treatment in acute myocardial infarction. A placebo-controlled, randomized trial. *Circulation.* 1997;96:183–191.

299. Freemantle N, Cleland J, Young P, Mason J, Harrison J. β-Blockade after myocardial infarction: systematic review and meta regression analysis. *BMJ.* 1999;318(7200):1730–1737.

300. Murray DP, Murray RG, Rafiqi E, Littler WA. Does acute-phase beta-blockade reduce mortality in acute myocardial infarction by limiting infarct size? *Int J Cardiol.* 1988;20:327–339.

301. Heidbuchel H, Tack J, Vanneste L, Ballet A, Ector H, Van de Werf F. Significance of arrhythmias during the first 24 hours of acute myocardial infarction treated with alteplase and effect of early administration of a

beta-blocker or a bradycardiac agent on their incidence. *Circulation.* 1994;89:1051–1059.

302. Herlitz J, Hjalmarson A, Swedberg K, Ryden L, Waagstein F. Effects on mortality during five years after early intervention with metoprolol in suspected acute myocardial infarction. *Acta Med Scand.* 1988;223: 227–231.

303. TIMI-11B Investigators, Antman EM, McCabe CH, Gurfinkel EP, Turpie AG, Bernink PJ, Salein D, Bayes De Luna A, Fox K, Lablanche JM, Radley D, Premmereur J, Braunwald E. Enoxaparin prevents death and cardiac ischemic events in unstable angina/non-Q-wave myocardial infarction. Results of the thrombolysis in myocardial infarction (TIMI) 11B trial. *Circulation.* 1999;100:1593–1601.

304. Campos JV, Juarez Herrera U, Rosas Peralta M, Lupi Herrera E, Gonzalez Pacheco H, Martinez Sanchez C, Chuquiure Valenzuela E, Vieyra Herrera G, Cardozo Zepeda C, Barrera Sanchez C, Reyes Corona J, Cortina de la Rosa E, de la Pena Diaz A, Izaguirre Avila R, de la Pena Fernandez A. [Decrease of total hemorrhage with reduced doses of enoxaparin in high risk unstable angina. ENHNFAI study. (Enoxaparin vs non-fractionated heparin in unstable angina). Preliminary report]. *Arch Cardiol Mex.* 2002;72:209–219.

305. Cohen M, Demers C, Gurfinkel EP, Turpie AG, Fromell GJ, Goodman S, Langer A, Califf RM, Fox KA, Premmereur J, Bigonzi F. A comparison of low-molecular-weight heparin with unfractionated heparin for unstable coronary artery disease. Efficacy and Safety of Subcutaneous Enoxaparin in Non-Q-Wave Coronary Events Study Group. *N Engl J Med.* 1997;337:447–452.

306. Cohen M, Theroux P, Borzak S, Frey MJ, White HD, Van Mieghem W, Senatore F, Lis J, Mukherjee R, Harris K, Bigonzi F. Randomized double-blind safety study of enoxaparin versus unfractionated heparin in patients with non-ST-segment elevation acute coronary syndromes treated with tirofiban and aspirin: the ACUTE II study. The Antithrombotic Combination Using Tirofiban and Enoxaparin. *Am Heart J.* 2002;144:470–477.

307. Goodman SG, Cohen M, Bigonzi F, Gurfinkel EP, Radley DR, Le Iouer V, Fromell GJ, Demers C, Turpie AG, Califf RM, Fox KA, Langer A. Randomized trial of low molecular weight heparin (enoxaparin) versus unfractionated heparin for unstable coronary artery disease: one-year results of the ESSENCE Study. Efficacy and Safety of Subcutaneous Enoxaparin in Non-Q Wave Coronary Events. *J Am Coll Cardiol.* 2000;36:693–698.

308. Goodman SG, Fitchett D, Armstrong PW, Tan M, Langer A. Randomized evaluation of the safety and efficacy of enoxaparin versus unfractionated heparin in high-risk patients with non-ST-segment elevation acute coronary syndromes receiving the glycoprotein IIb/IIIa inhibitor eptifibatide. *Circulation.* 2003;107:238–244.

309. Malhotra S, Bhargava VK, Grover A, Pandhi P, Sharma YP. A randomized trial to compare the efficacy, safety, cost and platelet aggregation effects of enoxaparin and unfractionated heparin (the ESCAPEU trial). *Int J Clin Pharmacol Ther.* 2001;39:110–115.

310. Blazing MA, de Lemos JA, White HD, Fox KA, Verheugt FW, Ardissino D, DiBattiste PM, Palmisano J, Bilheimer DW, Snapinn SM, Ramsey KE, Gardner LH, Hasselblad V, Pfeffer MA, Lewis EF, Braunwald E, Califf RM. Safety and efficacy of enoxaparin vs unfractionated heparin in patients who receive tirofiban and aspirin: a randomized controlled trial. *JAMA.* 2004;292:55–64.

311. Ferguson JJ, Califf RM, Antman EM, Cohen M, Grines CL, Goodman S, Kereiakes DJ, Langer A, Mahaffey KW, Nessel CC, Armstrong PW, Avezum A, Aylward P, Becker RC, Biasucci L, Borzak S, Col J, Frey MJ, Fry E, Gulba DC, Guneri S, Gurfinkel E, Harrington R, Hochman JS, Kleiman NS, Leon MB, Lopez-Sendon JL, Pepine CJ, Ruzyllo W, Steinhubl SR, Teirstein PS, Toro-Figueroa L, White H. Enoxaparin vs unfractionated heparin in high-risk patients with non-ST-segment elevation acute coronary syndromes managed with an intended early invasive strategy: primary results of the SYNERGY randomized trial. *JAMA.* 2004;292:45–54.

312. Mahaffey KW, Ferguson JJ. Exploring the role of enoxaparin in the management of high-risk patients with non-ST-elevation acute coronary syndromes: the SYNERGY trial. *Am heart journal.* 2005;149(4 Suppl): S81–S90.

313. Mitrovska S, Jovanova S. Low-molecular weight heparin enoxaparin in the treatment of acute coronary syndromes without ST segment elevation. *Bratislavske lekarske listy.* 2009;110:45–48.

314. Antman EM, Cohen M, Radley D, McCabe C, Rush J, Premmereur J, Braunwald E. Assessment of the treatment effect of enoxaparin for

unstable angina/non-Q-wave myocardial infarction: TIMI 11B-essence meta-analysis. *Circulation.* 1999;100:1602–1608.

315. Antman EM, Cohen M, McCabe C, Goodman SG, Murphy SA, Braunwald E. Enoxaparin is superior to unfractionated heparin for preventing clinical events at 1-year follow-up of TIMI 11B and ESSENCE. *Eur Heart J.* 2002;23:308–314.

316. Magee KD, Sevcik W, Moher D, Rowe BH Low molecular weight heparins versus unfractionated heparin for acute coronary syndromes. *Cochrane Database Syst Rev.* 2003:CD002132.

317. Petersen JL, Mahaffey KW, Hasselblad V, Antman EM, Cohen M, Goodman SG, Langer A, Blazing MA, Le-Moigne-Amrani A, de Lemos JA, Nessel CC, Harrington RA, Ferguson JJ, Braunwald E, Califf RM. Efficacy and bleeding complications among patients randomized to enoxaparin or unfractionated heparin for antithrombin therapy in non-ST-Segment elevation acute coronary syndromes: a systematic overview. *JAMA.* 2004;292:89–96.

318. Eikelboom JW, Anand SS, Malmberg K, Weitz JI, Ginsberg JS, Yusuf S. Unfractionated heparin and low-molecular-weight heparin in acute coronary syndrome without ST elevation: a meta-analysis. *Lancet.* 2000; 355(9219):1936–1942.

319. Le Nguyen MT, Spencer FA. Low molecular weight heparin and unfractionated heparin in the early pharmacologic management of acute coronary syndromes: a meta-analysis of randomized clinical trials. *J Thromb Thrombolysis.* 2001;12:289–295.

320. Murphy SA, Gibson CM, Morrow DA, Van de Werf F, Menown IB, Goodman SG, Mahaffey KW, Cohen M, McCabe CH, Antman EM, Braunwald E. Efficacy and safety of the low-molecular weight heparin enoxaparin compared with unfractionated heparin across the acute coronary syndrome spectrum: a meta-analysis. *Eur Heart J.* 2007;28: 2077–2086.

321. Joyner CD, Peters RJ, Afzal R, Chrolavicius S, Mehta SR, Fox KA, Granger CB, Franzosi MG, Flather M, Budaj A, Bassand JP, Yusuf S. Fondaparinux compared to enoxaparin in patients with acute coronary syndromes without ST-segment elevation: outcomes and treatment effect across different levels of risk. *Am Heart J.* 2009;157:502–508.

322. Mehta SR, Granger CB, Eikelboom JW, Bassand JP, Wallentin L, Faxon DP, Peters RJ, Budaj A, Afzal R, Chrolavicius S, Fox KA, Yusuf S. Efficacy and safety of fondaparinux versus enoxaparin in patients with acute coronary syndromes undergoing percutaneous coronary intervention: results from the OASIS-5 trial. *J Am Coll Cardiol.* 2007;50: 1742–1751.

323. Mehta SR, Steg PG, Granger CB, Bassand JP, Faxon DP, Weitz JI, Afzal R, Rush B, Peters RJ, Natarajan MK, Velianou JL, Goodhart DM, Labinaz M, Tanguay JF, Fox KA, Yusuf S. Randomized, blinded trial comparing fondaparinux with unfractionated heparin in patients undergoing contemporary percutaneous coronary intervention: Arixtra Study in Percutaneous Coronary Intervention: a Randomized Evaluation (ASPIRE) Pilot Trial. *Circulation.* 2005;111:1390–1397.

324. Yusuf S, Mehta SR, Chrolavicius S, Afzal R, Pogue J, Granger CB, Budaj A, Peters RJ, Bassand JP, Wallentin L, Joyner C, Fox KA. Comparison of fondaparinux and enoxaparin in acute coronary syndromes. *N Engl J Med.* 2006;354:1464–1476.

325. Mehta SR, Boden WE, Eikelboom JW, Flather M, Steg PG, Avezum A, Afzal R, Piegas LS, Faxon DP, Widimsky P, Budaj A, Chrolavicius S, Rupprecht HJ, Jolly S, Granger CB, Fox KA, Bassand JP, Yusuf S. Antithrombotic therapy with fondaparinux in relation to interventional management strategy in patients with ST- and non-ST-segment elevation acute coronary syndromes: an individual patient-level combined analysis of the Fifth and Sixth Organization to Assess Strategies in Ischemic Syndromes (OASIS 5 and 6) randomized trials. *Circulation.* 2008;118:2038–2046.

326. Feit F, Manoukian SV, Ebrahimi R, Pollack CV, Ohman EM, Attubato MJ, Mehran R, Stone GW. Safety and efficacy of bivalirudin monotherapy in patients with diabetes mellitus and acute coronary syndromes: a report from the ACUITY (Acute Catheterization and Urgent Intervention Triage Strategy) trial. *J Am Coll Cardiol.* 2008;51:1645–1652.

327. Lansky AJ, Mehran R, Cristea E, Parise H, Feit F, Ohman EM, White HD, Alexander KP, Bertrand ME, Desmet W, Hamon M, Stone GW. Impact of gender and antithrombin strategy on early and late clinical outcomes in patients with non-ST-elevation acute coronary syndromes (from the ACUITY trial). *Am J Cardiol.* 2009;103:1196–1203.

328. Lopes RD, Alexander KP, Manoukian SV, Bertrand ME, Feit F, White HD, Pollack CV Jr, Hoekstra J, Gersh BJ, Stone GW, Ohman EM. Advanced age, antithrombotic strategy, and bleeding in non-ST-segment elevation acute coronary syndromes: results from the ACUITY (Acute

Catheterization and Urgent Intervention Triage Strategy) trial. *Journal of the Am College of Cardiology*. 2009;53:1021–1030.

329. Singh S, Molnar J, Arora R. Efficacy and safety of bivalirudin versus heparins in reduction of cardiac outcomes in acute coronary syndrome and percutaneous coronary interventions. *J Cardiovasc Pharmacol Ther*. 2007;12:283–291.

330. Stone GW, Ware JH, Bertrand ME, Lincoff AM, Moses JW, Ohman EM, White HD, Feit F, Colombo A, McLaurin BT, Cox DA, Manoukian SV, Fahy M, Clayton TC, Mehran R, Pocock SJ. Antithrombotic strategies in patients with acute coronary syndromes undergoing early invasive management: one-year results from the ACUITY trial. *JAMA*. 2007;298:2497–2506.

331. Efficacy and safety of tenecteplase in combination with enoxaparin, abciximab, or unfractionated heparin: the ASSENT-3 randomised trial in acute myocardial infarction. *Lancet*. 2001;358(9282):605–613.

332. Antman EM, Louwerenburg HW, Baars HF, Wesdorp JC, Hamer B, Bassand JP, Bigonzi F, Pisapia G, Gibson CM, Heidbuchel H, Braunwald E, Van de Werf F. Enoxaparin as adjunctive antithrombin therapy for ST-elevation myocardial infarction: results of the ENTIRE-Thrombolysis in Myocardial Infarction (TIMI) 23 Trial. *Circulation*. 2002;105:1642–1649.

333. Antman EM, Morrow DA, McCabe CH, Murphy SA, Ruda M, Sadowski Z, Budaj A, Lopez-Sendon JL, Guneri S, Jiang F, White HD, Fox KA, Braunwald E. Enoxaparin versus unfractionated heparin with fibrinolysis for ST-elevation myocardial infarction. *N Engl J Med*. 2006;354:1477–1488.

334. Eikelboom JW, Quinlan DJ, Mehta SR, Turpie AG, Menown IB, Yusuf S. Unfractionated and low-molecular-weight heparin as adjuncts to thrombolysis in aspirin-treated patients with ST-elevation acute myocardial infarction: a meta-analysis of the randomized trials. *Circulation*. 2005;112:3855–3867.

335. Theroux P, Welsh RC. Meta-analysis of randomized trials comparing enoxaparin versus unfractionated heparin as adjunctive therapy to fibrinolysis in ST-elevation acute myocardial infarction. *Am J Cardiol*. 2003;91:860–864.

336. Ross AM, Molhoek P, Lundergan C, Knudtson M, Draoui Y, Regalado L, Le Louer V, Bigonzi F, Schwartz W, De Jong E, Coyne K. Randomized comparison of enoxaparin, a low-molecular-weight heparin, with unfractionated heparin adjunctive to recombinant tissue plasminogen activator thrombolysis and aspirin: Second Trial of Heparin and Aspirin Reperfusion Therapy (HART II). *Circulation*. 2001;104:648–652.

337. Sinnaeve PR, Alexander JH, Bogaerts K, Belmans A, Wallentin L, Armstrong P, Adgey JA, Tendera M, Diaz R, Soares-Piegas L, Vahanian A, Granger CB, Van De Werf FJ. Efficacy of tenecteplase in combination with enoxaparin, abciximab, or unfractionated heparin: one-year follow-up results of the Assessment of the Safety of a New Thrombolytic-3 (ASSENT-3) randomized trial in acute myocardial infarction. *Am Heart J*. 2004;147:993–998.

338. Wallentin L, Goldstein P, Armstrong PW, Granger CB, Adgey AA, Arntz HR, Bogaerts K, Danays T, Lindahl B, Makijarvi M, Verheugt F, Van de Werf F. Efficacy and safety of tenecteplase in combination with the low-molecular-weight heparin enoxaparin or unfractionated heparin in the prehospital setting: the Assessment of the Safety and Efficacy of a New Thrombolytic Regimen (ASSENT)-3 PLUS randomized trial in acute myocardial infarction. *Circulation*. 2003;108:135–142.

339. Armstrong PW, Chang WC, Wallentin L, Goldstein P, Granger CB, Bogaerts K, Danays T, Van de Werf F. Efficacy and safety of unfractionated heparin versus enoxaparin: a pooled analysis of ASSENT-3 and -3 PLUS data. *CMAJ*. 2006;174:1421–1426.

340. Yusuf S, Mehta SR, Chrolavicius S, Afzal R, Pogue J, Granger CB, Budaj A, Peters RJ, Bassand JP, Wallentin L, Joyner C, Fox KA. Effects of fondaparinux on mortality and reinfarction in patients with acute ST-segment elevation myocardial infarction: the OASIS-6 randomized trial. *JAMA*. 2006;295:1519–1530.

341. Ferguson J. Low-molecular-weight heparins and glycoprotein IIb/IIIa antagonists in acute coronary syndromes. *J Invasive Cardiol*. 2004;16:136–144.

342. Zeymer U, Gitt A, Junger C, Bauer T, Heer T, Koeth O, Wienbergen H, Zahn R, Senges J. Efficacy and safety of enoxaparin in unselected patients with ST-segment elevation myocardial infarction. *Thromb Haemost*. 2008;99:150–154.

343. Zeymer U, Gitt A, Zahn R, Junger C, Bauer T, Heer T, Koeth O, Senges J. Efficacy and safety of enoxaparin in combination with and without GP IIb/IIIa inhibitors in unselected patients with ST segment elevation

myocardial infarction treated with primary percutaneous coronary intervention. *EuroIntervention*. 2009;4:524–528.

344. Stone GW, Witzenbichler B, Guagliumi G, Peruga JZ, Brodie BR, Dudek D, Kornowski R, Hartmann F, Gersh BJ, Pocock SJ, Dangas G, Wong SC, Kirtane AJ, Parise H, Mehran R. Bivalirudin during primary PCI in acute myocardial infarction. *N Engl J Med*. 2008;358:2218–2230.

345. Mehran R, Lansky AJ, Witzenbichler B, Guagliumi G, Peruga JZ, Brodie BR, Dudek D, Kornowski R, Hartmann F, Gersh BJ, Pocock SJ, Wong SC, Nikolsky E, Gambone L, Vandertie L, Parise H, Dangas GD, Stone GW. Bivalirudin in patients undergoing primary angioplasty for acute myocardial infarction (HORIZONS-AMI): 1-year results of a randomised controlled trial. *Lancet*. 2009;374(9696):1149–1159.

346. GISSI-3: effects of lisinopril and transdermal glyceryl trinitrate singly and together on 6-week mortality and ventricular function after acute myocardial infarction. Gruppo Italiano per lo Studio della Sopravvivenza nell'infarto Miocardico. *Lancet*. 1994;343(8906):1115–1122.

347. Oral captopril versus placebo among 14,962 patients with suspected acute myocardial infarction: a multicenter, randomized, double-blind, placebo controlled clinical trial. Chinese Cardiac Study (CCS-1) Collaborative Group. *Chin Med J (Engl)*. 1997;110:834–838.

348. Ambrosioni E, Borghi C, Magnani B. The effect of the angiotensin-converting-enzyme inhibitor zofenopril on mortality and morbidity after anterior myocardial infarction: the Survival of Myocardial Infarction Long-Term Evaluation (SMILE) Study Investigators. *N Engl J Med*. 1995;332:80–85.

349. Borghi C, Marino P, Zardini P, Magnani B, Collatina S, Ambrosioni E. Short- and long-term effects of early fosinopril administration in patients with acute anterior myocardial infarction undergoing intravenous thrombolysis: results from the Fosinopril in Acute Myocardial Infarction Study. FAMIS Working Party. *Am Heart J*. 1998;136:213–225.

350. Oral captopril versus placebo among 13,634 patients with suspected acute myocardial infarction: interim report from the Chinese Cardiac Study (CCS-1). *Lancet*. 1995;345(8951):686–687.

351. Pfeffer MA, Greaves SC, Arnold JM, Glynn RJ, LaMotte FS, Lee RT, Menapace FJ Jr, Rapaport E, Ridker PM, Rouleau JL, Solomon SD, Hennekens CH. Early versus delayed angiotensin-converting enzyme inhibition therapy in acute myocardial infarction. The healing and early afterload reducing therapy trial. *Circulation*. 1997;95:2643–2651.

352. Indications for ACE inhibitors in the early treatment of acute myocardial infarction: systematic overview of individual data from 100,000 patients in randomized trials. ACE Inhibitor Myocardial Infarction Collaborative Group. *Circulation*. 1998;97:2202–2212.

353. Teo KK, Yusuf S, Pfeffer M, Torp-Pedersen C, Kober L, Hall A, Pogue J, Latini R, Collins R. Effects of long-term treatment with angiotensin-converting-enzyme inhibitors in the presence or absence of aspirin: a systematic review. *Lancet*. 2002;360(9339):1037–1043.

354. Latini R, Maggioni AP, Flather M, Sleight P, Tognoni G. ACE inhibitor use in patients with myocardial infarction. Summary of evidence from clinical trials. *Circulation*. 1995;92:3132–3137.

355. Latini R, Tognoni G, Maggioni AP, Baigent C, Braunwald E, Chen ZM, Collins R, Flather M, Franzosi MG, Kjekshus J, Kober L, Liu LS, Peto R, Pfeffer M, Pizzetti F, Santoro E, Sleight P, Swedberg K, Tavazzi L, Wang W, Yusuf S. Clinical effects of early angiotensin-converting enzyme inhibitor treatment for acute myocardial infarction are similar in the presence and absence of aspirin: systematic overview of individual data from 96,712 randomized patients. Angiotensin-converting Enzyme Inhibitor Myocardial Infarction Collaborative Group. *J Am Coll Cardiol*. 2000;35:1801–1807.

356. Lu CY [Treatment of acute myocardial infarction with oral captopril. A randomized, double blind and placebo controlled pilot study]. *Zhonghua Xin Xue Guan Bing Za Zhi*. 1993;21:74–76, 121–122.

357. Ray SG, Pye M, Oldroyd KG, Christie J, Connelly DT, Northridge DB, Ford I, Morton JJ, Dargie HJ, Cobbe SM. Early treatment with captopril after acute myocardial infarction. *Br Heart J*. 1993;69:215–222.

358. Di Pasquale P, Paterna S, Cannizzaro S, Bucca V. Does captopril treatment before thrombolysis in acute myocardial infarction attenuate reperfusion damage? Short-term and long-term effects. *Int J Cardiol*. 1994;43:43–50.

359. Spinar J, Vitovec J, Pluhacek L, Spinarova L, Fischerova B, Toman J. First dose hypotension after angiotensin converting enzyme inhibitor captopril and angiotensin II blocker losartan in patients with acute myocardial infarction. *Int J Cardiol*. 75(2–3):197–204, 2000.

360. Wagner A, Herkner H, Schreiber W, Bur A, Woisetschlager C, Stix G, Laggner AN, Hirschl MM. Ramipril prior to thrombolysis attenuates the early increase of PAI-1 in patients with acute myocardial infarction. *Thromb Haemost*. 2002;88:180–185.

361. Mehta PM, Przyklenk K, Kloner RA Cardioprotective effects of captopril in myocardial ischaemia, ischaemia/reperfusion and infarction. *Eur Heart J.* 1990;11 Suppl B:94–99.

362. Pfeffer MA, McMurray JJ, Velazquez EJ, Rouleau JL, Kober L, Maggioni AP, Solomon SD, Swedberg K, Van de Werf F, White H, Leimberger JD, Henis M, Edwards S, Zelenkofske S, Sellers MA, Califf RM. Valsartan, captopril, or both in myocardial infarction complicated by heart failure, left ventricular dysfunction, or both. *N Engl J Med.* 2003;349:1893–1906.

363. Di Pasquale P, Bucca V, Scalzo S, Cannizzaro S, Giubilato A, Paterna S. Does the addition of losartan improve the beneficial effects of ACE inhibitors in patients with anterior myocardial infarction? A pilot study. *Heart (British Cardiac Society).* 1999;81:606–611.

364. Kingma JH, van Gilst WH, Peels CH, Dambrink JH, Verheugt FW, Wielenga RP. Acute intervention with captopril during thrombolysis in patients with first anterior myocardial infarction. Results from the Captopril and Thrombolysis Study (CATS). *Eur Heart J.* 1994;15:898–907.

365. van Gilst WH, Kingma JH, Peels KH, Dambrink JH, St John Sutton M. Which patient benefits from early angiotensin-converting enzyme inhibition after myocardial infarction? Results of one-year serial echocardiographic follow-up from the Captopril and Thrombolysis Study (CATS). *J Am Coll Cardiol.* 1996;28:114–121.

366. de Kam PJ, Voors AA, van den Berg MP, van Veldhuisen DJ, Brouwer J, Crijns HJ, Borghi C, Ambrosioni E, Hochman JS, LeJemtel TH, Kingma JH, Sutton MS, van Gilst WH. Effect of very early angiotensin-converting enzyme inhibition on left ventricular dilation after myocardial infarction in patients receiving thrombolysis: results of a meta-analysis of 845 patients. FAMIS, CAPTIN and CATS Investigators. *Journal of the Am College of Cardiology.* 2000;36:2047–2053.

367. Voors AA, de Kam PJ, van den Berg MP, Borghi C, Hochman JS, van Veldhuisen DJ, van Gilst WH. Acute administration of angiotensin converting enzyme inhibitors in thrombolysed myocardial infarction patients is associated with a decreased incidence of heart failure, but an increased re-infarction risk. *Cardiovasc Drugs Ther.* 2005;19:119–124.

368. Kayikcioglu M, Can L, Kultursay H, Payzin S, Turkoglu C. Early use of pravastatin in patients with acute myocardial infarction undergoing coronary angioplasty. *Acta Cardiol.* 2002;57:295–302.

369. Kayikcioglu M, Can L, Evrengul H, Payzin S, Kultursay H. The effect of statin therapy on ventricular late potentials in acute myocardial infarction. *Int J Cardiol.* 2003;90:63–72.

370. Kinlay S, Schwartz GG, Olsson AG, Rifai N, Leslie SJ, Sasiela WJ, Szarek M, Libby P, Ganz P. High-dose atorvastatin enhances the decline in inflammatory markers in patients with acute coronary syndromes in the MIRACL study. *Circulation.* 2003;108:1560–1566.

371. Correia LC, Sposito AC, Lima JC, Magalhaes LP, Passos LC, Rocha MS, D'Oliveira A, Esteves JP. Anti-inflammatory effect of atorvastatin (80 mg) in unstable angina pectoris and non-Q-wave acute myocardial infarction. *Am J Cardiol.* 2003;92:298–301.

372. Heeschen C, Hamm CW, Laufs U, Snapinn S, Bohm M, White HD. Withdrawal of statins increases event rates in patients with acute coronary syndromes. *Circulation.* 2002;105:1446–1452.

373. Chan AW, Bhatt DL, Chew DP, Reginelli J, Schneider JP, Topol EJ, Ellis SG. Relation of inflammation and benefit of statins after percutaneous coronary interventions. *Circulation.* 2003;107:1750–1756.

374. Cuculi F, Radovanovic D, Eberli FR, Stauffer JC, Bertel O, Erne P. The impact of statin treatment on presentation mode and early outcomes in acute coronary syndromes. *Cardiology.* 2008;109:156–162.

375. Daskalopoulou SS, Delaney JA, Filion KB, Brophy JM, Mayo NE, Suissa S Discontinuation of statin therapy following an acute myocardial infarction: a population-based study. *Eur Heart J.* 2008.

376. Fonarow GC, Wright RS, Spencer FA, Fredrick PD, Dong W, Every N, French WJ. Effect of statin use within the first 24 hours of admission for acute myocardial infarction on early morbidity and mortality. *Am J Cardiol.* 2005;96:611–616.

377. Lenderink T, Boersma E, Gitt AK, Zeymer U, Wallentin L, Van de Werf F, Hasdai D, Behar S, Simoons ML. Patients using statin treatment within 24 h after admission for ST-elevation acute coronary syndromes had lower mortality than non-users: a report from the first Euro Heart Survey on acute coronary syndromes. *Eur Heart J.* 2006;27:1799–1804.

378. Saab FA, Petrina M, Kline-Rogers E, Fang J, Otten R, Mukherjee D, Eagle KA. Early statin therapy in elderly patients presenting with acute coronary syndrome causing less heart failure. *Indian Heart J.* 2006;58:321–324.

379. Spencer FA, Fonarow GC, Frederick PD, Wright RS, Every N, Goldberg RJ, Gore JM, Dong W, Becker RC, French W. Early withdrawal of statin therapy in patients with non-ST-segment elevation myocardial infarction: national registry of myocardial infarction. *Arch Intern Med.* 2004;164:2162–2168.

380. Kiyokuni M, Kosuge M, Ebina T, Hibi K, Tsukahara K, Okuda J, Iwahashi N, Maejima N, Kusama I, Komura N, Nakayama N, Umemura S, Kimura K. Effects of pretreatment with statins on infarct size in patients with acute myocardial infarction who receive fibrinolytic therapy. *Circ J.* 2009;73:330–335.

381. Wright RS, Bybee K, Miller WL, Laudon DA, Murphy JG, Jaffe AS. Reduced risks of death and CHF are associated with statin therapy administered acutely within the first 24 h of AMI. *Int J Cardiol.* 2006;108:314–319.

382. Pasceri V, Patti G, Nusca A, Pristipino C, Richichi G, Di Sciascio G. Randomized trial of atorvastatin for reduction of myocardial damage during coronary intervention: results from the ARMYDA (Atorvastatin for Reduction of MYocardial Damage during Angioplasty) study. *Circulation.* 2004;110:674–678.

383. Briguori C, Colombo A, Airoldi F, Violante A, Focaccio A, Balestrieri P, Paolo Elia P, Golia B, Lepore S, Riviezzo G, Scarpato P, Librera M, Bonizzoni E, Ricciardelli B. Statin administration before percutaneous coronary intervention: impact on periprocedural myocardial damage. *European heart journal.* 2004;25:1822–1828.

384. Patti G, Pasceri V, Colonna G, Miglionico M, Fischetti D, Sardella G, Montinaro A, Di Sciascio G. Atorvastatin pretreatment improves outcomes in patients with acute coronary syndromes undergoing early percutaneous coronary intervention: results of the ARMYDA-ACS randomized trial. *J Am Coll Cardiol.* 2007;49:1272–1278.

385. Mehta SR, Yusuf S, Diaz R, Zhu J, Pais P, Xavier D, Paolasso E, Ahmed R, Xie C, Kazmi K, Tai J, Orlandini A, Pogue J, Liu L. Effect of glucose-insulin-potassium infusion on mortality in patients with acute ST-segment elevation myocardial infarction: the CREATE-ECLA randomized controlled trial. *JAMA.* 2005;293:437–446.

386. Timmer J Glucose-insulin-potassium study in patients with ST-elevation myocardial infarction without signs of heart failure: The Gips-II Trial. paper presentated at Late-Breaking Clinical Trials III. Paper presented at: Am College of Cardiology Scientific Sessions;, March 9,2005; Orlando, Fla.

387. Pantridge JF, Geddes JS. A mobile intensive-care unit in the management of myocardial infarction. *Lancet.* 1967;2(7510):271–273.

388. Cohen MC, Rohtla KM, Lavery CE, Muller JE, Mittleman MA. Meta-analysis of the morning excess of acute myocardial infarction and sudden cardiac death [published correction appears in Am J Cardiol. 1998;81:260]. *Am J Cardiol.* 1997;79:1512–1516.

389. Colquhoun MC, Julien DG Sudden death in the community–the arrhythmia causing cardiac arrest and results of immediate resuscitation. *Resuscitation.* 1992;24:177A.

390. Campbell RW, Murray A, Julian DG. Ventricular arrhythmias in first 12 hours of acute myocardial infarction: natural history study. *Br Heart J.* 1981;46:351–357.

391. O'Doherty M, Tayler DI, Quinn E, Vincent R, Chamberlain DA. Five hundred patients with myocardial infarction monitored within one hour of symptoms. *BMJ.* 1983;286(6375):1405–1408.

392. Lie KI, Wellens HJ, Downar E, Durrer D. Observations on patients with primary ventricular fibrillation complicating acute myocardial infarction. *Circulation.* 1975;52:755–759.

393. MacMahon S, Collins R, Peto R, Koster RW, Yusuf S. Effects of prophylactic lidocaine in suspected acute myocardial infarction: an overview of results from the randomized, controlled trials. *JAMA.* 1988; 260:1910–1916.

394. Elizari MV, Martinez JM, Belziti C, Ciruzzi M, Perez de la Hoz R, Sinisi A, Carbajales J, Scapin O, Garguichevich J, Girotti L, Cagide A. Morbidity and mortality following early administration of amiodarone in acute myocardial infarction. GEMICA study investigators, GEMA Group, Buenos Aires, Argentina. Grupo de Estudios Multicentricos en Argentina. *Eur Heart J.* 2000;21:198–205. Copyright 2010 American Heart Association, Inc., European Resuscitation Council, and International Liaison Committee on Resuscitation.

KEY WORDS: acute coronary syndrome ■ myocardial infarction ■ non-ST-segment elevation acute coronary syndromes

# Part 11: Adult Stroke
## 2010 American Heart Association Guidelines for Cardiopulmonary Resuscitation and Emergency Cardiovascular Care

Edward C. Jauch, Co-Chair*; Brett Cucchiara, Co-Chair*; Opeolu Adeoye; William Meurer; Jane Brice; Yvonne (Yu-Feng) Chan; Nina Gentile; Mary Fran Hazinski

Nearly 15 years of increased stroke education and organization has produced significant strides in public awareness and development of stroke systems of care. Despite these successes, though, each year 795 000 people suffer a new or repeat stroke, and stroke remains the third leading cause of death in the United States.[1] Many advances have been made in stroke prevention, treatment, and rehabilitation, but arguably the greatest gains have been in the area of stroke systems of care. Integrating public education, 911 dispatch, prehospital detection and triage, hospital stroke system development, and stroke unit management have led to significant improvements in stroke care. Not only have the rates of appropriate fibrinolytic therapy increased over the past 5 years, but also overall stroke care has improved, in part through the creation of stroke centers.[2] To achieve further improvement in reducing the burden of stroke, healthcare providers, hospitals, and communities must continue to develop systems to increase the efficiency and effectiveness of stroke care.[3] The "D's of Stroke Care" remain the major steps in diagnosis and treatment of stroke and identify the key points at which delays can occur.[4,5]

- Detection: Rapid recognition of stroke symptoms
- Dispatch: Early activation and dispatch of emergency medical services (EMS) system by calling 911
- Delivery: Rapid EMS identification, management, and transport
- Door: Appropriate triage to stroke center
- Data: Rapid triage, evaluation, and management within the emergency department (ED)
- Decision: Stroke expertise and therapy selection
- Drug: Fibrinolytic therapy, intra-arterial strategies
- Disposition: Rapid admission to stroke unit, critical-care unit

This chapter summarizes the early management of acute ischemic stroke in adult patients. It describes care from out-of-hospital therapy through the first hours of in-hospital therapy. For additional information about the management of acute ischemic stroke, see the American Heart Association (AHA)/ American Stroke Association (ASA) guidelines for the management of acute ischemic stroke.[3,6,7]

## Management Goals

The overall goal of stroke care is to minimize acute brain injury and maximize patient recovery. The time-sensitive nature of stroke care is central to the establishment of successful stroke systems, hence the commonly used refrain "Time is Brain." The AHA and ASA have developed a community-oriented "Stroke Chain of Survival" that links specific actions to be taken by patients and family members with recommended actions by out-of-hospital healthcare responders, ED personnel, and in-hospital specialty services. These links, which are similar to those in the Adult Chain of Survival for victims of sudden cardiac arrest, include rapid recognition of stroke warning signs and activation of the emergency response system (call 911); rapid EMS dispatch, transport, and prehospital notification; triage to a stroke center; and rapid diagnosis, treatment, and disposition in the hospital.

The AHA ECC stroke guidelines focus on the initial out-of-hospital and ED assessment and management of the patient with acute stroke as depicted in the algorithm Goals for Management of Patients With Suspected Stroke (Figure). The time goals of the National Institute of Neurological Disorders and Stroke (NINDS)[8] are illustrated on the left side of the algorithm as clocks. A sweep hand depicts the goal in minutes from ED arrival to task completion to remind the clinician of the time-sensitive nature of management of acute ischemic stroke.

The sections below summarize the principles and goals of stroke system development and emergency assessment and management, as well as highlight new recommendations and training issues. The text refers to the numbered boxes in the algorithm.

## Stroke Systems of Care

The regionalization of stroke care was not widely considered in the era before availability of effective acute therapies. With the NINDS recombinant tissue plasminogen activator (rtPA) trial, the crucial need for local partnerships between academic medical centers and community hospitals became a reality.[9]

---

The American Heart Association requests that this document be cited as follows: Jauch EC, Cucchiara B, Adeoye O, Meurer W, Brice J, Chan Y-F, Gentile N, Hazinski MF. Part 11: adult stroke: 2010 American Heart Association Guidelines for Cardiopulmonary Resuscitation and Emergency Cardiovascular Care. *Circulation*. 2010;122(suppl 3):S818–S828.

*Co-chairs and equal first co-authors.

(*Circulation*. 2010;122[suppl 3]:S818–S828.)

*Circulation* is available at http://circ.ahajournals.org

DOI: 10.1161/CIRCULATIONAHA.110.971044

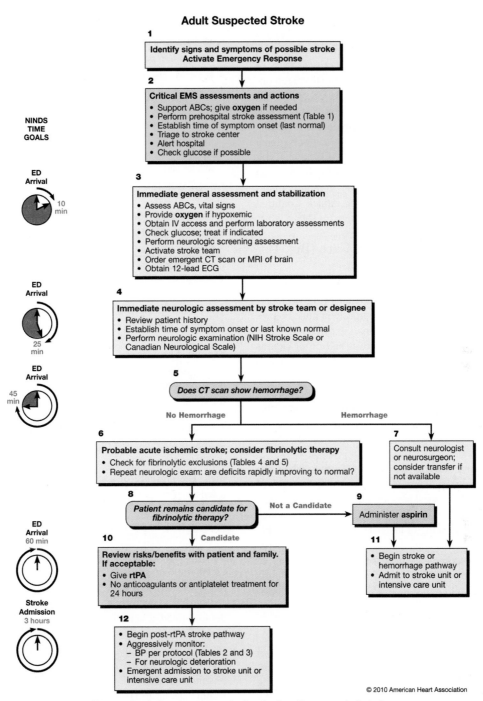

**Adult Suspected Stroke**

NINDS TIME GOALS

ED Arrival 10 min

ED Arrival 25 min

ED Arrival 45 min

ED Arrival 60 min

Stroke Admission 3 hours

1 — Identify signs and symptoms of possible stroke. Activate Emergency Response

2 — Critical EMS assessments and actions
- Support ABCs; give **oxygen** if needed
- Perform prehospital stroke assessment (Table 1)
- Establish time of symptom onset (last normal)
- Triage to stroke center
- Alert hospital
- Check glucose if possible

3 — Immediate general assessment and stabilization
- Assess ABCs, vital signs
- Provide **oxygen** if hypoxemic
- Obtain IV access and perform laboratory assessments
- Check glucose; treat if indicated
- Perform neurologic screening assessment
- Activate stroke team
- Order emergent CT scan or MRI of brain
- Obtain 12-lead ECG

4 — Immediate neurologic assessment by stroke team or designee
- Review patient history
- Establish time of symptom onset or last known normal
- Perform neurologic examination (NIH Stroke Scale or Canadian Neurological Scale)

5 — Does CT scan show hemorrhage?

No Hemorrhage    Hemorrhage

6 — Probable acute ischemic stroke; consider fibrinolytic therapy
- Check for fibrinolytic exclusions (Tables 4 and 5)
- Repeat neurologic exam: are deficits rapidly improving to normal?

7 — Consult neurologist or neurosurgeon; consider transfer if not available

8 — Patient remains candidate for fibrinolytic therapy?    Not a Candidate

9 — Administer **aspirin**

Candidate

10 — Review risks/benefits with patient and family. If acceptable:
- Give **rtPA**
- No anticoagulants or antiplatelet treatment for 24 hours

11 —
- Begin stroke or hemorrhage pathway
- Admit to stroke unit or intensive care unit

12 —
- Begin post-rtPA stroke pathway
- Aggressively monitor:
  – BP per protocol (Tables 2 and 3)
  – For neurologic deterioration
- Emergent admission to stroke unit or intensive care unit

© 2010 American Heart Association

**Figure.** Goals for management of patients with suspected stroke.

The time-sensitive nature of stroke requires such an approach, even in densely populated metropolitan centers. The idea of a "stroke-prepared" hospital emerged after the United States Food and Drug Administration (FDA) approved rtPA for stroke. In 2000 the Brain Attack Coalition provided a description of "primary stroke centers," which would ensure that best practices for stroke care (acute and beyond) would be offered in an organized fashion.[7] The logic of having a multitiered system such as that provided for trauma was evident. Therefore, in 2005 the Brain Attack Coalition followed the statement on primary stroke centers with recommendations for comprehensive stroke centers.[6] Following the establishment

of primary stroke centers and comprehensive stroke centers, the new concept of a stroke-prepared hospital has recently emerged. This stroke-prepared hospital can access stroke expertise via telemedicine. The comparison with a trauma system with Level 1, 2, and 3 centers is rational and quite intuitive to emergency care providers familiar with such configurations.

Substantial progress has been made toward regionalization of stroke care. Several states have passed legislation requiring prehospital providers to triage patients with suspected stroke to designated stroke centers. This is contingent on the accuracy of dispatch, an area where further improvement is needed.[10] The integration of EMS into regional stroke models is crucial for improvement of patient outcomes.[11] Efforts have been strong in many regions, especially in regions with relatively high population density and large critical mass of stroke centers to effectively create a model for stroke regionalization.[12] Although a large proportion of the US population is now within close proximity to a stroke center, it is not clear how many stroke patients arrive at stroke-prepared hospitals.

Additional work is needed to expand the reach of regional stroke networks. Healthcare professionals working in EMS, emergency medicine, or emergency nursing can also assist in this process by determining which hospitals in their community offer care concordant with the Brain Attack Coalition recommendations for primary stroke centers.[7,11,13,14]

## Stroke Recognition and EMS Care (Box 1)

### Stroke Warning Signs

Identifying clinical signs of possible stroke is important because recanalization strategies (intravenous [IV] fibrinolysis and intra-arterial/catheter-based approaches) must be provided within the first few hours from onset of symptoms.[9,15,16] Most strokes occur at home, and just over half of all victims of acute stroke use EMS for transport to the hospital.[17–21] Stroke knowledge among the lay public remains poor.[22,23] These factors can delay EMS access and treatment, resulting in increased morbidity and mortality. Community and professional education is essential[22,24] and has successfully increased the proportion of stroke patients treated with fibrinolytic therapy.[25–27]

Patient education efforts are most effective when the message is clear and succinct. The signs and symptoms of stroke include sudden weakness or numbness of the face, arm, or leg, especially on one side of the body; sudden confusion; trouble speaking or understanding; sudden trouble seeing in one or both eyes; sudden trouble walking, dizziness, loss of balance or coordination; or sudden severe headache with no known cause. Educational efforts need to couple the knowledge of the signs and symptoms of stroke with action—call 911.

### 911 and EMS Dispatch

EMS systems of care include both 911 emergency medical dispatch centers and EMS response personnel. It is imperative that the stroke system of care provide education and training to 911 and EMS personnel to minimize delays in prehospital dispatch, assessment, and transport. Emergency medical telecommunicators must identify and provide high-priority dispatch to patients with stroke symptoms. Current literature suggests that 911 telecommunicators do not recognize stroke well and that the use of scripted stroke-specific screens during a 911 call may be helpful.[10,28] Studies are ongoing to investigate the effectiveness of such a stroke assessment tool for 911 telecommunicators.[29,30]

In settings where ground transport to a stroke center is potentially long, air medical services may be used. Regional stroke resources work with EMS agencies to establish criteria for the use of air medical transport for patients with acute stroke and determine the most appropriate destination based on distance and the hospital's stroke capability. As with

**Table 1.**    **The Cincinnati Prehospital Stroke Scale**

Facial droop (have patient show teeth or smile)

- Normal—both sides of face move equally
- Abnormal—one side of face does not move as well as the other side

Arm drift (patient closes eyes and holds both arms straight out for 10 seconds)

- Normal—both arms move the same or both arms do not move at all (other findings, such as pronator drift, may be helpful)
- Abnormal—one arm does not move or one arm drifts down compared with the other

Abnormal speech (have the patient say "you can't teach an old dog new tricks")

- Normal—patient uses correct words with no slurring
- Abnormal—patient slurs words, uses the wrong words, or is unable to speak

Interpretation: If any 1 of these 3 signs is abnormal, the probability of a stroke is 72%.

ground transportation, prehospital notification should be performed to ensure appropriate activation of stroke resources.

### Stroke Assessment Tools

EMS providers can identify stroke patients with reasonable sensitivity and specificity, using abbreviated out-of-hospital tools such as the Cincinnati Prehospital Stroke Scale (CPSS)[31–34] (Table 1) or the Los Angeles Prehospital Stroke Screen (LAPSS).[35,36] The CPSS is based on physical examination only. The EMS provider checks for 3 physical findings: facial droop, arm weakness, and speech abnormalities. The presence of a single abnormality on the CPSS has a sensitivity of 59% and a specificity of 89% when scored by prehospital providers.[33] Another assessment tool, the LAPSS, requires that the provider rule out other causes of altered level of consciousness (eg, history of seizures, hypoglycemia) and then identify asymmetry in any of 3 examination categories: facial smile or grimace, grip, and arm strength. The LAPSS has a sensitivity of 93% and a specificity of 97%.[35,36]

With standard training in stroke recognition, paramedics demonstrated a sensitivity of 61% to 66% for identifying patients with stroke.[34,37,38] After receiving training in use of a stroke assessment tool, paramedic sensitivity for identifying patients with stroke increased to 86% to 97%.[36,39,40] We recommend that all paramedics and emergency medical technicians-basic (EMT-basic) be trained in recognition of stroke using a validated, abbreviated out-of-hospital screening tool such as the CPSS or LAPSS (Class I, LOE B).

### Prehospital Management and Triage (Box 2)

As with any other time-sensitive acute illness, prehospital providers must perform an initial assessment and intervene if necessary to provide cardiopulmonary support. In addition, for stroke, providers must clearly establish the *time of onset of symptoms*. This time represents time zero for the patient. If the patient wakes from sleep or is found with symptoms of a stroke, the time of onset of symptoms is defined as the last time the patient was observed to be normal. EMS providers must be able to support cardiopulmonary function, perform rapid stroke assessment, establish time of onset of symptoms (or the last time the patient was known to be normal), triage and transport the patient, and provide prearrival notification to the most appropriate receiving hospital.[31,41–44]

Patients with acute stroke are at risk for respiratory compromise from aspiration, upper airway obstruction, hypoventilation, and (rarely) neurogenic pulmonary edema. The combination of poor perfusion and hypoxemia will exacerbate and extend ischemic brain injury and has been associated with worse outcome from stroke.[45] Both out-of-hospital and in-hospital medical personnel should administer supplemental oxygen to hypoxemic (ie, oxygen saturation <94%) stroke patients (Class I, LOE C) or those with unknown oxygen saturation.

Although blood pressure management is a component of the ED care of stroke patients, there are no data to support initiation of hypertension intervention in the prehospital environment. Unless the patient is hypotensive (systolic blood pressure <90 mm Hg), prehospital intervention for blood pressure is not recommended (Class III, LOE C).

### Transport and Destination Hospital
EMS providers should consider transporting a witness, family member, or caregiver with the patient to verify the time of stroke symptom onset. En route to the facility, providers should continue to support cardiopulmonary function, monitor neurologic status, check blood glucose if possible, and provide prehospital notification.

Prearrival hospital notification by the transporting EMS unit has been found to significantly increase the percentage of patients with acute stroke who receive fibrinolytic therapy.[46–48] Bypass of community hospitals in favor of transporting patients directly to a stroke center has undergone investigations that merit attention. Investigators in New York, Canada, Italy, and Australia have performed before-and-after studies examining the difference in rates of rtPA administration after implementation of a hospital bypass protocol for EMS. All have found significantly larger percentages of patients with ischemic stroke treated with rtPA when patients are transported directly to stroke centers.[47,49,50] Recently investigators have begun to examine the impact of direct activation of stroke teams by EMS.[50,51]

EMS providers must rapidly deliver the patient to a medical facility capable of providing acute stroke care and provide prearrival notification to the receiving facility.[41,46,48] Each receiving hospital should define its capability for treating patients with acute stroke using the definitions established for stroke-prepared hospitals, primary stroke centers, and comprehensive stroke centers[3,6,7] and should communicate this information to the EMS system and the community. Although not every hospital is capable of organizing the necessary resources to safely administer fibrinolytic therapy, every hospital with an ED should have a written plan that is communicated to EMS systems describing how patients with acute stroke are to be managed in that institution. The plan should detail the roles of healthcare professionals in the care of patients with acute stroke and define which patients will be treated with fibrinolytic therapy at that facility and when transfer to another hospital with a dedicated stroke unit is appropriate.

The role of stroke centers and in particular stroke units continues to be defined, but a growing body of evidence[47,49,50,52–58] indicates a favorable benefit from triage of stroke patients directly to designated stroke centers (Class I, LOE B). EMS systems should establish a stroke destination preplan to enable EMS providers to direct patients with acute stroke to appropriate facilities. When multiple stroke hospitals are within similar transport distances, EMS personnel should consider triage to the stroke center with the highest capability of stroke care.

Multiple randomized clinical trials and meta-analyses in adults[50,59–62] document consistent improvement in 1-year survival rate, functional outcome, and quality of life when patients hospitalized with acute stroke are cared for in a dedicated stroke unit by a multidisciplinary team experienced in managing stroke. Although the studies reported were conducted outside the United States at in-hospital units that provided both acute care and rehabilitation, the improved outcomes were apparent very early in stroke care. These results should be relevant to the outcome of dedicated stroke units staffed with experienced multidisciplinary teams in the United States. When such a facility is available within a reasonable transport interval, stroke patients who require hospitalization should be admitted there (Class I, LOE B).

## In-Hospital Care

### Initial ED Assessment and Stabilization (Box 3)
Protocols should be used in the ED to minimize delay to definitive diagnosis and therapy: "Time is Brain."[43] As a goal, ED personnel should assess the patient with suspected stroke within 10 minutes of arrival in the ED. General care includes assessment, cardiopulmonary support (airway, breathing, circulation), and evaluation of baseline vital signs. Administration of oxygen to hypoxemic patients with stroke (oxygen saturation <94%) is recommended (Class I, LOE C).

On arrival ED personnel should establish or confirm IV access and obtain blood samples for baseline studies (eg, complete blood count, coagulation studies, blood glucose). If not already identified in the prehospital setting, ED staff should promptly identify and treat hypoglycemia. The ED physician should perform a neurologic screening assessment, order an emergent computed tomography (CT) scan of the brain, and activate the stroke team or arrange for consultation with a stroke expert.

A 12-lead electrocardiogram (ECG) does not take priority over the CT scan but may identify a recent acute myocardial infarction or arrhythmias (eg, atrial fibrillation) as the cause of an embolic stroke. If the patient is hemodynamically stable, treatment of other arrhythmias, including bradycardia, premature atrial or ventricular contractions, or asymptomatic atrioventricular conduction block, may not be necessary.[63] There is general agreement to recommend cardiac monitoring during the first 24 hours of evaluation in patients with acute ischemic stroke to detect atrial fibrillation and potentially life-threatening arrhythmias.[64]

### Assessment (Box 4)
The treating physician should review the patient's history and verify time of onset of symptoms.[65–67] This may require interviewing out-of-hospital providers, witnesses, and family members to establish the time that the patient was last known to be normal. Neurologic assessment is performed, incorpo-

**Table 2. Potential Approaches to Arterial Hypertension in Acute Ischemic Stroke Patients Who Are Potential Candidates for Acute Reperfusion Therapy**

Patient otherwise eligible for acute reperfusion therapy except that blood pressure is >185/110 mm Hg

- Labetalol 10–20 mg IV over 1–2 minutes, may repeat ×1, or
- Nicardipine IV 5 mg/hr, titrate up by 2.5 mg/hr every 5–15 minutes, maximum 15 mg/hr; when desired blood pressure reached, lower to 3 mg/hr, or
- Other agents (hydralazine, enalaprilat, etc) may be considered when appropriate

If blood pressure is not maintained at or below 185/110 mm Hg, do not administer rtPA

Management of blood pressure during and after rtPA or other acute reperfusion therapy:

- Monitor blood pressure every 15 minutes for 2 hours from the start of rtPA therapy; then every 30 minutes for 6 hours; and then every hour for 16 hours

If systolic BP 180–230 mm Hg or diastolic BP 105–120 mm Hg

- Labetalol 10 mg IV followed by continuous IV infusion 2–8 mg/min, or
- Nicardipine IV 5 mg/h, titrate up to desired effect by 2.5 mg/hr every 5–15 minutes, maximum 15 mg/h

If blood pressure not controlled or diastolic BP >140 mm Hg, consider sodium nitroprusside

rating either the National Institutes of Health Stroke Scale (NIHSS) or the Canadian Neurological Scale (CNS) (see the ASA website: *www.strokeassociation.org*).

Management of hypertension in the stroke patient is dependent on fibrinolytic eligibility. For patients potentially eligible for fibrinolytic therapy, blood pressure must be ≤185 mm Hg systolic and ≤110 mm Hg diastolic to limit the risk of bleeding complications. Because the maximum interval from onset of stroke until effective treatment of stroke with rtPA is limited, most patients with sustained hypertension above these levels (ie, systolic blood pressure >185 mm Hg or diastolic blood pressure >110 mm Hg) will not be eligible for IV rtPA (Tables 2 and 3).[68]

## Imaging (Box 5)

Ideally the CT scan should be completed within 25 minutes of the patient's arrival in the ED and should be interpreted within 45 minutes of ED arrival. Centers may perform more advanced neurologic imaging (multimodal magnetic reso-

**Table 3. Approach to Arterial Hypertension in Acute Ischemic Stroke Patients Who Are *Not* Potential Candidates for Acute Reperfusion Therapy**

Consider lowering blood pressure in patients with acute ischemic stroke if systolic blood pressure >220 mm Hg or diastolic blood pressure >120 mm Hg

Consider blood pressure reduction as indicated for other concomitant organ system injury

- Acute myocardial infarction
- Congestive heart failure
- Acute aortic dissection

A reasonable target is to lower blood pressure by 15% to 25% within the first day

nance imaging [MRI], CT perfusion, and CT angiography), but obtaining these studies should not delay initiation of IV rtPA in eligible patients. Emergent CT or MRI scans of patients with suspected stroke should be promptly evaluated by a physician with expertise in interpretation of these studies.[69] During the first few hours of an ischemic stroke the noncontrast CT scan may not indicate signs of brain ischemia. If the CT scan shows no evidence of intracerebral hemorrhage, the patient may be a candidate for fibrinolytic therapy (Boxes 6 and 8). If hemorrhage is noted on the CT scan, the patient is not a candidate for fibrinolytic therapy. Consult a neurologist or neurosurgeon and consider transfer as needed for appropriate care (Box 7).

If hemorrhage is not present on the initial CT scan and the patient is not a candidate for fibrinolytic therapy for other reasons, consider administration of aspirin (Box 9) either rectally or orally after the patient is screened for dysphagia (see below). Admit the patient to a stroke unit (if available) for careful monitoring (Box 11).

## Fibrinolytic Therapy (Boxes 6, 8, and 10)

The treating physician should review the inclusion and exclusion criteria for IV fibrinolytic therapy (Tables 4 and 5) and perform a repeat neurologic examination incorporating the NIHSS or CNS. If the patient's neurologic signs are spontaneously clearing (ie, function is rapidly improving to normal and is near baseline), administration of fibrinolytics may not be required (Box 6).[64]

As with all medications, fibrinolytics have potential adverse effects. The physician must verify that there are no exclusion criteria, consider the risks and benefits to the patient, and be prepared to monitor and treat any potential complications. The major complication of IV rtPA for stroke is symptomatic intracranial hemorrhage. This complication occurred in 6.4% of the 312 patients treated in the NINDS trials[9] and 4.6% of the 1135 patients treated in 60 Canadian centers.[70] A meta-analysis of 15 published case series on the open-label use of rtPA for acute ischemic stroke in general clinical practice showed a symptomatic hemorrhage rate of 5.2% of 2639 patients treated.[71] Other complications include orolingual angioedema (occurs in approximately 1.5% of patients), acute hypotension, and systemic bleeding. In one large prospective registry, major systemic bleeding was uncommon (0.4%) and usually occurred at the site of femoral puncture for acute angiography.[70,72]

If the patient remains a candidate for fibrinolytic therapy (Box 8), the physician should discuss the risks and potential benefits of the therapy with the patient or family if available (Box 10). After this discussion, if the patient/family elects to proceed with fibrinolytic therapy, begin the rtPA bolus and infusion as quickly as possible and begin the stroke pathway of care (see below). Careful dose calculation and removal of excess rtPA help prevent inadvertent administration of excess rtPA. Typically neither anticoagulant nor antiplatelet treatment may be administered for 24 hours after administration of rtPA until a repeat CT scan at 24 hours shows no hemorrhagic transformation.

Several studies[9,15,70] have documented a higher likelihood of good to excellent functional outcome when rtPA is

**Table 4.    Inclusion and Exclusion Characteristics of Patients With Ischemic Stroke Who Could Be Treated With rtPA Within 3 Hours From Symptom Onset**

Inclusion criteria

- Diagnosis of ischemic stroke causing measurable neurologic deficit
- Onset of symptoms <3 hours before beginning treatment
- Age ≥18 years

Exclusion criteria

- Head trauma or prior stroke in previous 3 months
- Symptoms suggest subarachnoid hemorrhage
- Arterial puncture at noncompressible site in previous 7 days
- History of previous intracranial hemorrhage
- Elevated blood pressure (systolic >185 mm Hg or diastolic >110 mm Hg)
- Evidence of active bleeding on examination
- Acute bleeding diathesis, including but not limited to
  –Platelet count <100 000/mm$^3$
  –Heparin received within 48 hours, resulting in aPTT >upper limit of normal
  –Current use of anticoagulant with INR >1.7 or PT >15 seconds
- Blood glucose concentration <50 mg/dL (2.7 mmol/L)
- CT demonstrates multilobar infarction (hypodensity >1/3 cerebral hemisphere)

Relative exclusion criteria

Recent experience suggests that under some circumstances—with careful consideration and weighing of risk to benefit—patients may receive fibrinolytic therapy despite 1 or more relative contraindications. Consider risk to benefit of rtPA administration carefully if any of these relative contraindications is present

- Only minor or rapidly improving stroke symptoms (clearing spontaneously)
- Seizure at onset with postictal residual neurologic impairments
- Major surgery or serious trauma within previous 14 days
- Recent gastrointestinal or urinary tract hemorrhage (within previous 21 days)
- Recent acute myocardial infarction (within previous 3 months)

rtPA indicates recombinant tissue plasminogen activator; aPTT, activated partial thromboplastin time; INR, international normalized ratio; and PT, partial thromboplastin time.

**Table 5.    Additional Inclusion and Exclusion Characteristics of Patients With Ischemic Stroke Who Could Be Treated With rtPA From 3 to 4.5 Hours From Symptom Onset**

Inclusion criteria

- Diagnosis of ischemic stroke causing measurable neurologic deficit
- Onset of symptoms 3 to 4.5 hours before beginning treatment

Exclusion criteria

- Age >80 years
- Severe stroke (NIHSS >25)
- Taking an oral anticoagulant regardless of INR
- History of both diabetes and prior ischemic stroke

Notes

- The checklist includes some FDA-approved indications and contraindications for administration of rtPA for acute ischemic stroke. Recent guideline revisions have modified the original FDA criteria. A physician with expertise in acute stroke care may modify this list
- Onset time is either witnessed or last known normal
- In patients without recent use of oral anticoagulants or heparin, treatment with rtPA can be initiated before availability of coagulation study results but should be discontinued if INR is >1.7 or PT is elevated by local laboratory standards
- In patients without history of thrombocytopenia, treatment with rtPA can be initiated before availability of platelet count but should be discontinued if platelet count is <100 000/mm$^3$

rtPA indicates recombinant tissue plasminogen activator; NIHSS, National Institutes of Health Stroke Scale; INR, international normalized ratio; FDA, Food and Drug Administration; and PT, partial thromboplastin time.

outcome, although the degree of clinical benefit is smaller than that achieved with treatment within 3 hours.[16,78] Data supporting treatment in this time window come from a large, randomized trial (ECASS-3) that specifically enrolled patients between 3 and 4.5 hours after symptom onset, as well as a meta-analysis of prior trials. Criteria for inclusion in ECASS-3 were similar to the NINDS criteria, except that ECASS-3 excluded patients older than 80 years of age, with a baseline NIHSS >25, taking oral anticoagulants, or who had a combination of diabetes and prior stroke. At present, use of IV rtPA within the 3- to 4.5-hour window has not yet been FDA approved, although it is recommended by a current AHA/ASA science advisory.[78] Administration of IV rtPA to patients with acute ischemic stroke who meet the NINDS or ECASS-3 eligibility criteria is recommended if rtPA is administered by physicians in the setting of a clearly defined protocol, a knowledgeable team, and institutional commitment (Class I, LOE B).

It is important to note that the superior outcomes reported in both community and tertiary care hospitals in clinical trials of rtPA may be difficult to replicate in hospitals with less experience in, and institutional commitment to, acute stroke care.[79,80] Failure to adhere to protocol is associated with an increased rate of complications, particularly the risk of symptomatic intracranial hemorrhage.[79,81] There is a relationship between violations of the NINDS treatment protocol and increased risk of symptomatic intracerebral hemorrhage and death.[71] In Germany there was an increased risk of death after administration of rtPA for acute ischemic stroke in hospitals that treated ≤5 patients per year, suggesting that clinical

administered to adult patients with acute ischemic stroke within 3 hours of onset of symptoms. These results are obtained when rtPA is administered by physicians in hospitals with a stroke protocol that rigorously adheres to the eligibility criteria and therapeutic regimen of the NINDS protocol. These results have been supported by a subsequent 1-year follow-up study,[73] reanalysis of the NINDS data,[74] and a meta-analysis.[75] Evidence from prospective randomized studies[9,15,74,76] in adults also documents a greater likelihood of benefit the earlier treatment is begun. Additional analyses of the original NINDS data by an independent group of investigators confirmed the validity of the results,[74] verifying that improved outcomes in the rtPA treatment arm persist even when imbalances in the baseline stroke severity among treatment groups is corrected.[77]

Treatment of carefully selected patients with acute ischemic stroke with IV rtPA between 3 and 4.5 hours after onset of symptoms has also been shown to improve clinical experience is an important factor in ensuring adherence to protocol.[72] Adding a dedicated stroke team to a community hospital can increase the number of patients with acute stroke treated with fibrinolytic therapy and produce excellent clinical outcomes.[82] There is also strong evidence to avoid all delays and treat patients as soon as possible. These findings show that it is important to have an institutional commitment to ensure optimal patient outcomes.

Evidence from 3 prospective randomized studies in adults and a meta-analysis[83–87] have demonstrated improved outcome from intra-arterial fibrinolysis. Thus, for patients with acute ischemic stroke who are not candidates for standard IV fibrinolysis, administration of intra-arterial fibrinolytics is reasonable (Class I, LOE B). To date, intra-arterial administration of fibrinolytics has not been FDA approved. In carefully selected patients, catheter-based thrombectomy is being performed at centers where resources and expertise are available. The pending ASA acute ischemic stroke guidelines will provide greater detail about intra-arterial strategies.

## General Stroke Care

Recent studies establish that stroke unit care is superior to care in general medical wards, and the positive effects of stroke unit care can persist for years. The benefits from treatment in a stroke unit are comparable to the effects achieved with IV rtPA. Patients should be admitted to a stroke unit (if available) for careful observation (Box 11), including monitoring of blood pressure and neurologic status and physiologic optimization. General stroke care, centered on physiologic optimization, includes prevention of hypoxia, management of hypertension, optimal glucose control, maintenance of euthermia, and nutritional support. Additional efforts center on prevention of complications associated with stroke (eg, aspiration pneumonia, deep venous thrombosis, urinary tract infections) and initiation of secondary stroke prevention.

Given the requirements for frequent neurologic assessment and vital sign measurements, especially after administration of IV rtPA, patients should be admitted as quickly as possible, ideally within 3 hours from arrival.[8] If the patient's neurologic status deteriorates, an emergent CT scan is required to determine if cerebral edema or hemorrhage is responsible for the deterioration. Treatment of hemorrhage or edema should be started immediately as indicated.

### Blood Pressure Management

Blood pressure management varies depending on whether or not fibrinolytic or intra-arterial therapies were used. Current recommendations for control of blood pressure in patients who receive IV rtPA or intra-arterial recanalization therapies are shown in Table 2. In those patients for whom recanalization is not planned, more liberal acceptance of hypertension is recommended, provided no other comorbid conditions require intervention (Table 3). Normal saline, administered at a rate of approximately 75 to 100 mL/h, is used to maintain euvolemia as needed. In stroke patients who may be relatively hypovolemic, careful administration of IV normal saline boluses may be appropriate.

### Glycemic Control

Hyperglycemia is associated with worse clinical outcome in patients with acute ischemic stroke,[88–95] but there is no direct evidence that active glucose control improves clinical outcome.[96,97] There is contradictory evidence for the benefit of insulin treatment of hyperglycemia in other critically ill patients.[98,99] Current AHA/ASA recommendations call for the use of insulin when the serum glucose level is greater than 185 mg/dL in patients with acute stroke (Class IIa, LOE C); however, the utility of administration of IV or subcutaneous insulin to lower blood glucose in patients with acute ischemic stroke when serum glucose is ≤185 mg/dL remains uncertain.

### Temperature Control

Hyperthermia in the setting of acute cerebral ischemia is associated with increased morbidity and mortality and should be managed aggressively (treat fever >37.5°C [99.5°F]).[100–103] Hypothermia has been shown to improve survival and functional outcome in patients following resuscitation from ventricular fibrillation (VF) sudden cardiac arrest; however, there are limited data on the role of hypothermia specific to acute ischemic stroke. At this time there is insufficient scientific evidence to recommend for or against the use of hypothermia in the treatment of acute ischemic stroke (Class IIb, LOE C).

### Dysphagia Screening

All patients with stroke should be screened for dysphagia before they are given anything by mouth. A simple bedside screening evaluation involves asking the patient to sip water from a cup. If the patient can sip and swallow without difficulty, the patient is asked to take a large gulp of water and swallow. If there are no signs of coughing or aspiration after 30 seconds, then it is safe for the patient to have a thickened diet until formally assessed by a speech pathologist. Medications may be given in applesauce or jam. Any patient who fails a swallow test may be given medications such as aspirin rectally or, if appropriate for the medication, intravenously, intramuscularly, or subcutaneously.

### Other Stroke Management

Additional stroke care includes support of the airway, oxygenation and ventilation, and nutritional support. Seizure prophylaxis is not recommended, but for patients who experience a seizure, administration of anticonvulsants is recommended to prevent more seizures.[104] In patients with severe stroke, posterior circulation stroke, and in younger patients, healthcare providers must observe for signs of increased intracranial pressure.

## Summary

Advances in stroke care will have the greatest effect on stroke outcome if care is delivered within a regional stroke system designed to improve both efficiency and effectiveness. The ultimate goal of stroke care is to minimize ongoing injury, emergently recanalize acute vascular occlusions, and begin secondary measures to maximize functional recovery. These efforts will provide stroke patients with the greatest opportunity for a return to previous quality of life and decrease the overall societal burden of stroke.

# Disclosures

**Guidelines Part 11: Stroke: Writing Group Disclosures**

| Writing Group Member | Employment | Research Grant | Other Research Support | Speakers' Bureau/ Honoraria | Ownership Interest | Consultant/ Advisory Board | Other |
|---|---|---|---|---|---|---|---|
| Edward C. Jauch | Medical University of South Carolina–Professor | NIH trials related to stroke | None | None | None | None | None |
| Brett Cucchiara | University of Pennsylvania–Assistant Professor of Neurology | †NIH RO1-migraine imaging research-significant | None | *Multiple CME talks at different institutions | None | None | *Occasionally serves as expert witness for medicolegal cases |
| Opeolu Adeoye | University of Cincinnati–Assistant Professor of Emergency Medicine and Neurosurgery | None | None | *Genentech EKR Therapeutics | None | None | None |
| William Meurer | University of Michigan–Assistant Professor | None | None | None | None | None | None |
| Jane Brice | University of North Carolina: Associate professor in the department of emergency medicine. Perform clinical work in the emergency department. Perform research in the areas of EMS and stroke. Teach in the School of Medicine–Associate Professor | None | None | None | None | None | None |
| Yvonne (Yu-Feng) Chan | The Mount Sinai School of Medicine–Assistant Professor of Emergency Medicine | None | None | None | None | None | None |
| Nina Gentile | Temple University–Professor, Department of Emergency Medicine | †Active Support: 5 NIH U01 NS044876–03. Insulin Resistance Intervention after Stroke (IRIS) Trial. Investigation of the effect of Pioglitazone on development of diabetes and stroke recurrence after ischemic stroke or TIA. Total Award to Temple, direct costs: $184,000 2005–2010 NIH NINDS U01 NS40406-04 Albumin in Acute Ischemic Stroke (ALIAS) Trial. Human Serum Albumin will be compared to placebo on improving the 3 month outcome of ischemic stroke patients when administered within 5 hours of symptom onset. Total Award to Temple, direct costs: $225,000 2008–2011 | None | None | None | None | None |
| Mary Fran Hazinski | Vanderbilt University School of Nursing—Professor; AHA ECC Product Development–Senior Science Editor †Substantial consulting fees as a senior science editor for the AHA ECC Product Development. | None | None | None | None | None | None |

This table represents the relationships of writing group members that may be perceived as actual or reasonably perceived conflicts of interest as reported on the Disclosure Questionnaire, which all members of the writing group are required to complete and submit. A relationship is considered to be "significant" if (a) the person receives $10 000 or more during any 12-month period, or 5% or more of the person's gross income; or (b) the person owns 5% or more of the voting stock or share of the entity, or owns $10 000 or more of the fair market value of the entity. A relationship is considered to be "modest" if it is less than "significant" under the preceding definition.

*Modest.

†Significant.

# References

1. Lloyd-Jones DM, Hong Y, Labarthe D, Mozaffarian D, Appel LJ, Van Horn L, Greenlund K, Daniels S, Nichol G, Tomaselli GF, Arnett DK, Fonarow GC, Ho PM, Lauer MS, Masoudi FA, Robertson RM, Roger V, Schwamm LH, Sorlie P, Yancy CW, Rosamond WD. Defining and setting national goals for cardiovascular health promotion and disease reduction: the American Heart Association's strategic Impact Goal through 2020 and beyond. *Circulation*. 2010;121:586–613.

2. Schwamm LH, Fonarow GC, Reeves MJ, Pan W, Frankel MR, Smith EE, Ellrodt G, Cannon CP, Liang L, Peterson E, Labresh KA. Get With the Guidelines–Stroke is associated with sustained improvement in care for patients hospitalized with acute stroke or transient ischemic attack. *Circulation*. 2009;119:107–115.

3. Schwamm LH, Pancioli A, Acker JE III, Goldstein LB, Zorowitz RD, Shephard TJ, Moyer P, Gorman M, Johnston SC, Duncan PW, Gorelick P, Frank J, Stranne SK, Smith R, Federspiel W, Horton KB, Magnis E, Adams RJ. Recommendations for the establishment of stroke systems of care: recommendations from the American Stroke Association's Task Force on the Development of Stroke Systems. *Circulation*. 2005;111: 1078–1091.

4. Hazinski M. D-mystifying recognition and management of stroke. *Curr Emerg Cardiac Care*. 1996;7:8.

5. Acute stroke: current treatment and paradigms. In: Cummins R, Field J, Hazinski M, eds. *ACLS: Principles and Practice*. Dallas, Tex: American Heart Association;2003:437–482.

6. Alberts MJ, Latchaw RE, Selman WR, Shephard T, Hadley MN, Brass LM, Koroshetz W, Marler JR, Booss J, Zorowitz RD, Croft JB, Magnis E, Mulligan D, Jagoda A, O'Connor R, Cawley CM, Connors JJ, Rose-DeRenzy JA, Emr M, Warren M, Walker MD. Recommendations for comprehensive stroke centers: a consensus statement from the Brain Attack Coalition. *Stroke*. 2005;36:1597–1616.

7. Alberts MJ, Hademenos G, Latchaw RE, Jagoda A, Marler JR, Mayberg MR, Starke RD, Todd HW, Viste KM, Girgus M, Shephard T, Emr M, Shwayder P, Walker MD. Recommendations for the establishment of primary stroke centers. Brain Attack Coalition. *JAMA*. 2000;283: 3102–3109.

8. Marler J, Jones P, Emr M, eds. *Setting New Directions for Stroke Care: Proceedings of a National Symposium on Rapid Identification and Treatment of Acute Stroke*. Bethesda, Md: National Institute of Neurological Disorders and Stroke; 1997.

9. Tissue plasminogen activator for acute ischemic stroke. The National Institute of Neurological Disorders and Stroke rt-PA Stroke Study Group. *N Engl J Med*. 1995;333:1581–1587.

10. Buck BH, Starkman S, Eckstein M, Kidwell CS, Haines J, Huang R, Colby D, Saver JL. Dispatcher recognition of stroke using the National Academy Medical Priority Dispatch System. *Stroke*. 2009;40: 2027–2030.

11. Acker JE III, Pancioli AM, Crocco TJ, Eckstein MK, Jauch EC, Larrabee H, Meltzer NM, Mergendahl WC, Munn JW, Prentiss SM, Sand C, Saver JL, Eigel B, Gilpin BR, Schoeberl M, Solis P, Bailey JR, Horton KB, Stranne SK. Implementation strategies for emergency medical services within stroke systems of care: a policy statement from the American Heart Association/American Stroke Association Expert Panel on Emergency Medical Services Systems and the Stroke Council. *Stroke*. 2007;38:3097–3115.

12. Gropen T, Magdon-Ismail Z, Day D, Melluzzo S, Schwamm LH. Regional implementation of the stroke systems of care model: recommendations of the northeast cerebrovascular consortium. *Stroke*. 2009; 40:1793–1802.

13. Park S, Schwamm LH. Organizing regional stroke systems of care. *Curr Opin Neurol*. 2008;21:43–55.

14. Summers D, Leonard A, Wentworth D, Saver JL, Simpson J, Spilker JA, Hock N, Miller E, Mitchell PH. Comprehensive overview of nursing and interdisciplinary care of the acute ischemic stroke patient: a scientific statement from the American Heart Association. *Stroke*. 2009;40: 2911–2944.

15. Hacke W, Donnan G, Fieschi C, Kaste M, von Kummer R, Broderick JP, Brott T, Frankel M, Grotta JC, Haley EC Jr, Kwiatkowski T, Levine SR, Lewandowski C, Lu M, Lyden P, Marler JR, Patel S, Tilley BC, Albers G, Bluhmki E, Wilhelm M, Hamilton S. Association of outcome with early stroke treatment: pooled analysis of ATLANTIS, ECASS, and NINDS rt-PA stroke trials. *Lancet*. 2004;363:768–774.

16. Hacke W, Kaste M, Bluhmki E, Brozman M, Davalos A, Guidetti D, Larrue V, Lees KR, Medeghri Z, Machnig T, Schneider D, von Kummer R, Wahlgren N, Toni D. Thrombolysis with alteplase 3 to 4.5 hours after acute ischemic stroke. *N Engl J Med*. 2008;359:1317–1329.

17. Barsan WG, Brott TG, Olinger CP, Adams HP Jr, Haley EC Jr, Levy DE. Identification and entry of the patient with acute cerebral infarction. *Ann Emerg Med*. 1988;17:1192–1195.

18. Barsan WG, Brott TG, Broderick JP, Haley EC, Levy DE, Marler JR. Time of hospital presentation in patients with acute stroke. *Arch Intern Med*. 1993;153:2558–2561.

19. Pepe PE, Zachariah BS, Sayre MR, Floccare D. Ensuring the chain of recovery for stroke in your community. Chain of Recovery Writing Group. *Prehosp Emerg Care*. 1998;2:89–95.

20. Evenson KR, Foraker RE, Morris DL, Rosamond WD. A comprehensive review of prehospital and in-hospital delay times in acute stroke care. *Int J Stroke*. 2009;4:187–199.

21. Adeoye O, Lindsell C, Broderick J, Alwell K, Jauch E, Moomaw CJ, Flaherty ML, Pancioli A, Kissela B, Kleindorfer D. Emergency medical services use by stroke patients: a population-based study. *Am J Emerg Med*. 2009;27:141–145.

22. Kleindorfer D, Khoury J, Broderick JP, Rademacher E, Woo D, Flaherty ML, Alwell K, Moomaw CJ, Schneider A, Pancioli A, Miller R, Kissela BM. Temporal trends in public awareness of stroke: warning signs, risk factors, and treatment. *Stroke*. 2009;40:2502–2506.

23. Jones SP, Jenkinson AJ, Leathley MJ, Watkins CL. Stroke knowledge and awareness: an integrative review of the evidence. *Age Ageing*. 2010;39:11–22.

24. Lyden P, Rapp K, Babcock T, et al. Ultra-rapid identification, triage, and enrollment of stroke patients into clinical trials. *J Stroke Cerebrovasc Dis*. 1994;2:106–113.

25. Morgenstern LB, Staub L, Chan W, Wein TH, Bartholomew LK, King M, Felberg RA, Burgin WS, Groff J, Hickenbottom SL, Saldin K, Demchuk AM, Kalra A, Dhingra A, Grotta JC. Improving delivery of acute stroke therapy: the TLL Temple Foundation Stroke Project. *Stroke*. 2002;33:160–166.

26. Morgenstern LB, Bartholomew LK, Grotta JC, Staub L, King M, Chan W. Sustained benefit of a community and professional intervention to increase acute stroke therapy. *Arch Intern Med*. 2003;163:2198–2202.

27. Scott PA. Enhancing community delivery of tissue plasminogen activator in stroke through community-academic collaborative clinical knowledge translation. *Emerg Med Clin North Am*. 2009;27:115–136.

28. Rosamond WD, Evenson KR, Schroeder EB, Morris DL, Johnson AM, Brice JH. Calling emergency medical services for acute stroke: a study of 9-1-1 tapes. *Prehosp Emerg Care*. 2005;9:19–23.

29. Liferidge AT, Brice JH, Overby BA, Evenson KR. Ability of laypersons to use the Cincinnati Prehospital Stroke Scale. *Prehosp Emerg Care*. 2004;8:384–387.

30. Hurwitz AS, Brice JH, Overby BA, Evenson KR. Directed use of the Cincinnati Prehospital Stroke Scale by laypersons. *Prehosp Emerg Care*. 2005;9:292–296.

31. Kothari R, Barsan W, Brott T, Broderick J, Ashbrock S. Frequency and accuracy of prehospital diagnosis of acute stroke. *Stroke*. 1995;26: 937–941.

32. Kothari R, Hall K, Brott T, Broderick J. Early stroke recognition: developing an out-of-hospital NIH Stroke Scale. *Acad Emerg Med*. 1997;4:986–990.

33. Kothari RU, Pancioli A, Liu T, Brott T, Broderick J. Cincinnati Prehospital Stroke Scale: reproducibility and validity. *Ann Emerg Med*. 1999;33:373–378.

34. Smith WS, Isaacs M, Corry MD. Accuracy of paramedic identification of stroke and transient ischemic attack in the field. *Prehosp Emerg Care*. 1998;2:170–175.

35. Kidwell CS, Saver JL, Schubert GB, Eckstein M, Starkman S. Design and retrospective analysis of the Los Angeles Prehospital Stroke Screen (LAPSS). *Prehosp Emerg Care*. 1998;2:267–273.

36. Kidwell CS, Starkman S, Eckstein M, Weems K, Saver JL. Identifying stroke in the field. Prospective validation of the Los Angeles prehospital stroke screen (LAPSS). *Stroke*. 2000;31:71–76.

37. Ellison SR, Gratton MC, Schwab RA, Ma OJ. Prehospital dispatch assessment of stroke. *Mo Med*. 2004;101:64–66.

38. Wojner AW, Morgenstern L, Alexandrov AV, Rodriguez D, Persse D, Grotta JC. Paramedic and emergency department care of stroke: baseline data from a citywide performance improvement study. *Am J Crit Care*. 2003;12:411–417.

39. Smith WS, Corry MD, Fazackerley J, Isaacs SM. Improved paramedic sensitivity in identifying stroke victims in the prehospital setting. *Prehosp Emerg Care*. 1999;3:207–210.

40. Zweifler RM, York D, et al. Accuracy of paramedic diagnosis of stroke. *J Stroke Cerebrovasc Dis.* 1998;7:446–448.

41. Sayre MR, Swor RA, Honeykutt LK. Prehospital identification and treatment. In: Emr M, ed. *Setting New Directions for Stroke Care: Proceedings of a National Symposium on Rapid Identification and Treatment of Acute Stroke.* Bethesda, Md: National Institute of Neurological Disorders and Stroke;1997:35–44.

42. Zachariah B, Dunford J, Van Cott CC. Dispatch life support and the acute stroke patient: making the right call. In: *Proceedings of the National Institute of Neurological Disorders and Stroke.* Bethesda, Md: National Institute of Neurological Disorders and Stroke; 1991:29–33.

43. A systems approach to immediate evaluation and management of hyperacute stroke. Experience at eight centers and implications for community practice and patient care. The National Institute of Neurological Disorders and Stroke (NINDS) rt-PA Stroke Study Group. *Stroke.* 1997;28:1530–1540.

44. Crocco TJ, Grotta JC, Jauch EC, Kasner SE, Kothari RU, Larmon BR, Saver JL, Sayre MR, Davis SM. EMS management of acute stroke–prehospital triage (resource document to NAEMSP position statement). *Prehosp Emerg Care.* 2007;11:313–317.

45. Langhorne P, Tong BL, Stott DJ. Association between physiological homeostasis and early recovery after stroke. *Stroke.* 2000;31: 2518–2519.

46. Kim SK, Lee SY, Bae HJ, Lee YS, Kim SY, Kang MJ, Cha JK. Pre-hospital notification reduced the door-to-needle time for IV t-PA in acute ischaemic stroke. *Eur J Neurol.* 2009;16:1331–1335.

47. Quain DA, Parsons MW, Loudfoot AR, Spratt NJ, Evans MK, Russell ML, Royan AT, Moore AG, Miteff F, Hullick CJ, Attia J, McElduff P, Levi CR. Improving access to acute stroke therapies: a controlled trial of organised pre-hospital and emergency care. *Med J Aust.* 2008;189: 429–433.

48. Abdullah AR, Smith EE, Biddinger PD, Kalenderian D, Schwamm LH. Advance hospital notification by EMS in acute stroke is associated with shorter door-to-computed tomography time and increased likelihood of administration of tissue-plasminogen activator. *Prehosp Emerg Care.* 2008;12:426–431.

49. Gropen TI, Gagliano PJ, Blake CA, Sacco RL, Kwiatkowski T, Richmond NJ, Leifer D, Libman R, Azhar S, Daley MB. Quality improvement in acute stroke: the New York State Stroke Center Designation Project. *Neurology.* 2006;67:88–93.

50. Gladstone DJ, Rodan LH, Sahlas DJ, Lee L, Murray BJ, Ween JE, Perry JR, Chenkin J, Morrison LJ, Beck S, Black SE. A citywide prehospital protocol increases access to stroke thrombolysis in Toronto. *Stroke.* 2009;40:3841–3844.

51. Douglas VC, Tong DC, Gillum LA, Zhao S, Brass LM, Dostal J, Johnston SC. Do the Brain Attack Coalition's criteria for stroke centers improve care for ischemic stroke? *Neurology.* 2005;64:422–427.

52. Chapman KM, Woolfenden AR, Graeb D, Johnston DC, Beckman J, Schulzer M, Teal PA. Intravenous tissue plasminogen activator for acute ischemic stroke: a Canadian hospital's experience. *Stroke.* 2000;31: 2920–2924.

53. Merino JG, Silver B, Wong E, Foell B, Demaerschalk B, Tamayo A, Poncha F, Hachinski V. Extending tissue plasminogen activator use to community and rural stroke patients. *Stroke.* 2002;33:141–146.

54. Riopelle RJ, Howse DC, Bolton C, Elson S, Groll DL, Holtom D, Brunet DG, Jackson AC, Melanson M, Weaver DF. Regional access to acute ischemic stroke intervention. *Stroke.* 2001;32:652–655.

55. Cross DT III, Tirschwell DL, Clark MA, Tuden D, Derdeyn CP, Moran CJ, Dacey RG Jr. Mortality rates after subarachnoid hemorrhage: variations according to hospital case volume in 18 states. *J Neurosurg.* 2003;99:810–817.

56. Domeier R, Scott P, Wagner C. From research to the road: the development of EMS specialty triage. *Air Med J.* 2004;23:28–31.

57. Pepe PE, Zachariah BS, Sayre MR, Floccare D. Ensuring the chain of recovery for stroke in your community. *Acad Emerg Med.* 1998;5: 352–358.

58. Wojner-Alexandrov AW, Alexandrov AV, Rodriguez D, Persse D, Grotta JC. Houston paramedic and emergency stroke treatment and outcomes study (HoPSTO). *Stroke.* 2005;36:1512–1518.

59. Collaborative systematic review of the randomised trials of organised inpatient (stroke unit) care after stroke. Stroke Unit Trialists' Collaboration. *BMJ.* 1997;314:1151–1159.

60. How do stroke units improve patient outcomes? A collaborative systematic review of the randomized trials. Stroke Unit Trialists Collaboration. *Stroke.* 1997;28:2139–2144.

61. Organised inpatient (stroke unit) care for stroke. *Cochrane Database Syst Rev.* 2002:CD000197.

62. Ma RH, Wang YJ, Zhao XQ, Wang CX, Yang ZH, Qu H. [The impact of stroke unit on early outcome of cerebral infarction patients]. *Zhonghua Nei Ke Za Zhi.* 2004;43:183–185.

63. Oppenheimer SM, Cechetto DF, Hachinski VC. Cerebrogenic cardiac arrhythmias: cerebral electrocardiographic influences and their role in sudden death. *Arch Neurol.* 1990;47:513–519.

64. Adams HP Jr, Adams RJ, Brott T, del Zoppo GJ, Furlan A, Goldstein LB, Grubb RL, Higashida R, Kidwell C, Kwiatkowski TG, Marler JR, Hademenos GJ. Guidelines for the early management of patients with ischemic stroke: a scientific statement from the Stroke Council of the American Stroke Association. *Stroke.* 2003;34:1056–1083.

65. LaMonte MP, Bahouth MN, Hu P, Pathan MY, Yarbrough KL, Gunawardane R, Crarey P, Page W. Telemedicine for acute stroke: triumphs and pitfalls. *Stroke.* 2003;34:725–728.

66. Rymer MM, Thurtchley D, Summers D. Expanded modes of tissue plasminogen activator delivery in a comprehensive stroke center increases regional acute stroke interventions. *Stroke.* 2003;34:e58–e60.

67. Audebert HJ, Kukla C, Clarmann von Claranau S, Kuhn J, Vatankhah B, Schenkel J, Ickenstein GW, Haberl RL, Horn M. Telemedicine for safe and extended use of thrombolysis in stroke: the Telemedic Pilot Project for Integrative Stroke Care (TEMPiS) in Bavaria. *Stroke.* 2005;36: 287–291.

68. Adams HP Jr, del Zoppo G, Alberts MJ, Bhatt DL, Brass L, Furlan A, Grubb RL, Higashida RT, Jauch EC, Kidwell C, Lyden PD, Morgenstern LB, Qureshi AI, Rosenwasser RH, Scott PA, Wijdicks EF. Guidelines for the early management of adults with ischemic stroke: a guideline from the American Heart Association/American Stroke Association Stroke Council, Clinical Cardiology Council, Cardiovascular Radiology and Intervention Council, and the Atherosclerotic Peripheral Vascular Disease and Quality of Care Outcomes in Research Interdisciplinary Working Groups. *Stroke.* 2007;38:1655–1711.

69. Latchaw RE, Alberts MJ, Lev MH, Connors JJ, Harbaugh RE, Higashida RT, Hobson R, Kidwell CS, Koroshetz WJ, Mathews V, Villablanca P, Warach S, Walters B. Recommendations for imaging of acute ischemic stroke: a scientific statement from the American Heart Association. *Stroke.* 2009;40:3646–3678.

70. Hill MD, Buchan AM. Thrombolysis for acute ischemic stroke: results of the Canadian Alteplase for Stroke Effectiveness Study. Canadian Alteplase for Stroke Effectiveness Study (CASES) Investigators. *CMAJ.* 2005;172:1307.

71. Graham GD. Tissue plasminogen activator for acute ischemic stroke in clinical practice: a meta-analysis of safety data. *Stroke.* 2003;34: 2847–2850.

72. Heuschmann PU, Berger K, Misselwitz B, Hermanek P, Leffmann C, Adelmann M, Buecker-Nott HJ, Rother J, Neundoerfer B, Kolominsky-Rabas PL. Frequency of thrombolytic therapy in patients with acute ischemic stroke and the risk of in-hospital mortality: the German Stroke Registers Study Group. *Stroke.* 2003;34:1106–1113.

73. Kwiatkowski TG, Libman RB, Frankel M, Tilley BC, Morgenstern LB, Lu M, Broderick JP, Lewandowski CA, Marler JR, Levine SR, Brott T. Effects of tissue plasminogen activator for acute ischemic stroke at one year. National Institute of Neurological Disorders and Stroke Recombinant Tissue Plasminogen Activator Stroke Study Group. *N Engl J Med.* 1999;340:1781–1787.

74. Ingall TJ, O'Fallon WM, Asplund K, Goldfrank LR, Hertzberg VS, Louis TA, Christianson TJ. Findings from the reanalysis of the NINDS tissue plasminogen activator for acute ischemic stroke treatment trial. *Stroke.* 2004;35:2418–2424.

75. Wardlaw JM, Zoppo G, Yamaguchi T, Berge E. Thrombolysis for acute ischaemic stroke. *Cochrane Database Syst Rev.* 2003:CD000213.

76. Marler JR, Tilley BC, Lu M, Brott TG, Lyden PC, Grotta JC, Broderick JP, Levine SR, Frankel MP, Horowitz SH, Haley EC Jr, Lewandowski CA, Kwiatkowski TP. Early stroke treatment associated with better outcome: the NINDS rt-PA stroke study. *Neurology.* 2000;55: 1649–1655.

77. Kwiatkowski T, Libman R, Tilley BC, Lewandowski C, Grotta JC, Lyden P, Levine SR, Brott T. The impact of imbalances in baseline stroke severity on outcome in the National Institute of Neurological Disorders and Stroke Recombinant Tissue Plasminogen Activator Stroke Study. *Ann Emerg Med.* 2005;45:377–384.

78. Del Zoppo GJ, Saver JL, Jauch EC, Adams HP Jr. Expansion of the time window for treatment of acute ischemic stroke with intravenous tissue

plasminogen activator: a science advisory from the American Heart Association/American Stroke Association. *Stroke.* 2009;40:2945–2948.

79. Katzan IL, Furlan AJ, Lloyd LE, Frank JI, Harper DL, Hinchey JA, Hammel JP, Qu A, Sila CA. Use of tissue-type plasminogen activator for acute ischemic stroke: the Cleveland area experience. *JAMA.* 2000;283: 1151–1158.

80. Bravata DM, Kim N, Concato J, Krumholz HM, Brass LM. Thrombolysis for acute stroke in routine clinical practice. *Arch Intern Med.* 2002;162:1994–2001.

81. Lopez-Yunez AM, Bruno A, Williams LS, Yilmaz E, Zurru C, Biller J. Protocol violations in community-based rTPA stroke treatment are associated with symptomatic intracerebral hemorrhage. *Stroke.* 2001;32: 12–16.

82. Lattimore SU, Chalela J, Davis L, DeGraba T, Ezzeddine M, Haymore J, Nyquist P, Baird AE, Hallenbeck J, Warach S. Impact of establishing a primary stroke center at a community hospital on the use of thrombolytic therapy: the NINDS Suburban Hospital Stroke Center experience. *Stroke.* 2003;34:e55–e57.

83. Furlan A, Higashida R, Wechsler L, Gent M, Rowley H, Kase C, Pessin M, Ahuja A, Callahan F, Clark WM, Silver F, Rivera F. Intra-arterial prourokinase for acute ischemic stroke. The PROACT II study: a randomized controlled trial. Prolyse in Acute Cerebral Thromboembolism. *JAMA.* 1999;282:2003–2011.

84. Combined intravenous and intra-arterial recanalization for acute ischemic stroke: the Interventional Management of Stroke Study. *Stroke.* 2004;35:904–911.

85. Ogawa A, Mori E, Minematsu K, Taki W, Takahashi A, Nemoto S, Miyamoto S, Sasaki M, Inoue T. Randomized trial of intraarterial infusion of urokinase within 6 hours of middle cerebral artery stroke: the middle cerebral artery embolism local fibrinolytic intervention trial (MELT) Japan. *Stroke.* 2007;38:2633–2639.

86. del Zoppo GJ, Higashida RT, Furlan AJ, Pessin MS, Rowley HA, Gent M. PROACT: a phase II randomized trial of recombinant pro-urokinase by direct arterial delivery in acute middle cerebral artery stroke. PROACT Investigators. Prolyse in Acute Cerebral Thromboembolism. *Stroke.* 1998;29:4–11.

87. Saver JL. Intra-arterial fibrinolysis for acute ischemic stroke: the message of melt. *Stroke.* 2007;38:2627–2628.

88. Alvarez-Sabin J, Molina CA, Montaner J, Arenillas JF, Huertas R, Ribo M, Codina A, Quintana M. Effects of admission hyperglycemia on stroke outcome in reperfused tissue plasminogen activator–treated patients. *Stroke.* 2003;34:1235–1241.

89. Baird TA, Parsons MW, Phanh T, Butcher KS, Desmond PM, Tress BM, Colman PG, Chambers BR, Davis SM. Persistent poststroke hyperglycemia is independently associated with infarct expansion and worse clinical outcome. *Stroke.* 2003;34:2208–2214.

90. Parsons MW, Barber PA, Desmond PM, Baird TA, Darby DG, Byrnes G, Tress BM, Davis SM. Acute hyperglycemia adversely affects stroke outcome: a magnetic resonance imaging and spectroscopy study. *Ann Neurol.* 2002;52:20–28.

91. Capes SE, Hunt D, Malmberg K, Pathak P, Gerstein HC. Stress hyperglycemia and prognosis of stroke in nondiabetic and diabetic patients: a systematic overview. *Stroke.* 2001;32:2426–2432.

92. Bhalla A, Sankaralingam S, Tilling K, Swaminathan R, Wolfe C, Rudd A. Effect of acute glycaemic index on clinical outcome after acute stroke. *Cerebrovasc Dis.* 2002;13:95–101.

93. Bruno A, Biller J, Adams HP Jr, Clarke WR, Woolson RF, Williams LS, Hansen MD. Acute blood glucose level and outcome from ischemic stroke. Trial of ORG 10172 in Acute Stroke Treatment (TOAST) Investigators. *Neurology.* 1999;52:280–284.

94. Celik Y, Utku U, Asil T, Balci K. Factors affecting haemorrhagic transformation in middle cerebral artery infarctions. *J Clin Neurosci.* 2004;11:656–658.

95. Williams LS, Rotich J, Qi R, Fineberg N, Espay A, Bruno A, Fineberg SE, Tierney WR. Effects of admission hyperglycemia on mortality and costs in acute ischemic stroke. *Neurology.* 2002;59:67–71.

96. Scott JF, Robinson GM, French JM, O'Connell JE, Alberti KG, Gray CS. Glucose potassium insulin infusions in the treatment of acute stroke patients with mild to moderate hyperglycemia: the Glucose Insulin in Stroke Trial (GIST). *Stroke.* 1999;30:793–799.

97. Gray CS, Hildreth AJ, Alberti GK, O'Connell JE. Poststroke hyperglycemia: natural history and immediate management. *Stroke.* 2004;35: 122–126.

98. van den Berghe G, Wouters P, Weekers F, Verwaest C, Bruyninckx F, Schetz M, Vlasselaers D, Ferdinande P, Lauwers P, Bouillon R. Intensive insulin therapy in the critically ill patients. *N Engl J Med.* 2001;345:1359–1367.

99. Finfer S, Chittock DR, Su SY, Blair D, Foster D, Dhingra V, Bellomo R, Cook D, Dodek P, Henderson WR, Hebert PC, Heritier S, Heyland DK, McArthur C, McDonald E, Mitchell I, Myburgh JA, Norton R, Potter J, Robinson BG, Ronco JJ. Intensive versus conventional glucose control in critically ill patients. *N Engl J Med.* 2009;360:1283–1297.

100. Hajat C, Hajat S, Sharma P. Effects of poststroke pyrexia on stroke outcome: a meta-analysis of studies in patients. *Stroke.* 2000;31: 410–414.

101. Azzimondi G, Bassein L, Nonino F, Fiorani L, Vignatelli L, Re G, D'Alessandro R. Fever in acute stroke worsens prognosis. A prospective study. *Stroke.* 1995;26:2040–2043.

102. Reith J, Jorgensen HS, Pedersen PM, Nakayama H, Raaschou HO, Jeppesen LL, Olsen TS. Body temperature in acute stroke: relation to stroke severity, infarct size, mortality, and outcome. *Lancet.* 1996;347: 422–425.

103. Boysen G, Christensen H. Stroke severity determines body temperature in acute stroke. *Stroke.* 2001;32:413–417.

104. Adams HJ, Brott T, Crowell R, Furlan A, Gomez C, Grotta J, Helgason C, Marler J, Woolson R, Zivin J, Feinberg W, Mayberg M. Guidelines for the management of patients with acute ischemic stroke: a statement for healthcare professionals from a special writing group of the Stroke Council, American Heart Association. *Stroke.* 1994;25:1901–1914.

KEY WORDS: emergency department ■ hemorrhage ■ ischemic stroke ■ stroke

# Part 12: Cardiac Arrest in Special Situations
## 2010 American Heart Association Guidelines for Cardiopulmonary Resuscitation and Emergency Cardiovascular Care

Terry L. Vanden Hoek, Chair; Laurie J. Morrison; Michael Shuster; Michael Donnino; Elizabeth Sinz; Eric J. Lavonas; Farida M. Jeejeebhoy; Andrea Gabrielli

This section of the *2010 AHA Guidelines for CPR and ECC* addresses cardiac arrest in situations that require special treatments or procedures beyond those provided during basic life support (BLS) and advanced cardiovascular life support (ACLS). We have included 15 specific cardiac arrest situations. The first several sections discuss cardiac arrest associated with internal physiological or metabolic conditions, such as asthma (12.1), anaphylaxis (12.2), pregnancy (12.3), morbid obesity (12.4), pulmonary embolism (PE) (12.5), and electrolyte imbalance (12.6).

The next several sections relate to resuscitation and treatment of cardiac arrest associated with external or environmentally related circumstances, such as ingestion of toxic substances (12.7), trauma (12.8), accidental hypothermia (12.9), avalanche (12.10), drowning (12.11), and electric shock/lightning strikes (12.12).

The last 3 sections review management of cardiac arrest that may occur during special situations affecting the heart, including percutaneous coronary intervention (PCI) (12.13), cardiac tamponade (12.14), and cardiac surgery (12.15).

## Part 12.1: Cardiac Arrest Associated With Asthma

Asthma is responsible for more than 2 million visits to the emergency department (ED) in the United States each year, with 1 in 4 patients requiring admission to a hospital.[1] Annually there are 5,000 to 6,000 asthma-related deaths in the United States, many occurring in the prehospital setting.[2] Severe asthma accounts for approximately 2% to 20% of admissions to intensive care units, with up to one third of these patients requiring intubation and mechanical ventilation.[3] This section focuses on the evaluation and treatment of patients with near-fatal asthma.

Several consensus groups have developed excellent guidelines for the management of asthma that are available on the World Wide Web:

- http://www.nhlbi.nih.gov/about/naepp
- http://www.ginasthma.com

### Pathophysiology
The pathophysiology of asthma consists of 3 key abnormalities:

- Bronchoconstriction
- Airway inflammation
- Mucous plugging

Complications of severe asthma, such as tension pneumothorax, lobar atelectasis, pneumonia, and pulmonary edema, can contribute to fatalities. Severe asthma exacerbations are commonly associated with hypercarbia and acidemia, hypotension due to decreased venous return, and depressed mental status, but the most common cause of death is asphyxia. Cardiac causes of death are less common.[4]

### Clinical Aspects of Severe Asthma
Wheezing is a common physical finding, although the severity of wheezing does not correlate with the degree of airway obstruction. The absence of wheezing may indicate critical airway obstruction, whereas increased wheezing may indicate a positive response to bronchodilator therapy.

Oxygen saturation ($SaO_2$) levels may not reflect progressive alveolar hypoventilation, particularly if oxygen is being administered. Note that $SaO_2$ may fall initially during therapy because $\beta_2$-agonists produce both bronchodilation and vasodilation and initially may increase intrapulmonary shunting.

Other causes of wheezing are pulmonary edema,[5] chronic obstructive pulmonary disease (COPD), pneumonia, anaphylaxis,[6] foreign bodies, PE, bronchiectasis, and subglottic mass.[7]

### Initial Stabilization
Patients with severe life-threatening asthma require urgent and aggressive treatment with simultaneous administration of oxygen, bronchodilators, and steroids. Healthcare providers must monitor these patients closely for deterioration. Although the pathophysiology of life-threatening asthma consists of bronchoconstriction, inflammation, and mucous plugging, only bronchoconstriction and inflammation are amenable to drug treatment.

The American Heart Association requests that this document be cited as follows: Vanden Hoek TL, Morrison LJ, Shuster M, Donnino M, Sinz E, Lavonas EJ, Jeejeebhoy FM, Gabrielli A. Part 12: cardiac arrest in special situations: 2010 American Heart Association guidelines for cardiopulmonary resuscitation and emergency cardiovascular care. *Circulation*. 2010;122(suppl 3):S829–S861.

(*Circulation*. 2010;122[suppl 3]:S829–S861.)

*Circulation* is available at http://circ.ahajournals.org

DOI: 10.1161/CIRCULATIONAHA.110.971069

# Primary Therapy

## Oxygen

Oxygen should be provided to all patients with severe asthma, even those with normal oxygenation. As noted above, successful treatment with $\beta_2$-agonists may cause an initial decrease in oxygen saturation because the resultant bronchodilation can initially increase the ventilation-perfusion mismatch.

## Inhaled $\beta_2$-Agonists

Short-acting $\beta$-agonists provide rapid, dose-dependent bronchodilation with minimal side effects. Because the dose delivered depends on the patient's lung volume and inspiratory flow rate, the same dose can be used in most patients regardless of age or size. Studies have shown no difference in the effects of continuous versus intermittent administration of nebulized albuterol[8,9]; however, continuous administration was more effective in a subset of patients with severe exacerbations of asthma.[8] A Cochrane meta-analysis showed no overall difference between the effects of albuterol delivered by metered-dose inhaler spacer or nebulizer.[10] If prior use of a metered-dose inhaler has not been effective, use of a nebulizer is reasonable.

Although albuterol is sometimes administered intravenously (IV) in severe asthma, a systematic review of 15 clinical trials found that IV $\beta_2$-agonists, administered by either bolus or infusion, did not lead to significant improvements in any clinical outcome measure.[9]

Levalbuterol is the R-isomer of albuterol. Comparisons with albuterol have produced mixed results, with some studies showing a slightly improved bronchodilator effect in the treatment of acute asthma in the ED.[11] There is no evidence that levalbuterol should be favored over albuterol.

One of the most common adjuncts used with $\beta$-agonist treatment, particularly in the first hours of treatment, include anticholinergic agents (see "Adjunctive Therapies" below for more detail). When combined with short-acting $\beta$-agonists, anticholinergic agents such as ipratropium can produce a clinically modest improvement in lung function compared with short-acting $\beta$-agonists alone.[12,13]

## Corticosteroids

Systemic corticosteroids are the only treatment for the inflammatory component of asthma proven to be effective for acute asthma exacerbations. Because the antiinflammatory effects after administration may not be apparent for 6 to 12 hours, corticosteroids should be administered early. The early use of systemic steroids hastens the resolution of airflow obstruction and may reduce admission to the hospital.[14] Although there may be no difference in clinical effects between oral and IV formulations of corticosteroids,[15,16] the IV route is preferable in patients with severe asthma. In adults a typical initial dose of methylprednisolone is 125 mg (dose range: 40 mg to 250 mg); a typical dose of dexamethasone is 10 mg.

# Adjunctive Therapies

## Anticholinergics

Ipratropium bromide is an anticholinergic bronchodilator pharmacologically related to atropine. The nebulizer dose is 500 mcg.[15,16] Ipratropium bromide has a slow onset of action (approximately 20 minutes), with peak effectiveness at 60 to 90 minutes and no systemic side effects. The drug is typically given only once because of its prolonged onset of action, but some studies have shown that repeat doses of 250 mcg or 500 mcg every 20 minutes may be beneficial.[17] A recent meta-analysis indicated a reduced number of hospital admissions associated with treatment with ipratropium bromide, particularly in patients with severe exacerbations.[18]

## Magnesium Sulfate

When combined with nebulized $\beta$-adrenergic agents and corticosteroids, IV magnesium sulfate can moderately improve pulmonary function in patients with asthma.[19] Magnesium causes relaxation of bronchial smooth muscle independent of serum magnesium level, with only minor side effects (flushing, lightheadedness). A Cochrane meta-analysis of 7 studies concluded that IV magnesium sulfate improves pulmonary function and reduces hospital admissions, particularly for patients with the most severe exacerbations of asthma.[20] The use of nebulized magnesium sulfate as an adjunct to nebulized $\beta$-adrenergic agents has been reported in a small case series to improve FEV1 and $SpO_2$,[21] although a prior meta-analysis demonstrated only a trend toward improved pulmonary function with nebulized magnesium.[22] For those with severe refractory asthma, providers may consider IV magnesium at the standard adult dose of 2 g administered over 20 minutes.

## Epinephrine or Terbutaline

Epinephrine and terbutaline are adrenergic agents that can be given subcutaneously to patients with acute severe asthma. The dose of subcutaneous epinephrine (concentration 1:1000) is 0.01 mg/kg, divided into 3 doses of approximately 0.3 mg administered at 20-minute intervals. Although the nonselective adrenergic properties of epinephrine may cause an increase in heart rate, myocardial irritability, and increased oxygen demand, its use is well-tolerated, even in patients >35 years of age.[23] Terbutaline is given in a subcutaneous dose of 0.25 mg, which can be repeated every 20 minutes for 3 doses. There is no evidence that subcutaneous epinephrine or terbutaline has advantages over inhaled $\beta_2$-agonists. Epinephrine has been administered IV (initiated at 0.25 mcg/min to 1 mcg/min continuous infusion) in severe asthma; however, 1 retrospective investigation indicated a 4% incidence of serious side effects. There is no evidence of improved outcomes with IV epinephrine compared with selective inhaled $\beta_2$-agonists.[24]

## Ketamine

Ketamine is a parenteral, dissociative anesthetic with bronchodilatory properties that also can stimulate copious bronchial secretions. One case series[25] suggested substantial efficacy, whereas 2 published randomized trials in children[26,27] found no benefit of ketamine when compared with standard care. Ketamine has sedative and analgesic properties that may be useful if intubation is planned.

## Heliox

Heliox is a mixture of helium and oxygen (usually a 70:30 helium to oxygen ratio mix) that is less viscous than ambient air. Heliox has been shown to improve the delivery and deposition of nebulized albuterol[28]; however, a recent meta-analysis of clinical trials did not support its use as initial treatment for patients with acute asthma.[29] Because the heliox mixture requires at least 70% helium for effect, it cannot be used if the patient requires >30% oxygen.

### Methylxanthines

Although once considered a mainstay in the treatment of acute asthma, methylxanthines are no longer recommended because of their erratic pharmacokinetics, known side effects, and lack of evidence of benefit.[30]

### Leukotriene Antagonists

Leukotriene antagonists improve lung function and decrease the need for short-acting $\beta_2$-agonists for long-term asthma therapy, but their effectiveness during acute exacerbations of asthma is unproven.

### Inhaled Anesthetics

Case reports in adults[31] and children[32] suggest a benefit of the potent inhalation anesthetics sevoflurane and isoflurane for patients with life-threatening asthma unresponsive to maximal conventional therapy. These agents may have direct bronchodilator effects. In addition, the anesthetic effect of these drugs increases the ease of mechanical ventilation and reduces oxygen demand and carbon dioxide production. This therapy requires expert consultation in an intensive care setting, and its effectiveness has not been evaluated in randomized clinical studies.

## Assisted Ventilation

### Noninvasive Positive-Pressure Ventilation

Noninvasive positive-pressure ventilation (NIPPV) may offer short-term support for patients with acute respiratory failure and may delay or eliminate the need for endotracheal intubation.[33–35] This therapy requires that the patient is alert and has adequate spontaneous respiratory effort. Bilevel positive airway pressure (BiPAP), the most common method of delivering NIPPV, allows for separate control of inspiratory and expiratory pressures.

### Endotracheal Intubation With Mechanical Ventilation

Endotracheal intubation is indicated for patients who present with apnea, coma, persistent or increasing hypercapnia, exhaustion, severe distress, and depression of mental status. Clinical judgment is necessary to assess the need for immediate endotracheal intubation for these critically ill patients. Endotracheal intubation does not solve the problem of small airway constriction in patients with severe asthma; thus, therapy directed toward relief of bronchoconstriction should be continued. Mechanical ventilation in the asthmatic patient can be difficult and associated risks require careful management. Intubation and positive-pressure ventilation can trigger further bronchoconstriction and complications such as breath stacking that result from incomplete expiration, air trapping, and buildup of positive end-expiratory pressure (ie, intrinsic or auto-PEEP). This breath stacking can cause barotrauma. Decreasing tidal volume may avoid auto-PEEP and high peak airway pressures. Optimal ventilator management requires expert consultation and ongoing careful review of ventilation flow and pressure curves. Although endotracheal intubation introduces risks, it should be performed when necessary based on clinical condition.

Rapid sequence intubation is the technique of choice and should be performed by an expert in airway management. The provider should use the largest endotracheal tube available (usually 8 or 9 mm) to decrease airway resistance. Immediately after intubation, endotracheal tube placement should be confirmed by clinical examination and waveform capnography. A chest radiograph should then be performed.

## Troubleshooting After Intubation

When severe bronchoconstriction is present, breath stacking (so-called auto-PEEP) can develop during positive-pressure ventilation, leading to complications such as hyperinflation, tension pneumothorax, and hypotension. During manual or mechanical ventilation, a slower respiratory rate should be used with smaller tidal volumes (eg, 6 to 8 mL/kg),[36] shorter inspiratory time (eg, adult inspiratory flow rate 80 to 100 mL/min), and longer expiratory time (eg, inspiratory to expiratory ratio 1:4 or 1:5) than generally would be provided to patients without asthma.[37] Management of mechanical ventilation will vary based on patient-ventilation characteristics. Expert consultation should be obtained.

Mild hypoventilation (permissive hypercapnia) reduces the risk of barotrauma. Hypercapnia is typically well tolerated.[38,39] Sedation is often required to optimize ventilation, decrease ventilator dyssynchrony (and therefore auto-PEEP), and minimize barotrauma after intubation. Because delivery of inhaled medications may be inadequate before intubation, the provider should continue to administer inhaled albuterol treatments through the endotracheal tube.

Four common causes of acute deterioration in any intubated patient are recalled by the mnemonic **DOPE** (tube **D**isplacement, tube **O**bstruction, **P**neumothorax, **E**quipment failure). Auto-PEEP is another common cause of deterioration in patients with asthma. If the asthmatic patient's condition deteriorates or if it is difficult to ventilate the patient, check the ventilator for leaks or malfunction; verify endotracheal tube position; eliminate tube obstruction (eliminate any mucous plugs and kinks); evaluate for auto-PEEP; and rule out a pneumothorax.

High-end expiratory pressure can be reduced quickly by separating the patient from the ventilator circuit; this will allow PEEP to dissipate during passive exhalation. If auto-PEEP results in significant hypotension, assisting with exhalation by pressing on the chest wall after disconnection of the ventilator circuit will allow active exhalation and should lead to immediate resolution of hypotension. To minimize auto-PEEP, decrease the respiratory rate or tidal volume or both. If auto-PEEP persists and the patient displays ventilator dyssynchrony despite adequate sedation, paralytic agents may be considered.

In exceedingly rare circumstances, aggressive treatment for acute respiratory failure due to severe asthma will not provide adequate gas exchange. There are case reports that describe successful use of extracorporeal membrane oxygenation (ECMO) in adult and pediatric patients[40–43] with severe asthma after other aggressive measures have failed to reverse hyoxemia and hypercarbia.

## BLS Modifications

BLS treatment of cardiac arrest in asthmatic patients is unchanged.

## ACLS Modifications

When cardiac arrest occurs in the patient with acute asthma, standard ACLS guidelines should be followed.

Case series and case reports describe a novel technique of cardiopulmonary resuscitation (CPR) termed "lateral chest compressions"; however, there is insufficient evidence to recommend this technique over standard techniques.[44–50]

The adverse effect of auto-PEEP on coronary perfusion pressure and capacity for successful defibrillation has been described in patients in cardiac arrest without asthma.[51,52] Moreover, the adverse effect of auto-PEEP on hemodynamics in asthmatic patients who are not in cardiac arrest has also been well-described.[53–56] Therefore, since the effects of auto-PEEP in an asthmatic patient with cardiac arrest are likely quite severe, a ventilation strategy of low respiratory rate and tidal volume is reasonable (Class IIa, LOE C). During arrest a brief disconnection from the bag mask or ventilator may be considered, and compression of the chest wall to relieve air-trapping can be effective (Class IIa, LOE C).

For all asthmatic patients with cardiac arrest, and especially for patients in whom ventilation is difficult, the possible diagnosis of a tension pneumothorax should be considered and treated (Class I, LOE C).

## Part 12.2: Cardiac Arrest Associated With Anaphylaxis

Anaphylaxis is an allergic reaction characterized by multisystem involvement, including skin, airway, vascular system, and gastrointestinal tract. Severe cases may result in complete obstruction of the airway and cardiovascular collapse from vasogenic shock. Anaphylaxis accounts for about 500 to 1000 deaths per year in the United States.[57]

The term *classic anaphylaxis* refers to hypersensitivity reactions mediated by the immunoglobulins IgE and IgG. Prior sensitization to an allergen produces antigen-specific immunoglobulins. Subsequent reexposure to the allergen provokes the anaphylactic reaction, although many anaphylactic reactions occur with no documented prior exposure. Pharmacological agents, latex, foods, and stinging insects are among the most common causes of anaphylaxis described.

## Signs and Symptoms

The initial symptoms of anaphylaxis are often nonspecific and include tachycardia, faintness, cutaneous flushing, urticaria, diffuse or localized pruritus, and a sensation of impending doom. Urticaria is the most common physical finding. The patient may be agitated or anxious and may appear either flushed or pale.

A common early sign of respiratory involvement is rhinitis. As respiratory compromise becomes more severe, serious upper airway (laryngeal) edema may cause stridor and lower airway edema (asthma) may cause wheezing. Upper airway edema can also be a sign in angiotensin converting enzyme inhibitor-induced angioedema or C1 esterase inhibitor deficiency with spontaneous laryngeal edema.[58–60]

Cardiovascular collapse is common in severe anaphylaxis. If not promptly corrected, vasodilation and increased capillary permeability, causing decreased preload and relative hypovolemia of up to 37% of circulating blood volume, can rapidly lead

to cardiac arrest.[61,62] Myocardial ischemia and acute myocardial infarction, malignant arrhythmias, and cardiovascular depression can also contribute to rapid hemodynamic deterioration and cardiac arrest.[63] Additionally, cardiac dysfunction may result from underlying disease or development of myocardial ischemia due to hypotension or following administration of epinephrine.[64,65]

There are no randomized controlled trials evaluating alternative treatment algorithms for cardiac arrest due to anaphylaxis. Evidence is limited to case reports and extrapolations from nonfatal cases, interpretation of pathophysiology, and consensus opinion. Providers must be aware that urgent support of airway, breathing, and circulation is essential in suspected anaphylactic reactions.

Because of limited evidence, the management of cardiac arrest secondary to anaphylaxis should be treated with standard BLS and ACLS. The following therapies are largely consensus-based but commonly used and widely accepted in the management of the patient with anaphylaxis who is not in cardiac arrest.

## BLS Modifications

### Airway

Early and rapid advanced airway management is critical and should not be unnecessarily delayed. Given the potential for the rapid development of oropharyngeal or laryngeal edema,[66] immediate referral to a health professional with expertise in advanced airway placement is recommended (Class I, LOE C).

### Circulation

The intramuscular (IM) administration of epinephrine (epinephrine autoinjectors, eg, the EpiPen™) in the anterolateral aspect of the middle third of the thigh provides the highest peak blood levels.[67] Absorption and subsequent achievement of maximum plasma concentration after subcutaneous administration is slower than the IM route and may be significantly delayed with shock.[67]

Epinephrine[68] should be administered early by IM injection to all patients with signs of a systemic allergic reaction, especially hypotension, airway swelling, or difficulty breathing (Class I, LOE C). The recommended dose is 0.2 to 0.5 mg (1:1000) IM to be repeated every 5 to 15 minutes in the absence of clinical improvement (Class I, LOE C).[69] The adult epinephrine IM auto-injector will deliver 0.3 mg of epinephrine and the pediatric epinephrine IM auto-injector will deliver 0.15 mg of epinephrine. In both anaphylaxis and cardiac arrest the immediate use of an epinephrine autoinjector is recommended if available (Class I, LOE C).

## ACLS Modifications

### Airway

Early recognition of the potential for a difficult airway in anaphylaxis is paramount in patients who develop hoarseness, lingual edema, stridor, or oropharyngeal swelling. Planning for advanced airway management, including a surgical airway,[70] is recommended (Class I, LOE C).

### Fluid Resuscitation

In a prospective evaluation of volume resuscitation after diagnostic sting challenge, repeated administration of 1000-mL bolus doses of isotonic crystalloid (eg, normal saline) titrated to systolic blood pressure above 90 mm Hg was used successfully in patients whose hypotension did not respond immediately to vasoactive drugs.[61,71] Vasogenic shock from anaphylaxis may require aggressive fluid resuscitation (Class IIa, LOE C).

### Vasopressors
There are no human trials establishing the role of epinephrine or preferred route of administration in anaphylactic shock managed by ACLS providers.[68] In an animal study of profound anaphylactic shock, IV epinephrine restored blood pressure to baseline; however, the effect was limited to the first 15 minutes after shock, and no therapeutic effect was observed with the same dose of epinephrine administered IM or subcutaneously.[72] Therefore, when an IV line is in place, it is reasonable to consider the IV route as an alternative to IM administration of epinephrine in anaphylactic shock (Class IIa, LOE C).

For patients not in cardiac arrest, IV epinephrine 0.05 to 0.1 mg (5% to 10% of the epinephrine dose used routinely in cardiac arrest) has been used successfully in patients with anaphylactic shock.[73] Because fatal overdose of epinephrine has been reported,[64,71,74,75] close hemodynamic monitoring is recommended (Class I, LOE B).

In a study of animals sensitized by ragweed, a continuous IV infusion of epinephrine maintained a mean arterial pressure at 70% of preshock levels better than no treatment or bolus epinephrine treatment (IV, subcutaneous, or IM).[76] Furthermore, a recent human study suggests that careful titration of a continuous infusion of IV epinephrine (5 to 15 mcg/min), based on severity of reaction and in addition to crystalloid infusion, may be considered in treatment of anaphylactic shock.[71] Therefore, IV infusion of epinephrine is a reasonable alternative to IV boluses for treatment of anaphylaxis in patients not in cardiac arrest (Class IIa, LOE C) and may be considered in postarrest management (Class IIb, LOE C).

Recently vasopressin has been used successfully in patients with anaphylaxis (with or without cardiac arrest) who did not respond to standard therapy.[77–79] Other small case series described successful results with administration of alternative α-agonists such as norepinephrine,[80] methoxamine,[81,82] and metaraminol.[83–85] Alternative vasoactive drugs (vasopressin, norepinephrine, methoxamine, and metaraminol) may be considered in cardiac arrest secondary to anaphylaxis that does not respond to epinephrine (Class IIb, LOE C). No randomized controlled trials have evaluated epinephrine versus the use of alternative vasoactive drugs for cardiac arrest due to anaphylaxis.

### Other Interventions
There are no prospective randomized clinical studies evaluating the use of other therapeutic agents in anaphylactic shock or cardiac arrest. Adjuvant use of antihistamines (H1 and H2 antagonist),[86,87] inhaled β-adrenergic agents,[88] and IV corticosteroids[89] has been successful in management of the patient with anaphylaxis and may be considered in cardiac arrest due to anaphylaxis (Class IIb, LOE C).

### Extracorporeal Support of Circulation
Cardiopulmonary bypass has been successful in isolated case reports of anaphylaxis followed by cardiac arrest.[90,91] Use of

these advanced techniques may be considered in clinical situations where the required professional skills and equipment are immediately available (Class IIb, LOE C).

## Part 12.3: Cardiac Arrest Associated With Pregnancy

### Scope of the Problem
The Confidential Enquiries into Maternal and Child Health (CEMACH) data set constitutes the largest population-based data set on this target population.[92] The overall maternal mortality rate was calculated at 13.95 deaths per 100 000 maternities. There were 8 cardiac arrests with a frequency calculated at 0.05 per 1000 maternities, or 1:20 000. The frequency of cardiac arrest in pregnancy is on the rise with previous reports estimating the frequency to be 1:30 000 maternities.[93] Despite pregnant women being younger than the traditional cardiac arrest patient, the survival rates are poorer, with one case series reporting a survival rate of 6.9%.[93,94]

During attempted resuscitation of a pregnant woman, providers have 2 potential patients: the mother and the fetus. The best hope of fetal survival is maternal survival. For the critically ill pregnant patient, rescuers must provide appropriate resuscitation based on consideration of the physiological changes caused by pregnancy.

### Key Interventions to Prevent Arrest
The following interventions are the standard of care for treating the critically ill pregnant patient (Class I, LOE C):

- Place the patient in the full left-lateral position to relieve possible compression of the inferior vena cava. Uterine obstruction of venous return can produce hypotension and may precipitate arrest in the critically ill patient.[95,96]
- Give 100% oxygen.
- Establish intravenous (IV) access above the diaphragm.
- Assess for hypotension; maternal hypotension that warrants therapy has been defined as a systolic blood pressure <100 mm Hg or <80% of baseline.[97,98] Maternal hypotension can result in reduced placental perfusion.[99–102] In the patient who is not in arrest, both crystalloid and colloid solutions have been shown to increase preload.[103]
- Consider reversible causes of critical illness and treat conditions that may contribute to clinical deterioration as early as possible.

### Resuscitation of the Pregnant Patient in Cardiac Arrest (Figure 1)
There are no randomized controlled trials evaluating the effect of specialized obstetric resuscitation versus standard care in pregnant patients in cardiac arrest. There are reports in the literature of patients not in arrest that describe the science behind important physiological changes that occur in pregnancy that may influence treatment recommendations and guidelines for resuscitation from cardiac arrest in pregnancy.

### BLS Modifications

#### Patient Positioning
Patient position has emerged as an important strategy to improve the quality of CPR and resultant compression force and output.

**Maternal Cardiac Arrest**

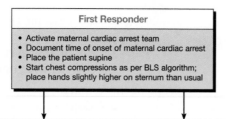

Figure 1. Maternal cardiac arrest algorithm.

The pregnant uterus can compress the inferior vena cava, impeding venous return and thereby reducing stroke volume and cardiac output. Reports of noncardiac arrest parturients indicate that left-lateral tilt results in improved maternal hemodynamics of blood pressure, cardiac output, and stroke volume[96,98,104]; and improved fetal parameters of oxygenation, nonstress test, and fetal heart rate.[100–102]

Although chest compressions in the left-lateral tilt position are feasible in a manikin study,[105] they result in less forceful chest compressions than are possible in the supine position.[106] Two studies found no improvement in maternal hemodynamic or fetal parameters with 10° to 20° left-lateral tilt in patients not in arrest.[107,108] One study reported more aortic compression at 15° left-lateral tilt compared with a full left-lateral tilt.[97] In addition, aortic compression has been found at >30° of tilt,[109] however the majority of these patients were in labor.

If left-lateral tilt is used to improve maternal hemodynamics during cardiac arrest, the degree of tilt should be maximized. However, at a tilt ≥30° the patient may slide or roll off the inclined plane,[106] so this degree of tilt may not be practical during resuscitation. Although important, the degree of tilt is difficult to estimate reliably; 1 study reported that the degree of table tilt is often overestimated.[110] Using a fixed, hard wedge of a predetermined angle may help.

Two studies in pregnant women not in arrest found that manual left uterine displacement, which is done with the patient supine, is as good as or better than left-lateral tilt in relieving aortocaval compression (as assessed by the incidence of hypotension and use of ephedrine).[111,112]

Therefore, to relieve aortocaval compression during chest compressions and optimize the quality of CPR, it is reasonable to perform manual left uterine displacement in the supine position first (Class IIa, LOE C). Left uterine displacement can be performed from either the patient's left side with the 2-handed technique (Figure 2) or the patient's right side with the 1-handed technique (Figure 3), depending on the positioning of the resuscitation team. If this technique is unsuccessful, and an appropriate wedge is readily available, then providers may consider placing the patient in a left-lateral tilt of 27° to 30°,[106] using a firm wedge to support the pelvis and thorax (Figure 4) (Class IIb, LOE C).

If chest compressions remain inadequate after lateral uterine displacement or left-lateral tilt, immediate emergency cesarean section should be considered. (See "Emergency Cesarean Section in Cardiac Arrest," below.)

### Airway

Airway management is more difficult during pregnancy (see "ACLS Modifications: Airway," below), and placing the

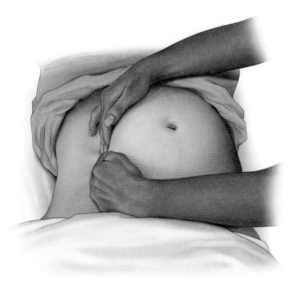

**Figure 2.** . Left uterine displacement with 2-handed technique.

patient in a tilt may increase the difficulty. In addition, altered airway anatomy increases the risks of aspiration and rapid desaturation. Therefore, optimal use of bag-mask ventilation and suctioning, while preparing for advanced airway placement (see "ACLS Modifications") is critical.

### Breathing
Pregnant patients can develop hypoxemia rapidly because of decreased functional residual capacity and increased oxygen demand. One study in normal pregnancy reported increased intrapulmonary shunting of 12.8% to 15.3% compared with the nonpregnant state, in which the normal value is 2% to 5%,[113] which further increases the risk of hypoxemia. Ventilation volumes may need to be reduced because the mother's diaphragm is elevated. Providers should be prepared to support oxygenation and ventilation and monitor oxygen saturation closely.

### Circulation
Chest compressions should be performed slightly higher on the sternum than normally recommended to adjust for the elevation

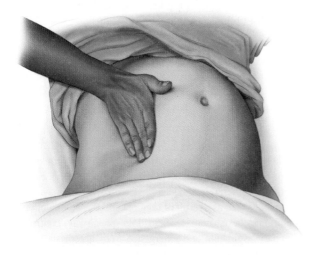

**Figure 3.** Left uterine displacement using 1-handed technique.

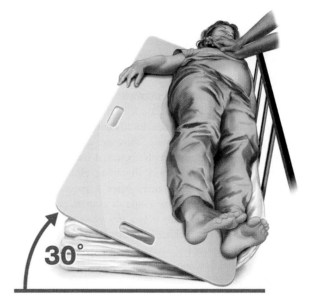

**Figure 4.** Patient in a 30° left-lateral tilt using a firm wedge to support pelvis and thorax.

of the diaphragm and abdominal contents caused by the gravid uterus.

### Defibrillation
Use of an AED on a pregnant victim has not been studied but is reasonable.

## ACLS Modifications
There should be no delay in delivering usual treatments during the management of cardiac arrest in pregnancy.

### Airway
Pregnancy results in changes in airway mucosa, including edema, friability, hypersecretion, and hyperemia.[114,115] In addition, 1 study found that the upper airway in the third trimester of pregnancy is smaller compared with that of nonpregnant women and women in the postpartum period.[116] Therefore, airway management of the pregnant patient may be more difficult than airway management of the nonpregnant patient.

There is significant literature recognizing the issue of failed intubation in obstetric anesthesia as a major cause of maternal morbidity and mortality.[117,118] All providers involved in a resuscitation attempt should be aware of the increased risk for pregnancy-related complications in airway management. Intubation with an endotracheal tube or supraglottic airway should be performed only by experienced providers if possible.

Cheun et al[119] found that during apnea desaturation in pregnant patients is significantly faster than in nonpregnant patients. Bag-mask ventilation with 100% oxygen before intubation is especially important in pregnancy (Class IIa, LOE B).[120]

### Circulation

#### Changes in Pharmacokinetics
One clinical pharmacokinetic study discovered an increase in the rate of glomerular filtration and volume of plasma during normal pregnancy.[121] There is no evidence, however, that current

medications or doses should be altered during management of cardiac arrest in pregnancy; therefore, current recommended drug dosages for use in resuscitation of adults should also be used in resuscitation of the pregnant patient.

### Defibrillation

Defibrillation should be performed at the recommended ACLS defibrillation doses (Class I, LOE C).[122]

Although there are no studies documenting maternal or fetal complications with defibrillation, there are case reports[123–130] and case series[131–133] that describe potential harm to the fetus when an accidental electric shock (lightning, electric circuit) is delivered directly to the mother. After a pregnant woman receives an electric shock, the range of clinical presentations varies from the mother feeling only a strange sensation with no fetal effects to fetal death either immediately or a few days after the shock. Risk factors for adverse fetal outcomes include the magnitude of current and duration of contact. The greatest predictor of risk for adverse fetal outcome is if the current travels through the uterus, because amniotic fluid most likely transmits current in a manner similar to that transmitted via other body fluids, which could increase the risk of fetal death or burns.

Although there is a small risk of inducing fetal arrhythmias, cardioversion and defibrillation on the external chest are considered safe at all stages of pregnancy.[134–136]

Some experts have raised concern that electric arcing may occur if fetal monitors are attached during defibrillation of a pregnant woman, but there is no evidence to support this. Overall it is reasonable to assume that if the shock is delivered to the mother's thorax, there is very low to no risk of electric arcing to fetal monitors. If internal or external fetal monitors are attached during cardiac arrest in a pregnant woman, it is reasonable to remove them (Class IIb, LOE C).

## Treatment of Reversible Causes

The same reversible causes of cardiac arrest that occur in nonpregnant women can occur during pregnancy. Providers should be familiar with pregnancy-specific diseases and procedural complications and during resuscitation attempts should try to identify common and reversible causes of cardiac arrest in pregnancy.[92]

### Cardiac Disease

Cardiac disease is the primary cause of maternal mortality, according to the *2003 to 2005 Confidential Enquiries into Maternal and Child Health* report.[92] For example, the number of deaths from cardiac disease was 2.27 per 100,000 pregnancies, whereas the number of deaths from thrombosis and thromboembolism was 1.94 per 100,000 pregnancies.[92] The number of cardiac deaths during pregnancy has increased steadily since 1991. The most common causes of maternal death from cardiac disease are myocardial infarction, followed by aortic dissection.[92] A study completed in California also found that the incidence of myocardial infarction in pregnancy increased throughout the 1990s.[137] In addition, a nationwide review of myocardial infarction in pregnancy in the United States found that the risk of myocardial infarction in pregnancy is 3 to 4 times that of nonpregnant women of reproductive age.[138]

Women are deferring pregnancy to older ages, increasing the chance that they will have atherosclerotic heart disease. Because fibrinolytics are relatively contraindicated in pregnancy, PCI is the reperfusion strategy of choice for ST-elevation myocardial infarction.

The number of babies born with congenital heart disease who now survive to adulthood has increased exponentially over the last 3 decades.[139,140] It is estimated that 85% of neonates born with congenital heart disease will survive to adulthood. Therefore, more women with congenital heart disease are surviving to have children, which translates into higher risk for a cardiac event during pregnancy. In fact, illnesses related to congenital heart disease and pulmonary hypertension are the third most common cause of maternal cardiac deaths.[92]

### Magnesium Sulfate Toxicity

Patients with magnesium toxicity present with cardiac effects ranging from ECG interval changes (prolonged PR, QRS and QT intervals) at magnesium levels of 2.5–5 mmol/L to AV nodal conduction block, bradycardia, hypotension and cardiac arrest at levels of 6–10 mmol/L. Neurological effects ranging from loss of tendon reflexes, sedation, severe muscular weakness, and respiratory depression are seen at levels of 4–5 mmol/L. Other signs of magnesium toxicity include gastrointestinal symptoms (nausea and vomiting), skin changes (flushing), and electrolyte/fluid abnormalities (hypophosphatemia, hyperosmolar dehydration). Patients with renal failure and metabolic derangements can develop toxicity after relatively lower magnesium doses.

Iatrogenic overdose is possible in the pregnant woman who receives magnesium sulfate, particularly if the woman becomes oliguric. Empirical calcium administration may be lifesaving in these cases.[141–143]

### Preeclampsia/Eclampsia

Preeclampsia/eclampsia develops after the 20th week of gestation and can produce severe hypertension and ultimately diffuse organ-system failure. If untreated, maternal and fetal morbidity and mortality may result.

### Life-Threatening Pulmonary Embolism (PE)

Successful use of fibrinolytics in pregnant women has been reported for massive, life-threatening PE[144–146] and ischemic stroke.[147] Pregnant women in cardiac arrest with suspected PE should be treated in accordance with the ACLS guidelines (see Part 12.5: "Cardiac Arrest Associated With Pulmonary Embolism").

### Amniotic Fluid Embolism

Clinicians have reported successful use of cardiopulmonary bypass for pregnant women with a life-threatening amniotic fluid embolism during labor and delivery.[148] The use of perimortem cesarean section has resulted in maternal and neonatal survival.[149]

### Anesthetic Complications

Anesthesia-related maternal morbidity and mortality continue to be a major concern, which has led to development of specialized obstetric anesthesia techniques.[118] Cardiac arrest may result from spinal shock as a result of regional anesthesia. Induction of general anesthesia may lead to loss of airway control or pulmonary aspiration, and emergence from anesthesia can be associated with hypoventilation or airway obstruction, leading to cardiac arrest.[150–155]

## Maternal Cardiac Arrest Not Immediately Reversed by BLS and ACLS

### Emergency Cesarean Section in Cardiac Arrest

Resuscitation team leaders should activate the protocol for an emergency cesarean delivery as soon as cardiac arrest is identified in a pregnant woman with an obviously gravid uterus. By the time the physician is ready to deliver the baby, standard ACLS should be underway and immediately reversible causes of cardiac arrest should be ruled out. When the gravid uterus is large enough to cause maternal hemodynamic changes due to aortocaval compression, emergency cesarean section should be considered, regardless of fetal viability.

### What Defines a Gravid Uterus With the Potential to Cause Aortocaval Compression?

A study found that maternal aortocaval compression can occur for singleton pregnancies at ≥20 weeks of gestational age.[156] However, the exact gestational age at which aortocaval compression occurs is not consistent, especially with multiple-gestation pregnancies or intrauterine growth retardation, and gestational age and number of fetuses may not always be known in the emergency situation. Fundal height is often used to estimate gestational age. In a singleton gestation, by 20 weeks fundal height is approximately at the level of the umbilicus[157]; however the fundus may reach the umbilicus between 15 and 19 weeks of gestation.[158] Fundal height may also be skewed by other factors such as abdominal distention[157] and increased body mass index; therefore fundal height may be a poor predictor of gestational age.

One review of emergency cesarean sections in maternal cardiac arrest before the third trimester concluded that if the fundus extends above the level of the umbilicus, aortocaval compression can occur, and emergency cesarean section should be performed regardless of gestational age.[158]

Two cases of maternal cardiac arrest in early pregnancy of 13 to 15 weeks were reported in which the mother was resuscitated without an emergency cesarean section being performed and the pregnancy continued to successful delivery of a live infant at term.[159,160] Not every pregnant woman in cardiac arrest is a candidate for an emergency cesarean section; the decision depends on whether or not the gravid uterus is thought to interfere with maternal hemodynamics.

### Why Perform an Emergency Cesarean Section in Cardiac Arrest?

Several case reports of emergency cesarean section in maternal cardiac arrest indicate a return of spontaneous circulation or improvement in maternal hemodynamic status only after the uterus has been emptied.[94–96,143,149,161–166] In a case series of 38 cases of perimortem cesarean section, 12 of 20 women for whom maternal outcome was recorded had return of spontaneous circulation immediately after delivery. No cases of worsened maternal status after cesarean section were reported.[166] The critical point to remember is that both mother and infant may die if the provider cannot restore blood flow to the mother's heart.[94]

### The Importance of Timing With Emergency Cesarean Section

The 5-minute window that providers have to determine if cardiac arrest can be reversed by BLS and ACLS was first described in 1986 and has been perpetuated in specialty guidelines.[143,166] The rescue team is not required to wait 5 minutes before initiating emergency hysterotomy, and there are circumstances that support an earlier start.[157] For instance, in an obvious nonsurvivable injury,[166,167–169] when the maternal prognosis is grave and resuscitative efforts appear futile, moving straight to an emergency cesarean section may be appropriate, especially if the fetus is viable.

Many reports document long intervals between an urgent decision for hysterotomy and actual delivery of the infant, far exceeding the obstetric guideline of 30 minutes for patients not in arrest.[170,171] Very few cases of perimortem cesarean section fall within the recommended 5-minute period.[94,166] Survival of the mother has been reported with perimortem cesarean section performed up to 15 minutes after the onset of maternal cardiac arrest.[94,172–174] If emergency cesarean section cannot be performed by the 5-minute mark, it may be advisable to prepare to evacuate the uterus while the resuscitation continues. (Class IIb, LOE C).

At >24 to 25 weeks of gestation, the best survival rate for the infant occurs when the infant is delivered no more than 5 minutes after the mother's heart stops beating.[175–178] Typically this requires that the provider begin the hysterotomy about 4 minutes after cardiac arrest. At gestational ages ≥30 weeks, infant survival has been seen even when delivery occurred after 5 minutes from onset of maternal cardiac arrest.[166] In a recent retrospective cohort series, neonatal survival was documented when delivery occurred within 30 minutes after onset of maternal cardiac arrest.[94]

When there is an obvious gravid uterus, the emergency cesarean section team should be activated at the onset of maternal cardiac arrest (Class I, LOE B). Emergency cesarean section may be considered at 4 minutes after onset of maternal cardiac arrest if there is no return of spontaneous circulation (Class IIb, LOE C).

## Institutional Preparation for Maternal Cardiac Arrest

Experts and organizations have emphasized the importance of preparation.[143,179] Providers at medical centers must review whether performance of an emergency hysterotomy is feasible, and if so, they must identify the best means of accomplishing this procedure rapidly. Team planning should be done in collaboration with the obstetric, neonatal, emergency, anesthesiology, intensive care, and cardiac arrest services (Class I, LOE C).

## Post–Cardiac Arrest Care

One case report showed that post–cardiac arrest hypothermia can be used safely and effectively in early pregnancy without emergency cesarean section (with fetal heart monitoring), with favorable maternal and fetal outcome after a term delivery.[159] No cases in the literature have reported the use of therapeutic hypothermia with perimortem cesarean section. Therapeutic hypothermia may be considered on an individual basis after cardiac arrest in a comatose pregnant patient based on current recommendations for the nonpregnant patient (Class IIb, LOE C). During therapeutic hypothermia of the pregnant patient, it is recommended that the fetus be continuously monitored for bradycardia as a potential complication, and obstetric and neonatal consultation should be sought (Class I, LOE C).

## Part 12.4: Cardiac Arrest in the Morbidly Obese

Morbid obesity can provide challenges during the resuscitation attempt. Airway management may be more challenging, and changes to the thorax may make resuscitative efforts more demanding. Evidence from 2 case studies,[180,181] 1 case series,[182] and 1 related clinical study[183] indicated no differences in survival based on patient weight. However, one large case series demonstrated lower survival for morbidly obese children who required in-hospital pediatric CPR.[184]

### BLS and ACLS Modifications

No modifications to standard BLS or ACLS care have been proven efficacious, although techniques may need to be adjusted due to the physical attributes of individual patients.

## Part 12.5: Cardiac Arrest Associated With Pulmonary Embolism

Pulmonary embolism (PE) can result in cardiovascular collapse and cardiac arrest. Although cardiac arrest caused by PE often presents as pulseless electric activity (PEA), not all cases of PEA are caused by PE.

### ACLS Modifications

In patients with cardiac arrest and without known PE, routine fibrinolytic treatment given during CPR shows no benefit[185,186] and is not recommended (Class III, LOE A).

In patients with cardiac arrest and presumed PE, however, the use of fibrinolytics during CPR may improve the patient's chance of survival.[187–194] Despite the potential to increase the risk of severe bleeding, fibrinolytics may improve survival to discharge and long-term neurological function in patients with presumed PE-induced cardiac arrest.[193–196] Emergency echocardiography may be helpful in determining the presence of thrombus or PE.

In a small number of patients, percutaneous mechanical thromboembolectomy during CPR has been performed successfully.[189] Surgical embolectomy has also been used successfully in some patients with PE-induced cardiac arrest.[191,197,198]

In patients with cardiac arrest due to presumed or known PE, it is reasonable to administer fibrinolytics (Class IIa, LOE B). Survival has been described with percutaneous mechanical thrombectomy or surgical embolectomy with or without prior treatment with fibrinolysis.

## Part 12.6: Cardiac Arrest Associated With Life-Threatening Electrolyte Disturbances

Electrolyte abnormalities can be associated with cardiovascular emergencies and may cause or contribute to cardiac arrest, hinder resuscitative efforts, and affect hemodynamic recovery after cardiac arrest. An evidence-based review in 2010 focused on electrolyte abnormalities most often associated with cardiac arrest.

Early consideration may be given to using selective methods of therapeutic management in addition to standard ACLS protocols that can be provided rapidly and have been shown to be effective in patients with cardiovascular instability as outlined below. Current BLS and ACLS should be used to manage cardiac arrest associated with all electrolyte disturbances.

### Potassium (K+)

Potassium is maintained mainly in the intracellular compartment through the action of the Na+/K+ ATPase pump. The magnitude of the potassium gradient across cell membranes determines excitability of nerve and muscle cells, including the myocardium.

Potassium is tightly regulated. Under normal conditions potential differences across membranes, especially cardiac, are not affected by alterations in potassium level. Rapid or significant changes in serum concentrations of potassium result from the shifting of potassium from one space to another and may have life-threatening consequences.

### Hyperkalemia

Hyperkalemia is one of the few potentially lethal electrolyte disturbances. Severe hyperkalemia (defined as a serum potassium concentration >6.5 mmol/L) occurs most commonly from renal failure or from release of potassium from cells and can cause cardiac arrhythmias and cardiac arrest. In 1 retrospective in-hospital study of 29 063 patients, hyperkalemia was found to be directly responsible for sudden cardiac arrest in 7 cases.[199] Acute kidney injury was present in all the arrest cases, accompanied by acute pancreatitis in 3 cases and acute hepatic failure in 2 cases. Overall renal failure and drug treatment were the most common causes of hyperkalemia, with the most severe cases occurring when excessive IV potassium was administered to a patient with renal insufficiency.

Although severe hyperkalemia may cause flaccid paralysis, paresthesia, depressed deep tendon reflexes, or respiratory difficulties,[200–202] the first indicator of hyperkalemia may be the presence of peaked T waves (tenting) on the electrocardiogram (ECG). As serum potassium rises, the ECG may progressively develop flattened or absent P waves, a prolonged PR interval, widened QRS complex, deepened S waves, and merging of S and T waves (Figure 5). If hyperkalemia is left untreated, a sine-wave pattern, idioventricular rhythms, and asystolic cardiac arrest may develop.[203,204]

#### ACLS Modifications in Management of Severe Cardiotoxicity or Cardiac Arrest Due to Hyperkalemia

Treatment of severe hyperkalemia aims at protecting the heart from the effects of hyperkalemia by antagonizing the effect of potassium on excitable cell membranes, forcing potassium into cells to remove it promptly from the circulation, and removing potassium from the body. Therapies that shift potassium will act rapidly but are temporary and thus may need to be repeated. In order of urgency, treatment includes the following:

- Stabilize myocardial cell membrane:
  - Calcium chloride (10%): 5 to 10 mL (500 to 1000 mg) IV over 2 to 5 minutes or calcium gluconate (10%): 15 to 30 mL IV over 2 to 5 minutes
- Shift potassium into cells:
  - Sodium bicarbonate: 50 mEq IV over 5 minutes

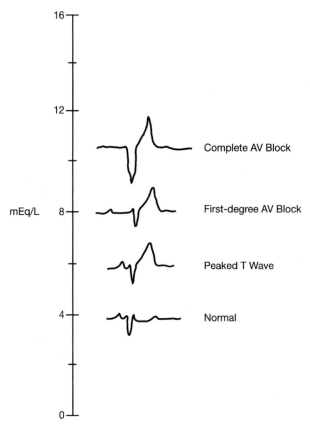

**Figure 5.** ECG changes in hyperkalemia.

· Glucose plus insulin: mix 25 g (50 mL of D50) glucose and 10 U regular insulin and give IV over 15 to 30 minutes
· Nebulized albuterol: 10 to 20 mg nebulized over 15 minutes
· Promote potassium excretion:
  · Diuresis: furosemide 40 to 80 mg IV
  · Kayexalate: 15 to 50 g plus sorbitol per oral or per rectum
  · Dialysis

When cardiac arrest occurs secondary to hyperkalemia, it may be reasonable to administer adjuvant IV therapy as outlined above for cardiotoxicity in addition to standard ACLS (Class IIb, LOE C).

### ACLS Modifications in Management of Severe Cardiotoxicity Due to Hypokalemia

Life-threatening hypokalemia is uncommon but can occur in the setting of gastrointestinal and renal losses and is associated with hypomagnesemia. Severe hypokalemia will alter cardiac tissue excitability and conduction. Hypokalemia can produce ECG changes such as U waves, T-wave flattening, and arrhythmias (especially if the patient is taking digoxin), particularly ventricular arrhythmias,[205,206] which, if left untreated, deteriorate to PEA or asystole.

Several studies reported an association with hypokalemia and development of ventricular fibrillation,[207–210] whereas a single animal study reported that hypokalemia lowered the ventricular fibrillation threshold.[211] However, the management of hypokalemia in the setting of cardiotoxicity, specifically torsades de pointes, is largely based on historical case reports that report slow infusion of potassium over hours.[212] The effect of bolus administration of potassium for cardiac arrest suspected to be secondary to hypokalemia is unknown and ill advised (Class III, LOE C).

### Sodium (Na⁺)

Sodium is the major intravascular ion that influences serum osmolality. Sodium abnormalities are unlikely to lead to cardiac arrest, and there are no specific recommendations for either checking or treating sodium during cardiac arrest. Disturbances in sodium level are unlikely to be the primary cause of severe cardiovascular instability.

### Magnesium (Mg⁺⁺)

Magnesium is an essential electrolyte and an important cofactor for multiple enzymes, including ATPase. Magnesium is necessary for the movement of sodium, potassium, and calcium into and out of cells and plays an important role in stabilizing excitable membranes. The presence of a low plasma magnesium concentration has been associated with poor prognosis in cardiac arrest patients.[208,213–216]

### Hypermagnesemia

Hypermagnesemia is defined as a serum magnesium concentration >2.2 mEq/L (normal: 1.3 to 2.2 mEq/L). Neurological symptoms of hypermagnesemia include muscular weakness, paralysis, ataxia, drowsiness, and confusion. Hypermagnesemia can produce vasodilation and hypotension.[217] Extremely high serum magnesium levels may produce a depressed level of consciousness, bradycardia, cardiac arrhythmias, hypoventilation, and cardiorespiratory arrest.[208,215,216]

### ACLS Modifications in Management of Cardiac Arrest and Severe Cardiotoxicity Due to Hypermagnesemia

Administration of calcium (calcium chloride [10%] 5 to 10 mL or calcium gluconate [10%] 15 to 30 mL IV over 2 to 5 minutes) may be considered during cardiac arrest associated with hypermagnesemia (Class IIb, LOE C).

### Hypomagnesemia

Hypomagnesemia, defined as a serum magnesium concentration <1.3 mEq/L, is far more common than hypermagnesemia. Hypomagnesemia usually results from decreased absorption or increased loss of magnesium from either the kidneys or intestines (diarrhea). Alterations in thyroid hormone function, certain medications (eg, pentamidine, diuretics, alcohol), and malnourishment can also induce hypomagnesemia.

### ACLS Modifications in Management of Cardiac Arrest and Severe Cardiotoxicity Due to Hypomagnesemia

Hypomagnesemia can be associated with polymorphic ventricular tachycardia, including torsades de pointes, a pulseless form (polymorphic) of ventricular tachycardia. For cardiotoxicity and cardiac arrest, IV magnesium 1 to 2 g of MgSO₄ bolus IV push is recommended (Class I, LOE C).

### Calcium (Ca⁺⁺)

Calcium abnormality as an etiology of cardiac arrest is rare. There are no studies evaluating the treatment of hypercalcemia or hypocalcemia during arrest. However, empirical use of calcium (calcium chloride [10%] 5 to 10 mL OR calcium gluconate [10%] 15 to 30 mL IV over 2 to 5 minutes) may be considered when hyperkalemia or hypermagnesemia is suspected as the cause of cardiac arrest (Class IIb, LOE C).

# Part 12.7: Cardiac Arrest Associated With Toxic Ingestions

Poisoning has been likened to trauma on the cellular level, destroying the natural workings of a victim's physiology.[218] Severe poisoning alters the function of a cellular receptor, ion channel, organelle, or chemical pathway to the extent that critical organ systems can no longer support life.

As with any patient in cardiac arrest, management of the patient with a toxic exposure begins with support of airway, breathing, and circulation. Cardiac arrest due to toxicity is managed in accordance with the current standards of BLS and ACLS. With few exceptions, there are no unique antidotes or toxin-specific interventions that are recommended during resuscitation from cardiac arrest.

Once return of spontaneous circulation is achieved, urgent consultation with a medical toxicologist or certified regional poison center is recommended, as the postarrest management of the critically poisoned patient may benefit from a thorough understanding of the toxic agent. Consultation is also recommended early in the management of a patient with potentially life-threatening poisoning, when appropriate interventions might prevent deterioration to cardiac arrest. In the United States a certified poison center can be reached by calling 1-800-222-1222; in Canada, call 1-800-268-9017.

It is extremely difficult to conduct clinical trials of acute life-threatening poisoning. Challenges include the infrequency with which most specific conditions occur, the heterogeneity of presentation, and ethical challenges related to withholding established care from patients who are unable to provide informed consent because the patient has an altered mental status, the patient is suicidal, or there is a lack of time to explain treatment alternatives.[219]

The majority of questions addressing cardiac arrest due to drug toxicity remain unanswered. Epidemiological studies are required to document the incidence rate of cardiac arrests secondary to drug toxicity and the safety and efficacy baseline rates for current therapeutic strategies. This section presents recommendations for the care of the patient with a toxicological problem causing cardiac arrest or severe cardiovascular instability (respiratory depression, hypotension, life-threatening alterations of cardiac conduction, etc). Some recommendations are evidence-based, but most research in this area consists of case reports, small case series, animal studies, and pharmacokinetic studies in healthy volunteers. Virtually no toxicology research involves human cardiac arrest. Thus, many of these recommendations are based on expert consensus, and further research is needed to validate them.

## Initial Approach to the Critically Poisoned Patient

Management of the critically poisoned patient begins with airway protection, support of respiration and circulation, and rapid assessment. Patients may or may not be able to provide an accurate history of exposure to a toxic substance. Whenever possible, history gathering should include questioning of persons who accompany the patient, evaluation of containers, review of pharmacy records, and examination of the patient's prior medical record.[220] Many patients who ingest medications in a suicide attempt take more than 1 substance, and the number of substances ingested is greater in fatal than in nonfatal suicide attempts.[221] Comprehensive toxicology laboratory testing is virtually never available in a time frame that supports early resuscitation decisions.[222]

Poisoned patients may deteriorate rapidly. Care for all adult patients who are critically ill or under evaluation for possible toxin exposure or ingestion, particularly when the history is uncertain, should begin in a monitored treatment area where the development of central nervous system depression, hemodynamic instability, or seizures can be rapidly recognized and addressed.[223]

Gastrointestinal decontamination, once a mainstay in the management of ingested toxins, has a less significant role in poisoning treatment today. With rare exceptions, gastric lavage, whole bowel irrigation, and administration of syrup of ipecac are no longer recommended.[224–226] Administration of single-dose activated charcoal to adsorb ingested toxins is generally recommended for the ingestion of life-threatening poisons for which no adequate antidotal therapy is available and when the charcoal can be administered within 1 hour of poisoning.[228] Multiple-dose activated charcoal should be considered for patients who have ingested a life-threatening amount of specific toxins (eg, carbamazepine, dapsone, phenobarbital, quinine, or theophylline) for which a benefit of this strategy has been established.[229] Charcoal should not be administered for ingestions of caustic substances, metals, or hydrocarbons.[228]

Charcoal should only be administered to patients with an intact or protected airway. In patients who are at risk for aspiration, endotracheal intubation and head-of-bed elevation should be performed before charcoal administration.[229,230] Because the decision to perform gastrointestinal decontamination is complex, multifactorial, and associated with risk, expert advice can be helpful.

### Toxidromes

A "toxidrome" is a clinical syndrome—a constellation of signs, symptoms, and laboratory findings—suggestive of the effects of a specific toxin. By recognizing these presentations, the clinician can establish a working diagnosis that guides initial management. Some common toxidromes are presented in the Table. Practically every sign and symptom observed in poisoning can be produced by natural disease, and many clinical presentations associated with natural disease can be mimicked by some poison.[231] It is important to maintain a broad differential diagnosis, particularly when the history of toxic chemical exposure is unclear.

### Opioid Toxicity

There are no data to support the use of specific antidotes in the setting of cardiac arrest due to opioid overdose. Resuscitation from cardiac arrest should follow standard BLS and ACLS algorithms.

Naloxone is a potent antagonist of the binding of opioid medications to their receptors in the brain and spinal cord. Administration of naloxone can reverse central nervous system

**Table. Common Toxidromes\***

| Cardiac Signs | | |
| --- | --- | --- |
| Tachycardia and/or Hypertension | Bradycardia and/or Hypotension | Cardiac Conduction Delays (Wide QRS) |
| Amphetamines | Beta blockers | Cocaine |
| Anticholinergic drugs | Calcium channel blockers | Cyclic antidepressants |
| Antihistamines | Clonidine | Local anesthetics |
| Cocaine | Digoxin and related glycosides | Propoxyphene |
| Theophylline/caffeine | Organophosphates and carbamates | Antiarrhythmics (e.g., quinidine, flecainide) |
| Withdrawal states | | |

| CNS/Metabolic Signs | | |
| --- | --- | --- |
| Seizures | CNS and/or Respiratory Depression | Metabolic Acidosis |
| Cyclic antidepressants | Antidepressants (several classes) | Cyanide |
| Isoniazid | Benzodiazepines | Ethylene glycol |
| Selective and non-selective norepinephrine reuptake inhibitors (eg, bupropion) | Carbon monoxide | Metformin |
| Withdrawal states | Ethanol | Methanol |
| | Methanol | Salicylates |
| | Opioids | |
| | Oral hypoglycemics | |

\*Differential diagnosis lists are partial.

and respiratory depression caused by opioid overdose. Naloxone has no role in the management of cardiac arrest.

In the patient with known or suspected opioid overdose with respiratory depression who is not in cardiac arrest, ventilation should be assisted by a bag mask,[232–238] followed by administration of naloxone and placement of an advanced airway if there is no response to naloxone (Class I, LOE A).

Administration of naloxone can produce fulminate opioid withdrawal in opioid-dependent individuals, leading to agitation, hypertension, and violent behavior. For this reason, naloxone administration should begin with a low dose (0.04 to 0.4 mg), with repeat dosing or dose escalation to 2 mg if the initial response is inadequate.[239] Some patients may require much higher doses to reverse intoxication with atypical opioids, such as propoxyphene, or following massive overdose ingestions.[240,241] Naloxone can be given IV,[235,236,242,243] IM,[232,235,236] intranasally,[232,242] and into the trachea.[244]

The duration of action of naloxone is approximately 45 to 70 minutes, but respiratory depression caused by ingestion of a long-acting opioid (eg, methadone) may last longer. Thus, the clinical effects of naloxone may not last as long as those of the opioid, and repeat doses of naloxone may be needed.

Patients with life-threatening central nervous system or respiratory depression reversed by naloxone administration should be observed for resedation. Although a brief period of observation may be appropriate for patients with morphine or heroin overdose,[245] a longer period of observation may be required to safely discharge a patient with life-threatening overdose of a long-acting or sustained-release opioid.[239,246]

## Benzodiazepines

There are no data to support the use of specific antidotes in the setting of cardiac arrest due to benzodiazepine overdose. Resuscitation from cardiac arrest should follow standard BLS and ACLS algorithms.

Flumazenil is a potent antagonist of the binding of benzodiazepines to their central nervous system receptors. Administration of flumazenil can reverse central nervous system and respiratory depression caused by benzodiazepine overdose. Flumazenil has no role in the management of cardiac arrest.

The administration of flumazenil to patients with undifferentiated coma confers risk and is not recommended (Class III, LOE B). Flumazenil administration can precipitate seizures in benzodiazepine-dependent patients and has been associated with seizures, arrhythmia, and hypotension in patients with co-ingestion of certain medications, such as tricyclic antidepressants.[247,248] However, flumazenil may be used safely to reverse excessive sedation known to be due to the use of benzodiazepines in a patient without known contraindications (eg, procedural sedation).[249]

## β-Blockers

There are no data to support the use of specific antidotes in the setting of cardiac arrest due to β-blocker overdose. Resuscitation from cardiac arrest should follow standard BLS and ACLS algorithms.

β-Blocker medication overdose may cause such severe inhibition of β-adrenergic receptors that high-dose vasopressors cannot effectively restore blood pressure, cardiac output, or perfusion. Therapeutic options in the treatment of refractory hemodynamic instability due to β-blocker overdose include administration of glucagon, high-dose insulin, or IV calcium salts.

### Glucagon

Administration of glucagon may be helpful for severe cardiovascular instability associated with β-blocker toxicity that is refractory to standard measures, including vasopressors. The recommended dose of glucagon is a bolus of 3 to 10 mg, administered slowly over 3 to 5 minutes, followed by an infusion of 3 to 5 mg/h (0.05 to 0.15 mg/kg followed by an infusion of 0.05 to 0.10 mg/kg per hour) (Class IIb, LOE C).[250–262] The infusion rate is titrated to achieve an adequate hemodynamic response (appropriate mean arterial pressure and evidence of good perfusion). Because the amount of glucagon required to sustain this therapy may exceed 100 mg in a 24-hour period, plans should be made early to ensure that an adequate supply of glucagon is available. Glucagon commonly causes vomiting. In patients with central nervous system depression, the airway must be protected before glucagon administration. Animal studies have suggested that the concomitant use of dopamine alone or in combination with isoproterenol and milrinone may decrease the effectiveness of glucagon.[263–265]

### Insulin

Animal studies suggest that high-dose IV insulin, accompanied by IV dextrose supplementation and electrolyte monitoring, may improve hemodynamic stability and survival in β-blocker overdose by improving myocardial energy utilization.[266,267] A single human case report[268] showed improved hemodynamic stability and survival to discharge following administration of high-dose insulin in refractory shock due to a massive overdose of metoprolol. Administration of high-dose insulin in patients with shock refractory to other measures may be considered (Class IIb, LOE C).

Although the ideal human dose has not been determined, a commonly used protocol calls for IV administration of 1 U/kg regular insulin as a bolus, accompanied by 0.5 g/kg dextrose, followed by continuous infusions of 0.5 to 1 U/kg per hour of insulin and 0.5 g/kg per hour of dextrose.[269] The insulin infusion is titrated as needed to achieve adequate hemodynamic response, whereas the dextrose infusion is titrated to maintain serum glucose concentrations of 100 to 250 mg/dL (5.5 to 14 mmol/L). Very frequent serum glucose monitoring (up to every 15 minutes) may be needed during the initial phase of dextrose titration. Sustained infusions of concentrated dextrose solutions (<10%) require central venous access. Insulin causes potassium to shift into the cells. Moderate hypokalemia is common during high-dose insulin-euglycemia therapy, and animals treated with aggressive potassium repletion developed asystole.[266] To avoid overly aggressive potassium repletion, 1 human protocol targets potassium levels of 2.5 to 2.8 mEq/L.[269]

### Calcium

One human case report[270] and a large-animal study[271] suggest that calcium may be helpful in β-blocker overdose. Administration of calcium in patients with shock refractory to other measures may be considered (Class IIb, LOE C).

One approach is to administer 0.3 mEq/kg of calcium (0.6 mL/kg of 10% calcium gluconate solution or 0.2 mL/kg of 10% calcium chloride solution) IV over 5 to 10 minutes, followed by an infusion of 0.3 mEq/kg per hour.[269] The infusion rate is titrated to adequate hemodynamic response. Serum ionized calcium levels should be monitored, and severe hypercalcemia (ionized calcium levels greater than twice the upper limits of normal) should be avoided. Sustained infusions of IV calcium require central venous access.

### Other Therapies

Case reports have suggested that in patients who remain critically hypotensive despite maximal vasopressor therapy, specific interventions using intra-aortic balloon counterpulsation, ventricular assist devices, and extracorporeal membrane oxygenation or other extra corporeal life support (ECLS) devices may be lifesaving.[272–274] While evidence remains weak, at least two human case reports indicate a possible benefit from lipid emulsion infusion for overdose by β-blockers.[275,276] Animal studies are mixed.[277–280] Because this area of therapy is rapidly evolving,[281–283] prompt consultation with a medical toxicologist or other specialists with up-to-date knowledge is recommended when managing treatment-refractory hypotension from β-blocker overdosage.

## Calcium Channel Blockers

There are no data to support the use of specific antidotes in the setting of cardiac arrest due to calcium channel blocker overdose. Resuscitation from cardiac arrest should follow standard BLS and ACLS algorithms.

Calcium channel blocker overdose also may cause life-threatening hypotension and bradycardia that are refractory to

standard agents. Treatment with high-dose insulin has been described in a number of clinical case reports[284–295] and animal studies.[296–299] High-dose insulin, in the doses listed in the β-blocker section above, may be effective for restoring hemodynamic stability and improving survival in the setting of severe cardiovascular toxicity associated with toxicity from a calcium channel blocker overdose (Class IIb, LOE B).

Limited evidence supports the use of calcium in the treatment of hemodynamically unstable calcium channel blocker overdose refractory to other treatments.[285,286,289,290,292–294,297,300–303] Administration of calcium in patients with shock refractory to other measures may be considered (Class IIb, LOE C).

There is insufficient and conflicting evidence to recommend the use of glucagon[289,290,294,296,297,300,303–306] in the treatment of hemodynamically unstable calcium channel blocker overdose.

## Digoxin and Related Cardiac Glycosides

Digoxin poisoning can cause severe bradycardia and life-threatening arrhythmias, including ventricular tachycardia, ventricular fibrillation, and high degrees of AV nodal blockade. Other plant- and animal-derived cardiac glycosides may produce similar effects, including those found in oleander, lily-of-the-valley, toad skin, and some herbal medications. There are no data to support the use of specific antidotes in the setting of cardiac arrest due to digoxin overdose. Resuscitation from cardiac arrest should follow standard BLS and ACLS algorithms, with specific antidotes used in the post-cardiac arrest phase if severe cardiotoxicity is encountered.

Antidigoxin Fab antibodies should be administered to patients with severe life-threatening cardiac glycoside toxicity (Class I, LOE B).[307–316] One vial of antidigoxin Fab is standardized to neutralize 0.5 mg of digoxin. Although the ideal dose is unknown, a reasonable strategy is as follows:

- If the ingested dose of digoxin is known, administer 2 vials of Fab for every milligram of digoxin ingested.
- In cases of chronic digoxin toxicity or when the ingested dose is not known, calculate the number of vials to administer by using the following formula: serum digoxin concentration (ng/mL)×weight (kg)/100.
- In critical cases in which therapy is required before a serum digoxin level can be obtained or in cases of life-threatening toxicity due to cardiac glycosides, administer empirically 10 to 20 vials.

Hyperkalemia is a marker of severity in acute cardiac glycoside poisoning and is associated with poor prognosis.[317] Antidigoxin Fab may be administered empirically to patients with acute poisoning from digoxin or related cardiac glycosides whose serum potassium level exceeds 5.0 mEq/L.[318]

## Cocaine

There are no data to support the use of cocaine-specific interventions in the setting of cardiac arrest due to cocaine overdose. Resuscitation from cardiac arrest should follow standard BLS and ACLS algorithms, with specific antidotes used in the postresuscitation phase if severe cardiotoxicity or neurotoxicity is encountered. A single case series demonstrated excellent overall and neurologically intact survival (55%) in patients with cardiac arrest associated with cocaine overdose who were treated with standard therapy.[319]

Cocaine-induced tachycardia and hypertension are predominantly caused by central nervous system stimulation. Treatment strategies are extrapolated from acute coronary syndrome studies, small case series, and experiments in cocaine-naïve human volunteers. It may be reasonable to try agents that have shown efficacy in the management of acute coronary syndrome in patients with severe cardiovascular toxicity. α-Blockers (phentolamine),[320] benzodiazepines (lorazepam, diazepam),[321] calcium channel blockers (verapamil),[322] morphine,[323] and sublingual nitroglycerin[324,325] may be used as needed to control hypertension, tachycardia, and agitation (Class IIb, LOE B). The available data do not support the use of 1 agent over another in the treatment of cardiovascular toxicity due to cocaine (Class IIb, LOE B).

There is clear evidence that cocaine can precipitate acute coronary syndromes.[326] For cocaine-induced hypertension or chest discomfort, benzodiazepines, nitroglycerin, and/or morphine can be beneficial (Class IIa, LOE B).[321,324,327] Because the effects of cocaine and other stimulant medications are transient, drugs and doses should be chosen carefully to minimize the risk of producing hypotension after the offending agent has been metabolized. Catheterization laboratory studies demonstrate that cocaine administration leads to reduced coronary artery diameter. This effect is reversed by morphine,[323] nitroglycerin,[325] phentolamine,[320] and verapamil[322]; is not changed by labetalol[328]; and is exacerbated by propranolol.[329] Several studies suggest that administration of β-blockers may worsen cardiac perfusion and/or produce paradoxical hypertension when cocaine is present.[329,330] Although contradictory evidence exists,[331,332] current recommendations are that pure β-blocker medications in the setting of cocaine are not indicated (Class IIb, LOE C).[333]

In severe overdose, cocaine acts as a Vaughan-Williams class Ic antiarrhythmic, producing wide-complex tachycardia through several mechanisms, including blockade of cardiac sodium channels.[107] Although there is no human evidence in cocaine poisoning, extrapolation from evidence in the treatment of wide-complex tachycardia caused by other class Ic agents (flecainide) and tricyclic antidepressants suggests that administration of hypertonic sodium bicarbonate may be beneficial.[334] A typical treatment strategy used for these other sodium channel blockers involves administration of 1 mL/kg of sodium bicarbonate solution (8.4%, 1 mEq/mL) IV as a bolus, repeated as needed until hemodynamic stability is restored and QRS duration is ≤120 ms.[335–342] Current evidence neither supports nor refutes a role for lidocaine in the management of wide-complex tachycardia caused by cocaine.

## Cyclic Antidepressants

Many drugs can prolong the QRS interval in overdose. These include Vaughan-Williams class Ia and Ic antiarrhythmics (eg, procainamide, quinidine, flecainide), cyclic antidepressants (eg, amitriptyline), and cocaine. Type Ia and Ic antiarrhythmics were not reviewed in 2010. Similar to the type Ia antiarrhythmics, cyclic antidepressants block cardiac sodium channels, leading to hypotension and wide-complex arrhythmia in overdose.

Cardiac arrest caused by cyclic antidepressant toxicity should be managed by current BLS and ACLS treatment guidelines. A small case series of cardiac arrest patients demonstrated improvement with sodium bicarbonate and epinephrine,[343] but the concomitant use of physostigmine in the prearrest period in this study reduces the ability to generalize this study. Administration of sodium bicarbonate for cardiac arrest due to cyclic antidepressant overdose may be considered (Class IIb, LOE C).

Therapeutic strategies for treatment of severe cyclic antidepressant cardiotoxicity include increasing serum sodium, increasing serum pH, or doing both simultaneously. The relative contributions of hypernatremia and alkalemia are controversial, but in practice most experience involves administration of hypertonic sodium bicarbonate solution (8.4% solution, 1 mEq/mL). Sodium bicarbonate boluses of 1 mL/kg may be administered as needed to achieve hemodynamic stability (adequate mean arterial blood pressure and perfusion) and QRS narrowing (Class IIb, LOE C).[335–342] Serum sodium levels and pH should be monitored, and severe hypernatremia (sodium >155 mEq/L) and alkalemia (pH >7.55) should be avoided. A number of vasopressors and inotropes have been associated with improvement in the treatment of tricyclic-induced hypotension, ie, epinephrine,[239,344,345] norepinephrine,[345–348] dopamine,[348–350] and dobutamine.[349]

## Local Anesthetic Toxicity

Inadvertent intravascular administration of local anesthetics, such as bupivacaine, mepivacaine, or lidocaine, can produce refractory seizures and rapid cardiovascular collapse leading to cardiac arrest. Clinical case reports[351–355] and controlled animal studies[356–360] have suggested that rapid IV infusion of lipids may reverse this toxicity either by redistributing the local anesthetic away from its site of action or by augmenting metabolic pathways within the cardiac myocyte.

Case reports have shown return of spontaneous circulation in patients with prolonged cardiac arrest unresponsive to standard ACLS measures,[361,362] suggesting a role for administration of IV lipids during cardiac arrest. Although ideal dosing has not been determined, because dosage varied across all studies, it may be reasonable to consider 1.5 mL/kg of 20% long-chain fatty acid emulsion as an initial bolus, repeated every 5 minutes until cardiovascular stability is restored (Class IIb, LOE C).[363] After the patient is stabilized, some papers suggest a maintenance infusion of 0.25 mL/kg per minute for at least 30 to 60 minutes. A maximum cumulative dose of 12 mL/kg has been proposed.[363]

Some animal data suggest that lipid infusion alone may be more effective than standard doses of epinephrine or vasopressin.[357,360] Although there is limited evidence to change routine care for severe cardiotoxicity, several professional societies advocate protocolized clinical use.[364–366] Because this is a rapidly evolving clinical area,[367,368] prompt consultation with a medical toxicologist, anesthesiologist, or other specialist with up-to-date knowledge is strongly recommended.

## Carbon Monoxide

Apart from complications from deliberate drug abuse, carbon monoxide is the leading cause of unintentional poisoning death in the United States.[369] In addition to reducing the ability of hemoglobin to deliver oxygen, carbon monoxide causes direct cellular damage to the brain and myocardium.[370] Survivors of carbon monoxide poisoning are at risk for lasting neurological injury.[370]

Several studies have suggested that very few patients who develop cardiac arrest from carbon monoxide poisoning survive to hospital discharge, regardless of treatment administered following return of spontaneous circulation.[371–373] Routine care of patients in cardiac arrest and severe cardiotoxicity from carbon monoxide poisoning should comply with standard BLS and ACLS recommendations.

### *Hyperbaric Oxygen*

Two studies suggest that neurological outcomes were improved in patients with carbon monoxide toxicity of all severity (excluding "moribund" patients)[374] and mild to moderate severity (excluding loss of consciousness and cardiac instability)[375] who received hyperbaric oxygen therapy for carbon monoxide poisoning. Other studies found no difference in neurologically intact survival.[376,377] A systematic review[378,379] and a recent evidence-based clinical policy review[380] concluded that, based on the available evidence, improvement in neurologically intact survival following treatment for carbon monoxide poisoning with hyperbaric oxygen is possible but unproven.

Hyperbaric oxygen therapy is associated with a low incidence of severe side effects. Because hyperbaric oxygen therapy appears to confer little risk,[380] the available data suggest that hyperbaric oxygen therapy may be helpful in treatment of acute carbon monoxide poisoning in patients with severe toxicity (Class IIb, LOE C).

Patients with carbon monoxide poisoning who develop a cardiac injury have an increased risk of cardiovascular and all-cause mortality for at least 7 years after the event, even if hyperbaric oxygen is administered.[381,382] Although data about effective interventions in this population are lacking, it is reasonable to advise enhanced follow-up for these patients.

On the basis of this conflicting evidence, the routine transfer of patients to a hyperbaric treatment facility following resuscitation from severe cardiovascular toxicity should be carefully considered, weighing the risk of transport against the possible improvement in neurologically intact survival.

## Cyanide

Cyanide is a surprisingly common chemical. In addition to industrial sources, cyanide can be found in jewelry cleaners, electroplating solutions, and as a metabolic product of the putative antitumor drug amygdalin (laetrile). Cyanide is a major component of fire smoke, and cyanide poisoning must be considered in victims of smoke inhalation who have hypotension, central nervous system depression, metabolic acidosis, or soot in the nares or respiratory secretions.[383] Cyanide poisoning causes rapid cardiovascular collapse, which manifests as hypotension, lactic acidosis, central apnea, and seizures.

Patients in cardiac arrest[383–385] or those presenting with cardiovascular instability[383–389] caused by known or suspected cyanide poisoning should receive cyanide-antidote therapy with a cyanide scavenger (either IV hydroxocobalamin or a nitrate such as IV sodium nitrite and/or inhaled amyl nitrite), followed as soon as possible by IV sodium thiosulfate.[387,390,391]

Both hydroxocobalamin[383–389] and sodium nitrite[387,390,391] serve to rapidly and effectively bind cyanide in the serum and reverse the effects of cyanide toxicity. Because nitrites induce methemoglobin formation[390] and can cause hypotension,[392] hydroxocobalamin has a safety advantage, particularly in children and victims of smoke inhalation who might also have carbon monoxide poisoning. A detailed comparison of these measures has been recently published.[393]

Sodium thiosulfate serves as a metabolic cofactor, enhancing the detoxification of cyanide to thiocyanate. Thiosulfate administration enhances the effectiveness of cyanide scavengers in animal experimentation[394–397] and has been used successfully in humans with both hydroxocobalamin[383,389] and sodium nitrite.[387,390,391] Sodium thiosulfate is associated with vomiting but has no other significant toxicity.[398] Therefore, based on the best evidence available, a treatment regimen of 100% oxygen and hydroxocobalamin, with or without sodium thiosulfate, is recommended (Class I, LOE B).

## Part 12.8: Cardiac Arrest Associated With Trauma

BLS and ACLS for the trauma patient are fundamentally the same as that for the patient with primary cardiac arrest, with focus on support of airway, breathing, and circulation. In addition, reversible causes of cardiac arrest need to considered. While CPR in the pulseless trauma patient has overall been considered futile, several reversible causes of cardiac arrest in the context of trauma are correctible and their prompt treatment could be life-saving. These include hypoxia, hypovolemia, diminished cardiac output secondary to pneumothorax or pericardial tamponade, and hypothermia.

### BLS Modifications

When multisystem trauma is present or trauma involves the head and neck, the cervical spine must be stabilized. A jaw thrust should be used instead of a head tilt–chin lift to establish a patent airway. If breathing is inadequate and the patient's face is bloody, ventilation should be provided with a barrier device, a pocket mask, or a bag-mask device while maintaining cervical spine stabilization. Stop any visible hemorrhage using direct compression and appropriate dressings. If the patient is completely unresponsive despite rescue breathing, provide standard CPR and defibrillation as indicated.

### ACLS Modifications

After initiation of BLS care, if bag-mask ventilation is inadequate, an advanced airway should be inserted while maintaining cervical spine stabilization. If insertion of an advanced airway is not possible and ventilation remains inadequate, experienced providers should consider a cricothyrotomy.

A unilateral decrease in breath sounds during positive-pressure ventilation should prompt the rescuer to consider the possibility of pneumothorax, hemothorax, or rupture of the diaphragm.

When the airway, oxygenation, and ventilation are adequate, evaluate and support circulation. Control ongoing bleeding where possible and replace lost volume if the losses appear to have significantly compromised circulating blood volume. Cardiac arrest resuscitation will likely be ineffective in the presence of uncorrected severe hypovolemia.

Treatment of PEA requires identification and treatment of reversible causes, such as severe hypovolemia, hypothermia, cardiac tamponade, or tension pneumothorax.[399] Development of bradyasystolic rhythms often indicates the presence of severe hypovolemia, severe hypoxemia, or cardiorespiratory failure. Ventricular fibrillation (VF) and pulseless ventricular tachycardia (VT) are treated with CPR and defibrillation. For treatment recommendations regarding cardiac tamponade in traumatic cardiac arrest, see Part 12.14: "Cardiac Arrest Caused by Cardiac Tamponade."

Resuscitative thoracotomy may be indicated in selected patients. A review of the literature from 1966 to 1999, carried out by the American College of Surgeons Committee on Trauma, found a survival rate of 7.8% (11.2% for penetrating injuries and 1.6% for blunt lesions) in trauma victims who would otherwise have 100% mortality.[400] Practitioners should consult the guidelines for withholding or terminating resuscitation, which were developed for victims of traumatic cardiac arrest by a joint committee of the National Association of EMS Physicians and the American College of Surgeons Committee on Trauma.[401,402]

## Commotio Cordis

Commotio cordis is VF triggered by a blow to the anterior chest during a cardiac repolarization.[403,404] Blunt cardiac injury may result in cardiac contusion with injured myocardium and risk of ECG changes and arrhythmias. Even a small blow to the anterior chest during a cardiac repolarization, such as that imparted by the strike of a baseball or hockey puck, may trigger VF, so-called commotio cordis.[405] Events causing commotio cordis are most commonly seen in young persons up to 18 years of age who are engaged in sports but may occur during daily activities. Prompt recognition that a precordial blow may cause VF is critical. Rapid defibrillation is often life-saving for these frequently young victims of cardiac arrest. Provision of immediate BLS care using an automated external defibrillator (AED) and ACLS for VF in this setting is appropriate.

# Part 12.9: Cardiac Arrest in Accidental Hypothermia

Unintentional or accidental hypothermia is a serious and preventable health problem. Severe hypothermia (body temperature <30°C [86°F]) is associated with marked depression of critical body functions, which may make the victim appear clinically dead during the initial assessment. Therefore, life-saving procedures should be initiated unless the victim is obviously dead (eg, rigor mortis, decomposition, hemisection, decapitation). The victim should be transported as soon as possible to a center where aggressive rewarming during resuscitation is possible.

## Initial Care for Victims of Accidental Hypothermia

When the victim is extremely cold but has maintained a perfusing rhythm, the rescuer should focus on interventions that prevent further loss of heat and begin to rewarm the victim immediately. Additional interventions include the following:

- Preventing additional evaporative heat loss by removing wet garments and insulating the victim from further environmental exposures. Passive rewarming is generally adequate for patients with mild hypothermia (temperature >34°C [93.2°F]).
- For patients with moderate (30°C to 34°C [86°F to 93.2°F]) hypothermia with a perfusing rhythm, external warming techniques are appropriate.[406] Passive rewarming alone will be inadequate for these patients.[407]
- For patients with severe hypothermia (<30°C [86°F]) with a perfusing rhythm, core rewarming is often used, although some have reported successful rewarming with active external warming techniques.[408,409] Active external warming techniques include forced air or other efficient surface-warming devices.
- Patients with severe hypothermia and cardiac arrest can be rewarmed most rapidly with cardiopulmonary bypass.[406,410–415] Alternative effective core rewarming techniques include warm-water lavage of the thoracic cavity[413,416–420] and extracorporeal blood warming with partial bypass.[421–423]
- Adjunctive core rewarming techniques include warmed IV or intraosseous (IO) fluids and warm humidified oxygen.[424] Heat transfer with these measures is not rapid, and should be considered supplementary to active warming techniques.
- Do not delay urgent procedures such as airway management and insertion of vascular catheters. Although these patients may exhibit cardiac irritability, this concern should not delay necessary interventions.

Beyond these critical initial steps, the treatment of severe hypothermia (temperature <30°C [86°F]) in the field remains controversial. Many providers do not have the time or equipment to assess core body temperature or to institute aggressive rewarming techniques, although these methods should be initiated when available.

### BLS Modifications

When the victim is hypothermic, pulse and respiratory rates may be slow or difficult to detect,[425,426] and the ECG may even show asystole. If the hypothermic victim has no signs of life, begin CPR without delay. If the victim is not breathing, start rescue breathing immediately.

The temperature at which defibrillation should first be attempted in the severely hypothermic patient and the number of defibrillation attempts that should be made have not been established. There are case reports of refractory ventricular arrhythmias with severe hypothermia; however, in a recent animal model it was found that an animal with a temperature of as low as 30°C had a better response to defibrillation than did normothermic animals in arrest.[427,428]

If VT or VF is present, defibrillation should be attempted. If VT or VF persists after a single shock, the value of deferring subsequent defibrillations until a target temperature is achieved is uncertain. It may be reasonable to perform further defibrillation attempts according to the standard BLS algorithm concurrent with rewarming strategies (Class IIb, LOE C).

To prevent further loss of core heat, remove wet garments and protect the victim from additional environmental exposure. Insofar as possible, this should be done while providing initial BLS therapies. Rewarming should be attempted when feasible.

### ACLS Modifications

For unresponsive patients or those in arrest, advanced airway insertion is appropriate as recommended in the standard ACLS guidelines. Advanced airway management enables effective ventilation with warm, humidified oxygen and reduces the likelihood of aspiration in patients in periarrest.

ACLS management of cardiac arrest due to hypothermia focuses on aggressive active core rewarming techniques as the primary therapeutic modality. Conventional wisdom indicates that the hypothermic heart may be unresponsive to cardiovascular drugs, pacemaker stimulation, and defibrillation; however, the data to support this are essentially theoretical.[429] In addition, drug metabolism may be reduced, and there is a theoretical concern that medications could accumulate to toxic levels in the peripheral circulation if given repeatedly to the severely hypothermic victim. For these reasons, previous guidelines suggest withholding IV drugs if the victim's core body temperature is <30°C (86°F).

In the last decade a number of animal investigations have been performed evaluating both vasopressors and antiarrhythmic medications that could challenge some of this conventional wisdom.[430–435] In a meta-analysis of these studies, Wira et al[436] found that vasopressor medications (ie, epinephrine or vasopressin) increased rates of return of spontaneous circulation (ROSC) when compared with placebo (62% versus 17%; $P<0.0001$, n=77). Coronary perfusion pressures were increased in groups that received vasopressors compared with placebo. But groups given antiarrhythmics showed no improvement in ROSC when compared with control groups, although sample sizes were relatively small (n=34 and n=40, respectively).

One small-animal investigation suggested that the application of standard normothermic ACLS algorithms using both drugs (ie, epinephrine and amiodarone) and defibrillation improved ROSC compared with a placebo arm of defibrillation only (91% versus 30%; $P<0.01$; n=21). Human trials of medication use in accidental hypothermia do not exist, although case reports of survival with use of intra-arrest medication have been reported.[414,418,437]

Given the lack of human evidence and relatively small number of animal investigations, the recommendation for administration or withholding of medications is not clear. It may be reasonable to consider administration of a vasopressor during cardiac arrest according to the standard ACLS algorithm concurrent with rewarming strategies (Class IIb, LOE C).

### After ROSC

After ROSC, patients should continue to be warmed to a goal temperature of approximately 32° to 34°C; this can be maintained according to standard postarrest guidelines for mild to moderate hypothermia in patients for whom induced hypothermia is appropriate. For those with contraindications to induced hypothermia, rewarming can continue to normal temperatures.

Because severe hypothermia is frequently preceded by other disorders (eg, drug overdose, alcohol use, or trauma), the clinician must look for and treat these underlying conditions while simultaneously treating hypothermia.

### Withholding and Cessation of Resuscitative Efforts

Multiple case reports indicate survival from accidental hypothermia even with prolonged CPR and downtimes.[410,422] Thus, patients with severe accidental hypothermia and cardiac arrest may benefit from resuscitation even in cases of prolonged downtime and prolonged CPR. Low serum potassium may indicate hypothermia, and not hypoxemia, as the primary cause of the arrest.[438] Patients should not be considered dead before warming has been provided.

## Part 12.10: Cardiac Arrest in Avalanche Victims

Avalanche-related deaths are on the rise in North America due to winter recreational activities, including backcountry skiing and snowboarding, helicopter and snowcat skiing, snowmobiling, out-of-bounds skiing, ice climbing, mountaineering, and snowshoeing. The most common causes of avalanche-related death are asphyxia, trauma, and hypothermia, or combinations of the 3. Rescue and resuscitation strategies focus on management of asphyxia and hypothermia, because most field research has been done on these 2 conditions.

Avalanches occur in areas that are difficult to access by rescuers in a timely manner, and burials frequently involve multiple victims. The decision to initiate full resuscitative measures should be determined by the number of victims, resources available, and likelihood of survival. Studies of avalanche victims demonstrate a progressive nonlinear reduction in survival as the time of avalanche burial lengthens.[439–442] The likelihood of survival is minimal when avalanche victims are buried >35 minutes with an obstructed airway and in cardiac arrest on extrication[440,441,443–449] or are buried for any length of time and in cardiac arrest on extrication with an obstructed airway and an initial core temperature of <32°C.[441–443,447,450]

It may be difficult to know with any certainty how long an avalanche victim has been buried. The core temperature at time of extrication provides a proxy for duration of burial. A case series[450] of buried avalanche victims showed a maximum cooling rate of 8°C per hour, whereas a case report[447] described a maximum cooling rate of 9°C per hour. These cooling rates suggest that at 35 minutes of burial, the core temperature may drop as low as 32°C.

If information on the duration of burial or the state of the airway on extrication is not available to the receiving physician, a serum potassium level of <8 mmol/L on hospital admission is a prognostic marker for ROSC[444] and survival to hospital discharge.[443,450] High potassium values are associated with asphyxia,[443,450–452] and there is an inverse correlation between admission K+ and survival to discharge in all-cause hypothermic patients.[443,453–456] In a series of 32 avalanche survivors the highest serum K+ was 6.4 mmol/L,[450] but there is a single case report of a 31- month-old child with a K+ of 11.8 mmol/L presenting with hypothermia from exposure unrelated to an avalanche who survived.[457] This suggests that the upper survivable limit of potassium is unknown for children who are hypothermic and victims of avalanche.

Full resuscitative measures, including extracorporeal rewarming when available, are recommended for all avalanche victims without the characteristics outlined above that deem them unlikely to survive or with any obvious lethal traumatic injury (Class I, LOE C).

## Part 12.11: Drowning

Each year drowning is responsible for more than 500 000 deaths worldwide.[458] Drowning is a leading preventable cause of unintentional morbidity and mortality.[459,460] All victims of drowning who require any form of resuscitation (including rescue breathing alone) should be transported to the hospital for evaluation and monitoring, even if they appear to be alert and demonstrate effective cardiorespiratory function at the scene (Class I, LOE C).

A number of terms are used to describe drowning.[461] To aid in use of consistent terminology and uniform reporting of data, use of the Utstein definitions and style of data reporting specific to drowning is recommended.[462,463]

Although survival is uncommon in victims who have undergone prolonged submersion and require prolonged resuscitation,[464,465] successful resuscitation with full neurological recovery has occurred occasionally after prolonged submersion in icy water[466–469] and, in some instances, warm water.[470,471] For this reason, scene resuscitation should be initiated and the victim transported to the ED unless there is obvious death (eg, rigor mortis, decomposition, hemisection, decapitation, lividity).

### BLS Modifications

The most important and detrimental consequence of submersion is hypoxia; therefore, oxygenation, ventilation, and perfusion should be restored as rapidly as possible. This will require immediate bystander CPR plus activation of the EMS system. With the *2010 AHA Guidelines for CPR and ECC*, CPR now begins with chest compressions in a C-A-B sequence. However, the guidelines recommend individualization in sequence based upon the presumed etiology of the arrest. CPR for drowning victims should use the traditional A-B-C approach in view of the hypoxic nature of the arrest. Victims with only respiratory arrest usually respond after a few artificial breaths are given.

### Recovery From the Water

When attempting to rescue a drowning victim, the rescuer should get to the victim as quickly as possible. It is crucial, however, that the rescuer pays constant attention to his or her own personal safety during the rescue process.

The reported incidence of cervical spine injury in drowning victims is low (0.009%).[472,473] Unnecessary cervical spine immobilization can impede adequate opening of the airway and delay delivery of rescue breaths. Routine stabilization of the cervical spine in the absence of circumstances that suggest a spinal injury is not recommended (Class III, LOE B).[473,474]

### Rescue Breathing

The first and most important treatment of the drowning victim is the immediate provision of ventilation. Prompt initiation of rescue breathing increases the victim's chance of survival.[475] Rescue breathing is usually performed once the unresponsive victim is in shallow water or out of the water. Mouth-to-nose ventilation may be used as an alternative to mouth-to-mouth ventilation if it is difficult for the rescuer to pinch the victim's nose, support the head, and open the airway in the water.

Management of the drowning victim's airway and breathing is similar to that recommended for any victim of cardiopulmonary arrest. Some victims aspirate no water because they develop laryngospasm or breath-holding.[465,476] Even if water is aspirated, there is no need to clear the airway of aspirated water, because only a modest amount of water is aspirated by the majority of drowning victims, and aspirated water is rapidly absorbed into the central circulation.[465,477] Attempts to remove water from the breathing passages by any means other than suction (eg, abdominal thrusts or the Heimlich maneuver) are unnecessary and potentially dangerous.[477] The routine use of abdominal thrusts or the Heimlich maneuver for drowning victims is not recommended (Class III, LOE C).

### Chest Compressions

As soon as the unresponsive victim is removed from the water, the rescuer should open the airway, check for breathing, and if there is no breathing, give 2 rescue breaths that make the chest rise (if this was not done previously in the water). After delivery of 2 effective breaths, the lay rescuer should immediately begin chest compressions and provide cycles of compressions and ventilations according to the BLS guidelines. Once the victim is out of the water, if he or she is unresponsive and not breathing after delivery of 2 rescue breaths, rescuers should attach an AED and attempt defibrillation if a shockable rhythm is identified. It is only necessary to dry the chest area before applying the defibrillation pads and using the AED. If hypothermia is present, follow the recommendations in Part 12.9: "Cardiac Arrest in Accidental Hypothermia."

### Vomiting by the Victim During Resuscitation

The victim may vomit when the rescuer performs chest compressions or rescue breathing. In fact, in a 10-year study in Australia, two thirds of victims who received rescue breathing and 86% of those who required compressions and ventilations vomited.[478] If vomiting occurs, turn the victim to the side and remove the vomitus using your finger, a cloth, or suction. If spinal cord injury is suspected, the victim should be logrolled so that the head, neck, and torso are turned as a unit to protect the cervical spine.

## ACLS Modifications

Victims in cardiac arrest may present with asystole, PEA, or pulseless VT/VF. For treatment of these rhythms, follow the appropriate PALS or ACLS guidelines. Case reports of pediatric patients document the use of surfactant for fresh water–induced respiratory distress, but further research is needed.[479–482] The use of extracorporeal membrane oxygenation in patients with severe hypothermia after submersion has been documented in case reports.[468,469,483]

# Part 12.12: Cardiac Arrest Associated With Electric Shock and Lightning Strikes

Injuries from electric shock and lightning strike result from the direct effects of current on the heart and brain, cell membranes, and vascular smooth muscle. Additional injuries result from the conversion of electric energy into heat energy as current passes through body tissues.[484]

## Electric Shock

Fatal electrocutions may occur with household current; however, high-tension current generally causes the most serious injuries.[485] Contact with alternating current (the type of current commonly present in most North American households and commercial settings) may cause tetanic skeletal muscle contractions, "locking" the victim to the source of the electricity and thereby leading to prolonged exposure. The frequency of alternating current increases the likelihood of current flow through the heart during the relative refractory period, which is the "vulnerable period" of the cardiac cycle. This exposure can precipitate VF, which is analogous to the R-on-T phenomenon that occurs in nonsynchronized cardioversion.[486]

## Lightning Strike

The National Weather Service estimates that an average of 70 deaths and 630 injuries occur due to lightning strikes in the United States each year.[487] Lightning strike injuries can vary widely, even among groups of people struck at the same time. Symptoms are mild in some victims, whereas fatal injuries occur in others.[488,489]

The primary cause of death in victims of lightning strike is cardiac arrest, which may be associated with primary VF or asystole.[488–491] Lightning acts as an instantaneous, massive direct-current shock, simultaneously depolarizing the entire myocardium.[489,492] In many cases intrinsic cardiac automaticity may spontaneously restore organized cardiac activity and a perfusing rhythm. However, concomitant respiratory arrest due to thoracic muscle spasm and suppression of the respiratory center may continue after ROSC. Unless ventilation is supported, a secondary hypoxic (asphyxial) cardiac arrest will develop.[493]

Lightning also can have myriad effects on the cardiovascular system, producing extensive catecholamine release or autonomic stimulation. The victim may develop hypertension, tachycardia, nonspecific ECG changes (including prolongation of the QT interval and transient T-wave inversion), and myocardial necrosis with release of creatinine kinase-MB fraction.

Lightning can produce a wide spectrum of peripheral and central neurological injuries. The current can produce brain hemorrhages, edema, and small-vessel and neuronal injury. Hypoxic encephalopathy can result from cardiac arrest.

Victims are most likely to die of lightning injury if they experience immediate respiratory or cardiac arrest and no treatment is provided. Patients who do not suffer respiratory or cardiac arrest, and those who respond to immediate treatment, have an excellent chance of recovery. Therefore, when multiple victims are struck simultaneously by lightning, rescuers should give the highest priority to patients in respiratory or cardiac arrest.

For victims in cardiac arrest, treatment should be early, aggressive, and persistent. Victims with respiratory arrest may require only ventilation and oxygenation to avoid secondary hypoxic cardiac arrest. Resuscitation attempts may have high success rates and efforts may be effective even when the interval before the resuscitation attempt is prolonged.[493]

## BLS Modifications

The rescuer must first be certain that rescue efforts will not put him or her in danger of electric shock. When the scene is safe (ie, the danger of shock has been removed), determine the victim's cardiorespiratory status. If spontaneous respiration or circulation is absent, immediately initiate standard BLS resuscitation care, including the use of an AED to identify and treat VT or VF.

Maintain spinal stabilization during extrication and treatment if there is a likelihood of head or neck trauma.[494,495] Both lightning and electric shock often cause multiple trauma, including injury to the spine,[495] muscular strains, internal injuries from being thrown, and fractures caused by the tetanic response of skeletal muscles.[496] Remove smoldering clothing, shoes, and belts to prevent further thermal damage.

## ACLS Modifications

No modification of standard ACLS care is required for victims of electric injury or lightning strike, with the exception of paying attention to possible cervical spine injury. Establishing an airway may be difficult for patients with electric burns of the face, mouth, or anterior neck. Extensive soft-tissue swelling may develop rapidly, complicating airway control measures. Thus, early intubation should be performed for patients with evidence of extensive burns even if the patient has begun to breathe spontaneously.

For victims with significant tissue destruction and in whom a pulse is regained, rapid IV fluid administration is indicated to counteract distributive/hypovolemic shock and to correct ongoing fluid losses due to third spacing. Fluid administration should be adequate to maintain diuresis and facilitate excretion of myoglobin, potassium, and other byproducts of tissue destruction (this is particularly true for patients with electric injury).[492] Regardless of the extent of external injuries after electrothermal shock, the underlying tissue damage can be far more extensive.

## Part 12.13: Cardiac Arrest During Percutaneous Coronary Intervention

During both elective and emergent percutaneous coronary intervention (PCI), there is risk of cardiac arrest. Although high-quality chest compressions improve the chance of successful resuscitation and survival, it is difficult to perform effective, high-quality chest compressions during PCI. Therefore, resuscitation adjuncts have been explored for the treatment of cardiac arrest during PCI. There are no randomized controlled trials evaluating alternative treatment strategies as opposed to standard care for cardiac arrest during PCI.

### Mechanical CPR During PCI

Mechanical chest compression devices have been used successfully in an animal model[497] and adult humans[497–501] to provide maintenance of circulation in cardiac arrest while continuing a percutaneous coronary procedure. It is reasonable to use mechanical CPR during PCI (Class IIa, LOE C).

### Emergency Cardiopulmonary Bypass

One case series[502] describes the use of emergency cardiopulmonary bypass to stabilize and facilitate emergency coronary angioplasty in patients with cardiac arrest unresponsive to ACLS during PCI. It is reasonable to use emergency cardiopulmonary bypass during PCI (Class IIb, LOE C).

### Cough CPR

Multiple case reports[503–507] describe the use of cough CPR to temporarily maintain adequate blood pressure and level of consciousness in patients who develop ventricular arrhythmias during PCI while definitive therapy for malignant arrhythmias is instituted. It is reasonable to use cough CPR during PCI (Class IIa, LOE C).

### Intracoronary Verapamil

One large case series[508] describes the successful use of intracoronary verapamil to terminate reperfusion-induced VT following mechanical revascularization therapy. Verapamil was not successful in terminating VF.

## Part 12.14: Cardiac Arrest Caused by Cardiac Tamponade

Cardiac tamponade can be a life-threatening event. Increasing fluid and pressure in the pericardium reduces atrial and ventricular filling. As filling is reduced, stroke volume and cardiac output fall, with associated hypotension leading to cardiac arrest. Rapid diagnosis and drainage of the pericardial fluid are required to avoid cardiovascular collapse.

Pericardiocentesis guided by echocardiography is a safe and effective method of relieving tamponade in a nonarrest setting, especially when used in conjunction with a pericardial drain, and may obviate the need for subsequent operating room treatment.[509–513] In the arrest setting, in the absence of echocardiography, emergency pericardiocentesis without imaging guidance can be beneficial (Class IIa, LOE C).

Emergency department thoracotomy may improve survival compared with pericardiocentesis in patients with pericardial tamponade secondary to trauma who are in cardiac arrest or who are prearrest,[514–516] especially if gross blood causes clotting that blocks a pericardiocentesis needle (Class IIb, LOE C).[517]

## Part 12.15: Cardiac Arrest Following Cardiac Surgery

The incidence of cardiac arrest following cardiac surgery is in the range of 1–3%. Causes include conditions that may be readily reversed such as ventricular fibrillation, hypovolemia, cardiac tamponade, or tension pneumothorax. Pacing wires, if present, may reverse symptomatic bradycardia or asystole. A recent review may be helpful for those seeking additional information.[518]

### Resternotomy

Studies of patients with cardiac arrest after cardiac surgery who are treated with resternotomy and internal cardiac compression have reported improved outcome compared with a standard protocol[519–529] when patients are treated by experienced personnel in intensive care units. Findings of similar quality studies[530–534] reported no difference in outcomes when resternotomy was compared with standard management of cardiac arrest after cardiac surgery. Resternotomy performed outside an intensive care unit generally has a very poor outcome.[519,526,533]

For patients with cardiac arrest following cardiac surgery, it is reasonable to perform resternotomy in an appropriately staffed and equipped intensive care unit (Class IIa, LOE B). Despite rare case reports describing damage to the heart possibly due to external chest compressions,[535,536] chest compressions should not be withheld if emergency resternotomy is not immediately available (Class IIa, LOE C).

### Mechanical Circulatory Support

Nine case series have reported survival of some post–cardiac surgery patients during cardiac arrest refractory to standard resuscitation measures following the use of extracorporeal membrane oxygenation[537–541] and cardiopulmonary bypass.[529,542–544] In post–cardiac surgery patients who are refractory to standard resuscitation procedures, mechanical circulatory support (eg, extracorporeal membrane oxygenation and cardiopulmonary bypass) may be effective in improving outcome (Class IIb, LOE B).

### Pharmacological Intervention

Rebound hypertension following administration of pressors during resuscitation has the potential to induce significant bleeding in this group of patients. Results from a single study of epinephrine[545] and another study evaluating the choice of antiarrhythmics[546] in patients with cardiac arrest following cardiac surgery were neutral. There is insufficient evidence on epinephrine dose, antiarrhythmic use, and other routine pharmacological interventions to recommend deviating from standard resuscitation guidelines when cardiac arrest occurs after cardiac surgery.

# Disclosures

## Guidelines Part 12: Cardiac Arrest in Special Situations: Writing Group Disclosures

| Writing Group Member | Employment | Research Grant | Other Research Support | Speakers' Bureau/ Honoraria | Ownership Interest | Consultant/ Advisory Board | Other |
|---|---|---|---|---|---|---|---|
| Terry L. Vanden Hoek | The University of Chicago–Associate Professor | *Vanden Hoek, Principal Investigator, Department of Defense, Office of Naval Research, "Proteomic Development of Molecular Vital Signs: Mapping a Mitochondrial Injury Severity Score to Triage and Guide Resuscitation of Hemorrhagic Shock." Research grant awarded to the University of Chicago | None | None | None | None | None |
| Laurie J. Morrison | St. Michaels Clinician scientist | None | None | None | None | None | None |
| Michael Shuster | Self-employed–emergency physician | None | None | None | None | None | None |
| Michael Donnino | Harvard Medical Faculty Physicians–Physician | †Corticosteroids in Post-arrest Shock (American Heart Association, Scientist Development Grant); Thiamine as a Metabolic Resuscitator in Septic Shock (NIH pending); *Statins in Sepsis (Eleanor Shore) Clinical Correlates to Influenza Genome (NIH); Thiamine Deficiency in Critically Ill (Harvard Medical School/NIH); Thiamine for Congestive Heart Failure (Baystate Incubator Fund-NON-industry, academic hospital funding) | None | None | None | None | None |
| Elizabeth Sinz | Penn State Hershey Medical Center–Professor of Anesthesiology and Neurosurgery; AHA–Associate Science Editor | None | None | None | None | None | None |
| Eric J. Lavonas | Rocky Mountain Poison & Drug Center; (RMPDC) Denver, Colo. Associate Director | †RMPDC performed research related to hydroxocobalamin prior to its licensure in the United States. This occurred prior to my arrival at RMPDC. RMPDC-DH performed work related to the development of hydroxocobalamin (CyanoKit, Dey LP) as a cyanide antidote. Various projects were completed in 2001, 2005, and 2006. Some of the sponsors of this research (EMD; Merck KGA) either no longer exist or no longer have an interest in hydroxocobalamin. I was not involved in this research, which was performed long before my arrival. RMPDC-DH does not have any current or pending hydroxocobalamin-related projects. Neither I nor any other DHHA employee derives personal financial benefit from these relationships. I don't get a bonus of any sort. My salary is supported by general institutional funds and an unrelated research endowment. Also, my performance evaluation is not related the performance of any of these contracts. My role: PI on one portion of the project, collaborator on the rest 2008–2009 (ongoing) | None | None | None | None | None |
| Farida M. Jeejeebhoy | Self employed cardiologist, affiliate with University Health Network/Mt Sinai and University of Toronto | None | None | None | None | None | None |
| Andrea Gabrielli | University of Florida–Professor of Anesthesiology and Surgery | †NIH-Biomarkers in Traumatic Brain Injury | None | None | None | None | None |

This table represents the relationships of writing group members that may be perceived as actual or reasonably perceived conflicts of interest as reported on the Disclosure Questionnaire, which all members of the writing group are required to complete and submit. A relationship is considered to be "significant" if (a) the person receives $10 000 or more during any 12-month period, or 5% or more of the person's gross income; or (b) the person owns 5% or more of the voting stock or share of the entity, or owns $10 000 or more of the fair market value of the entity. A relationship is considered to be "modest" if it is less than "significant" under the preceding definition.

*Modest.

†Significant.

# References

1. Kenyon N, Albertson TE. Status asthmaticus: from the emergency department to the intensive care unit. *Clin Rev Allergy Immunol.* 2001; 20:271–292.

2. Division of Data Services. *New Asthma Estimates: Tracking Prevalence, Health Care, and Mortality.* Hyattsville, Md: National Center for Health Statistics; 2001.

3. McFadden ER Jr. Acute severe asthma. *Am J Respir Crit Care Med.* 2003;168:740–759.

4. McFadden ER Jr, Warren EL. Observations on asthma mortality. *Ann Intern Med.* 1997;127:142–147.

5. Jorge S, Becquemin MH, Delerme S, Bennaceur M, Isnard R, Achkar R, Riou B, Boddaert J, Ray P. Cardiac asthma in elderly patients: incidence, clinical presentation and outcome. *BMC Cardiovasc Disord.* 2007;7:16.

6. Rainbow J, Browne GJ. Fatal asthma or anaphylaxis? *Emerg Med J.* 2002;19:415–417.

7. Kokturk N, Demir N, Kervan F, Dinc E, Koybasioglu A, Turktas H. A subglottic mass mimicking near-fatal asthma: a challenge of diagnosis. *J Emerg Med.* 2004;26:57–60.

8. Camargo CA Jr, Spooner CH, Rowe BH. Continuous versus intermittent beta-agonists in the treatment of acute asthma. *Cochrane Database Syst Rev.* 2003;No. 4:CD001115.

9. Travers A, Jones AP, Kelly K, Barker SJ, Camargo CA, Rowe BH. Intravenous beta2-agonists for acute asthma in the emergency department. *Cochrane Database Syst Rev.* 2001:CD002988.

10. Cates CJ, Crilly JA, Rowe BH. Holding chambers (spacers) versus nebulisers for beta-agonist treatment of acute asthma. *Cochrane Database Syst Rev.* 2006;No. 2:CD000052.

11. Kelly HW. Levalbuterol for asthma: a better treatment? *Curr Allergy Asthma Rep.* 2007;7:310–314.

12. Aaron SD. The use of ipratropium bromide for the management of acute asthma exacerbation in adults and children: a systematic review. *J Asthma.* 2001;38:521–530.

13. Rodrigo G, Rodrigo C, Burschtin O. A meta-analysis of the effects of ipratropium bromide in adults with acute asthma. *Am J Med.* 1999;107: 363–370.

14. Edmonds ML, Camargo CA Jr, Pollack CV Jr, Rowe BH. Early use of inhaled corticosteroids in the emergency department treatment of acute asthma. *Cochrane Database Syst Rev.* 2003;No. 3:CD002308.

15. Harrison BD, Stokes TC, Hart GJ, Vaughan DA, Ali NJ, Robinson AA. Need for intravenous hydrocortisone in addition to oral prednisolone in patients admitted to hospital with severe asthma without ventilatory failure. *Lancet.* 1986;1:181–184.

16. Ratto D, Alfaro C, Sipsey J, Glovsky MM, Sharma OP. Are intravenous corticosteroids required in status asthmaticus? *JAMA.* 1988;260: 527–529.

17. Plotnick LH, Ducharme FM. Acute asthma in children and adolescents: should inhaled anticholinergics be added to beta(2)-agonists? *Am J Respir Med.* 2003;2:109–115.

18. Rodrigo GJ, Castro-Rodriguez JA. Anticholinergics in the treatment of children and adults with acute asthma: a systematic review with meta-analysis. *Thorax.* 2005;60:740–746.

19. Silverman RA, Osborn H, Runge J, Gallagher EJ, Chiang W, Feldman J, Gaeta T, Freeman K, Levin B, Mancherje N, Scharf S. IV magnesium sulfate in the treatment of acute severe asthma: a multicenter randomized controlled trial. *Chest.* 2002;122:489–497.

20. Rowe BH, Bretzlaff JA, Bourdon C, Bota GW, Camargo CA Jr. Magnesium sulfate for treating exacerbations of acute asthma in the emergency department. *Cochrane Database Syst Rev.* 2000;No. 1:CD001490.

21. Gallegos-Solórzanó MC, Pérez-Padilla R, Hernández-Zenteno RJ. "Usefulness of inhaled magnesium sulfate in the coadjuvant management of severe asthma crisis in an emergency department. *Pulm Pharmacol Ther.* 2010;23:432–437.

22. Blitz M, Blitz S, Hughes R, Diner B, Beasley R, Knopp J, Rowe BH. Aerosolized magnesium sulfate for acute asthma: a systematic review. *Chest.* 2005;128:337–344.

23. Cydulka R, Davison R, Grammer L, Parker M, Mathews JIV. The use of epinephrine in the treatment of older adult asthmatics. *Ann Emerg Med.* 1988;17:322–326.

24. Putland M, Kerr D, Kelly AM. Adverse events associated with the use of intravenous epinephrine in emergency department patients presenting with severe asthma. *Ann Emerg Med.* 2006;47:559–563.

25. Petrillo TM, Fortenberry JD, Linzer JF, Simon HK. Emergency department use of ketamine in pediatric status asthmaticus. *J Asthma.* 2001;38:657–664.

26. Howton JC, Rose J, Duffy S, Zoltanski T, Levitt MA. Randomized, double-blind, placebo-controlled trial of intravenous ketamine in acute asthma. *Ann Emerg Med.* 1996;27:170–175.

27. Allen JY, Macias CG. The efficacy of ketamine in pediatric emergency department patients who present with acute severe asthma. *Ann Emerg Med.* 2005;46:43–50.

28. Hess DR, Acosta FL, Ritz RH, Kacmarek RM, Camargo CA Jr. The effect of heliox on nebulizer function using a beta-agonist bronchodilator. *Chest.* 1999;115:184–189.

29. Rodrigo G, Pollack C, Rodrigo C, Rowe BH. Heliox for nonintubated acute asthma patients. *Cochrane Database Syst Rev.* 2006;No. 4:CD002884.

30. Parameswaran K, Belda J, Rowe BH. Addition of intravenous aminophylline to $\beta_2$-agonists in adults with acute asthma. *Cochrane Database Syst Rev.* 2000;No. 4:CD002742.

31. Schultz TE. Sevoflurane administration in status asthmaticus: a case report. *AANA J.* 2005;73:35–36.

32. Wheeler DS, Clapp CR, Ponaman ML, Bsn HM, Poss WB. Isoflurane therapy for status asthmaticus in children: a case series and protocol. *Pediatr Crit Care Med.* 2000;1:55–59.

33. British Thoracic Society Standards of Care Committee. Non-invasive ventilation in acute respiratory failure. *Thorax.* 2002;57:192–211.

34. Soroksky A, Stav D, Shpirer I. A pilot prospective, randomized, placebo-controlled trial of bilevel positive airway pressure in acute asthmatic attack. *Chest.* 2003;123:1018–1025.

35. Ram FS, Wellington S, Rowe BH, Wedzicha JA. Non-invasive positive pressure ventilation for treatment of respiratory failure due to severe acute exacerbations of asthma. *Cochrane Database Syst Rev.* 2005;No. 3:CD004360.

36. Marik PE, Varon J, Fromm R Jr. The management of acute severe asthma. *J Emerg Med.* 2002;23:257–268.

37. Brenner B, Corbridge T, Kazzi A. Intubation and mechanical ventilation of the asthmatic patient in respiratory failure. *Proc Am Thorac Soc.* 2009;6:371–379.

38. Darioli R, Perret C. Mechanical controlled hypoventilation in status asthmaticus. *Am Rev Respir Dis.* 1984;129:385–387.

39. Tuxen DV. Permissive hypercapnic ventilation. *Am J Respir Crit Care Med.* 1994;150:870–874.

40. Mikkelsen ME, Woo YJ, Sager JS, Fuchs BD, Christie JD. Outcomes using extracorporeal life support for adult respiratory failure due to status asthmaticus. *Asaio J.* 2009;55(1):47–52.

41. Leiba A, Bar-Yosef S, Bar-Dayan Y, Weiss Y, Segal E, Paret G, Vardi A. Early administration of extracorporeal life support for near fatal asthma. *Isr Med Assoc J.* 2003;5(8):600–602.

42. Conrad SA, Green R, Scott LK. Near-fatal pediatric asthma managed with pumpless arteriovenous carbon dioxide removal. *Criti Care Med.* 2007;35:2624–2629.

43. Elliot SC, Paramasivam K, Oram J, Bodenham AR, Howell SJ, Mallick A. Pumpless extracorporeal carbon dioxide removal for life-threatening asthma. *Crit Care Med.* 2007;35:945–948.

44. Barker P. Resuscitation in status asthmaticus. *Med J Aust.* 1985; 142:238.

45. Diament RH, Sloan JP. Failed resuscitation in acute severe asthma: a medical indication for emergency thoracotomy? *Arch Emerg Med.* 1987; 4:233–235.

46. Eason J, Tayler D, Cottam S, Edwards R, Beard C, Peachey T, Lanigan C, Knibb A, Dimond J. Manual chest compression for total bronchospasm. *Lancet.* 1991;337:366.

47. Fisher MM, Bowey CJ, Ladd-Hudson K. External chest compression in acute asthma: a preliminary study. *Crit Care Med.* 1989;17:686–687.

48. Fisher MM, Whaley AP, Pye RR. External chest compression in the management of acute severe asthma: a technique in search of evidence. *Prehosp Disaster Med.* 2001;16:124–127.

49. Mostert JW. Lung massage for total bronchospasm: a case report. *S Afr Med J.* 1960;34:703–704.

50. Smolnikoff VP. Total bronchospasm and lung massage. *Anaesthesia.* 1960;15:40–44.

51. Deakin CD, McLaren RM, Petley GW, Clewlow F, Dalrymple-Hay MJ. Effects of positive end-expiratory pressure on transthoracic impedance: implications for defibrillation. *Resuscitation.* 1998;37:9–12.

52. Voelckel WG, Lurie KG, Zielinski T, McKnite S, Plaisance P, Wenzel V, Lindner KH. The effects of positive end-expiratory pressure during

active compression decompression cardiopulmonary resuscitation with the inspiratory threshold valve. *Anesth Analg.* 2001;92:967–974.

53. Tuxen DV. Detrimental effects of positive end-expiratory pressure during controlled mechanical ventilation of patients with severe airflow obstruction. *Am Rev Respir Dis.* 1989;140:5–9.

54. Myles PS, Madder H, Morgan EB. Intraoperative cardiac arrest after unrecognized dynamic hyperinflation. *Br J Anaesth.* 1995;74:340–342.

55. Mercer M. Cardiac arrest after unrecognized dynamic inflation. *Br J Anaesth.* 1995;75:252.

56. Rosengarten PL, Tuxen DV, Dziukas L, Scheinkestel C, Merrett K, Bowes G. Circulatory arrest induced by intermittent positive pressure ventilation in a patient with severe asthma. *Anaesth Intensive Care.* 1991;19:118–121.

57. Neugut AI, Ghatak AT, Miller RL. Anaphylaxis in the United States: an investigation into its epidemiology. *Arch Intern Med.* 2001;161:15–21.

58. Banerji A, Clark S, Blanda M, LoVecchio F, Snyder B, Camargo CA Jr. Multicenter study of patients with angiotensin-converting enzyme inhibitor-induced angioedema who present to the emergency department. *Ann Allergy Asthma Immunol.* 2008;100:327–332.

59. Agah R, Bandi V, Guntupalli KK. Angioedema: the role of ACE inhibitors and factors associated with poor clinical outcome. *Intensive Care Med.* 1997;23:793–796.

60. Bork K, Hardt J, Schickketanz KH, Ressel N. Clinical studies of sudden upper airway obstruction in patients with hereditary angioedema due to C1 esterase inhibitor deficiency. *Arch Intern Med.* 2003;163:1229–1235.

61. Fisher M. Blood volume replacement in acute anaphylactic cardiovascular collapse related to anaesthesia. *Br J Anaesth.* 1977;49:1023–1026.

62. Nicolas F, Villers D, Blanloeil Y. Hemodynamic pattern in anaphylactic shock with cardiac arrest. *Crit Care Med.* 1984;12:144–145.

63. Raper RF, Fisher MM. Profound reversible myocardial depression after anaphylaxis. *Lancet.* 1988;1:386–388.

64. Pumphrey RS. Lessons for management of anaphylaxis from a study of fatal reactions. *Clin Exp Allergy.* 2000;30:1144–1150.

65. Pumphrey RS. Fatal anaphylaxis in the UK, 1992–2001. *Novartis Found Symp.* 2004;257:116–128.

66. Yilmaz R, Yuksekbas O, Erkol Z, Bulut ER, Arslan MN. Postmortem findings after anaphylactic reactions to drugs in Turkey. *Am J Forensic Med Pathol.* 2009;30:346–349.

67. Simons FE, Gu X, Simons KJ. Epinephrine absorption in adults: intramuscular versus subcutaneous injection. *J Allergy Clin Immunol.* 2001;108:871–873.

68. Sheikh A, Shehata YA, Brown SG, Simons FE. Adrenaline (epinephrine) for the treatment of anaphylaxis with and without shock. *Cochrane Database Syst Rev.* 2008;No. 4:CD006312.

69. Korenblat P, Lundie MJ, Dankner RE, Day JH. A retrospective study of epinephrine administration for anaphylaxis: how many doses are needed? *Allergy Asthma Proc.* 1999;20:383–386.

70. Yunginger JW, Sweeney KG, Sturner WQ, Giannandrea LA, Teigland JD, Bray M, Benson PA, York JA, Biedrzycki L, Squillace DL, Helm RM. Fatal food-induced anaphylaxis. *JAMA.* 1988;260:1450–1452.

71. Brown SG, Blackman KE, Stenlake V, Heddle RJ. Insect sting anaphylaxis; prospective evaluation of treatment with intravenous adrenaline and volume resuscitation. *Emerg Med J.* 2004;21:149–154.

72. Bautista E, Simons FE, Simons KJ, Becker AB, Duke K, Tillett M, Kepron W, Mink SN. Epinephrine fails to hasten hemodynamic recovery in fully developed canine anaphylactic shock. *Int Arch Allergy Immunol.* 2002;128:151–164.

73. Bochner BS, Lichtenstein LM. Anaphylaxis. *N Engl J Med.* 1991;324:1785–1790.

74. Pumphrey R. Anaphylaxis: can we tell who is at risk of a fatal reaction? *Curr Opin Allergy Clin Immunol.* 2004;4:285–290.

75. Johnston SL, Unsworth J, Gompels MM. Adrenaline given outside the context of life threatening allergic reactions. *BMJ.* 2003;326:589–590.

76. Mink SN, Simons FE, Simons KJ, Becker AB, Duke K. Constant infusion of epinephrine, but not bolus treatment, improves haemodynamic recovery in anaphylactic shock in dogs. *Clin Exp Allergy.* 2004;34:1776–1783.

77. Kill C, Wranze E, Wulf H. Successful treatment of severe anaphylactic shock with vasopressin: two case reports. *Int Arch Allergy Immunol.* 2004;134:260–261.

78. Williams SR, Denault AY, Pellerin M, Martineau R. Vasopressin for treatment of shock following aprotinin administration. *Can J Anaesth.* 2004;51:169–172.

79. Schummer C, Wirsing M, Schummer W. The pivotal role of vasopressin in refractory anaphylactic shock. *Anesth Analg.* 2008;107:620–624.

80. Kluger MT. The Bispectral Index during an anaphylactic circulatory arrest. *Anaesth Intensive Care.* 2001;29:544–547.

81. McBrien ME, Breslin DS, Atkinson S, Johnston JR. Use of methoxamine in the resuscitation of epinephrine-resistant electromechanical dissociation. *Anaesthesia.* 2001;56:1085–1089.

82. Rocq N, Favier JC, Plancade D, Steiner T, Mertes PM. Successful use of terlipressin in post-cardiac arrest resuscitation after an epinephrine-resistant anaphylactic shock to suxamethonium. *Anesthesiology.* 2007;107:166–167.

83. Green R, Ball A. Alpha-agonists for the treatment of anaphylactic shock. *Anaesthesia.* 2005;60:621–622.

84. Heytman M, Rainbird A. Use of alpha-agonists for management of anaphylaxis occurring under anaesthesia: case studies and review. *Anaesthesia.* 2004;59:1210–1215.

85. Higgins DJ, Gayatri P. Methoxamine in the management of severe anaphylaxis. *Anaesthesia.* 1999;54:1126.

86. Simons FE. Advances in H1-antihistamines. *N Engl J Med.* 2004;351:2203–2217.

87. Sheikh A, Ten Broek V, Brown SG, Simons FE. H1-antihistamines for the treatment of anaphylaxis: Cochrane systematic review. *Allergy.* 2007;62:830–837.

88. Gibbs MW, Kuczkowski KM, Benumof JL. Complete recovery from prolonged cardio-pulmonary resuscitation following anaphylactic reaction to readministered intravenous cefazolin. *Acta Anaesthesiol Scand.* 2003;47:230–232.

89. Choo KJ, Simons FE, Sheikh A. Glucocorticoids for the treatment of anaphylaxis. *Cochrane Database Syst Rev.* 2010;3:CD007596.

90. Allen SJ, Gallagher A, Paxton LD. Anaphylaxis to rocuronium. *Anaesthesia.* 2000;55:1223–1224.

91. Lafforgue E, Sleth JC, Pluskwa F, Saizy C. Successful extracorporeal resuscitation of a probable perioperative anaphylactic shock due to atracurium [in French]. *Ann Fr Anesth Reanim.* 2005;24:551–555.

92. Lewis G, ed. The Confidential Enquiry into Maternal and Child Health (CEMACH). Saving mothers' lives: reviewing maternal deaths to make motherhood safer—2003–2005. The Seventh Report on Confidential Enquiries into Maternal Deaths in the United Kingdom. London: CEMACH. 2007.

93. Department of Health, Welsh Office, Scottish Office Department of Health, Department of Health and Social Services, Northern Ireland. Why mothers die. Report on confidential enquiries into maternal deaths in the United Kingdom 2000–2002. London (UK): The Stationery Office; 2004.

94. Dijkman A, Huisman CM, Smit M, Schutte JM, Zwart JJ, van Roosmalen JJ, Oepkes D. Cardiac arrest in pregnancy: increasing use of perimortem caesarean section due to emergency skills training? *BJOG.* 2010;117:282–287.

95. Page-Rodriguez A, Gonzalez-Sanchez JA. Perimortem cesarean section of twin pregnancy: case report and review of the literature. *Acad Emerg Med.* 1999;6:1072–1074.

96. Cardosi RJ, Porter KB. Cesarean delivery of twins during maternal cardiopulmonary arrest. *Obstet Gynecol.* 1998;92(pt 2):695–697.

97. Rees SG, Thurlow JA, Gardner IC, Scrutton MJ, Kinsella SM. Maternal cardiovascular consequences of positioning after spinal anaesthesia for Caesarean section: left 15 degree table tilt vs. left lateral. *Anaesthesia.* 2002;57:15–20.

98. Mendonca C, Griffiths J, Ateleanu B, Collis RE. Hypotension following combined spinal-epidural anaesthesia for Caesarean section: left lateral position vs. tilted supine position. *Anaesthesia.* 2003;58:428–431.

99. Alahuhta S, Jouppila P. How to maintain uteroplacental perfusion during obstetric anaesthesia. *Acta Anaesthesiol Scand.* 1997;110:106–108.

100. Carbonne B, Benachi A, Leveque ML, Cabrol D, Papiernik E. Maternal position during labor: effects on fetal oxygen saturation measured by pulse oximetry. *Obstet Gynecol.* 1996;88:797–800.

101. Tamas P, Szilagyi A, Jeges S, Vizer M, Csermely T, Ifi Z, Balint A, Szabo I. Effects of maternal central hemodynamics on fetal heart rate patterns. *Acta Obstet Gynecol Scand.* 2007;86:711–714.

102. Abitbol MM. Supine position in labor and associated fetal heart rate changes. *Obstet Gynecol.* 1985;65:481–486.

103. Tamilselvan P, Fernando R, Bray J, Sodhi M, Columb M. The effects of crystalloid and colloid preload on cardiac output in the parturient undergoing planned cesarean delivery under spinal anesthesia: a randomized trial. *Anesth Analg.* 2009;109:1916–1921.

104. Bamber JH, Dresner M. Aortocaval compression in pregnancy: the effect of changing the degree and direction of lateral tilt on maternal cardiac output. *Anesth Analg.* 2003;97:256–258.

105. Goodwin AP, Pearce AJ. The human wedge: a manoeuvre to relieve aortocaval compression during resuscitation in late pregnancy. *Anaesthesia.* 1992;47:433–434.

106. Rees GA, Willis BA. Resuscitation in late pregnancy. *Anaesthesia.* 1988;43:347–349.

107. Ellington C, Katz VL, Watson WJ, Spielman FJ. The effect of lateral tilt on maternal and fetal hemodynamic variables. *Obstet Gynecol.* 1991; 77:201–203.

108. Matorras R, Tacuri C, Nieto A, Gutierrez de Teran G, Cortes J. Lack of benefits of left tilt in emergent cesarean sections: a randomized study of cardiotocography, cord acid-base status and other parameters of the mother and the fetus. *J Perinat Med.* 1998;26:284–292.

109. Kinsella SM, Whitwam JG, Spencer JA. Aortic compression by the uterus: identification with the Finapres digital arterial pressure instrument. *Br J Obstet Gynaecol.* 1990;97:700–705.

110. Jones SJ, Kinsella SM, Donald FA. Comparison of measured and estimated angles of table tilt at Caesarean section. *Br J Anaesth.* 2003; 90:86–87.

111. Kundra P, Khanna S, Habeebullah S, Ravishankar M. Manual displacement of the uterus during Caesarean section. *Anaesthesia.* 2007; 62:460–465.

112. Amaro A, Capelli E, Cardoso M, Rosa M, Carvalho J. Manual left uterine displacement or modified Crawford's edge: a comparative study in spinal anesthesia for cesarean delivery. *Rev Bras Anest.* 1998;48: 99–104.

113. Hankins GD, Harvey CJ, Clark SL, Uckan EM, Van Hook JW. The effects of maternal position and cardiac output on intrapulmonary shunt in normal third-trimester pregnancy. *Obstet Gynecol.* 1996;88:327–330.

114. Elkus R, Popovich J Jr. Respiratory physiology in pregnancy. *Clin Chest Med.* 1992;13:555–565.

115. Lapinsky SE, Kruczynski K, Slutsky AS. Critical care in the pregnant patient. *Am J Respir Crit Care Med.* 1995;152:427–455.

116. Izci B, Vennelle M, Liston WA, Dundas KC, Calder AA, Douglas NJ. Sleep-disordered breathing and upper airway size in pregnancy and post-partum. *Eur Respir J.* 2006;27:321–327.

117. Vasdev GM, Harrison BA, Keegan MT, Burkle CM. Management of the difficult and failed airway in obstetric anesthesia. *J Anesth.* 2008;22: 38–48.

118. Marx GF, Berman JA. Anesthesia-related maternal mortality. *Bull N Y Acad Med.* 1985;61:323–330.

119. Cheun JK, Choi KT. Arterial oxygen desaturation rate following obstructive apnea in parturients. *J Korean Med Sci.* 1992;7:6–10.

120. Norris MC, Dewan DM. Preoxygenation for cesarean section: a comparison of two techniques. *Anesthesiology.* 1985;62:827–829.

121. Varga I, Rigo J Jr, Somos P, Joo JG, Nagy B. Analysis of maternal circulation and renal function in physiologic pregnancies: parallel examinations of the changes in the cardiac output and the glomerular filtration rate. *J Matern Fetal Med.* 2000;9:97–104.

122. Nanson J, Elcock D, Williams M, Deakin CD. Do physiological changes in pregnancy change defibrillation energy requirements? *Br J Anaesth.* 2001;87:237–239.

123. Toongsuwan S. Post mortem caesarean section following death by electrocution. *Aust N Z J Obstet Gynaecol.* 1972;12:265–266.

124. Hrozek D. Intrauterine death of the fetus in a mother shocked by an electric current (case report) [in German]. *Zentralbl Gynakol.* 1963;85: 203–204.

125. Esteve H. Abortion and electrocution: an exceptional industrial accident [in French]. *Arch Mal Prof.* 1971;32:559–562.

126. Steer RG. Delayed fetal death following electrical injury in the first trimester. *Aust N Z J Obstet Gynaecol.* 1992;32:377–378.

127. Mehl LE. Electrical injury from Tasering and miscarriage. *Acta Obstet Gynecol Scand.* 1992;71:118–123.

128. Peppler RD, Labranche FJ Jr, Comeaux JJ. Intrauterine death of a fetus in a mother shocked by an electrical current: a case report. *J La State Med Soc.* 1973;124:37–38.

129. Jaffe R, Fejgin M, Ben Aderet N. Fetal death in early pregnancy due to electric current. *Acta Obstet Gynecol Scand.* 1986;65:283.

130. Yoong AF. Electrical shock sustained in pregnancy followed by placental abruption. *Postgrad Med J.* 1990;66:563–564.

131. Rees WD. Pregnant woman struck by lightning. *BMJ.* 1965;1:103–104.

132. Fatovich DM. Electric shock in pregnancy. *J Emerg Med.* 1993;11: 175–177.

133. Leiberman JR, Mazor M, Molcho J, Haiam E, Maor E, Insler V. Electrical accidents during pregnancy. *Obstet Gynecol.* 1986;67: 861–863.

134. Brown O, Davidson N, Palmer J. Cardioversion in the third trimester of pregnancy. *Aust N Z J Obstet Gynaecol.* 2001;41:241–242.

135. Adamson DL, Nelson-Piercy C. Managing palpitations and arrhythmias during pregnancy. *Heart.* 2007;93:1630–1636.

136. Goldman RD, Einarson A, Koren G. Electric shock during pregnancy. *Can Fam Physician.* 2003;49:297–298.

137. Ladner HE, Danielsen B, Gilbert WM. Acute myocardial infarction in pregnancy and the puerperium: a population-based study. *Obstet Gynecol.* 2005;105:480–484.

138. James AH, Jamison MG, Biswas MS, Brancazio LR, Swamy GK, Myers ER. Acute myocardial infarction in pregnancy: a United States population-based study. *Circulation.* 2006;113:1564–1571.

139. Marelli AJ, Therrien J, Mackie AS, Ionescu-Ittu R, Pilote L. Planning the specialized care of adult congenital heart disease patients: from numbers to guidelines; an epidemiologic approach. *Am Heart J.* 2009; 157:1–8.

140. Warnes CA, Williams RG, Bashore TM, Child JS, Connolly HM, Dearani JA, Del Nido P, Fasules JW, Graham TP Jr, Hijazi ZM, Hunt SA, King ME, Landzberg MJ, Miner PD, Radford MJ, Walsh EP, Webb GD. ACC/AHA 2008 guidelines for the management of adults with congenital heart disease: executive summary: a report of the American College of Cardiology/American Heart Association Task Force on Practice Guidelines (writing committee to develop guidelines for the management of adults with congenital heart disease). *Circulation.* 2008; 118:2395–2451.

141. Poole JH, Long J. Maternal mortality: a review of current trends. *Crit Care Nurs Clin North Am.* 2004;16:227–230.

142. Munro PT. Management of eclampsia in the accident and emergency department. *J Accid Emerg Med.* 2000;17:7–11.

143. McDonnell NJ. Cardiopulmonary arrest in pregnancy: two case reports of successful outcomes in association with perimortem Caesarean delivery. *Br J Anaesth.* 2009;103:406–409.

144. Turrentine MA, Braems G, Ramirez MM. Use of thrombolytics for the treatment of thromboembolic disease during pregnancy. *Obstet Gynecol Surv.* 1995;50:534–541.

145. Thabut G, Thabut D, Myers RP, Bernard-Chabert B, Marrash-Chahla R, Mal H, Fournier M. Thrombolytic therapy of pulmonary embolism: a meta-analysis. *J Am Coll Cardiol.* 2002;40:1660–1667.

146. Patel RK, Fasan O, Arya R. Thrombolysis in pregnancy. *Thromb Haemost.* 2003;90:1216–1217.

147. Dapprich M, Boessenecker W. Fibrinolysis with alteplase in a pregnant woman with stroke. *Cerebrovasc Dis.* 2002;13:290.

148. Stanten RD, Iverson LI, Daugharty TM, Lovett SM, Terry C, Blumenstock E. Amniotic fluid embolism causing catastrophic pulmonary vasoconstriction: diagnosis by transesophageal echocardiogram and treatment by cardiopulmonary bypass. *Obstet Gynecol.* 2003;102: 496–498.

149. Stehr SN, Liebich I, Kamin G, Koch T, Litz RJ. Closing the gap between decision and delivery: amniotic fluid embolism with severe cardiopulmonary and haemostatic complications with a good outcome. *Resuscitation.* 2007;74:377–381.

150. Mhyre JM, Riesner MN, Polley LS, Naughton NN. A series of anesthesia-related maternal deaths in Michigan, 1985–2003. *Anesthesiology.* 2007;106: 1096–1104.

151. D'Angelo R. Anesthesia-related maternal mortality: a pat on the back or a call to arms? *Anesthesiology.* 2007;106:1082–1084.

152. Hawkins JL, Koonin LM, Palmer SK, Gibbs CP. Anesthesia-related deaths during obstetric delivery in the United States, 1979–1990. *Anesthesiology.* 1997;86:277–284.

153. Fisher RS, Roberts GS, Grabowski CJ, Cohen S. Altered lower esophageal sphincter function during early pregnancy. *Gastroenterology.* 1978;74: 1233–1237.

154. Dodds WJ, Dent J, Hogan WJ. Pregnancy and the lower esophageal sphincter. *Gastroenterology.* 1978;74:1334–1336.

155. Baron TH, Ramirez B, Richter JE. Gastrointestinal motility disorders during pregnancy. *Ann Intern Med.* 1993;118:366–375.

156. Ueland K, Novy MJ, Peterson EN, Metcalfe J. Maternal cardiovascular dynamics, IV: the influence of gestational age on the maternal cardiovascular response to posture and exercise. *Am J Obstet Gynecol.* 1969; 104:856–864.

157. Stallard TC, Burns B. Emergency delivery and perimortem C-section. *Emerg Med Clin North Am.* 2003;21:679–693.

158. Mackway-Jones K. Towards evidence based emergency medicine: best BETs from the Manchester Royal Infirmary. *Emerg Med J.* 2003; 20:464.

159. Rittenberger JC, Kelly E, Jang D, Greer K, Heffner A. Successful outcome utilizing hypothermia after cardiac arrest in pregnancy: a case report. *Crit Care Med.* 2008;36:1354–1356.

160. Selden BS, Burke TJ. Complete maternal and fetal recovery after prolonged cardiac arrest. *Ann Emerg Med.* 1988;17:346–349.

161. McCartney CJL, Dark A. Caesarean delivery during cardiac arrest in late pregnancy. *Anaesthesia.* 1998;53:310–311.

162. Lurie S, Mamet Y. Caesarean delivery during maternal cardiopulmonary resuscitation for status asthmaticus. *Emerg Med J.* 2003;20:296–297.

163. O'Connor RL, Sevarino FB. Cardiopulmonary arrest in the pregnant patient: a report of a successful resuscitation. *J Clin Anesth.* 1994;6: 66–68.

164. Finegold H, Darwich A, Romeo R, Vallejo M, Ramanathan S. Successful resuscitation after maternal cardiac arrest by immediate cesarean section in the labor room. *Anesthesiology.* 2002;96:1278.

165. Parker J, Balis N, Chester S, Adey D. Cardiopulmonary arrest in pregnancy: successful resuscitation of mother and infant following immediate caesarean section in labour ward. *Aust N Z J Obstet Gynaecol.* 1996;36:207–210.

166. Katz V, Balderston K, DeFreest M. Perimortem cesarean delivery: were our assumptions correct? *Am J Obstet Gynecol.* 2005;192:1916–1920.

167. Lanoix R, Akkapeddi V, Goldfeder B. Perimortem cesarean section: case reports and recommendations. *Acad Emerg Med.* 1995;2: 1063–1067.

168. Tang G, Nada W, Gyaneshwar R, Crooke D. Perimortem Caesarean section: two case reports and a management protocol. *Aust N Z J Obstet Gynaecol.* 2000;40:405–408.

169. Lopez-Zeno JA, Carlo WA, O'Grady JP, Fanaroff AA. Infant survival following delayed postmortem cesarean delivery. *Obstet Gynecol.* 1990;76(pt 2):991–992.

170. MacKenzie IZ, Cooke I. What is a reasonable time from decision-to-delivery by caesarean section? Evidence from 415 deliveries. *BJOG.* 2002;109:498–504.

171. Helmy WH, Jolaoso AS, Ifaturoti OO, Afify SA, Jones MH. The decision-to-delivery interval for emergency caesarean section: is 30 minutes a realistic target? *BJOG.* 2002;109:505–508.

172. Kam CW. Perimortem caesarean sections (PMCS). *J Accid Emerg Med.* 1994;11:57–58.

173. Kupas DF, Harter SC, Vosk A. Out-of-hospital perimortem cesarean section. *Prehosp Emerg Care.* 1998;2:206–208.

174. Kazandi M, Mgoyi L, Gundem G, Haciveliolglu S, Yucebilgin S, Ozkinay E. Post-mortem Caesarean section performed 30 minutes after maternal cardiopulmonary arrest. *Aust N Z J Obstet Gynaecol.* 2004;44: 351–353.

175. Katz VL, Dotters DJ, Droegemueller W. Perimortem cesarean delivery. *Obstet Gynecol.* 1986;68:571–576.

176. Oates S, Williams GL, Rees GA. Cardiopulmonary resuscitation in late pregnancy. *BMJ.* 1988;297:404–405.

177. Strong THJ, Lowe RA. Perimortem cesarean section. *Am J Emerg Med.* 1989;7:489–494.

178. Boyd R, Teece S. Towards evidence based emergency medicine: best BETs from the Manchester Royal Infirmary: perimortem caesarean section. *Emerg Med J.* 2002;19:324–325.

179. Morris S, Stacey M. Resuscitation in pregnancy. *BMJ.* 2003;327: 1277–1279.

180. Bunch TJ, White RD, Lopez-Jimenez F, Thomas RJ. Association of body weight with total mortality and with ICD shocks among survivors of ventricular fibrillation in out-of-hospital cardiac arrest. *Resuscitation.* 2008;77:351–355.

181. White RD, Blackwell TH, Russell JK, Jorgenson DB. Body weight does not affect defibrillation, resuscitation, or survival in patients with out-of-hospital cardiac arrest treated with a nonescalating biphasic waveform defibrillator. *Crit Care Med.* 2004;32:S387–S392.

182. DeSilva RA, Lown B. Energy requirement for defibrillation of a markedly overweight patient. *Circulation.* 1978;57:827–830.

183. White RD, Blackwell TH, Russell JK, Snyder DE, Jorgenson DB. Transthoracic impedance does not affect defibrillation, resuscitation or survival in patients with out-of-hospital cardiac arrest treated with a non-escalating biphasic waveform defibrillator. *Resuscitation.* 2005;64: 63–69.

184. Srinivasan V, Nadkarni VM, Helfaer MA, Carey SM, Berg RA. Childhood obesity and survival after in-hospital pediatric cardiopulmonary resuscitation. *Pediatrics.* 2010:125:e481–e488.

185. Bottiger BW, Arntz HR, Chamberlain DA, Bluhmki E, Belmans A, Danays T, Carli PA, Adgey JA, Bode C, Wenzel V. Thrombolysis during resuscitation for out-of-hospital cardiac arrest. *N Engl J Med.* 2008;359:2651–2662.

186. Abu-Laban RB, Christenson JM, Innes GD, van Beek CA, Wanger KP, McKnight RD, MacPhail IA, Puskaric J, Sadowski RP, Singer J, Schechter MT, Wood VM. Tissue plasminogen activator in cardiac arrest with pulseless electrical activity. *N Engl J Med.* 2002;346: 1522–1528.

187. Bottiger BW, Bode C, Kern S, Gries A, Gust R, Glatzer R, Bauer H, Motsch J, Martin E. Efficacy and safety of thrombolytic therapy after initially unsuccessful cardiopulmonary resuscitation: a prospective clinical trial. *Lancet.* 2001;357:1583–1585.

188. Fatovich DM, Dobb GJ, Clugston RA. A pilot randomised trial of thrombolysis in cardiac arrest (the TICA trial). *Resuscitation.* 2004;61: 309–313.

189. Fava M, Loyola S, Bertoni H, Dougnac A. Massive pulmonary embolism: percutaneous mechanical thrombectomy during cardiopulmonary resuscitation. *J Vasc Interv Radiol.* 2005;16:119–123.

190. Janata K, Holzer M, Kurkciyan I, Losert H, Riedmuller E, Pikula B, Laggner AN, Laczika K. Major bleeding complications in cardiopulmonary resuscitation: the place of thrombolytic therapy in cardiac arrest due to massive pulmonary embolism. *Resuscitation.* 2003;57:49–55.

191. Konstantinov IE, Saxena P, Koniuszko MD, Alvarez J, Newman MA. Acute massive pulmonary embolism with cardiopulmonary resuscitation: management and results. *Tex Heart Inst J.* 2007;34:41–45.

192. Lederer W, Lichtenberger C, Pechlaner C, Kroesen G, Baubin M. Recombinant tissue plasminogen activator during cardiopulmonary resuscitation in 108 patients with out-of-hospital cardiac arrest. *Resuscitation.* 2001;50:71–76.

193. Lederer W, Lichtenberger C, Pechlaner C, Kinzl J, Kroesen G, Baubin M. Long-term survival and neurological outcome of patients who received recombinant tissue plasminogen activator during out-of-hospital cardiac arrest. *Resuscitation.* 2004;61:123–129.

194. Zahorec R. Rescue systemic thrombolysis during cardiopulmonary resuscitation. *Bratisl Lek Listy.* 2002;103:266–269.

195. Li X, Fu QL, Jing XL, Li YJ, Zhan H, Ma ZF, Liao XX. A meta-analysis of cardiopulmonary resuscitation with and without the administration of thrombolytic agents. *Resuscitation.* 2006;70:31–36.

196. Varriale P, Maldonado JM. Echocardiographic observations during in hospital cardiopulmonary resuscitation. *Critical Care Medicine.* 1997; 25:1717–1720.

197. Schmid C, Zietlow S, Wagner TO, Laas J, Borst HG. Fulminant pulmonary embolism: symptoms, diagnostics, operative technique, and results. *Ann Thorac Surg.* 1991;52:1102–1105.

198. Dauphine C, Omari B. Pulmonary embolectomy for acute massive pulmonary embolism. *Ann Thorac Surg.* 2005;79:1240–1244.

199. Paice B, Gray JM, McBride D, Donnelly T, Lawson DH. Hyperkalaemia in patients in hospital. *Br Med J (Clin Res Ed).* 1983;286:1189–1192.

200. Weiner ID, Wingo CS. Hyperkalemia: a potential silent killer. *J Am Soc Nephrol.* 1998;9:1535–1543.

201. Weiner M, Epstein FH. Signs and symptoms of electrolyte disorders. *Yale J Biol Med.* 1970;43:76–109.

202. Rastegar A, Soleimani M. Hypokalaemia and hyperkalaemia. *Postgrad Med J.* 2001;77:759–764.

203. Mattu A, Brady WJ, Robinson DA. Electrocardiographic manifestations of hyperkalemia. *Am J Emerg Med.* 2000;18:721–729.

204. Frohnert PP, Giuliani ER, Friedberg M, Johnson WJ, Tauxe WN. Statistical investigation of correlations between serum potassium levels and electrocardiographic findings in patients on intermittent hemodialysis therapy. *Circulation.* 1970;41:667–676.

205. Gennari FJ. Hypokalemia. *N Engl J Med.* 1998;339:451–458.

206. Slovis C, Jenkins R. ABC of clinical electrocardiography: conditions not primarily affecting the heart [published corrections appear in *BMJ.* 2007;334(7603) doi: 10.1136/bmj.39219.615243.AE and *BMJ.* 2002; 325:259]. *BMJ.* 2002;324:1320–1323.

207. Clausen TG, Brocks K, Ibsen H. Hypokalemia and ventricular arrhythmias in acute myocardial infarction. *Acta Med Scand.* 1988;224: 531–537.

208. Higham PD, Adams PC, Murray A, Campbell RW. Plasma potassium, serum magnesium and ventricular fibrillation: a prospective study. *Q J Med.* 1993;86:609–617.

209. Nordrehaug JE. Malignant arrhythmia in relation to serum potassium in acute myocardial infarction. *Am J Cardiol.* 1985;56:20D–23D.

210. Nordrehaug JE, von der Lippe G. Hypokalaemia and ventricular fibrillation in acute myocardial infarction. *Br Heart J.* 1983;50:525–529.

211. Obeid AI, Verrier RL, Lown B. Influence of glucose, insulin, and potassium on vulnerability to ventricular fibrillation in the canine heart. *Circ Res.* 1978;43:601–608.

212. Curry P, Fitchett D, Stubbs W, Krikler D. Ventricular arrhythmias and hypokalaemia. *Lancet.* 1976;2:231–233.

213. Buylaert WA, Calle PA, Houbrechts HN. Serum electrolyte disturbances in the post-resuscitation period. *Resuscitation.* 1989;17(suppl): S189–S196.

214. Cannon LA, Heiselman DE, Dougherty JM, Jones J. Magnesium levels in cardiac arrest victims: relationship between magnesium levels and successful resuscitation. *Ann Emerg Med.* 1987;16:1195–1199.

215. McDonnell NJ, Muchatuta NA, Paech MJ. Acute magnesium toxicity in an obstetric patient undergoing general anaesthesia for caesarean delivery. *Int J Obstet Anesth.* 2010;19:226–231.

216. James MF. Cardiopulmonary arrest in pregnancy. *Br J Anaesth.* 2010; 104:115.

217. Mordes JP, Swartz R, Arky RA. Extreme hypermagnesemia as a cause of refractory hypotension. *Ann Intern Med.* 1975;83:657–658.

218. Trestrail JH. *Criminal Poisoning: Investigational Guide for Law Enforcement, Toxicologists, Forensic Scientists, and Attorneys.* 2nd ed. Totowa, NJ: Humana; 2007.

219. Courtney DM, Neumar RW, Venkatesh AK, Kaji AH, Cairns CB, Lavonas E, Richardson LD. Unique characteristics of emergency care research: scope, populations, and infrastructure. *Acad Emerg Med.* 2009; 16:990–994.

220. Matsika MD, Tournier M, Lagnaoui R, Pehourcq F, Molimard M, Begaud B, Verdoux H, Moore N. Comparison of patient questionnaires and plasma assays in intentional drug overdoses. *Basic Clin Pharmacol Toxicol.* 2004;95:31–37.

221. Neeleman J, Wessely S. Drugs taken in fatal and non-fatal self-poisoning: a study in south London. *Acta Psychiatr Scand.* 1997;95: 283–287.

222. Wu AH, McKay C, Broussard LA, Hoffman RS, Kwong TC, Moyer TP, Otten EM, Welch SL, Wax P. National Academy of Clinical Biochemistry Laboratory Medicine Practice Guidelines: recommendations for the use of laboratory tests to support poisoned patients who present to the emergency department. *Clin Chem.* 2003;49:357–379.

223. Shannon MW. A general approach to poisoning. In: Shannon MW, Borron SW, Burns MJ, eds. *Haddad and Winchester's Clinical Management of Poisoning and Drug Overdose.* 4th ed. Philadelphia, Pa: Saunders/Elsevier; 2007:13–30.

224. Position paper: ipecac syrup. *J Toxicol Clin Toxicol.* 2004;42:133–143.

225. Vale JA, Kulig K; American Academy of Clinical Toxicology; European Association of Poisons Centres and Clinical Toxicologists. Position paper: gastric lavage. *J Toxicol Clin Toxicol.* 2004;42:933–943.

226. Position paper: whole bowel irrigation. *J Toxicol Clin Toxicol.* 2004; 42:843–854.

227. Deleted in proof.

228. Chyka PA, Seger D, Krenzelok EP, Vale JA; American Academy of Clinical Toxicology; European Association of Poisons Centres and Clinical Toxicologists. Position paper: single-dose activated charcoal. *Clin Toxicol (Phila).* 2005;43:61–87.

229. American Academy of Clinical Toxicology; European Association of Poisons Centres and Clinical Toxicologists. Position statement and practice guidelines on the use of multi-dose activated charcoal in the treatment of acute poisoning. *J Toxicol Clin Toxicol.* 1999;37:731–751.

230. Metheny NA. Preventing respiratory complications of tube feedings: evidence-based practice. *Am J Crit Care.* 2006;15:360–369.

231. Adelson L. Poison and the pathologist. *JAMA.* 1964;187:918–920.

232. Kelly AM, Kerr D, Dietze P, Patrick I, Walker T, Koutsogiannis Z. Randomised trial of intranasal versus intramuscular naloxone in prehospital treatment for suspected opioid overdose. *Med J Aust.* 2005;182: 24–27.

233. Rupreht J, Dworacek B, Oosthoek H, Dzoljic MR, Valkenburg M. Physostigmine versus naloxone in heroin-overdose. *J Toxicol Clin Toxicol.* 1983;21:387–397.

234. Wanger K, Brough L, Macmillan I, Goulding J, MacPhail I, Christenson JM. Intravenous vs subcutaneous naloxone for out-of-hospital management of presumed opioid overdose. *Acad Emerg Med.* 1998;5: 293–299.

235. Leach M. Naloxone: a new therapeutic and diagnostic agent for emergency use. *JACEP.* 1973;2:21–23.

236. Sporer KA, Firestone J, Isaacs SM. Out-of-hospital treatment of opioid overdoses in an urban setting. *Acad Emerg Med.* 1996;3:660–667.

237. Yealy DM, Paris PM, Kaplan RM, Heller MB, Marini SE. The safety of prehospital naloxone administration by paramedics. *Ann Emerg Med.* 1990;19:902–905.

238. Mills CA, Flacke JW, Flacke WE, Bloor BC, Liu MD. Narcotic reversal in hypercapnic dogs: comparison of naloxone and nalbuphine. *Can J Anaesth.* 1990;37:238–244.

239. Clarke SF, Dargan PI, Jones AL. Naloxone in opioid poisoning: walking the tightrope. *Emerg Med J.* 2005;22:612–616.

240. Moore RA, Rumack BH, Conner CS, Peterson RG. Naloxone: underdosage after narcotic poisoning. *Am J Dis Child.* 1980;134:156–158.

241. Schneir AB, Vadeboncoeur TF, Offerman SR, Barry JD, Ly BT, Williams SR, Clark RF. Massive OxyContin ingestion refractory to naloxone therapy. *Ann Emerg Med.* 2002;40:425–428.

242. Robertson TM, Hendey GW, Stroh G, Shalit M. Intranasal naloxone is a viable alternative to intravenous naloxone for prehospital narcotic overdose. *Prehosp Emerg Care.* 2009;13:512–515.

243. Evans LE, Swainson CP, Roscoe P, Prescott LF. Treatment of drug overdosage with naloxone, a specific narcotic antagonist. *Lancet.* 1973; 1:452–455.

244. Greenberg MI, Roberts JR, Baskin SI. Endotracheal naloxone reversal of morphine-induced respiratory depression in rabbits. *Ann Emerg Med.* 1980;9:289–292.

245. Vilke GM, Sloane C, Smith AM, Chan TC. Assessment for deaths in out-of-hospital heroin overdose patients treated with naloxone who refuse transport. *Acad Emerg Med.* 2003;10:893–896.

246. Etherington J, Christenson J, Innes G, Grafstein E, Pennington S, Spinelli JJ, Gao M, Lahiffe B, Wanger K, Fernandes C. Is early discharge safe after naloxone reversal of presumed opioid overdose? *CJEM.* 2000;2:156–162.

247. The Flumazenil in Benzodiazepine Intoxication Multicenter Study Group. Treatment of benzodiazepine overdose with flumazenil. *Clin Ther.* 1992;14:978–995.

248. Lheureux P, Vranckx M, Leduc D, Askenasi R. Flumazenil in mixed benzodiazepine/tricyclic antidepressant overdose: a placebo-controlled study in the dog. *Am J Emerg Med.* 1992;10:184–188.

249. Pitetti RD, Singh S, Pierce MC. Safe and efficacious use of procedural sedation and analgesia by nonanesthesiologists in a pediatric emergency department. *Arch Pediatr Adolesc Med.* 2003;157:1090–1096.

250. Fahed S, Grum DF, Papadimos TJ. Labetalol infusion for refractory hypertension causing severe hypotension and bradycardia: an issue of patient safety. *Patient Saf Surg.* 2008;2:13.

251. Fernandes CM, Daya MR. Sotalol-induced bradycardia reversed by glucagon. *Can Fam Physician.* 1995;41:659–660, 663–665.

252. Frishman W, Jacob H, Eisenberg E, Ribner H. Clinical pharmacology of the new beta-adrenergic blocking drugs, part 8: self-poisoning with beta-adrenoceptor blocking agents: recognition and management. *Am Heart J.* 1979;98:798–811.

253. Gabry AL, Pourriat JL, Hoang TD, Lapandry C. Cardiogenic shock caused by metoprolol poisoning: reversibility with high doses of glucagon and isoproterenol [in French]. *Presse Med.* 1985;14:229.

254. Hazouard E, Ferrandiere M, Lesire V, Joye F, Perrotin D, de Toffol B. Peduncular hallucinosis related to propranolol self-poisoning: efficacy of intravenous glucagon. *Intensive Care Med.* 1999;25:336–337.

255. Khan MI, Miller MT. Beta-blocker toxicity: the role of glucagon: report of 2 cases. *S Afr Med J.* 1985;67:1062–1063.

256. Moller BH. Massive intoxication with metoprolol. *BMJ.* 1976;1:222. Letter.

257. O'Mahony D, O'Leary P, Molloy MG. Severe oxprenolol poisoning: the importance of glucagon infusion. *Hum Exp Toxicol.* 1990;9:101–103.

258. Wallin CJ, Hulting J. Massive metoprolol poisoning treated with prenalterol. *Acta Med Scand.* 1983;214:253–255.

259. Weinstein RS. Recognition and management of poisoning with beta-adrenergic blocking agents. *Ann Emerg Med.* 1984;13:1123–1131.

260. Alderfliegel F, Leeman M, Demaeyer P, Kahn RJ. Sotalol poisoning associated with asystole. *Intensive Care Med.* 1993;19:57–58.

261. Kenyon CJ, Aldinger GE, Joshipura P, Zaid GJ. Successful resuscitation using external cardiac pacing in beta adrenergic antagonist-induced bradyasystolic arrest. *Ann Emerg Med.* 1988;17:711–713.

262. Freestone S, Thomas HM, Bhamra RK, Dyson EH. Severe atenolol poisoning: treatment with prenalterol. *Hum Toxicol.* 1986;5:343–345.

263. Toet AE, Wemer J, Vleeming W, te Biesebeek JD, Meulenbelt J, de Wildt DJ. Experimental study of the detrimental effect of dopamine/glucagon combination in d,l-propranolol intoxication. *Hum Exp Toxicol.* 1996;15:411–421.

264. Toet AE, te Biesebeek JD, Vleeming W, Wemer J, Meulenbelt J, de Wildt DJ. Reduced survival after isoprenaline/dopamine in d,l-propranolol intoxicated rats. *Hum Exp Toxicol.* 1996;15:120–128.

265. Sato S, Tsuji MH, Okubo N, Nishimoto C, Naito H. Combined use of glucagon and milrinone may not be preferable for severe propranolol poisoning in the canine model. *J Toxicol Clin Toxicol.* 1995;33:337–342.

266. Kerns W II, Schroeder D, Williams C, Tomaszewski C, Raymond R. Insulin improves survival in a canine model of acute beta-blocker toxicity. *Ann Emerg Med.* 1997;29:748–757.

267. Holger JS, Engebretsen KM, Fritzlar SJ, Patten LC, Harris CR, Flottemesch TJ. Insulin versus vasopressin and epinephrine to treat beta-blocker toxicity. *Clin Toxicol (Phila).* 2007;45:396–401.

268. Page C, Hacket LP, Isbister GK. The use of high-dose insulin-glucose euglycemia in beta-blocker overdose: a case report. *J Med Toxicol.* 2009;5:139–143.

269. Kerns W II. Management of beta-adrenergic blocker and calcium channel antagonist toxicity. *Emerg Med Clin North Am.* 2007;25:309–331.

270. Pertoldi F, D'Orlando L, Mercante WP. Electromechanical dissociation 48 hours after atenolol overdose: usefulness of calcium chloride. *Ann Emerg Med.* 1998;31:777–781.

271. Love JN, Hanfling D, Howell JM. Hemodynamic effects of calcium chloride in a canine model of acute propranolol intoxication. *Ann Emerg Med.* 1996;28:1–6.

272. McVey FK, Corke CF. Extracorporeal circulation in the management of massive propranolol overdose. *Anaesthesia.* 1991;46:744–746.

273. Lane AS, Woodward AC, Goldman MR. Massive propranolol overdose poorly responsive to pharmacologic therapy: use of the intra-aortic balloon pump. *Ann Emerg Med.* 1987;16:1381–1383.

274. Rooney M, Massey KL, Jamali F, Rosin M, Thomson D, Johnson DH. Acebutolol overdose treated with hemodialysis and extracorporeal membrane oxygenation. *J Clin Pharmacol.* 1996;36:760–763.

275. Stellpflug SJ, Harris CR, Engebretsen KM, Cole JB, Holger JS. Intentional overdose with cardiac arrest treated with intravenous fat emulsion and high-dose insulin. *Clin Toxicol.* 2010:48:227–229.

276. Zimmer BW, Marcus RJ, Sawyer K, Harchelroad F. Salicylate intoxication as a cause of pseudohyperchloremia. *Am J Kidney Dis.* 2008;51(2):346–347.

277. Cave G, Harvey M. Lipid emulsion may augment early blood pressure recovery in a rabbit model of atenolol toxicity. *J Med Toxicol.* 2009;5:50–51.

278. Cave G, Harvey MG, Castle CD. The role of fat emulsion therapy in a rodent model of propranolol toxicity: a preliminary study. *J Med Toxicol.* 2006;2(1):4–7.

279. Harvey MG, Cave GR. Intralipid infusion ameliorates propranolol-induced hypotension in rabbits. *J Med Toxicol.* 2008;4:71–76.

280. Browne A, Harvey M, Cave G. Intravenous lipid emulsion does not augment blood pressure recovery in a rabbit model of metoprolol toxicity. *J Med Toxicol.* 2010:ePub.

281. Turner-Lawrence DE, Kerns Ii W. Intravenous fat emulsion: a potential novel antidote. *J Med Toxicol.* 2008;4:109–114.

282. Cave G, Harvey M. Intravenous lipid emulsion as antidote beyond local anesthetic toxicity: a systematic review. *Acad Emerg Med.* 2009;16:815–824.

283. Jamaty C, Bailey B, Larocque A, Notebaert E, Sanogo K, Chauny JM. Lipid emulsions in the treatment of acute poisoning: a systematic review of human and animal studies. *Clin Toxicol.* 2010:48:1–27.

284. Boyer EW, Duic PA, Evans A. Hyperinsulinemia/euglycemia therapy for calcium channel blocker poisoning. *Pediatr Emerg Care.* 2002;18:36–37.

285. Cohen E, Du D, Joyce D, Kapernick EA, Volovik Y, Kelly JW, Dillin A. Temporal requirements of insulin/IGF-1 signaling for proteotoxicity protection. *Aging Cell.* 2010;9:126–134.

286. Greene SL, Gawarammana I, Wood DM, Jones AL, Dargan PI. Relative safety of hyperinsulinaemia/euglycaemia therapy in the management of calcium channel blocker overdose: a prospective observational study. *Intensive Care Med.* 2007;33:2019–2024.

287. Harris NS. Case records of the Massachusetts General Hospital: case 24–2006: a 40-year-old woman with hypotension after an overdose of amlodipine. *N Engl J Med.* 2006;355:602–611.

288. Johansen KK, Belhage B. A 48-year-old woman's survival from a massive verapamil overdose [in Danish]. *Ugeskr Laeger.* 2007;169:4074–4075.

289. Kanagarajan K, Marraffa JM, Bouchard NC, Krishnan P, Hoffman RS, Stork CM. The use of vasopressin in the setting of recalcitrant hypotension due to calcium channel blocker overdose. *Clin Toxicol (Phila).* 2007;45:56–59.

290. Marques M, Gomes E, de Oliveira J. Treatment of calcium channel blocker intoxication with insulin infusion: case report and literature review. *Resuscitation.* 2003;57:211–213.

291. Ortiz-Munoz L, Rodriguez-Ospina LF, Figueroa-Gonzalez M. Hyperinsulinemic-euglycemic therapy for intoxication with calcium channel blockers. *Bol Asoc Med P R.* 2005;97(pt 2):182–189.

292. Patel NP, Pugh ME, Goldberg S, Eiger G. Hyperinsulinemic euglycemia therapy for verapamil poisoning: case report. *Am J Crit Care.* 2007;16:518–529.

293. Rasmussen L, Husted SE, Johnsen SP. Severe intoxication after an intentional overdose of amlodipine. *Acta Anaesthesiol Scand.* 2003;47:1038–1040.

294. Smith SW, Ferguson KL, Hoffman RS, Nelson LS, Greller HA. Prolonged severe hypotension following combined amlodipine and valsartan ingestion. *Clin Toxicol (Phila).* 2008;46:470–474.

295. Yuan TH, Kerns WPI, Tomaszewski CA, Ford MD, Kline JA. Insulin-glucose as adjunctive therapy for severe calcium channel antagonist poisoning. *J Toxicol Clin Toxicol.* 1999;37:463–474.

296. Kline JA, Tomaszewski CA, Schroeder JD, Raymond RM. Insulin is a superior antidote for cardiovascular toxicity induced by verapamil in the anesthetized canine. *J Pharmacol Exp Ther.* 1993;267:744–750.

297. Kline JA, Leonova E, Raymond RM. Beneficial myocardial metabolic effects of insulin during verapamil toxicity in the anesthetized canine. *Crit Care Med.* 1995;23:1251–1263.

298. Kline JA, Leonova E, Williams TC, Schroeder JD, Watts JA. Myocardial metabolism during graded intraportal verapamil infusion in awake dogs. *J Cardiovasc Pharmacol.* 1996;27:719–726.

299. Kline JA, Raymond RM, Schroeder JD, Watts JA. The diabetogenic effects of acute verapamil poisoning. *Toxicol Appl Pharmacol.* 1997;145:357–362.

300. Durward A, Guerguerian AM, Lefebvre M, Shemie SD. Massive diltiazem overdose treated with extracorporeal membrane oxygenation. *Pediatr Crit Care Med.* 2003;4:372–376.

301. Fiszer M, Kolacinski Z, Rechcinski T. The application of 4-aminopyridine in calcium channel inhibitors acute poisoning [in Polish]. *Przegl Lek.* 2007;64:293–297.

302. Pfaender M, Casetti PG, Azzolini M, Baldi ML, Valli A. Successful treatment of a massive atenolol and nifedipine overdose with CVVHDF. *Minerva Anestesiol.* 2008;74:97–100.

303. Sabatier J, Pouyet T, Shelvey G, Cavero I. Antagonistic effects of epinephrine, glucagon and methylatropine but not calcium chloride against atrio-ventricular conduction disturbances produced by high doses of diltiazem, in conscious dogs. *Fundam Clin Pharmacol.* 1991;5:93–106.

304. Stone CK, May WA, Carroll R. Treatment of verapamil overdose with glucagon in dogs. *Ann Emerg Med.* 1995;25:369–374.

305. Stone CK, Thomas SH. Cardiopulmonary resuscitation (CPR) performance. *Prehosp Disaster Med.* 1996;11:120.

306. Tuncok Y, Apaydin S, Kalkan S, Ates M, Guven H. The effects of amrinone and glucagon on verapamil-induced cardiovascular toxicity in anaesthetized rats. *Int J Exp Pathol.* 1996;77:207–212.

307. Eddleston M, Rajapakse S, Rajakanthan, Jayalath S, Sjostrom L, Santharaj W, Thenabadu PN, Sheriff MH, Warrell DA. Anti-digoxin Fab fragments in cardiotoxicity induced by ingestion of yellow oleander: a randomised controlled trial. *Lancet.* 2000;355:967–972.

308. Smith TW, Butler VP Jr, Haber E, Fozzard H, Marcus FI, Bremner WF, Schulman IC, Phillips A. Treatment of life-threatening digitalis intoxication with digoxin-specific Fab antibody fragments: experience in 26 cases. *N Engl J Med.* 1982;307:1357–1362.

309. Wenger TL, Butler VPJ, Haber E, Smith TW. Treatment of 63 severely digitalis-toxic patients with digoxin-specific antibody fragments. *J Am Coll Cardiol.* 1985;5(suppl):118A–123A.

310. Antman EM, Wenger TL, Butler VP Jr, Haber E, Smith TW. Treatment of 150 cases of life-threatening digitalis intoxication with digoxin-specific Fab antibody fragments: final report of a multicenter study. *Circulation.* 1990;81:1744–1752.

311. Woolf AD, Wenger T, Smith TW, Lovejoy FHJ. The use of digoxin-specific Fab fragments for severe digitalis intoxication in children. *N Engl J Med.* 1992;326:1739–1744.

312. Hickey AR, Wenger TL, Carpenter VP, Tilson HH, Hlatky MA, Furberg CD, Kirkpatrick CH, Strauss HC, Smith TW. Digoxin immune Fab therapy in the management of digitalis intoxication: safety and efficacy results of an observational surveillance study. *J Am Coll Cardiol.* 1991; 17:590–598.

313. Wenger TL. Experience with digoxin immune Fab (ovine) in patients with renal impairment. *Am J Emerg Med.* 1991;9(suppl 1):21–23.

314. Woolf AD, Wenger TL, Smith TW, Lovejoy FHJ. Results of multicenter studies of digoxin-specific antibody fragments in managing digitalis intoxication in the pediatric population. *Am J Emerg Med.* 1991;9(suppl 1):16–20.

315. Taboulet P, Baud FJ, Bismuth C, Vicaut E. Acute digitalis intoxication: is pacing still appropriate? *J Toxicol Clin Toxicol.* 1993;31:261–273.

316. Lapostolle F, Borron SW, Verdier C, Taboulet P, Guerrier G, Adnet F, Clemessy JL, Bismuth C, Baud FJ. Digoxin-specific Fab fragments as single first-line therapy in digitalis poisoning. *Crit Care Med.* 2008;36: 3014–3018.

317. Bismuth C, Gaultier M, Conso F, Efthymiou ML. Hyperkalemia in acute digitalis poisoning: prognostic significance and therapeutic implications. *Clin Toxicol.* 1973;6:153–162.

318. Lapostolle F, Borron SW. Digitalis. In: Shannon MW, Borron SW, Burns MJ, eds. *Haddad and Winchester's Clinical Management of Poisoning and Drug Overdose.* Philadelphia, Pa: Saunders/Elsevier; 2007:949–962.

319. Hsue PY, McManus D, Selby V, Ren X, Pillutla P, Younes N, Goldschlager N, Waters DD. Cardiac arrest in patients who smoke crack cocaine. *Am J Cardiol.* 2007;99:822–824.

320. Lange RA, Cigarroa RG, Yancy CW Jr, Willard JE, Popma JJ, Sills MN, McBride W, Kim AS, Hillis LD. Cocaine-induced coronary-artery vasoconstriction. *N Engl J Med.* 1989;321:1557–1562.

321. Baumann BM, Perrone J, Hornig SE, Shofer FS, Hollander JE. Randomized, double-blind, placebo-controlled trial of diazepam, nitroglycerin, or both for treatment of patients with potential cocaine-associated acute coronary syndromes. *Acad Emerg Med.* 2000;7:878–885.

322. Negus BH, Willard JE, Hillis LD, Glamann DB, Landau C, Snyder RW, Lange RA. Alleviation of cocaine-induced coronary vasoconstriction with intravenous verapamil. *Am J Cardiol.* 1994;73:510–513.

323. Saland KE, Hillis LD, Lange RA, Cigarroa JE. Influence of morphine sulfate on cocaine-induced coronary vasoconstriction. *Am J Cardiol.* 2002;90:810–811.

324. Hollander JE, Hoffman RS, Gennis P, Fairweather P, DiSano MJ, Schumb DA, Feldman JA, Fish SS, Dyer S, Wax P, Whelan C, Schwarzwald E. Nitroglycerin in the treatment of cocaine associated chest pain: clinical safety and efficacy. *J Toxicol Clin Toxicol.* 1994; 32:243–256.

325. Brogan WCI, Lange RA, Kim AS, Moliterno DJ, Hillis LD. Alleviation of cocaine-induced coronary vasoconstriction by nitroglycerin. *J Am Coll Cardiol.* 1991;18:581–586.

326. Mittleman MA, Mintzer D, Maclure M, Tofler GH, Sherwood JB, Muller JE. Triggering of myocardial infarction by cocaine. *Circulation.* 1999;99:2737–2741.

327. Honderick T, Williams D, Seaberg D, Wears R. A prospective, randomized, controlled trial of benzodiazepines and nitroglycerine or nitroglycerine alone in the treatment of cocaine-associated acute coronary syndromes. *Am J Emerg Med.* 2003;21:39–42.

328. Boehrer JD, Moliterno DJ, Willard JE, Hillis LD, Lange RA. Influence of labetalol on cocaine-induced coronary vasoconstriction in humans. *Am J Med.* 1993;94:608–610.

329. Lange RA, Cigarroa RG, Flores ED, McBride W, Kim AS, Wells PJ, Bedotto JB, Danziger RS, Hillis LD. Potentiation of cocaine-induced coronary vasoconstriction by beta-adrenergic blockade. *Ann Intern Med.* 1990;112:897–903.

330. Sand IC, Brody SL, Wrenn KD, Slovis CM. Experience with esmolol for the treatment of cocaine-associated cardiovascular complications. *Am J Emerg Med.* 1991;9:161–163.

331. Dattilo PB, Hailpern SM, Fearon K, Sohal D, Nordin C. Beta-blockers are associated with reduced risk of myocardial infarction after cocaine use. *Ann Emerg Med.* 2008;51:117–125.

332. Vongpatanasin W, Mansour Y, Chavoshan B, Arbique D, Victor RG. Cocaine stimulates the human cardiovascular system via a central mechanism of action. *Circulation.* 1999;100:497–502.

333. McCord J, Jneid H, Hollander JE, de Lemos JA, Cercek B, Hsue P, Gibler WB, Ohman EM, Drew B, Philippides G, Newby LK. Management of cocaine-associated chest pain and myocardial infarction: a scientific statement from the American Heart Association Acute Cardiac Care Committee of the Council on Clinical Cardiology. *Circulation.* 2008;117:1897–1907.

334. Wood DM, Dargan PI, Hoffman RS. Management of cocaine-induced cardiac arrhythmias due to cardiac ion channel dysfunction. *Clin Toxicol (Phila).* 2009;47:14–23.

335. Hoffman JR, Votey SR, Bayer M, Silver L. Effect of hypertonic sodium bicarbonate in the treatment of moderate-to-severe cyclic antidepressant overdose. *Am J Emerg Med.* 1993;11:336–341.

336. Koppel C, Wiegreffe A, Tenczer J. Clinical course, therapy, outcome and analytical data in amitriptyline and combined amitriptyline/chlordiazepoxide overdose. *Hum Exp Toxicol.* 1992;11:458–465.

337. Brown TC. Tricyclic antidepressant overdosage: experimental studies on the management of circulatory complications. *Clin Toxicol.* 1976;9: 255–272.

338. Hedges JR, Baker PB, Tasset JJ, Otten EJ, Dalsey WC, Syverud SA. Bicarbonate therapy for the cardiovascular toxicity of amitriptyline in an animal model. *J Emerg Med.* 1985;3:253–260.

339. Knudsen K, Abrahamsson J. Epinephrine and sodium bicarbonate independently and additively increase survival in experimental amitriptyline poisoning. *Crit Care Med.* 1997;25:669–674.

340. Nattel S, Mittleman M. Treatment of ventricular tachyarrhythmias resulting from amitriptyline toxicity in dogs. *J Pharmacol Exp Ther.* 1984;231:430–435.

341. Pentel P, Benowitz N. Efficacy and mechanism of action of sodium bicarbonate in the treatment of desipramine toxicity in rats. *J Pharmacol Exp Ther.* 1984;230:12–19.

342. Sasyniuk BI, Jhamandas V, Valois M. Experimental amitriptyline intoxication: treatment of cardiac toxicity with sodium bicarbonate. *Ann Emerg Med.* 1986;15:1052–1059.

343. Pentel P, Peterson CD. Asystole complicating physostigmine treatment of tricyclic antidepressant overdose. *Ann Emerg Med.* 1980;9:588–590.

344. Knudsen K, Abrahamsson J. Effects of epinephrine and norepinephrine on hemodynamic parameters and arrhythmias during a continuous infusion of amitriptyline in rats. *J Toxicol Clin Toxicol.* 1993;31: 461–471.

345. Knudsen K, Abrahamsson J. Effects of epinephrine, norepinephrine, magnesium sulfate, and milrinone on survival and the occurrence of arrhythmias in amitriptyline poisoning in the rat. *Crit Care Med.* 1994; 22:1851–1855.

346. Tran TP, Panacek EA, Rhee KJ, Foulke GE. Response to dopamine vs norepinephrine in tricyclic antidepressant-induced hypotension. *Acad Emerg Med.* 1997;4:864–868.

347. Tobis JM, Aronow WS. Effect of amitriptyline antidotes on repetitive extrasystole threshold. *Clin Pharmacol Ther.* 1980;27:602–606.

348. Vernon DD, Banner W Jr, Garrett JS, Dean JM. Efficacy of dopamine and norepinephrine for treatment of hemodynamic compromise in amitriptyline intoxication. *Crit Care Med.* 1991;19:544–549.

349. Follmer CH, Lum BK. Protective action of diazepam and of sympathomimetic amines against amitryptyline-induced toxicity. *J Pharmacol Exp Ther.* 1982;222:424–429.

350. Sangster B, de Groot G, Borst C, de Wildt D. Dopamine and isoproterenol in imipramine intoxication in the dog. *J Toxicol Clin Toxicol.* 1985;23:407–420.

351. Foxall GL, Hardman JG, Bedforth NM. Three-dimensional, multiplanar, ultrasound-guided, radial nerve block. *Reg Anesth Pain Med.* 2007;32: 516–521.

352. Shah S, Gopalakrishnan S, Apuya J, Martin T. Use of Intralipid in an infant with impending cardiovascular collapse due to local anesthetic toxicity. *J Anesth.* 2009;23:439–441.

353. Zimmer C, Piepenbrink K, Riest G, Peters J. Cardiotoxic and neurotoxic effects after accidental intravascular bupivacaine administration: therapy with lidocaine propofol and lipid emulsion [in German]. *Anaesthesist.* 2007;56:449–453.

354. Litz RJ, Roessel T, Heller AR, Stehr SN. Reversal of central nervous system and cardiac toxicity after local anesthetic intoxication by lipid emulsion injection. *Anesth Analg.* 2008;106:1575–1577.

355. Ludot H, Tharin JY, Belouadah M, Mazoit JX, Malinovsky JM. Successful resuscitation after ropivacaine and lidocaine-induced ventricular arrhythmia following posterior lumbar plexus block in a child. *Anesth Analg.* 2008;106:1572–1574.

356. Cave G, Harvey MG, Winterbottom T. Evaluation of the Association of Anaesthetists of Great Britain and Ireland lipid infusion protocol in bupivacaine induced cardiac arrest in rabbits. *Anaesthesia.* 2009;64: 732–737.

357. DiGregorio RV, Fung HB. Rapid dosing of critical care infusions: the dopamine and norepinephrine "clocks." *J Emerg Nurs.* 2009;35: 165–168.

358. Weinberg GL, VadeBoncouer T, Ramaraju GA, Garcia-Amaro MF, Cwik MJ. Pretreatment or resuscitation with a lipid infusion shifts the dose-response to bupivacaine-induced asystole in rats. *Anesthesiology.* 1998;88:1071–1075.

359. Weinberg G, Ripper R, Feinstein DL, Hoffman W. Lipid emulsion infusion rescues dogs from bupivacaine-induced cardiac toxicity. *Reg Anesth Pain Med.* 2003;28:198–202.

360. Weinberg GL, Di Gregorio G, Ripper R, Kelly K, Massad M, Edelman L, Schwartz D, Shah N, Zheng S, Feinstein DL. Resuscitation with lipid versus epinephrine in a rat model of bupivacaine overdose. *Anesthesiology.* 2008;108:907–913.

361. Litz RJ, Popp M, Stehr SN, Koch T. Successful resuscitation of a patient with ropivacaine-induced asystole after axillary plexus block using lipid infusion. *Anaesthesia.* 2006;61:800–801.

362. Rosenblatt MA, Abel M, Fischer GW, Itzkovich CJ, Eisenkraft JB. Successful use of a 20% lipid emulsion to resuscitate a patient after a presumed bupivacaine-related cardiac arrest. *Anesthesiology.* 2006;105: 217–218.

363. Civetta JM, Gabel JC. Flow directed-pulmonary artery catheterization in surgical patients: indications and modifications of technic. *Ann Surg.* 1972;176:753–756.

364. Association of Anaesthetists of Great Britain and Ireland. Guidelines for the Management of Severe Local Anaesthetic Toxicity. 2010. Available from: http://www.aagbi.org/publications/guidelines/docs/la_toxicity_2010.pdf. Accessed January 31, 2010.

365. United Kingdom Resuscitation Council. Cardiac arrest or cardiovascular collapse caused by local anaesthetic 2008; Available from: http://www.resus.org.uk/pages/caLocalA.htm.

366. Neal JM, Bernards CM, Butterworth JF, DiGregorio G, Drasner K, Hejtmanek MR, Mulroy MF, Rosenquist RW, Weinberg GL. ASRA Practice Advisory on Local Anesthetic Systemic Toxicity. *Regional Anesthesia and Pain Medicine* 2010;35:152–161. Available at: http://journals.lww.com/rapm/Fulltext/2010/03000/ASRA_Practice_Advisory_on_Local_Anesthetic.7.aspx. Accessed July 14, 2010.

367. Turner-Lawrence DE, Kerns W II. Intravenous fat emulsion: a potential novel antidote. *J Med Toxicol.* 2008;4:109–114.

368. Picard J, Ward SC, Zumpe R, Meek T, Barlow J, Harrop-Griffiths W. Guidelines and the adoption of 'lipid rescue' therapy for local anaesthetic toxicity. *Anaesthesia.* 2009;64(2):122–125.

369. Centers for Disease Control and Prevention. Unintentional poisoning deaths: United States, 1999–2004. *MMWR Morb Mortal Wkly Rep.* 2007;56:93–96.

370. Weaver LK. Clinical practice: carbon monoxide poisoning. *N Engl J Med.* 2009;360:1217–1225.

371. Hampson NB, Zmaeff JL. Outcome of patients experiencing cardiac arrest with carbon monoxide poisoning treated with hyperbaric oxygen. *Ann Emerg Med.* 2001;38:36–41.

372. Sloan EP, Murphy DG, Hart R, Cooper MA, Turnbull T, Barreca RS, Ellerson B. Complications and protocol considerations in carbon monoxide-poisoned patients who require hyperbaric oxygen therapy: report from a ten-year experience. *Ann Emerg Med.* 1989;18:629–634.

373. Chou KJ, Fisher JL, Silver EJ. Characteristics and outcome of children with carbon monoxide poisoning with and without smoke exposure referred for hyperbaric oxygen therapy. *Pediatr Emerg Care.* 2000;16: 151–155.

374. Weaver LK, Hopkins RO, Chan KJ, Churchill S, Elliott CG, Clemmer TP, Orme JF Jr, Thomas FO, Morris AH. Hyperbaric oxygen for acute carbon monoxide poisoning. *N Engl J Med.* 2002;347:1057–1067.

375. Thom SR, Taber RL, Mendiguren II, Clark JM, Hardy KR, Fisher AB. Delayed neuropsychologic sequelae after carbon monoxide poisoning: prevention by treatment with hyperbaric oxygen. *Ann Emerg Med.* 1995;25:474–480.

376. Scheinkestel CD, Bailey M, Myles PS, Jones K, Cooper DJ, Millar IL, Tuxen DV. Hyperbaric or normobaric oxygen for acute carbon monoxide poisoning: a randomised controlled clinical trial. *Med J Aust.* 1999;170:203–210.

377. Raphael JC, Elkharrat D, Jars-Guincestre MC, Chastang C, Chasles V, Vercken JB, Gajdos P. Trial of normobaric and hyperbaric oxygen for acute carbon monoxide intoxication. *Lancet.* 1989;2:414–419.

378. Juurlink DN, Buckley NA, Stanbrook MB, Isbister GK, Bennett M, McGuigan MA. Hyperbaric oxygen for carbon monoxide poisoning. *Cochrane Database Syst Rev.* 2005;No. 1:CD002041.

379. Buckley NA, Isbister GK, Stokes B, Juurlink DN. Hyperbaric oxygen for carbon monoxide poisoning: a systematic review and critical analysis of the evidence. *Toxicol Rev.* 2005;24:75–92.

380. Wolf SJ, Lavonas EJ, Sloan EP, Jagoda AS. Clinical policy: critical issues in the management of adult patients presenting to the emergency department with acute carbon monoxide poisoning. *Ann Emerg Med.* 2008;51:138–152.

381. Satran D, Henry CR, Adkinson C, Nicholson CI, Bracha Y, Henry TD. Cardiovascular manifestations of moderate to severe carbon monoxide poisoning. *J Am Coll Cardiol.* 2005;45:1513–1516.

382. Henry CR, Satran D, Lindgren B, Adkinson C, Nicholson CI, Henry TD. Myocardial injury and long-term mortality following moderate to severe carbon monoxide poisoning. *JAMA.* 2006;295:398–402.

383. Baud FJ, Barriot P, Toffis V, Riou B, Vicaut E, Lecarpentier Y, Bourdon R, Astier A, Bismuth C. Elevated blood cyanide concentrations in victims of smoke inhalation. *N Engl J Med.* 1991;325:1761–1766.

384. Borron SW, Baud FJ, Barriot P, Imbert M, Bismuth C. Prospective study of hydroxocobalamin for acute cyanide poisoning in smoke inhalation. *Ann Emerg Med.* 2007;49:794–801, 801.e1–e2.

385. Fortin JL, Giocanti JP, Ruttimann M, Kowalski JJ. Prehospital administration of hydroxocobalamin for smoke inhalation-associated cyanide poisoning: 8 years of experience in the Paris Fire Brigade. *Clin Toxicol (Phila).* 2006;44(suppl 1):37–44.

386. Borron SW, Baud FJ, Megarbane B, Bismuth C. Hydroxocobalamin for severe acute cyanide poisoning by ingestion or inhalation. *Am J Emerg Med.* 2007;25:551–558.

387. Espinoza OB, Perez M, Ramirez MS. Bitter cassava poisoning in eight children: a case report. *Vet Hum Toxicol.* 1992;34:65.

388. Houeto P, Hoffman JR, Imbert M, Levillain P, Baud FJ. Relation of blood cyanide to plasma cyanocobalamin concentration after a fixed dose of hydroxocobalamin in cyanide poisoning. *Lancet.* 1995;346: 605–608.

389. Pontal P, Bismuth C, Garnier R. Therapeutic attitude in cyanide poisoning: retrospective study of 24 non-lethal cases. *Vet Hum Toxicol.* 1982;24:286–287.

390. Kirk MA, Gerace R, Kulig KW. Cyanide and methemoglobin kinetics in smoke inhalation victims treated with the cyanide antidote kit. *Ann Emerg Med.* 1993;22:1413–1418.

391. Chen KK, Rose CL. Nitrite and thiosulfate therapy in cyanide poisoning. *JAMA.* 1952;149:113–119.

392. Kiese M, Weger N. Formation of ferrihaemoglobin with aminophenols in the human for the treatment of cyanide poisoning. *Eur J Pharmacol.* 1969;7:97–105.

393. Hall AH, Saiers J, Baud F. Which cyanide antidote? *Critical Reviews in Toxicology.* 2009;39:541–552.

394. Hobel M, Engeser P, Nemeth L, Pill J. The antidote effect of thiosulphate and hydroxocobalamin in formation of nitroprusside intoxication of rabbits. *Arch Toxicol.* 1980;46:207–213.

395. Mengel K, Kramer W, Isert B, Friedberg KD. Thiosulphate and hydroxocobalamin prophylaxis in progressive cyanide poisoning in guinea-pigs. *Toxicology.* 1989;54:335–342.

396. Friedberg KD, Shukla UR. The efficiency of aquocobalamine as an antidote in cyanide poisoning when given alone or combined with sodium thiosulfate. *Arch Toxicol.* 1975;33:103–113.

397. Hall AH, Rumack BH. Hydroxycobalamin/sodium thiosulfate as a cyanide antidote. *J Emerg Med.* 1987;5:115–121.

398. Forsyth JC, Mueller PD, Becker CE, Osterloh J, Benowitz NL, Rumack BH, Hall AH. Hydroxocobalamin as a cyanide antidote: safety, efficacy and pharmacokinetics in heavily smoking normal volunteers. *J Toxicol Clin Toxicol.* 1993;31:277–294.

399. Kloeck WG. A practical approach to the aetiology of pulseless electrical activity: a simple 10-step training mnemonic. *Resuscitation.* 1995;30: 157–159.

400. Working Group, Ad Hoc Subcommittee on Outcomes, American College of Surgeons–Committee on Trauma. Practice management guidelines for emergency department thoracotomy. *J Am Coll Surg.* 2001;193:303–309.

401. Hopson LR, Hirsh E, Delgado J, Domeier RM, McSwain NE, Krohmer J. Guidelines for withholding or termination of resuscitation in pre-

hospital traumatic cardiopulmonary arrest: joint position statement of the National Association of EMS Physicians and the American College of Surgeons Committee on Trauma. *J Am Coll Surg.* 2003;196:106–112.

402. *Advanced Trauma Life Support for Doctors.* 7th Ed. Chicago: American College of Surgeons; 2004.

403. Maron BJ, Estes NA III. Commotio cordis. *N Engl J Med.* 2010;362:917–927.

404. Maron BJ, Doerer JJ, Haas TS, Estes NA, Hodges JS, Link MS. Commotio cordis and the epidemiology of sudden death in competitive lacrosse. *Pediatrics.* 2009;124:966–971.

405. Link MS, Maron BJ, Wang PJ, VanderBrink BA, Zhu W, Estes NA III. Upper and lower limits of vulnerability to sudden arrhythmic death with chest-wall impact (commotio cordis). *J Am Coll Cardiol.* 2003;41:99–104.

406. Sheridan RL, Goldstein MA, Stoddard FJ Jr, Walker TG. Case records of the Massachusetts General Hospital: case 41–2009: a 16-year-old boy with hypothermia and frostbite. *N Engl J Med.* 2009;361:2654–2662.

407. Larach MG. Accidental hypothermia. *Lancet.* 1995;345:493–498.

408. Kornberger E, Schwarz B, Lindner KH, Mair P. Forced air surface rewarming in patients with severe accidental hypothermia. *Resuscitation.* 1999;41:105–111.

409. Roggla M, Frossard M, Wagner A, Holzer M, Bur A, Roggla G. Severe accidental hypothermia with or without hemodynamic instability: rewarming without the use of extracorporeal circulation. *Wien Klin Wochenschr.* 2002;114:315–320.

410. Gilbert M, Busund R, Skagseth A, Nilsen PÅ, Solbø JP. Resuscitation from accidental hypothermia of 13.7°C with circulatory arrest. *Lancet.* 2000;355:375–376.

411. Coleman E, Doddakula K, Meeke R, Marshall C, Jahangir S, Hinchion J. An atypical case of successful resuscitation of an accidental profound hypothermia patient, occurring in a temperate climate. *Perfusion.* 2010;25:103–106.

412. Walpoth BH, Walpoth-Aslan BN, Mattle HP, Radanov BP, Schroth G, Schaeffler L, Fischer AP, von Segesser L, Althaus U. Outcome of survivors of accidental deep hypothermia and circulatory arrest treated with extracorporeal blood warming. *N Engl J Med.* 1997;337:1500–1505.

413. Althaus U, Aeberhard P, Schupbach P, Nachbur BH, Muhlemann W. Management of profound accidental hypothermia with cardiorespiratory arrest. *Ann Surg.* 1982;195:492–495.

414. Dobson JA, Burgess JJ. Resuscitation of severe hypothermia by extracorporeal rewarming in a child. *J Trauma.* 1996;40:483–485.

415. Farstad M, Andersen KS, Koller ME, Grong K, Segadal L, Husby P. Rewarming from accidental hypothermia by extracorporeal circulation: a retrospective study. *Eur J Cardiothorac Surg.* 2001;20:58–64.

416. Kangas E, Niemela H, Kojo N. Treatment of hypothermic circulatory arrest with thoracotomy and pleural lavage. *Ann Chir Gynaecol.* 1994;83:258–260.

417. Plaisier BR. Thoracic lavage in accidental hypothermia with cardiac arrest: report of a case and review of the literature. *Resuscitation.* 2005;66:99–104.

418. Winegard C. Successful treatment of severe hypothermia and prolonged cardiac arrest with closed thoracic cavity lavage. *J Emerg Med.* 1997;15:629–632.

419. Walters DT. Closed thoracic cavity lavage for hypothermia with cardiac arrest. *Ann Emerg Med.* 1991;20:439–440.

420. Hall KN, Syverud SA. Closed thoracic cavity lavage in the treatment of severe hypothermia in human beings. *Ann Emerg Med.* 1990;19:204–206.

421. Oberhammer R, Beikircher W, Hormann C, Lorenz I, Pycha R, Adler-Kastner L, Brugger H. Full recovery of an avalanche victim with profound hypothermia and prolonged cardiac arrest treated by extracorporeal re-warming. *Resuscitation.* 2008;76:474–480.

422. Tiruvoipati R, Balasubramanian SK, Khoshbin E, Hadjinikolaou L, Sosnowski AW, Firmin RK. Successful use of venovenous extracorporeal membrane oxygenation in accidental hypothermic cardiac arrest. *ASAIO J.* 2005;51:474–476.

423. Scaife ER, Connors RC, Morris SE, Nichol PF, Black RE, Matlak ME, Hansen K, Bolte RG. An established extracorporeal membrane oxygenation protocol promotes survival in extreme hypothermia. *J Pediatr Surg.* 2007;42:2012–2016.

424. Weinberg AD. The role of inhalation rewarming in the early management of hypothermia. *Resuscitation.* 1998;36:101–104.

425. Steinman AM. Cardiopulmonary resuscitation and hypothermia. *Circulation.* 1986;74(pt 2):IV-29–IV-32.

426. Danzl DF, Pozos RS, Auerbach PS, Glazer S, Goetz W, Johnson E, Jui J, Lilja P, Marx JA, Miller J, Mills W Jr, Nowak R, Shields R, Vicario S, Wayne M. Multicenter hypothermia survey. *Ann Emerg Med.* 1987;16:1042–1055.

427. Incagnoli P, Bourgeois B, Teboul A, Laborie JM. Resuscitation from accidental hypothermia of 22 degrees C with circulatory arrest: importance of prehospital management [in French]. *Ann Fr Anesth Reanim.* 2006;25:535–538.

428. Boddicker KA, Zhang Y, Zimmerman MB, Davies LR, Kerber RE. Hypothermia improves defibrillation success and resuscitation outcomes from ventricular fibrillation. *Circulation.* 2005;111:3195–3201.

429. Reuler JB. Hypothermia: pathophysiology, clinical settings, and management. *Ann Intern Med.* 1978;89:519–527.

430. Elenbaas RM, Mattson K, Cole H, Steele M, Ryan J, Robinson W. Bretylium in hypothermia-induced ventricular fibrillation in dogs. *Ann Emerg Med.* 1984;13:994–999.

431. Kornberger E, Lindner KH, Mayr VD, Schwarz B, Rackwitz KS, Wenzel V, Krismer AC, Mair P. Effects of epinephrine in a pig model of hypothermic cardiac arrest and closed-chest cardiopulmonary resuscitation combined with active rewarming. *Resuscitation.* 2001;50:301–308.

432. Schwarz B, Mair P, Raedler C, Deckert D, Wenzel V, Lindner KH. Vasopressin improves survival in a pig model of hypothermic cardiopulmonary resuscitation. *Crit Care Med.* 2002;30:1311–1314.

433. Schwarz B, Mair P, Wagner-Berger H, Stadlbauer KH, Girg S, Wenzel V, Lindner KH. Neither vasopressin nor amiodarone improve CPR outcome in an animal model of hypothermic cardiac arrest. *Acta Anaesthesiol Scand.* 2003;47:1114–1118.

434. Stoner J, Martin G, O'Mara K, Ehlers J, Tomlanovich M. Amiodarone and bretylium in the treatment of hypothermic ventricular fibrillation in a canine model. *Acad Emerg Med.* 2003;10:187–191.

435. Wira C, Martin G, Stoner J, Margolis K, Donnino M. Application of normothermic cardiac arrest algorithms to hypothermic cardiac arrest in a canine model. *Resuscitation.* 2006;69:509–516.

436. Wira CR, Becker JU, Martin G, Donnino MW. Anti-arrhythmic and vasopressor medications for the treatment of ventricular fibrillation in severe hypothermia: a systematic review of the literature. *Resuscitation.* 2008;78:21–29.

437. Lienhart HG, John W, Wenzel V. Cardiopulmonary resuscitation of a near-drowned child with a combination of epinephrine and vasopressin. *Pediatr Crit Care Med.* 2005;6:486–488.

438. Kjaergaard B, Jakobsen LK, Nielsen C, Knudsen PJ, Kristensen SR, Larsson A. Low plasma potassium in deep hypothermic cardiac arrest indicates that cardiac arrest is secondary to hypothermia: a porcine study. *Eur J Emerg Med.* 2010;17:131–135.

439. Falk M, Brugger H, Adler-Kastner L. Avalanche survival chances. *Nature.* 1994;368:21.

440. Buser O, Etter HJ, Jaccard C. Probability of dying in an avalanche [in German]. *Z Unfallchir Versicherungsmed.* 1993;suppl 1:263–271.

441. Brugger H, Falk M. New perspectives of avalanche disasters: phase classification using pathophysiologic considerations [in German]. *Wien Klin Wochenschr.* 1992;104:167–173.

442. Brugger H, Durrer B, Adler-Kastner L, Falk M, Tschirky F. Field management of avalanche victims. *Resuscitation.* 2001;51:7–15.

443. Locher T, Walpoth B, Pfluger D, Althaus U. Accidental hypothermia in Switzerland (1980–1987): case reports and prognostic factors [in German]. *Schweiz Med Wochenschr.* 1991;121:1020–1028.

444. Mair P, Kornberger E, Furtwaengler W, Balogh D, Antretter H. Prognostic markers in patients with severe accidental hypothermia and cardiocirculatory arrest. *Resuscitation.* 1994;27:47–54.

445. Grosse AB, Grosse CA, Steinbach LS, Zimmermann H, Anderson S. Imaging findings of avalanche victims. *Skeletal Radiol.* 2007;36:515–521.

446. Stalsberg H, Albretsen C, Gilbert M, Kearney M, Moestue E, Nordrum I, Rostrup M, Orbo A. Mechanism of death in avalanche victims. *Virchows Arch A Pathol Anat Histopathol.* 1989;414:415–422.

447. Oberhammer R, Beikircher W, Hormann C, Lorenz I, Pycha R, Adler-Kastner L, Brugger H. Full recovery of an avalanche victim with profound hypothermia and prolonged cardiac arrest treated by extracorporeal re-warming. *Resuscitation.* 2008;76:474–480.

448. Radwin MI, Grissom CK. Technological advances in avalanche survival. *Wilderness Environ Med.* 2002;13:143–152.

449. Paal P, Ellerton J, Sumann G, Demetz F, Mair P, Brugger H. Basic life support ventilation in mountain rescue: official recommendations of the International Commission for Mountain Emergency Medicine (ICAR MEDCOM). *High Alt Med Biol.* 2007;8:147–154.

450. Locher T, Walpoth BH. Differential diagnosis of circulatory failure in hypothermic avalanche victims: retrospective analysis of 32 avalanche accidents [in German]. *Praxis (Bern 1994)*. 1996;85:1275–1282.

451. Farstad M, Andersen KS, Koller ME, Grong K, Segadal L, Husby P. Rewarming from accidental hypothermia by extracorporeal circulation: a retrospective study. *Eur J Cardiothorac Surg*. 2001;20:58–64.

452. Schaller MD, Fischer AP, Perret CH. Hyperkalemia: a prognostic factor during acute severe hypothermia. *JAMA*. 1990;264:1842–1845.

453. Danzl DF, Pozos RS, Auerbach PS, Glazer S, Goetz W, Johnson E, Jui J, Lilja P, Marx JA, Miller J, Mills W Jr, Nowak R, Shields R, Vicario S, Wayne M. Multicenter hypothermia survey. *Ann Emerg Med*. 1987;16: 1042–1055.

454. Ruttmann E, Weissenbacher A, Ulmer H, Muller L, Hofer D, Kilo J, Rabl W, Schwarz B, Laufer G, Antretter H, Mair P. Prolonged extra-corporeal membrane oxygenation-assisted support provides improved survival in hypothermic patients with cardiocirculatory arrest. *J Thorac Cardiovasc Surg*. 2007;134:594–600.

455. Silfvast T, Pettila V. Outcome from severe accidental hypothermia in Southern Finland: a 10-year review. *Resuscitation*. 2003;59:285–290.

456. Hauty MG, Esrig BC, Hill JG, Long WB. Prognostic factors in severe accidental hypothermia: experience from the Mt. Hood tragedy. *J Trauma*. 1987;27:1107–1112.

457. Dobson JA, Burgess JJ. Resuscitation of severe hypothermia by extra-corporeal rewarming in a child. *J Trauma*. 1996;40:483–485.

458. Peden MM, McGee K. The epidemiology of drowning worldwide. *Inj Control Saf Promot*. 2003;10:195–199.

459. Warner DS, Bierens JJ, Beerman SB, Katz LM. Drowning: a cry for help. *Anesthesiology*. 2009;110:1211–1213.

460. Joost, JLM *Handbook on Drowning*. Berlin: Springer; 2004.

461. Papa L, Hoelle R, Idris A. Systematic review of definitions for drowning incidents. *Resuscitation*. 2005;65:255–264.

462. Idris AH, Berg RA, Bierens J, Bossaert L, Branche CM, Gabrielli A, Graves SA, Handley AJ, Hoelle R, Morley PT, Papa L, Pepe PE, Quan L, Szpilman D, Wigginton JG, Modell JH. Recommended guidelines for uniform reporting of data from drowning: the "Utstein style." *Resuscitation*. 2003; 59:45–57.

463. Youn CS, Choi SP, Yim HW, Park KN. Out-of-hospital cardiac arrest due to drowning: an Utstein Style report of 10 years of experience from St. Mary's Hospital. *Resuscitation*. 2009;80:778–783.

464. Quan L, Wentz KR, Gore EJ, Copass MK. Outcome and predictors of outcome in pediatric submersion victims receiving prehospital care in King County, Washington. *Pediatrics*. 1990;86:586–593.

465. Modell JH, Davis JH. Electrolyte changes in human drowning victims. *Anesthesiology*. 1969;30:414–420.

466. Southwick FS, Dalglish PH Jr. Recovery after prolonged asystolic cardiac arrest in profound hypothermia: a case report and literature review. *JAMA*. 1980;243:1250–1253.

467. Siebke H, Rød T, Breivik H, Lind B. Survival after 40 minutes' sub-mersion without cerebral sequelae. *Lancet*. 1975;1:1275–1277.

468. Bolte RG, Black PG, Bowers RS, Thorne JK, Corneli HM. The use of extracorporeal rewarming in a child submerged for 66 minutes. *JAMA*. 1988;260:377–379.

469. Gilbert M, Busund R, Skagseth A, Nilsen PÅ, Solbø JP. Resuscitation from accidental hypothermia of 13.7°C with circulatory arrest. *Lancet*. 2000;355:375–376.

470. Szpilman D, Soares M. In-water resuscitation: is it worthwhile? *Resuscitation*. 2004;63:25–31.

471. Allman FD, Nelson WB, Pacentine GA, McComb G. Outcome fol-lowing cardiopulmonary resuscitation in severe pediatric near-drowning. *Am J Dis Child*. 1986;140:571–575.

472. Weinstein MD, Krieger BP. Near-drowning: epidemiology, pathophys-iology, and initial treatment. *J Emerg Med*. 1996;14:461–467.

473. Watson RS, Cummings P, Quan L, Bratton S, Weiss NS. Cervical spine injuries among submersion victims. *J Trauma*. 2001;51:658–662.

474. Hwang V, Shofer FS, Durbin DR, Baren JM. Prevalence of traumatic injuries in drowning and near drowning in children and adolescents. *Arch Pediatr Adolesc Med*. 2003;157:50–53.

475. Kyriacou DN, Arcinue EL, Peek C, Kraus JF. Effect of immediate resuscitation on children with submersion injury. *Pediatrics*. 1994;94(pt 1):137–142.

476. Modell JH. Drowning. *N Engl J Med*. 1993;328:253–256.

477. Rosen P, Stoto M, Harley J. The use of the Heimlich maneuver in near-drowning: Institute of Medicine report. *J Emerg Med*. 1995;13: 397–405.

478. Manolios N, Mackie I. Drowning and near-drowning on Australian beaches patrolled by life-savers: a 10-year study, 1973–1983. *Med J Aust*. 1988;148:165–167, 170–171.

479. Onarheim H, Vik V. Porcine surfactant (Curosurf) for acute respiratory failure after near-drowning in 12 year old. *Acta Anaesthesiol Scand*. 2004;48:778–781.

480. Staudinger T, Bankier A, Strohmaier W, Weiss K, Locker GJ, Knapp S, Roggla M, Laczika K, Frass M. Exogenous surfactant therapy in a patient with adult respiratory distress syndrome after near drowning. *Resuscitation*. 1997;35:179–182.

481. Suzuki H, Ohta T, Iwata K, Yamaguchi K, Sato T. Surfactant therapy for respiratory failure due to near-drowning. *Eur J Pediatr*. 1996;155: 383–384.

482. Cubattoli L, Franchi F, Coratti G. Surfactant therapy for acute respi-ratory failure after drowning: two children victim of cardiac arrest. *Resuscitation*. 2009;80:1088–1089.

483. Thalmann M, Trampitsch E, Haberfellner N, Eisendle E, Kraschl R, Kobinia G. Resuscitation in near drowning with extracorporeal membrane oxygenation. *Ann Thorac Surg*. 2001;72:607–608.

484. Fish RM, Geddes LA. Conduction of electrical current to and through the human body: a review. *Eplasty*. 2009;9:e44.

485. Budnick LD. Bathtub-related electrocutions in the United States, 1979 to 1982. *JAMA*. 1984;252:918–920.

486. Geddes LA, Bourland JD, Ford G. The mechanism underlying sudden death from electric shock. *Med Instrum*. 1986;20:303–315.

487. Medical aspects of lightning. National Weather Service Web site. Available at: www.lightningsafety.noaa.gov/medical.html. Accessed May 7, 2010.

488. Patten BM. Lightning and electrical injuries. *Neurol Clin*. 1992;10: 1047–1058.

489. Browne BJ, Gaasch WR. Electrical injuries and lightning. *Emerg Med Clin North Am*. 1992;10:211–229.

490. Kleiner JP, Wilkin JH. Cardiac effects of lightning stroke. *JAMA*. 1978;240:2757–2759.

491. Lichtenberg R, Dries D, Ward K, Marshall W, Scanlon P. Cardio-vascular effects of lightning strikes. *J Am Coll Cardiol*. 1993;21: 531–536.

492. Cooper MA. Emergent care of lightning and electrical injuries. *Semin Neurol*. 1995;15:268–278.

493. Milzman DP, Moskowitz L, Hardel M. Lightning strikes at a mass gathering. *South Med J*. 1999;92:708–710.

494. Duclos PJ, Sanderson LM. An epidemiological description of lightning-related deaths in the United States. *Int J Epidemiol*. 1990;19:673–679.

495. Epperly TD, Stewart JR. The physical effects of lightning injury. *J Fam Pract*. 1989;29:267–272.

496. Whitcomb D, Martinez JA, Daberkow D. Lightning injuries. *South Med J*. 2002;95:1331–1334.

497. Grogaard HK, Wik L, Eriksen M, Brekke M, Sunde K. Continuous mechanical chest compressions during cardiac arrest to facilitate resto-ration of coronary circulation with percutaneous coronary intervention. *J Am Coll Cardiol*. 2007;50:1093–1094.

498. Agostoni P, Cornelis K, Vermeersch P. Successful percutaneous treatment of an intraprocedural left main stent thrombosis with the support of an automatic mechanical chest compression device. *Int J Cardiol*. 2008;124:e19–e21.

499. Steen S, Sjoberg T, Olsson P, Young M. Treatment of out-of-hospital cardiac arrest with LUCAS, a new device for automatic mechanical compression and active decompression resuscitation. *Resuscitation*. 2005;67:25–30.

500. Larsen AI, Hjornevik AS, Ellingsen CL, Nilsen DW. Cardiac arrest with continuous mechanical chest compression during percutaneous coronary intervention: a report on the use of the LUCAS device. *Resuscitation*. 2007;75:454–459.

501. Wagner H, Terkelsen CJ, Friberg H, Harnek J, Kern K, Lassen JF, Olivecrona GK. Cardiac arrest in the catheterisation laboratory: a 5-year experience of using mechanical chest compressions to facilitate PCI during prolonged resuscitation efforts. *Resuscitation*. 2010;81:383–387.

502. Shawl FA, Domanski MJ, Wish MH, Davis M, Punja S, Hernandez TJ. Emergency cardiopulmonary bypass support in patients with cardiac arrest in the catheterization laboratory. *Cathet Cardiovasc Diagn*. 1990; 19:8–12.

503. Criley JM, Blaufuss AH, Kissel GL. Cough-induced cardiac com-pression: self-administered form of cardiopulmonary resuscitation. *JAMA*. 1976;236:1246–1250.

504. Criley JM, Blaufuss AH, Kissel GL. Self-administered cardiopulmonary resuscitation by cough-induced cardiac compression. *Trans Am Clin Climatol Assoc*. 1976;87:138–146.

505. Miller B, Lesnefsky E, Heyborne T, Schmidt B, Freeman K, Breckinridge S, Kelley K, Mann D, Reiter M. Cough-cardiopulmonary resuscitation in the cardiac catheterization laboratory: hemodynamics during an episode of prolonged hypotensive ventricular tachycardia. *Cathet Cardiovasc Diagn*. 1989;18:168–171.

506. Keeble W, Tymchak WJ. Triggering of the Bezold Jarisch reflex by reperfusion during primary PCI with maintenance of consciousness by cough CPR: a case report and review of pathophysiology. *J Invasive Cardiol*. 2008;20:E239–E242.

507. Saba SE, David SW. Sustained consciousness during ventricular fibrillation: case report of cough cardiopulmonary resuscitation. *Cathet Cardiovasc Diagn*. 1996;37:47–48.

508. Kato M, Dote K, Sasaki S, Takemoto H, Habara S, Hasegawa D. Intracoronary verapamil rapidly terminates reperfusion tachyarrhythmias in acute myocardial infarction. *Chest*. 2004;126:702–708.

509. Maggiolini S, Bozzano A, Russo P, Vitale G, Osculati G, Cantu E, Achilli F, Valagussa F. Echocardiography-guided pericardiocentesis with probe-mounted needle: report of 53 cases. *J Am Soc Echocardiogr*. 2001;14:821–824.

510. Salem K, Mulji A, Lonn E. Echocardiographically guided pericardiocentesis: the gold standard for the management of pericardial effusion and cardiac tamponade. *Can J Cardiol*. 1999;15:1251–1255.

511. Susini G, Pepi M, Sisillo E, Bortone F, Salvi L, Barbier P, Fiorentini C. Percutaneous pericardiocentesis versus subxiphoid pericardiotomy in cardiac tamponade due to postoperative pericardial effusion. *J Cardiothorac Vasc Anesth*. 1993;7:178–183.

512. Tsang TS, Barnes ME, Gersh BJ, Bailey KR, Seward JB. Outcomes of clinically significant idiopathic pericardial effusion requiring intervention. *Am J Cardiol*. 2003;91:704–707.

513. Tsang TS, Enriquez-Sarano M, Freeman WK, Barnes ME, Sinak LJ, Gersh BJ, Bailey KR, Seward JB. Consecutive 1127 therapeutic echocardiographically guided pericardiocenteses: clinical profile, practice patterns, and outcomes spanning 21 years. *Mayo Clin Proc*. 2002;77: 429–436.

514. Coats TJ, Keogh S, Clark H, Neal M. Prehospital resuscitative thoracotomy for cardiac arrest after penetrating trauma: rationale and case series. *J Trauma*. 2001;50:670–673.

515. Powell DW, Moore EE, Cothren CC, Ciesla DJ, Burch JM, Moore JB, Johnson JL. Is emergency department resuscitative thoracotomy futile care for the critically injured patient requiring prehospital cardiopulmonary resuscitation? *J Am Coll Surg*. 2004;199:211–215.

516. Lewis G, Knottenbelt JD. Should emergency room thoracotomy be reserved for cases of cardiac tamponade? *Injury*. 1991;22:5–6.

517. Wang JC, Jiang P, Huang J, Qian GS. The protective effects and mechanisms of peroxisome proliferator-activated receptor-gamma agonist in rats with acute lung injury [in Chinese]. *Zhonghua Jie He He Hu Xi Za Zhi*. 2008;31:425–430.

518. Dunning J, Fabbri A, Kohl PH, Levine A, Lockowandt U, Mackay J, Pavie AJ, Strang T, Versteegh MI, Nashef SA, EACTS Clinical Guidelines Committee. Guideline for resuscitation in cardiac arrest after cardiac surgery. *Eur J Cardiothorac Surg*. 2009;36:3–28.

519. Mackay JH, Powell SJ, Charman SC, Rozario C. Resuscitation after cardiac surgery: are we ageist? *Eur J Anaesthesiol*. 2004;21:66–71.

520. Raman J, Saldanha RF, Branch JM, Esmore DS, Spratt PM, Farnsworth AE, Harrison GA, Chang VP, Shanahan MX. Open cardiac compression in the postoperative cardiac intensive care unit. *Anaesth Intensive Care*. 1989;17:129–135.

521. Karhunen JP, Sihvo EI, Suojaranta-Ylinen RT, Ramo OJ, Salminen US. Predictive factors of hemodynamic collapse after coronary artery bypass grafting: a case-control study. *J Cardiothorac Vasc Anesth*. 2006;20: 143–148.

522. Anthi A, Tzelepis GE, Alivizatos P, Michalis A, Palatianos GM, Geroulanos S. Unexpected cardiac arrest after cardiac surgery: incidence, predisposing causes, and outcome of open chest cardiopulmonary resuscitation. *Chest*. 1998;113:15–19.

523. Dimopoulou I, Anthi A, Michalis A, Tzelepis GE. Functional status and quality of life in long-term survivors of cardiac arrest after cardiac surgery. *Crit Care Med*. 2001;29:1408–1411.

524. el-Banayosy A, Brehm C, Kizner L, Hartmann D, Kortke H, Korner MM, Minami K, Reichelt W, Korfer R. Cardiopulmonary resuscitation after cardiac surgery: a two-year study. *J Cardiothorac Vasc Anesth*. 1998;12:390–392.

525. Fairman RM, Edmunds LH Jr. Emergency thoracotomy in the surgical intensive care unit after open cardiac operation. *Ann Thorac Surg*. 1981;32:386–391.

526. Mackay JH, Powell SJ, Osgathorp J, Rozario CJ. Six-year prospective audit of chest reopening after cardiac arrest. *Eur J Cardiothorac Surg*. 2002;22:421–425.

527. Ngaage DL, Cowen ME. Survival of cardiorespiratory arrest after coronary artery bypass grafting or aortic valve surgery. *Ann Thorac Surg*. 2009;88:64–68.

528. Kriaras I, Anthi A, Michelopoulos A, Karakatsani A, Tzelepis G, Papadimitriou L, Geroulanos S. Antimicrobial protection in cardiac surgery patients undergoing open chest CPR. *Resuscitation*. 1996;31:10–11.

529. Rousou JA, Engelman RM, Flack JE III, Deaton DW, Owen SG. Emergency cardiopulmonary bypass in the cardiac surgical unit can be a lifesaving measure in postoperative cardiac arrest. *Circulation*. 1994;90(pt 2):II-280–II-284.

530. Beyersdorf F, Kirsh M, Buckberg GD, Allen BS. Warm glutamate/aspartate-enriched blood cardioplegic solution for perioperative sudden death. *J Thorac Cardiovasc Surg*. 1992;104:1141–1147.

531. Feng WC, Bert AA, Browning RA, Singh AK. Open cardiac massage and periresuscitative cardiopulmonary bypass for cardiac arrest following cardiac surgery. *J Cardiovasc Surg*. 1995;36:319–321.

532. Wahba A, Gotz W, Birnbaum DE. Outcome of cardiopulmonary resuscitation following open heart surgery. *Scand Cardiovasc J*. 1997;31: 147–149.

533. Pottle A, Bullock I, Thomas J, Scott L. Survival to discharge following open chest cardiac compression (OCCC): a 4-year retrospective audit in a cardiothoracic specialist centre: Royal Brompton and Harefield NHS Trust, United Kingdom. *Resuscitation*. 2002;52:269–272.

534. Kaiser GC, Naunheim KS, Fiore AC, Harris HH, McBride LR, Pennington DG, Barner HB, Willman VL. Reoperation in the intensive care unit. *Ann Thorac Surg*. 1990;49:903–907.

535. Bohrer H, Gust R, Bottiger BW. Cardiopulmonary resuscitation after cardiac surgery. *J Cardiothorac Vasc Anesth*. 1995;9:352.

536. Ricci M, Karamanoukian HL, D'Ancona G, Jajkowski MR, Bergsland J, Salerno TA. Avulsion of an H graft during closed-chest cardiopulmonary resuscitation after minimally invasive coronary artery bypass graft surgery. *J Cardiothorac Vasc Anesth*. 2000;14:586–587.

537. Chen YS, Chao A, Yu HY, Ko WJ, Wu IH, Chen RJ, Huang SC, Lin FY, Wang SS. Analysis and results of prolonged resuscitation in cardiac arrest patients rescued by extracorporeal membrane oxygenation. *J Am Coll Cardiol*. 2003;41:197–203.

538. Dalton HJ, Siewers RD, Fuhrman BP, Del Nido P, Thompson AE, Shaver MG, Dowhy M. Extracorporeal membrane oxygenation for cardiac rescue in children with severe myocardial dysfunction. *Crit Care Med*. 1993;21:1020–1028.

539. Ghez O, Feier H, Ughetto F, Fraisse A, Kreitmann B, Metras D. Postoperative extracorporeal life support in pediatric cardiac surgery: recent results. *ASAIO J*. 2005;51:513–516.

540. del Nido PJ, Dalton HJ, Thompson AE, Siewers RD. Extracorporeal membrane oxygenator rescue in children during cardiac arrest after cardiac surgery. *Circulation*. 1992;86(suppl):II-300–II-304.

541. Duncan BW, Ibrahim AE, Hraska V, del Nido PJ, Laussen PC, Wessel DL, Mayer JE Jr, Bower LK, Jonas RA. Use of rapid-deployment extracorporeal membrane oxygenation for the resuscitation of pediatric patients with heart disease after cardiac arrest. *J Thorac Cardiovasc Surg*. 1998;116:305–311.

542. Newsome LR, Ponganis P, Reichman R, Nakaji N, Jaski B, Hartley M. Portable percutaneous cardiopulmonary bypass: use in supported coronary angioplasty, aortic valvuloplasty, and cardiac arrest. *J Cardiothorac Vasc Anesth*. 1992;6:328–331.

543. Parra DA, Totapally BR, Zahn E, Jacobs J, Aldousany A, Burke RP, Chang AC. Outcome of cardiopulmonary resuscitation in a pediatric cardiac intensive care unit. *Crit Care Med*. 2000;28:3296–3300.

544. Overlie PA. Emergency use of cardiopulmonary bypass. *J Interv Cardiol*. 1995;8:239–247.

545. Cipolotti G, Paccagnella A, Simini G. Successful cardiopulmonary resuscitation using high doses of epinephrine. *Int J Cardiol*. 1991;33: 430–431.

546. Kron IL, DiMarco JP, Harman PK, Crosby IK, Mentzer RM Jr, Nolan SP, Wellons HA Jr. Unanticipated postoperative ventricular tachyarrhythmias. *Ann Thorac Surg*. 1984;38:317–322.

KEY WORDS: cardiac arrest ■ defibrillation ■ emergency

# Part 13: Pediatric Basic Life Support

## 2010 American Heart Association Guidelines for Cardiopulmonary Resuscitation and Emergency Cardiovascular Care

Marc D. Berg, Chair; Stephen M. Schexnayder; Leon Chameides; Mark Terry; Aaron Donoghue; Robert W. Hickey; Robert A. Berg; Robert M. Sutton; Mary Fran Hazinski

For best survival and quality of life, pediatric basic life support (BLS) should be part of a community effort that includes prevention, early cardiopulmonary resuscitation (CPR), prompt access to the emergency response system, and rapid pediatric advanced life support (PALS), followed by integrated post–cardiac arrest care. These 5 links form the American Heart Association (AHA) pediatric Chain of Survival (Figure 1), the first 3 links of which constitute pediatric BLS.

Rapid and effective bystander CPR can be associated with successful return of spontaneous circulation (ROSC) and neurologically intact survival in children following out-of-hospital cardiac arrest.[1–3] Bystander resuscitation may have the greatest impact for out-of-hospital respiratory arrest,[4] because survival rates >70% have been reported with good neurologic outcome.[5,6] Bystander resuscitation may also have substantial impact on survival from primary ventricular fibrillation (VF), because survival rates of 20% to 30% have been documented in children with sudden out-of-hospital witnessed VF.[7]

Overall about 6%[8] of children who suffer an out-of-hospital cardiac arrest and 8% of those who receive prehospital emergency response resuscitation survive, but many suffer serious permanent brain injury as a result of their arrest.[7,9–14] Out-of-hospital survival rates and neurological outcome can be improved with prompt bystander CPR,[3,6,15–17] but only about one third to one half of infants and children who suffer cardiac arrest receive bystander CPR.[3,9,12,18] Infants are less likely to survive out-of-hospital cardiac arrest (4%) than children (10%) or adolescents (13%), presumably because many infants included in the arrest figure are found dead after a substantial period of time, most from sudden infant death syndrome (SIDS).[8] As in adults, survival is greater in pediatric patients with an initial rhythm of VF or pulseless ventricular tachycardia (VT) than in those with asystole or pulseless electric activity.[7,8]

Results of in-hospital resuscitation are better with an overall survival of 27%.[19–21] The 2008 pediatric data from the National Registry of CardioPulmonary Resuscitation (NRCPR) recorded an overall survival of 33% for pulseless arrests among the 758 cases of in-hospital pediatric arrests that occurred in the participating hospitals. Pediatric patients with VF/pulseless VT had a 34% survival to discharge, while patients with pulseless electric activity had a 38% survival. The worst outcome was in patients with asystole, only 24% of whom survived to hospital discharge. Infants and children with a pulse, but poor perfusion and bradycardia who required CPR, had the best survival (64%) to discharge. Children are more likely to survive in-hospital arrests than adults,[19] and infants have a higher survival rate than children.[20]

## Prevention of Cardiopulmonary Arrest

In infants, the leading causes of death are congenital malformations, complications of prematurity, and SIDS. In children over 1 year of age, injury is the leading cause of death. Survival from traumatic cardiac arrest is rare, emphasizing the importance of injury prevention in reducing deaths.[22,23] Motor vehicle crashes are the most common cause of fatal childhood injuries; targeted interventions, such as the use of child passenger safety seats, can reduce the risk of death. Resources for the prevention of motor vehicle-related injuries are detailed on the US National Highway Traffic Safety Administration's website at www.nhtsa.gov. The World Health Organization provides information on the prevention of violence and injuries at www.who.int/violence_injury_prevention/en/.

## ABC or CAB?

The recommended sequence of CPR has previously been known by the initials "ABC": Airway, Breathing/ventilation, and Chest compressions (or Circulation). The *2010 AHA Guidelines for CPR and ECC* recommend a CAB sequence (chest compressions, airway, breathing/ventilations). This section will review some of the rationale for making the change for children as well as for adults.

During cardiac arrest high-quality CPR, particularly high-quality chest compressions are essential to generate

---

The American Heart Association requests that this document be cited as follows: Berg MD, Schexnayder SM, Chameides L, Terry M, Donoghue A, Hickey RW, Berg RA, Sutton RM, Hazinski MF. Part 13: pediatric basic life support: 2010 American Heart Association Guidelines for Cardiopulmonary Resuscitation and Emergency Cardiovascular Care. *Circulation*. 2010;122(suppl 3):S862–S875.

(*Circulation*. 2010;122[suppl 3]:S862–S875.)

*Circulation* is available at http://circ.ahajournals.org

DOI: 10.1161/CIRCULATIONAHA.110.971085

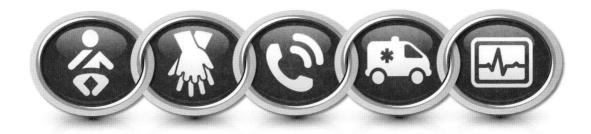

**Figure 1.** Pediatric Chain of Survival.

blood flow to vital organs and to achieve ROSC. The arguments in favor of starting with chest compressions are as follows:

- The vast majority of victims who require CPR are adults with VF cardiac arrest in whom compressions are more important than ventilations.[24] They have a better outcome if chest compressions are started as early as possible with minimal interruptions. Beginning CPR with 30 compressions rather than 2 ventilations leads to a shorter delay to first compression in adult studies.[25–27]
- All rescuers should be able to start chest compressions almost immediately. In contrast, positioning the head and attaining a seal for mouth-to-mouth or a bag-mask apparatus for rescue breathing take time and delays the initiation of chest compressions.

Asphyxial cardiac arrest is more common than VF cardiac arrest in infants and children, and ventilations are extremely important in pediatric resuscitation. Animal studies[28–30] and a recent large pediatric study[3] show that resuscitation results for asphyxial arrest are better with a combination of ventilations and chest compressions. It is, however, unknown whether it makes a difference if the sequence begins with ventilations (ABC) or with chest compressions (CAB). Starting CPR with 30 compressions followed by 2 ventilations should theoretically delay ventilations by only about 18 seconds for the lone rescuer and by an even a shorter interval for 2 rescuers. The CAB sequence for infants and children is recommended in order to simplify training with the hope that more victims of sudden cardiac arrest will receive bystander CPR. It offers the advantage of consistency in teaching rescuers, whether their patients are infants, children, or adults.

For the purposes of these guidelines

- Infant BLS guidelines apply to infants<approximately 1 year of age.
- Child BLS guidelines apply to children approximately 1 year of age until puberty. For teaching purposes puberty is defined as breast development in females and the presence of axillary hair in males.
- Adult BLS guidelines (see Part 5) apply at and beyond puberty.

## BLS Sequence for Lay Rescuers

These guidelines delineate a series of skills as a *sequence* of distinct steps depicted in the Pediatric BLS Algorithm,

but they should be performed *simultaneously* (eg, starting CPR and activating the emergency response system) when there is more than 1 rescuer.

### Safety of Rescuer and Victim

Always make sure that the area is safe for you and the victim. Although provision of CPR carries a theoretical risk of transmitting infectious disease, the risk to the rescuer is very low.[31]

### Assess Need for CPR

To assess the need for CPR, the lay rescuer should assume that cardiac arrest is present if the victim is unresponsive and not breathing or only gasping.

### Check for Response

Gently tap the victim and ask loudly, "Are you okay?" Call the child's name if you know it. If the child is responsive, he or she will answer, move, or moan. Quickly check to see if the child has any injuries or needs medical assistance. If you are alone and the child is breathing, leave the child to phone the emergency response system, but return quickly and recheck the child's condition frequently. Children with respiratory distress often assume a position that maintains airway patency and optimizes ventilation. Allow the child with respiratory distress to remain in a position that is most comfortable. If the child is unresponsive, shout for help.

### Check for Breathing

If you see regular breathing, the victim does not need CPR. If there is no evidence of trauma, turn the child onto the side (recovery position), which helps maintain a patent airway and decreases risk of aspiration.

If the victim is unresponsive and not breathing (or only gasping), begin CPR. Sometimes victims who require CPR will gasp, which may be misinterpreted as breathing. Treat the victim with gasps as though there is no breathing and begin CPR. Formal training as well as "just in time" training, such as that provided by an emergency response system dispatcher, should emphasize how to recognize the difference between gasping and normal breathing; rescuers should be instructed to provide CPR even when the unresponsive victim has occasional gasps (Class IIa, LOE C).

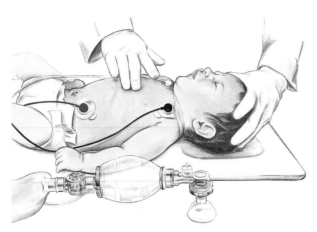

**Figure 2.** Two-finger chest compression technique in infant (1 rescuer).

## Start Chest Compressions

During cardiac arrest, high-quality chest compressions generate blood flow to vital organs and increase the likelihood of ROSC. If the infant or child is unresponsive and not breathing, give 30 chest compressions.

The following are characteristics of high-quality CPR:

- Chest compressions of appropriate rate and depth. "Push fast": push at a rate of at least 100 compressions per minute. "Push hard": push with sufficient force to depress at least one third the anterior-posterior (AP) diameter of the chest or approximately 1 ½ inches (4 cm) in infants and 2 inches (5 cm) in children (Class I, LOE C). Inadequate compression depth is common[32–34] even by health care providers.
- Allow complete chest recoil after each compression to allow the heart to refill with blood.
- Minimize interruptions of chest compressions.
- Avoid excessive ventilation.

For best results, deliver chest compressions on a firm surface.[35,36]

For an *infant,* lone rescuers (whether lay rescuers or healthcare providers) should compress the sternum with 2 fingers (Figure 2) placed just below the intermammary line (Class IIb, LOE C).[37–41] Do not compress over the xiphoid or ribs. Rescuers should compress at least one third the depth of the chest, or about 4 cm (1.5 inches).

For a *child,* lay rescuers and healthcare providers should compress the lower half of the sternum *at least* one third of the AP dimension of the chest or approximately 5 cm (2 inches) with the heel of 1 or 2 hands. Do not press on the xiphoid or the ribs. There are no data to determine if the 1- or 2-hand method produces better compressions and better outcome (Class IIb, LOE C). In a child manikin study, higher chest compression pressures were obtained[42] with less rescuer fatigue[43] with the 2-hand technique. Because children and rescuers come in all sizes, rescuers may use either 1 or 2 hands to compress the child's chest. Whichever you use, make sure to achieve an adequate compression depth with complete release after each compression.

After each compression, allow the chest to recoil completely (Class IIb, LOE B) because complete chest re-

expansion improves the flow of blood returning to the heart and thereby blood flow to the body during CPR.[44–46] During pediatric CPR incomplete chest wall recoil is common, particularly when rescuers become fatigued.[32,47,48] Incomplete recoil during CPR is associated with higher intrathoracic pressures and significantly decreased venous return, coronary perfusion, blood flow, and cerebral perfusion.[45,46] Manikin studies suggest that techniques to lift the heel of the hand slightly, but completely, off the chest can improve chest recoil, but this technique has not been studied in humans.[44,49] Automated CPR feedback devices hold promise as monitors of CPR quality parameters, including chest recoil, by providing real-time, corrective feedback to the rescuer. However, there is currently insufficient evidence for or against their use in infants and children.

Rescuer fatigue can lead to inadequate compression rate, depth, and recoil.[32,47,50] The quality of chest compressions may deteriorate within minutes even when the rescuer denies feeling fatigued.[51,52] Rescuers should therefore rotate the compressor role approximately every 2 minutes to prevent compressor fatigue and deterioration in quality and rate of chest compressions. Recent data suggest that when feedback devices are used and compressions are effective, some rescuers may be able to effectively continue past the 2-minute interval.[47] The switch should be accomplished as quickly as possible (ideally in less than 5 seconds) to minimize interruptions in chest compressions.

Resuscitation outcomes in infants and children are best if chest compressions are combined with ventilations (see below), but if a rescuer is not trained in providing ventilations, or is unable to do so, the lay rescuer should continue with chest compressions ("Hands-Only" or compression-only CPR) until help arrives.

## Open the Airway and Give Ventilations

For the lone rescuer a compression-to-ventilation ratio of 30:2 is recommended. After the initial set of 30 compressions, open the airway and give 2 breaths. In an unresponsive infant or child, the tongue may obstruct the airway and interfere with ventilations.[53–55] Open the airway using a head tilt–chin lift maneuver for both injured and noninjured victims (Class I, LOE B).

To give breaths to an infant, use a mouth-to-mouth-and-nose technique; to give breaths to a child, use a mouth-to-mouth technique.[56] Make sure the breaths are effective (ie, the chest rises). Each breath should take about 1 second. If the chest does not rise, reposition the head, make a better seal, and try again.[56] It may be necessary to move the child's head through a range of positions to provide optimal airway patency and effective rescue breathing.

In an infant, if you have difficulty making an effective seal over the mouth and nose, try either mouth-to-mouth or mouth-to-nose ventilation (Class IIb, LOE C).[57–59] If you use the mouth-to-mouth technique, pinch the nose closed. If you use the mouth-to-nose technique, close the mouth. In either case make sure the chest rises when you give a breath. If you are the only rescuer, provide 2 effective ventilations using as short a pause in chest compressions as possible after each set of 30 compressions (Class IIa, LOE C).

## Coordinate Chest Compressions and Breathing

After giving 2 breaths, immediately give 30 compressions. The lone rescuer should continue this cycle of 30 compressions and 2 breaths for approximately 2 minutes (about 5 cycles) before leaving the victim to activate the emergency response system and obtain an automated external defibrillator (AED) if one is nearby.

The ideal compression-to-ventilation ratio in infants and children is unknown. The following have been considered in recommending a compression-to-ventilation ratio of 30:2 for single rescuers:

- Evidence from manikin studies shows that lone rescuers cannot deliver the desired number of compressions per minute with the compression-to-ventilation ratio of 5:1 that was previously recommended (2000 and earlier).[60-63] For the lone rescuer, manikin studies show that a ratio of 30:2 yields more chest compressions than a 15:2 ratio with no, or minimal, increase in rescuer fatigue.[64-68]
- Volunteers recruited at an airport to perform single-rescuer layperson CPR on an adult manikin had less "no flow time" (ie, arrest time without chest compressions, when no blood flow is generated) with 30:2 compared with a 15:2 ratio.[69]
- An observational human study[70] comparing resuscitations by firefighters prior to and following the change from 15:2 to 30:2 compression-to-ventilation ratio reported more chest compressions per minute with a 30:2 ratio; ROSC was unchanged.
- Animal studies[71-73] show that coronary perfusion pressure, a major determinant of success in resuscitation, rapidly declines when chest compressions are interrupted; once compressions are resumed, several chest compressions are needed to restore coronary perfusion pressure. Thus, frequent interruptions of chest compressions prolong the duration of low coronary perfusion pressure and flow.
- Manikin studies,[25,69,74] as well as in- and out-of-hospital adult human studies,[33,34,75] have documented long interruptions in chest compressions. Adult studies[76-78] have also demonstrated that these interruptions reduce the likelihood of ROSC.

## Activate Emergency Response System

If there are 2 rescuers, one should start CPR immediately and the other should activate the emergency response system (in most locales by phoning 911) and obtain an AED, if one is available. Most infants and children with cardiac arrest have an asphyxial rather than a VF arrest[3,9,12]; therefore 2 minutes of CPR are recommended before the lone rescuer activates the emergency response system and gets an AED if one is nearby. The lone rescuer should then return to the victim as soon as possible and use the AED (if available) or resume CPR, starting with chest compressions. Continue with cycles of 30 compressions to 2 ventilations until emergency response rescuers arrive or the victim starts breathing spontaneously.

## BLS Sequence for Healthcare Providers and Others Trained in 2-Rescuer CPR

For the most part the sequence of BLS for healthcare providers is similar to that for laypeople with some variation as indicated below (see Figure 3). Healthcare providers are more likely to work in teams and less likely to be lone rescuers. Activities described as a series of individual sequences are often performed simultaneously (eg, chest compressions and preparing for rescue breathing) so there is less significance regarding which is performed first.

It is reasonable for healthcare providers to tailor the sequence of rescue actions to the most likely cause of arrest. For example, if the arrest is witnessed and sudden (eg, sudden collapse in an adolescent or a child identified at high risk for arrhythmia or during an athletic event), the healthcare provider may assume that the victim has suffered a sudden VF–cardiac arrest and as soon as the rescuer verifies that the child is unresponsive and not breathing (or only gasping) the rescuer should immediately phone the emergency response system, get the AED and then begin CPR and use the AED. (Class IIa LOE C).[2,7,79]

### Assess the Need for CPR (BOX 1)

If the victim is unresponsive and is not breathing (or only gasping), send someone to activate the emergency response system.

### Pulse Check (BOX 3)

If the infant or child is unresponsive and not breathing (gasps do not count as breathing), healthcare providers may take up to 10 seconds to attempt to feel for a pulse (brachial in an infant and carotid or femoral in a child). If, within 10 seconds, you don't feel a pulse or are not sure if you feel a pulse, begin chest compressions (Class IIa, LOE C). It can be difficult to feel a pulse, especially in the heat of an emergency, and studies show that healthcare providers,[80] as well as lay rescuers, are unable to reliably detect a pulse.[81-95]

### Inadequate Breathing With Pulse

If there is a palpable pulse ≥60 per minute but there is inadequate breathing, give rescue breaths at a rate of about 12 to 20 breaths per minute (1 breath every 3 to 5 seconds) until spontaneous breathing resumes (Box 3A). Reassess the pulse about every 2 minutes (Class IIa, LOE B) but spend no more than 10 seconds doing so.

### Bradycardia With Poor Perfusion

If the pulse is <60 per minute and there are signs of poor perfusion (ie, pallor, mottling, cyanosis) despite support of oxygenation and ventilation, begin chest compressions. Because cardiac output in infancy and childhood largely depends on heart rate, profound bradycardia with poor perfusion is an indication for chest compressions because cardiac arrest is imminent and beginning CPR prior to full cardiac arrest results in improved survival.[96] The absolute heart rate at which chest compressions should be initiated is unknown; the recommendation to provide chest compressions for a heart rate <60 per minute with signs of

**Pediatric BLS Healthcare Providers**

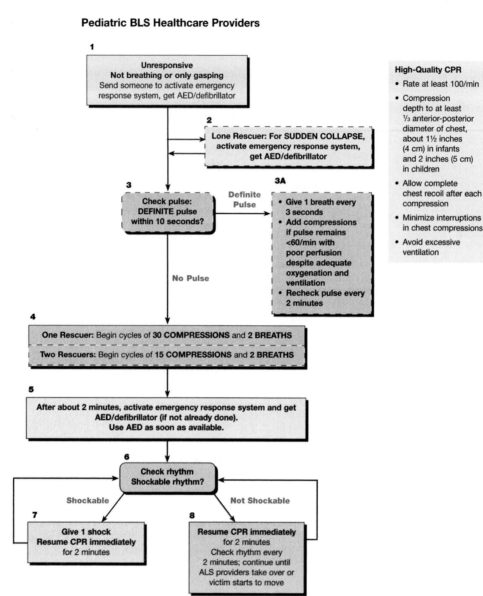

**Figure 3.** Pediatric BLS Algorithm.

poor perfusion is based on ease of teaching and retention of skills. For additional information see "Bradycardia" in Part 14: "Pediatric Advanced Life Support."

## Chest Compressions (BOX 4)

If the infant or child is unresponsive, not breathing, and has no pulse (or you are unsure whether there is a pulse), start chest compressions (see "Start Chest Compressions" in "BLS Sequence for Lay Rescuers"). The only difference in chest compressions for the healthcare provider is in chest compression for infants.

The lone healthcare provider should use the 2-finger chest compression technique for infants. The 2-thumb–encircling hands technique (Figure 4) is recommended when CPR is provided by 2 rescuers. Encircle the infant's chest with both hands; spread your fingers around the thorax, and place your thumbs together over the lower third of the sternum.[37–41,97–103] Forcefully compress the sternum with your thumbs. In the past, it has been recommended that the thorax be squeezed at the time of chest compression, but there is no data that show benefit from a circumferential squeeze. The 2-thumb–encircling hands technique is preferred over the 2-finger technique because it produces higher coronary artery perfusion pressure, results more consistently in appropriate depth or force of compression,[99–102] and may generate higher systolic and diastolic pressures.[97,98,103,104] If you cannot physically encircle the victim's chest, compress the chest with 2 fingers (see "Chest Compressions" above).

## Ventilations (Box 4)

After 30 compressions (15 compressions if 2 rescuers), open the airway with a head tilt–chin lift and give 2

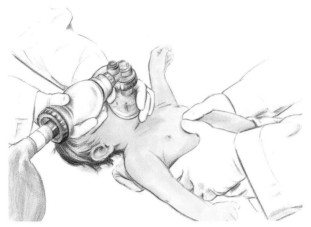

**Figure 4.** Two thumb-encircling hands chest compression in infant (2 rescuers).

breaths. If there is evidence of trauma that suggests spinal injury, use a jaw thrust without head tilt to open the airway (Class IIb LOE C).[55,105,106] Because maintaining a patent airway and providing adequate ventilation is important in pediatric CPR, use a head tilt–chin lift maneuver if the jaw thrust does not open the airway.

## Coordinate Chest Compressions and Ventilations

A lone rescuer uses a compression-to-ventilation ratio of 30:2. For 2-rescuer infant and child CPR, one provider should perform chest compressions while the other keeps the airway open and performs ventilations at a ratio of 15:2. Deliver ventilations with minimal interruptions in chest compressions (Class IIa, LOE C). If an advanced airway is in place, cycles of compressions and ventilations are no longer delivered. Instead the compressing rescuer should deliver at least 100 compressions per minute continuously without pauses for ventilation. The ventilation rescuer delivers 8 to 10 breaths per minute (a breath every 6 to 8 seconds), being careful to avoid excessive ventilation in the stressful environment of a pediatric arrest.

## Defibrillation (Box 6)

VF can be the cause of sudden collapse[7,107] or may develop during resuscitation attempts.[19,108] Children with sudden witnessed collapse (eg, a child collapsing during an athletic event) are likely to have VF or pulseless VT and need immediate CPR and rapid defibrillation. VF and pulseless VT are referred to as "shockable rhythms" because they respond to electric shocks (defibrillation).

Many AEDs have high specificity in recognizing pediatric shockable rhythms, and some are equipped to decrease (or attenuate) the delivered energy to make them suitable for infants and children <8 years of age.[109–111] For infants a manual defibrillator is preferred when a shockable rhythm is identified by a trained healthcare provider (Class IIb, LOE C). The recommended first energy dose for defibrillation is 2 J/kg. If a second dose is required, it should be doubled to 4 J/kg. If a manual defibrillator is not available, an AED equipped with a pediatric attenuator is

preferred for infants. An AED with a pediatric attenuator is also preferred for children <8 year of age. If neither is available, an AED without a dose attenuator may be used (Class IIb, LOE C). AEDs that deliver relatively high energy doses have been successfully used in infants with minimal myocardial damage and good neurological outcomes.[112,113]

Rescuers should coordinate chest compressions and shock delivery to minimize the time between compressions and shock delivery and to resume CPR, beginning with compressions, immediately after shock delivery. The AED will prompt the rescuer to re-analyze the rhythm about every 2 minutes. Shock delivery should ideally occur as soon as possible after compressions.

## Defibrillation Sequence Using an AED

Turn the AED on.

- Follow the AED prompts.
- End CPR cycle (for analysis and shock) with compressions, if possible
- Resume chest compressions immediately after the shock. Minimize interruptions in chest compressions.

## Hands-Only (Compression-Only) CPR

Optimal CPR for infants and children includes both compressions and ventilations (Class I LOE B). Animal studies[71–73,114,115] demonstrated that chest compressions alone, without ventilations, are sufficient to resuscitate VF-induced cardiac arrest. In contrast, in asphyxial cardiac arrest, 3 animal studies[28–30] showed that ventilations, when added to chest compressions, improved outcome. One large pediatric study demonstrated that bystander CPR with chest compressions and mouth-to-mouth rescue breathing is more effective than compressions alone when the arrest was from a noncardiac etiology.[3] In fact, although the numbers are small, outcomes from chest compressions-only CPR were no better than if no bystander resuscitation was provided for asphyxial arrest. In contrast, bystander CPR with compressions-only was as effective as compressions plus mouth-to-mouth rescue breathing for the 29% of arrests of cardiac etiology.[3] Thus ventilations are more important during resuscitation from asphyxia-induced arrest, the most common etiology in infants and children, than during resuscitation from VF or pulseless VT. But even in asphyxial arrest, fewer ventilations are needed to maintain an adequate ventilation-perfusion ratio in the presence of reduced cardiac output and, consequently, low pulmonary blood flow, achieved by chest compressions. Optimal CPR in infants and children includes both compressions and ventilations, but compressions alone are preferable to no CPR (Class 1 LOE B).

## Breathing Adjuncts

### Barrier Devices

Despite its safety,[31] some healthcare providers[116–118] and lay rescuers[9,119,120] may hesitate to give mouth-to-mouth rescue breathing without a barrier device. Barrier devices have not reduced the low risk of transmission of infec-

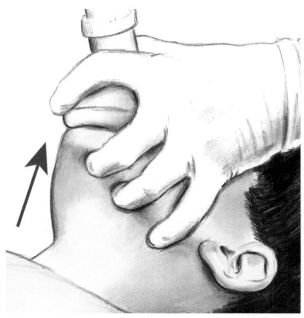

**Figure 5.** The EC clamp technique of bag-mask ventilations. Three fingers of one hand lift the jaw (they form the "E") while the thumb and index finger hold the mask to the face (making a "C").

tion,[31] and some may increase resistance to air flow.[121,122] If you use a barrier device, do not delay rescue breathing. If there is any delay in obtaining a barrier device or ventilation equipment, give mouth-to-mouth ventilation (if willing and able) or continue chest compressions alone.

### Bag-Mask Ventilation (Healthcare Providers)

Bag-mask ventilation is an essential CPR technique for healthcare providers. Bag-mask ventilation requires training and periodic retraining in the following skills: selecting the correct mask size, opening the airway, making a tight seal between the mask and face, delivering effective ventilation, and assessing the effectiveness of that ventilation.

Use a self-inflating bag with a volume of at least 450 to 500 mL[123] for infants and young children, as smaller bags may not deliver an effective tidal volume or the longer inspiratory times required by full-term neonates and infants.[124] In older children or adolescents, an adult self-inflating bag (1000 mL) may be needed to reliably achieve chest rise.

A self-inflating bag delivers only room air unless supplementary oxygen is attached, but even with an oxygen inflow of 10 L/min, the concentration of delivered oxygen varies from 30% to 80% and is affected by the tidal volume and peak inspiratory flow rate.[125] To deliver a high oxygen concentration (60% to 95%), attach an oxygen reservoir to the self-inflating bag. Maintain an oxygen flow of 10 to 15 L/min into a reservoir attached to a pediatric bag[125] and a flow of at least 15 L/min into an adult bag.

Effective bag-mask ventilation requires a tight seal between the mask and the victim's face. Open the airway by lifting the jaw toward the mask making a tight seal and squeeze the bag until the chest rises (see Figure 5). Because effective bag-mask ventilation requires complex steps, bag-mask ventilation is not recommended for a lone rescuer during CPR. During CPR the lone rescuer should use mouth-

to-barrier device techniques for ventilation. Bag-mask ventilation can be provided effectively during 2-person CPR.

### Precautions

Healthcare providers often deliver excessive ventilation during CPR,[34,126,127] particularly when an advanced airway is in place. Excessive ventilation is harmful because it

- Increases intrathoracic pressure and impedes venous return and therefore decreases cardiac output, cerebral blood flow, and coronary perfusion.[127]
- Causes air trapping and barotrauma in patients with small-airway obstruction.
- Increases the risk of regurgitation and aspiration in patients without an advanced airway.

Avoid excessive ventilation (Class III, LOE C); use only the force and tidal volume necessary to just make the chest rise. Give each breath slowly, over approximately 1 second, and watch for chest rise. If the chest does not rise, reopen the airway, verify that there is a tight seal between the mask and the face (or between the bag and the advanced airway), and reattempt ventilation.

Because effective bag-mask ventilation requires complex steps, bag-mask ventilation is not recommended for ventilation by a lone rescuer during CPR.

Patients with airway obstruction or poor lung compliance may require high inspiratory pressures to be properly ventilated (sufficient to produce chest rise). A pressure-relief valve may prevent the delivery of a sufficient tidal volume in these patients.[125] Make sure that the bag-mask device allows you to bypass the pressure-relief valve and use high pressures, if necessary, to achieve visible chest expansion.[128]

### Two-Person Bag-Mask Ventilation

If skilled rescuers are available, a 2-person technique may provide more effective bag-mask-ventilation than a single-person technique.[129] A 2-person technique may be required to provide effective bag-mask ventilation when there is significant airway obstruction, poor lung compliance,[128] or difficulty in creating a tight seal between the mask and the face. One rescuer uses both hands to open the airway and maintain a tight mask-to-face seal while the other compresses the ventilation bag. Both rescuers should observe the chest to ensure chest rise. Because the 2-person technique may be more effective, be careful to avoid delivering too high a tidal volume that may contribute to excessive ventilation.

### Gastric Inflation and Cricoid Pressure

Gastric inflation may interfere with effective ventilation[130] and cause regurgitation. To minimize gastric inflation

- Avoid creation of excessive peak inspiratory pressures by delivering each breath over approximately 1 second.[131]
- Cricoid pressure may be considered, but only in an unresponsive victim if there is an additional healthcare provider.[132–134] Avoid excessive cricoid pressure so as not to obstruct the trachea.[135]

### Oxygen

Animal and theoretical data suggest possible adverse effects of 100% oxygen,[136–139] but studies comparing various concentrations of oxygen during resuscitation have been performed only in the newborn period.[137,139–145] Until additional information becomes available, it is reasonable for healthcare providers to use 100% oxygen during resuscitation. Once circulation is restored, monitor systemic oxygen saturation, It may be reasonable, when appropriate equipment is available, to titrate oxygen administration to maintain the oxyhemoglobin saturation ≥94%. Provided appropriate equipment is available, once ROSC is achieved, adjust the $FIO_2$ to the minimum concentration needed to achieve transcutaneous or arterial oxygen saturation of at least 94% with the goal of avoiding hyperoxia while ensuring adequate oxygen delivery. Since an oxygen saturation of 100% may correspond to a $PaO_2$ anywhere between ~80 and 500 mm Hg, in general it is appropriate to wean the $FIO_2$ for a saturation of 100%, provided the oxyhemoglobin saturation can be maintained ≥94% (Class IIb, LOE C). Whenever possible, humidify oxygen to prevent mucosal drying and thickening of pulmonary secretions.

### Oxygen Masks

Simple oxygen masks can provide an oxygen concentration of 30% to 50% to a victim who is breathing spontaneously. To deliver a higher concentration of oxygen, use a tight-fitting nonrebreathing mask with an oxygen inflow rate of approximately 15 L/min to maintain inflation of the reservoir bag.

### Nasal Cannulas

Infant- and pediatric-size nasal cannulas are suitable for children with spontaneous breathing. The concentration of delivered oxygen depends on the child's size, respiratory rate, and respiratory effort,[146] but the concentration of inspired oxygen is limited unless a high-flow device is used.

## Other CPR Techniques and Adjuncts

There is insufficient data in infants and children to recommend for or against the use of the following: mechanical devices to compress the chest, active compression-decompression CPR, interposed abdominal compression CPR (IAC-CPR), the impedance threshold device, or pressure sensor accelerometer (feedback) devices. For further information, see Part 7: "CPR Devices" for adjuncts in adults.

## Foreign-Body Airway Obstruction (Choking)

### Epidemiology and Recognition

More than 90% of childhood deaths from foreign-body aspiration occur in children <5 years of age; 65% of the victims are infants. Liquids are the most common cause of choking in infants,[147] whereas balloons, small objects, and foods (eg, hot dogs, round candies, nuts, and grapes) are the most common causes of foreign-body airway obstruction (FBAO) in children.[148–151]

Signs of FBAO include a *sudden* onset of respiratory distress with coughing, gagging, stridor, or wheezing. Sudden onset of respiratory distress in the absence of fever or other respiratory symptoms (eg, antecedent cough, congestion) suggests FBAO rather than an infectious cause of respiratory distress, such as croup.

### Relief of FBAO

FBAO may cause mild or severe airway obstruction. When the airway obstruction is mild, the child can cough and make some sounds. When the airway obstruction is severe, the victim cannot cough or make any sound.

- If FBAO is mild, do not interfere. Allow the victim to clear the airway by coughing while you observe for signs of severe FBAO.
- If the FBAO is severe (ie, the victim is unable to make a sound) you must act to relieve the obstruction.

For a child perform subdiaphragmatic abdominal thrusts (Heimlich maneuver)[152,153] until the object is expelled or the victim becomes unresponsive. For an infant, deliver repeated cycles of 5 back blows (slaps) followed by 5 chest compressions[154–156] until the object is expelled or the victim becomes unresponsive. Abdominal thrusts are not recommended for infants because they may damage the infant's relatively large and unprotected liver.

If the victim becomes unresponsive, start CPR with chest compressions (do not perform a pulse check). After 30 chest compressions, open the airway. If you see a foreign body, remove it but do not perform blind finger sweeps because they may push obstructing objects farther into the pharynx and may damage the oropharynx.[157–159] Attempt to give 2 breaths and continue with cycles of chest compressions and ventilations until the object is expelled. After 2 minutes, if no one has already done so, activate the emergency response system.

## Special Resuscitation Situations

### Children With Special Healthcare Needs

Children with special healthcare needs may require emergency care for complications of chronic conditions (eg, obstruction of a tracheostomy), failure of support technology (eg, ventilator malfunction), progression of underlying disease, or events unrelated to those special needs.[160] Care is often complicated by a lack of medical information, a comprehensive plan of medical care, a list of current medications, and lack of clarity in limitation of resuscitation orders such as "Do Not Attempt Resuscitation (DNAR)" or "Allow Natural Death (AND)." Parents and child-care providers of children with special healthcare needs are encouraged to keep copies of medical information at home, with the child, and at the child's school or child-care facility. School nurses should have copies and should maintain a readily available list of children with DNAR/AND orders.[160,161] An Emergency Information Form (EIF) developed by the American Academy of Pediatrics and the

American College of Emergency Physicians[162] is available online (www.aap.org/advocacy/EIFTemp09.pdf).

### Advanced Directives

If a decision to limit or withhold resuscitative efforts is made, the physician must write an order clearly detailing the limits of any attempted resuscitation. A separate order must be written for the out-of-hospital setting. Regulations regarding out-of-hospital DNAR or AND directives vary from state to state.

When a child with a chronic or potentially life-threatening condition is discharged from the hospital, parents, school nurses, and home healthcare providers should be informed about the reason for hospitalization, a summary of the hospital course, and how to recognize signs of deterioration. They should receive specific instructions about CPR and whom to contact.[161]

### Ventilation With a Tracheostomy or Stoma

Everyone involved with the care of a child with a tracheostomy (parents, school nurses, and home healthcare providers) should know how to assess patency of the airway, clear the airway, change the tracheostomy tube, and perform CPR using the artificial airway.

Use the tracheostomy tube for ventilation and verify adequacy of airway and ventilation by watching for chest expansion. If the tracheostomy tube does not allow effective ventilation even after suctioning, replace it. If you are still unable to achieve chest rise, remove the tracheostomy tube and attempt alternative ventilation methods, such as mouth-to-stoma ventilation or bag-mask ventilation through the nose and mouth (while you or someone else occludes the tracheal stoma).

### Trauma

The principles of BLS resuscitation for the injured child are the same as those for the ill child, but some aspects require emphasis.

The following are important aspects of resuscitation of pediatric victims of trauma:

- Anticipate airway obstruction by dental fragments, blood, or other debris. Use a suction device if necessary.
- Stop all external bleeding with direct pressure.
- When the mechanism of injury is compatible with spinal injury, minimize motion of the cervical spine and movement of the head and neck.
- Professional rescuers should open and maintain the airway with a jaw thrust and try not to tilt the head. If a jaw thrust does not open the airway, use a head tilt–chin lift, because a patent airway is necessary. If there are 2 rescuers, 1 can manually restrict cervical spine motion while the other rescuer opens the airway.
- To limit spine motion, secure at least the thighs, pelvis, and shoulders to the immobilization board. Because of the disproportionately large size of the head in infants and young children, optimal positioning may require recessing the occiput[163] or elevating the torso to avoid undesirable backboard-induced cervical flexion.[163,164]
- If possible, transport children with potential for serious trauma to a trauma center with pediatric expertise.

### Drowning

Outcome after drowning is determined by the duration of submersion, the water temperature, and how promptly and effectively CPR is provided.[1,16,165] Neurologically intact survival has been reported after prolonged submersion in icy waters.[166,167] Start resuscitation by safely removing the victim from the water as rapidly as possible. If you have special training, start rescue breathing while the victim is still in the water[168] if doing so will not delay removing the victim from the water. Do not attempt chest compressions in the water.

After removing the victim from the water start CPR if the victim is unresponsive and is not breathing. If you are alone, continue with 5 cycles (about 2 minutes) of compressions and ventilations before activating the emergency response system and getting an AED. If 2 rescuers are present, send the second rescuer to activate the emergency response system immediately and get the AED while you continue CPR.

## The Quality of BLS

Immediate CPR can improve survival from cardiac arrest in children, but not enough children receive high-quality CPR. We must increase the number of laypersons who learn, remember, and perform CPR, and must improve the quality of CPR provided by lay rescuers and healthcare providers alike.

Healthcare systems that deliver CPR should implement processes of performance improvement. These include monitoring the time required for recognition and activation of the emergency response system, the quality of CPR delivered at the scene of cardiac arrest, other process-of-care measures (eg, initial rhythm, bystander CPR, and response intervals), and patient outcome up to hospital discharge (see Part 4: "Overview of CPR"). This evidence should be used to optimize the quality of CPR delivered.

# Disclosures

### Guidelines Part 13: Pediatric BLS Writing Group Disclosures

| Writing Group Member | Employment | Research Grant | Other Research Support | Speakers' Bureau/Honoraria | Ownership Interest | Consultant/ Advisory Board | Other |
|---|---|---|---|---|---|---|---|
| Marc D. Berg | University of Arizona/University Physician's Healthcare (UPH)–Associate Professor of Clinical Pediatrics and Member, Board of Directors | None | None | None | None | None | None |
| Stephen M. Schexnayder | University of Arkansas for Medical Sciences—Professor/Division Chief; AHA Compensated Consultant as Associate Senior Science Editor.† | *Pharmacokinetics of Proton Pump Inhibitors | None | *Contemporary Forums | None | None | |
| Leon Chameides | Emeritus Director Pediatric Cardiology, Connecticut Children's Medical Center Clinical Professor, University of Connecticut | None | None | None | None | None | None |
| Mark Terry | Johnson County Med-Act–Deputy Chief Operations | None | None | None | None | None | None |
| Aaron Donoghue | University of Pennsylvania–Assistant Professor of Pediatrics | None | None | None | None | None | None |
| Robert W. Hickey | University of Pittsburgh—MD | †Salary support on NIH grant to investigate the role of cylcopentenone prostaglandins in hypoxic-ischemic brain injury | None | None | None | None | |
| Robert A. Berg | University of Pennsylvania Professor | None | None | None | None | None | None |
| Robert M. Sutton | The Children's Hospital of Philadelphia–Critical Care Attending | None | None | None | None | None | None |
| Mary Fran Hazinski | Vanderbilt University School of Nursing—Professor; AHA ECC Product Development—Senior Science Editor. †Significant compensation from the AHA to provide protected time to edit, review, write for the development of the 2010 AHA Guidelines for CPR and ECC and the 2010 International Liaison Committee on Resuscitation Consensus on CPR and ECC Science with Treatment Recommendation | None | None | None | None | None | None |

This table represents the relationships of writing group members that may be perceived as actual or reasonably perceived conflicts of interest as reported on the Disclosure Questionnaire, which all members of the writing group are required to complete and submit. A relationship is considered to be "significant" if (a) the person receives $10 000 or more during any 12-month period, or 5% or more of the person's gross income; or (b) the person owns 5% or more of the voting stock or share of the entity, or owns $10 000 or more of the fair market value of the entity. A relationship is considered to be "modest" if it is less than "significant" under the preceding definition.

*Modest.
†Significant.

# References

1. Kyriacou DN, Arcinue EL, Peek C, Kraus JF. Effect of immediate resuscitation on children with submersion injury. *Pediatrics*. 1994;94(pt 1):137–142.
2. Hickey RW, Cohen DM, Strausbaugh S, Dietrich AM. Pediatric patients requiring CPR in the prehospital setting. *Ann Emerg Med*. 1995;25:495–501.
3. Kitamura T, Iwami T, Kawamura T, Nagao K, Tanaka H, Nadkarni VM, Berg RA, Hiraide A. Conventional and chest-compression-only cardiopulmonary resuscitation by bystanders for children who have out-of-hospital cardiac arrests: a prospective, nationwide, population-based cohort study. *Lancet*. 2010;375(9723):1347–1354.
4. Kuisma M, Alaspaa A. Out-of-hospital cardiac arrests of non-cardiac origin: epidemiology and outcome. *Eur Heart J*. 1997;18:1122–1128.
5. Friesen RM, Duncan P, Tweed WA, Bristow G. Appraisal of pediatric cardiopulmonary resuscitation. *Can Med Assoc J*. 1982; 126:1055–1058.
6. Lopez-Herce J, Garcia C, Rodriguez-Nunez A, Dominguez P, Carrillo A, Calvo C, Delgado MA. Long-term outcome of paediatric cardiorespiratory arrest in Spain. *Resuscitation*. 2005;64:79–85.
7. Mogayzel C, Quan L, Graves JR, Tiedeman D, Fahrenbruch C, Herndon P. Out-of-hospital ventricular fibrillation in children and adolescents: causes and outcomes. *Ann Emerg Med*. 1995;25:484–491.
8. Atkins DL, Everson-Stewart S, Sears GK, Daya M, Osmond MH, Warden CR, Berg RA. Epidemiology and outcomes from out-of-hospital cardiac arrest in children: the Resuscitation Outcomes Consortium Epistry-Cardiac Arrest. *Circulation*. 2009;119:1484–1491.

9. Sirbaugh PE, Pepe PE, Shook JE, Kimball KT, Goldman MJ, Ward MA, Mann DM. A prospective, population-based study of the demographics, epidemiology, management, and outcome of out-of-hospital pediatric cardiopulmonary arrest. *Ann Emerg Med.* 1999;33: 174–184.

10. Schindler MB, Bohn D, Cox PN, McCrindle BW, Jarvis A, Edmonds J, Barker G. Outcome of out-of-hospital cardiac or respiratory arrest in children. *N Engl J Med.* 1996;335:1473–1479.

11. O'Rourke PP. Outcome of children who are apneic and pulseless in the emergency room. *Crit Care Med.* 1986;14:466–468.

12. Young KD, Seidel JS. Pediatric cardiopulmonary resuscitation: a collective review. *Ann Emerg Med.* 1999;33:195–205.

13. Dieckmann RA, Vardis R. High-dose epinephrine in pediatric out-of-hospital cardiopulmonary arrest. *Pediatrics.* 1995;95:901–913.

14. Herlitz J, Engdahl J, Svensson L, Young M, Angquist KA, Holmberg S. Characteristics and outcome among children suffering from out of hospital cardiac arrest in Sweden. *Resuscitation.* 2005;64:37–40.

15. Lopez-Herce J, Garcia C, Dominguez P, Carrillo A, Rodriguez-Nunez A, Calvo C, Delgado MA. Characteristics and outcome of cardiorespiratory arrest in children. *Resuscitation.* 2004;63:311–320.

16. Suominen P, Baillie C, Korpela R, Rautanen S, Ranta S, Olkkola KT. Impact of age, submersion time and water temperature on outcome in near-drowning. *Resuscitation.* 2002;52:247–254.

17. Kuisma M, Suominen P, Korpela R. Paediatric out-of-hospital cardiac arrests: epidemiology and outcome. *Resuscitation.* 1995;30:141–150.

18. Pell JP, Sirel JM, Marsden AK, Ford I, Walker NL, Cobbe SM. Presentation, management, and outcome of out of hospital cardiopulmonary arrest: comparison by underlying aetiology. *Heart.* 2003;89:839–842.

19. Nadkarni VM, Larkin GL, Peberdy MA, Carey SM, Kaye W, Mancini ME, Nichol G, Lane-Truitt T, Potts J, Ornato JP, Berg RA. First documented rhythm and clinical outcome from in-hospital cardiac arrest among children and adults. *JAMA.* 2006;295:50–57.

20. Meaney PA, Nadkarni VM, Cook EF, Testa M, Helfaer M, Kaye W, Larkin GL, Berg RA. Higher survival rates among younger patients after pediatric intensive care unit cardiac arrests. *Pediatrics.* 2006;118: 2424–2433.

21. Tibballs J, Kinney S. A prospective study of outcome of in-patient paediatric cardiopulmonary arrest. *Resuscitation.* 2006;71:310–318.

22. Crewdson K, Lockey D, Davies G. Outcome from paediatric cardiac arrest associated with trauma. *Resuscitation.* 2007;75:29–34.

23. Donoghue AJ, Nadkarni V, Berg RA, Osmond MH, Wells G, Nesbitt L, Stiell IG. Out-of-hospital pediatric cardiac arrest: an epidemiologic review and assessment of current knowledge. *Ann Emerg Med.* 2005; 46:512–522.

24. Rea TD, Cook AJ, Stiell IG, Powell J, Bigham B, Callaway CW, Chugh S, Aufderheide TP, Morrison L, Terndrup TE, Beaudoin T, Wittwer L, Davis D, Idris A, Nichol G. Predicting survival after out-of-hospital cardiac arrest: role of the Utstein data elements. *Ann Emerg Med.* 2010;55:249–257.

25. Assar D, Chamberlain D, Colquhoun M, Donnelly P, Handley AJ, Leaves S, Kern KB. Randomised controlled trials of staged teaching for basic life support, 1: skill acquisition at bronze stage. *Resuscitation.* 2000;45:7–15.

26. Heidenreich JW, Higdon TA, Kern KB, Sanders AB, Berg RA, Niebler R, Hendrickson J, Ewy GA. Single-rescuer cardiopulmonary resuscitation: 'two quick breaths'–an oxymoron. *Resuscitation.* 2004;62: 283–289.

27. Kobayashi M, Fujiwara A, Morita H, Nishimoto Y, Mishima T, Nitta M, Hayashi T, Hotta T, Hayashi Y, Hachisuka E, Sato K. A manikin-based observational study on cardiopulmonary resuscitation skills at the Osaka Senri medical rally. *Resuscitation.* 2008;78:333–339.

28. Berg RA, Hilwig RW, Kern KB, Babar I, Ewy GA. Simulated mouth-to-mouth ventilation and chest compressions (bystander cardiopulmonary resuscitation) improves outcome in a swine model of prehospital pediatric asphyxial cardiac arrest. *Crit Care Med.* 1999;27:1893–1899.

29. Berg RA, Hilwig RW, Kern KB, Ewy GA. "Bystander" chest compressions and assisted ventilation independently improve outcome from piglet asphyxial pulseless "cardiac arrest." *Circulation.* 2000;101: 1743–1748.

30. Iglesias JM, Lopez-Herce J, Urbano J, Solana MJ, Mencia S, Del Castillo J. Chest compressions versus ventilation plus chest compressions in a pediatric asphyxial cardiac arrest animal model. *Intensive Care Med.* 2010;36:712–716.

31. Mejicano GC, Maki DG. Infections acquired during cardiopulmonary resuscitation: estimating the risk and defining strategies for prevention. *Ann Intern Med.* 1998;129:813–828.

32. Sutton RM, Niles D, Nysaether J, Abella BS, Arbogast KB, Nishisaki A, Maltese MR, Donoghue A, Bishnoi R, Helfaer MA, Myklebust H, Nadkarni V. Quantitative analysis of CPR quality during in-hospital resuscitation of older children and adolescents. *Pediatrics.* 2009;124: 494–499.

33. Wik L, Kramer-Johansen J, Myklebust H, Sorebo H, Svensson L, Fellows B, Steen PA. Quality of cardiopulmonary resuscitation during out-of-hospital cardiac arrest. *JAMA.* 2005;293:299–304.

34. Abella BS, Alvarado JP, Myklebust H, Edelson DP, Barry A, O'Hearn N, Vanden Hoek TL, Becker LB. Quality of cardiopulmonary resuscitation during in-hospital cardiac arrest. *JAMA.* 2005;293:305–310.

35. Nishisaki A, Nysaether J, Sutton R, Maltese M, Niles D, Donoghue A, Bishnoi R, Helfaer M, Perkins GD, Berg R, Arbogast K, Nadkarni V. Effect of mattress deflection on CPR quality assessment for older children and adolescents. *Resuscitation.* 2009;80:540–545.

36. Noordergraaf GJ, Paulussen IW, Venema A, van Berkom PF, Woerlee PH, Scheffer GJ, Noordergraaf A. The impact of compliant surfaces on in-hospital chest compressions: effects of common mattresses and a backboard. *Resuscitation.* 2009;80:546–552.

37. Clements F, McGowan J. Finger position for chest compressions in cardiac arrest in infants. *Resuscitation.* 2000;44:43–46.

38. Finholt DA, Kettrick RG, Wagner HR, Swedlow DB. The heart is under the lower third of the sternum: implications for external cardiac massage. *Am J Dis Child.* 1986;140:646–649.

39. Phillips GW, Zideman DA. Relation of infant heart to sternum: its significance in cardiopulmonary resuscitation. *Lancet.* 1986;1: 1024–1025.

40. Orlowski JP. Optimum position for external cardiac compression in infants and young children. *Ann Emerg Med.* 1986;15:667–673.

41. Shah NM, Gaur HK. Position of heart in relation to sternum and nipple line at various ages. *Indian Pediatr.* 1992;29:49–53.

42. Stevenson AG, McGowan J, Evans AL, Graham CA. CPR for children: one hand or two? *Resuscitation.* 2005;64:205–208.

43. Peska E, Kelly AM, Kerr D, Green D. One-handed versus two-handed chest compressions in paediatric cardio-pulmonary resuscitation. *Resuscitation.* 2006;71:65–69.

44. Aufderheide TP, Pirrallo RG, Yannopoulos D, Klein JP, von Briesen C, Sparks CW, Deja KA, Conrad CJ, Kitscha DJ, Provo TA, Lurie KG. Incomplete chest wall decompression: a clinical evaluation of CPR performance by EMS personnel and assessment of alternative manual chest compression-decompression techniques. *Resuscitation.* 2005;64: 353–362.

45. Yannopoulos D, McKnite S, Aufderheide TP, Sigurdsson G, Pirrallo RG, Benditt D, Lurie KG. Effects of incomplete chest wall decompression during cardiopulmonary resuscitation on coronary and cerebral perfusion pressures in a porcine model of cardiac arrest. *Resuscitation.* 2005;64:363–372.

46. Zuercher M, Hilwig RW, Ranger-Moore J, Nysaether J, Nadkarni VM, Berg MD, Kern KB, Sutton R, Berg RA. Leaning during chest compressions impairs cardiac output and left ventricular myocardial blood flow in piglet cardiac arrest. *Crit Care Med.* 2010;38:1141–1146.

47. Sutton RM, Maltese MR, Niles D, French B, Nishisaki A, Arbogast KB, Donoghue A, Berg RA, Helfaer MA, Nadkarni V. Quantitative analysis of chest compression interruptions during in-hospital resuscitation of older children and adolescents. *Resuscitation.* 2009;80:1259–1263.

48. Niles D, Nysaether J, Sutton R, Nishisaki A, Abella BS, Arbogast K, Maltese MR, Berg RA, Helfaer M, Nadkarni V. Leaning is common during in-hospital pediatric CPR, and decreased with automated corrective feedback. *Resuscitation.* 2009;80:553–557.

49. Aufderheide TP, Pirrallo RG, Yannopoulos D, Klein JP, von Briesen C, Sparks CW, Deja KA, Kitscha DJ, Provo TA, Lurie KG. Incomplete chest wall decompression: A clinical evaluation of CPR performance by trained laypersons and an assessment of alternative manual chest compression-decompression techniques. *Resuscitation.* 2006;71: 341–351.

50. Ashton A, McCluskey A, Gwinnutt CL, Keenan AM. Effect of rescuer fatigue on performance of continuous external chest compressions over 3 min. *Resuscitation.* 2002;55:151–155.

51. Ochoa FJ, Ramalle-Gomara E, Lisa V, Saralegui I. The effect of rescuer fatigue on the quality of chest compressions. *Resuscitation.* 1998;37: 149–152.

52. Hightower D, Thomas SH, Stone CK, Dunn K, March JA. Decay in quality of closed-chest compressions over time. *Ann Emerg Med*. 1995; 26:300–303.

53. Ruben HM, Elam JO, et al. Investigations of pharyngeal xrays and perfomance by laymen. *Anesthesiology*. 1961;22:271–279.

54. Safar P, Aguto-Escarraga L. Compliance in apneic anesthetized adults. *Anesthesiology*. 1959;20:283–289.

55. Elam JO, Greene DG, Schneider MA, Ruben HM, Gordon AS, Hustead RF, Benson DW, Clements JA, Ruben A. Head-tilt method of oral resuscitation. *JAMA*. 1960;172:812–815.

56. Zideman DA. Paediatric and neonatal life support. *Br J Anaesth*. 1997; 79:178–187.

57. Tonkin SL, Davis SL, Gunn TR. Nasal route for infant resuscitation by mothers. *Lancet*. 1995;345:1353–1354.

58. Segedin E, Torrie J, Anderson B. Nasal airway versus oral route for infant resuscitation. *Lancet*. 1995;346:382.

59. Tonkin SL, Gunn AJ. Failure of mouth-to-mouth resuscitation in cases of sudden infant death. *Resuscitation*. 2001;48:181–184.

60. Dorph E, Wik L, Steen PA. Effectiveness of ventilation-compression ratios 1:5 and 2:15 in simulated single rescuer paediatric resuscitation. *Resuscitation*. 2002;54:259–264.

61. Greingor JL. Quality of cardiac massage with ratio compression-ventilation 5/1 and 15/2. *Resuscitation*. 2002;55:263–267.

62. Kinney SB, Tibballs J. An analysis of the efficacy of bag-valve-mask ventilation and chest compression during different compression-ventilation ratios in manikin-simulated paediatric resuscitation. *Resuscitation*. 2000;43: 115–120.

63. Srikantan SK, Berg RA, Cox T, Tice L, Nadkarni VM. Effect of one-rescuer compression/ventilation ratios on cardiopulmonary resuscitation in infant, pediatric, and adult manikins. *Pediatr Crit Care Med*. 2005;6:293–297.

64. Betz AE, Callaway CW, Hostler D, Rittenberger JC. Work of CPR during two different compression to ventilation ratios with real-time feedback. *Resuscitation*. 2008;79:278–282.

65. Haque IU, Udassi JP, Udassi S, Theriaque DW, Shuster JJ, Zaritsky AL. Chest compression quality and rescuer fatigue with increased compression to ventilation ratio during single rescuer pediatric CPR. *Resuscitation*. 2008;79:82–89.

66. Bjorshol CA, Soreide E, Torsteinbo TH, Lexow K, Nilsen OB, Sunde K. Quality of chest compressions during 10 min of single-rescuer basic life support with different compression: ventilation ratios in a manikin model. *Resuscitation*. 2008;77:95–100.

67. Deschilder K, De Vos R, Stockman W. The effect on quality of chest compressions and exhaustion of a compression–ventilation ratio of 30:2 versus 15:2 during cardiopulmonary resuscitation–a randomised trial. *Resuscitation*. 2007;74:113–118.

68. Yannopoulos D, Aufderheide TP, Gabrielli A, Beiser DG, McKnite SH, Pirrallo RG, Wigginton J, Becker L, Vanden Hoek T, Tang W, Nadkarni VM, Klein JP, Idris AH, Lurie KG. Clinical and hemodynamic comparison of 15:2 and 30:2 compression-to-ventilation ratios for cardiopulmonary resuscitation. *Crit Care Med*. 2006;34:1444–1449.

69. Odegaard S, Saether E, Steen PA, Wik L. Quality of lay person CPR performance with compression: ventilation ratios 15:2, 30:2 or continuous chest compressions without ventilations on manikins. *Resuscitation*. 2006;71:335–340.

70. Hostler D, Rittenberger JC, Roth R, Callaway CW. Increased chest compression to ventilation ratio improves delivery of CPR. *Resuscitation*. 2007;74:446–452.

71. Berg RA, Sanders AB, Kern KB, Hilwig RW, Heidenreich JW, Porter ME, Ewy GA. Adverse hemodynamic effects of interrupting chest compressions for rescue breathing during cardiopulmonary resuscitation for ventricular fibrillation cardiac arrest. *Circulation*. 2001;104: 2465–2470.

72. Kern KB, Hilwig RW, Berg RA, Sanders AB, Ewy GA. Importance of continuous chest compressions during cardiopulmonary resuscitation: improved outcome during a simulated single lay-rescuer scenario. *Circulation*. 2002;105:645–649.

73. Ewy GA, Zuercher M, Hilwig RW, Sanders AB, Berg RA, Otto CW, Hayes MM, Kern KB. Improved neurological outcome with continuous chest compressions compared with 30:2 compressions-to-ventilations cardiopulmonary resuscitation in a realistic swine model of out-of-hospital cardiac arrest. *Circulation*. 2007;116:2525–2530.

74. Heidenreich JW, Sanders AB, Higdon TA, Kern KB, Berg RA, Ewy GA. Uninterrupted chest compression CPR is easier to perform and remember than standard CPR. *Resuscitation*. 2004;63:123–130.

75. Valenzuela TD, Kern KB, Clark LL, Berg RA, Berg MD, Berg DD, Hilwig RW, Otto CW, Newburn D, Ewy GA. Interruptions of chest compressions during emergency medical systems resuscitation. *Circulation*. 2005;112: 1259–1265.

76. Abella BS, Sandbo N, Vassilatos P, Alvarado JP, O'Hearn N, Wigder HN, Hoffman P, Tynus K, Vanden Hoek TL, Becker LB. Chest compression rates during cardiopulmonary resuscitation are suboptimal: a prospective study during in-hospital cardiac arrest. *Circulation*. 2005; 111:428–434.

77. Eftestol T, Sunde K, Steen PA. Effects of interrupting precordial compressions on the calculated probability of defibrillation success during out-of-hospital cardiac arrest. *Circulation*. 2002;105:2270–2273.

78. Christenson J, Andrusiek D, Everson-Stewart S, Kudenchuk P, Hostler D, Powell J, Callaway CW, Bishop D, Vaillancourt C, Davis D, Aufderheide TP, Idris A, Stouffer JA, Stiell I, Berg R. Chest compression fraction determines survival in patients with out-of-hospital ventricular fibrillation. *Circulation*. 2009;120:1241–1247.

79. Appleton GO, Cummins RO, Larson MP, Graves JR. CPR and the single rescuer: at what age should you "call first" rather than "call fast"? *Ann Emerg Med*. 1995;25:492–494.

80. Tibballs J, Russell P. Reliability of pulse palpation by healthcare personnel to diagnose paediatric cardiac arrest. *Resuscitation*. 2009;80: 61–64.

81. Bahr J, Klingler H, Panzer W, Rode H, Kettler D. Skills of lay people in checking the carotid pulse. *Resuscitation*. 1997;35:23–26.

82. Brearley S, Shearman CP, Simms MH. Peripheral pulse palpation: an unreliable physical sign. *Ann R Coll Surg Engl*. 1992;74:169–171.

83. Cavallaro DL, Melker RJ. Comparison of two techniques for detecting cardiac activity in infants. *Crit Care Med*. 1983;11:189–190.

84. Inagawa G, Morimura N, Miwa T, Okuda K, Hirata M, Hiroki K. A comparison of five techniques for detecting cardiac activity in infants. *Paediatr Anaesth*. 2003;13:141–146.

85. Kamlin CO, O'Donnell CP, Everest NJ, Davis PG, Morley CJ. Accuracy of clinical assessment of infant heart rate in the delivery room. *Resuscitation*. 2006;71:319–321.

86. Lee CJ, Bullock LJ. Determining the pulse for infant CPR: time for a change? *Mil Med*. 1991;156:190–193.

87. Mather C, O'Kelly S. The palpation of pulses. *Anaesthesia*. 1996;51: 189–191.

88. Ochoa FJ, Ramalle-Gomara E, Carpintero JM, Garcia A, Saralegui I. Competence of health professionals to check the carotid pulse. *Resuscitation*. 1998;37:173–175.

89. Owen CJ, Wyllie JP. Determination of heart rate in the baby at birth. *Resuscitation*. 2004;60:213–217.

90. Sarti A, Savron F, Casotto V, Cuttini M. Heartbeat assessment in infants: a comparison of four clinical methods. *Pediatr Crit Care Med*. 2005;6:212–215.

91. Sarti A, Savron F, Ronfani L, Pelizzo G, Barbi E. Comparison of three sites to check the pulse and count heart rate in hypotensive infants. *Paediatr Anaesth*. 2006;16:394–398.

92. Tanner M, Nagy S, Peat JK. Detection of infant's heart beat/pulse by caregivers: a comparison of 4 methods. *J Pediatr*. 2000;137:429–430.

93. Whitelaw CC, Goldsmith LJ. Comparison of two techniques for determining the presence of a pulse in an infant. *Acad Emerg Med*. 1997;4: 153–154.

94. Dick WF, Eberle B, Wisser G, Schneider T. The carotid pulse check revisited: what if there is no pulse? *Crit Care Med*. 2000;28(11 Suppl): N183–185.

95. Eberle B, Dick WF, Schneider T, Wisser G, Doetsch S, Tzanova I. Checking the carotid pulse check: diagnostic accuracy of first responders in patients with and without a pulse. *Resuscitation*. 1996;33: 107–116.

96. Donoghue A, Berg RA, Hazinski MF, Praestgaard AH, Roberts K, Nadkarni VM. Cardiopulmonary resuscitation for bradycardia with poor perfusion versus pulseless cardiac arrest. *Pediatrics*. 2009;124: 1541–1548.

97. David R. Closed chest cardiac massage in the newborn infant. *Pediatrics*. 1988;81:552–554.

98. Todres ID, Rogers MC. Methods of external cardiac massage in the newborn infant. *J Pediatr*. 1975;86:781–782.

99. Menegazzi JJ, Auble TE, Nicklas KA, Hosack GM, Rack L, Goode JS. Two-thumb versus two-finger chest compression during CRP in a swine infant model of cardiac arrest. *Ann Emerg Med*. 1993;22:240–243.

100. Houri PK, Frank LR, Menegazzi JJ, Taylor R. A randomized, controlled trial of two-thumb vs two-finger chest compression in a swine infant model of cardiac arrest. *Prehosp Emerg Care.* 1997;1:65–67.

101. Dorfsman ML, Menegazzi JJ, Wadas RJ, Auble TE. Two-thumb vs two-finger chest compression in an infant model of prolonged cardiopulmonary resuscitation. *Acad Emerg Med.* 2000;7:1077–1082.

102. Whitelaw CC, Slywka B, Goldsmith LJ. Comparison of a two-finger versus two-thumb method for chest compressions by healthcare providers in an infant mechanical model. *Resuscitation.* 2000;43:213–216.

103. Thaler MM, Stobie GH. An improved technique of external cardiac compression in infants and young children. *N Engl J Med.* 1963;269:606–610.

104. Ishimine P, Menegazzi J, Weinstein D. Evaluation of two-thumb chest compression with thoracic squeeze in a swine model of infant cardiac arrest. *Acad Emerg Med.* 1998;5:397.

105. Roth B, Magnusson J, Johansson I, Holmberg S, Westrin P. Jaw lift: a simple and effective method to open the airway in children. *Resuscitation.* 1998;39:171–174.

106. Bruppacher H, Reber A, Keller JP, Geiduschek J, Erb TO, Frei FJ. The effects of common airway maneuvers on airway pressure and flow in children undergoing adenoidectomies. *Anesth Analg.* 2003;97:29–34.

107. Atkins DL, Jorgenson DB. Attenuated pediatric electrode pads for automated external defibrillator use in children. *Resuscitation.* 2005;66:31–37.

108. Samson RA, Nadkarni VM, Meaney PA, Carey SM, Berg MD, Berg RA. Outcomes of in-hospital ventricular fibrillation in children. *N Engl J Med.* 2006;354:2328–2339.

109. Atkinson E, Mikysa B, Conway JA, Parker M, Christian K, Deshpande J, Knilans TK, Smith J, Walker C, Stickney RE, Hampton DR, Hazinski MF. Specificity and sensitivity of automated external defibrillator rhythm analysis in infants and children. *Ann Emerg Med.* 2003;42:185–196.

110. Cecchin F, Jorgenson DB, Berul CI, Perry JC, Zimmerman AA, Duncan BW, Lupinetti FM, Snyder D, Lyster TD, Rosenthal GL, Cross B, Atkins DL. Is arrhythmia detection by automatic external defibrillator accurate for children? Sensitivity and specificity of an automatic external defibrillator algorithm in 696 pediatric arrhythmias. *Circulation.* 2001;103:2483–2488.

111. Atkins DL, Scott WA, Blaufox AD, Law IH, Dick M II, Geheb F, Sobh J, Brewer JE. Sensitivity and specificity of an automated external defibrillator algorithm designed for pediatric patients. *Resuscitation.* 2008;76:168–174.

112. Bar-Cohen Y, Walsh EP, Love BA, Cecchin F. First appropriate use of automated external defibrillator in an infant. *Resuscitation.* 2005;67:135–137.

113. Konig B, Benger J, Goldsworthy L. Automatic external defibrillation in a 6 year old. *Arch Dis Child.* 2005;90:310–311.

114. Dorph E, Wik L, Stromme TA, Eriksen M, Steen PA. Oxygen delivery and return of spontaneous circulation with ventilation:compression ratio 2:30 versus chest compressions only CPR in pigs. *Resuscitation.* 2004;60:309–318.

115. Kern KB, Hilwig RW, Berg RA, Ewy GA. Efficacy of chest compression-only BLS CPR in the presence of an occluded airway. *Resuscitation.* 1998;39:179–188.

116. Ornato JP, Hallagan LF, McMahan SB, Peeples EH, Rostafinski AG. Attitudes of BCLS instructors about mouth-to-mouth resuscitation during the AIDS epidemic. *Ann Emerg Med.* 1990;19:151–156.

117. Brenner BE, Van DC, Cheng D, Lazar EJ. Determinants of reluctance to perform CPR among residents and applicants: the impact of experience on helping behavior. *Resuscitation.* 1997;35:203–211.

118. Hew P, Brenner B, Kaufman J. Reluctance of paramedics and emergency medical technicians to perform mouth-to-mouth resuscitation. *J Emerg Med.* 1997;15:279–284.

119. Locke CJ, Berg RA, Sanders AB, Davis MF, Milander MM, Kern KB, Ewy GA. Bystander cardiopulmonary resuscitation. Concerns about mouth-to-mouth contact. *Arch Intern Med.* 1995;155:938–943.

120. Shibata K, Taniguchi T, Yoshida M, Yamamoto K. Obstacles to bystander cardiopulmonary resuscitation in Japan. *Resuscitation.* 2000;44:187–193.

121. Terndrup TE, Warner DA. Infant ventilation and oxygenation by basic life support providers: comparison of methods. *Prehosp Disaster Med.* 1992;7:35–40.

122. Hess D, Ness C, Oppel A, Rhoads K. Evaluation of mouth-to-mask ventilation devices. *Respir Care.* 1989;34:191–195.

123. Terndrup TE, Kanter RK, Cherry RA. A comparison of infant ventilation methods performed by prehospital personnel. *Ann Emerg Med.* 1989;18:607–611.

124. Field D, Milner AD, Hopkin IE. Efficiency of manual resuscitators at birth. *Arch Dis Child.* 1986;61:300–302.

125. Finer NN, Barrington KJ, Al-Fadley F, Peters KL. Limitations of self-inflating resuscitators. *Pediatrics.* 1986;77:417–420.

126. Kern KB, Sanders AB, Raife J, Milander MM, Otto CW, Ewy GA. A study of chest compression rates during cardiopulmonary resuscitation in humans: the importance of rate-directed chest compressions. *Arch Intern Med.* 1992;152:145–149.

127. Aufderheide TP, Sigurdsson G, Pirrallo RG, Yannopoulos D, McKnite S, von Briesen C, Sparks CW, Conrad CJ, Provo TA, Lurie KG. Hyperventilation-induced hypotension during cardiopulmonary resuscitation. *Circulation.* 2004;109:1960–1965.

128. Hirschman AM, Kravath RE. Venting vs ventilating. A danger of manual resuscitation bags. *Chest.* 1982;82:369–370.

129. Davidovic L, LaCovey D, Pitetti RD. Comparison of 1- versus 2-person bag-valve-mask techniques for manikin ventilation of infants and children. *Ann Emerg Med.* 2005;46:37–42.

130. Berg MD, Idris AH, Berg RA. Severe ventilatory compromise due to gastric distention during pediatric cardiopulmonary resuscitation. *Resuscitation.* 1998;36:71–73.

131. Gausche M, Lewis RJ, Stratton SJ, Haynes BE, Gunter CS, Goodrich SM, Poore PD, McCollough MD, Henderson DP, Pratt FD, Seidel JS. Effect of out-of-hospital pediatric endotracheal intubation on survival and neurological outcome: a controlled clinical trial. *JAMA.* 2000;283:783–790.

132. Moynihan RJ, Brock-Utne JG, Archer JH, Feld LH, Kreitzman TR. The effect of cricoid pressure on preventing gastric insufflation in infants and children. *Anesthesiology.* 1993;78:652–656.

133. Salem MR, Wong AY, Mani M, Sellick BA. Efficacy of cricoid pressure in preventing gastric inflation during bag- mask ventilation in pediatric patients. *Anesthesiology.* 1974;40:96–98.

134. Sellick BA. Cricoid pressure to control regurgitation of stomach contents during induction of anaesthesia. *Lancet.* 1961;2:404–406.

135. Hartsilver EL, Vanner RG. Airway obstruction with cricoid pressure. *Anaesthesia.* 2000;55:208–211.

136. Lipinski CA, Hicks SD, Callaway CW. Normoxic ventilation during resuscitation and outcome from asphyxial cardiac arrest in rats. *Resuscitation.* 1999;42:221–229.

137. Liu Y, Rosenthal RE, Haywood Y, Miljkovic-Lolic M, Vanderhoek JY, Fiskum G. Normoxic ventilation after cardiac arrest reduces oxidation of brain lipids and improves neurological outcome. *Stroke.* 1998;29:1679–1686.

138. Lefkowitz W. Oxygen and resuscitation: beyond the myth. *Pediatrics.* 2002;109:517–519.

139. Zwemer CF, Whitesall SE, D'Alecy LG. Cardiopulmonary-cerebral resuscitation with 100% oxygen exacerbates neurological dysfunction following nine minutes of normothermic cardiac arrest in dogs. *Resuscitation.* 1994;27:159–170.

140. Balan IS, Fiskum G, Hazelton J, Cotto-Cumba C, Rosenthal RE. Oximetry-guided reoxygenation improves neurological outcome after experimental cardiac arrest. *Stroke.* 2006;37:3008–3013.

141. Marsala J, Marsala M, Vanicky I, Galik J, Orendacova J. Post cardiac arrest hyperoxic resuscitation enhances neuronal vulnerability of the respiratory rhythm generator and some brainstem and spinal cord neuronal pools in the dog. *Neurosci Lett.* 1992;146:121–124.

142. Richards EM, Rosenthal RE, Kristian T, Fiskum G. Postischemic hyperoxia reduces hippocampal pyruvate dehydrogenase activity. *Free Radic Biol Med.* 2006;40:1960–1970.

143. Richards EM, Fiskum G, Rosenthal RE, Hopkins I, McKenna MC. Hyperoxic reperfusion after global ischemia decreases hippocampal energy metabolism. *Stroke.* 2007;38:1578–1584.

144. Vereczki V, Martin E, Rosenthal RE, Hof PR, Hoffman GE, Fiskum G. Normoxic resuscitation after cardiac arrest protects against hippocampal oxidative stress, metabolic dysfunction, and neuronal death. *J Cereb Blood Flow Metab.* 2006;26:821–835.

145. Feet BA, Yu XQ, Rootwelt T, Oyasaeter S, Saugstad OD. Effects of hypoxemia and reoxygenation with 21% or 100% oxygen in newborn piglets: extracellular hypoxanthine in cerebral cortex and femoral muscle. *Crit Care Med.* 1997;25:1384–1391.

146. Finer NN, Bates R, Tomat P. Low flow oxygen delivery via nasal cannula to neonates. *Pediatr Pulmonol.* 1996;21:48–51.

147. Vilke GM, Smith AM, Ray LU, Steen PJ, Murrin PA, Chan TC. Airway obstruction in children aged less than 5 years: the prehospital experience. *Prehosp Emerg Care.* 2004;8:196–199.

148. Morley RE, Ludemann JP, Moxham JP, Kozak FK, Riding KH. Foreign body aspiration in infants and toddlers: recent trends in British Columbia. *J Otolaryngol.* 2004;33:37–41.

149. Harris CS, Baker SP, Smith GA, Harris RM. Childhood asphyxiation by food. A national analysis and overview. *JAMA.* 1984;251:2231–2235.

150. Rimell FL, Thome AJ, Stool S, Reilly JS, Rider G, Stool D, Wilson CL. Characteristics of objects that cause choking in children. *JAMA.* 1995; 274:1763–1766.

151. Prevention of choking among children. *Pediatrics.* 2010;125:601–607.

152. Heimlich HJ. A life-saving maneuver to prevent food-choking. *JAMA.* 1975;234:398–401.

153. Sternbach G, Kiskaddon RT. Henry Heimlich: a life-saving maneuver for food choking. *J Emerg Med.* 1985;3:143–148.

154. Langhelle A, Sunde K, Wik L, Steen PA. Airway pressure with chest compressions versus Heimlich manoeuvre in recently dead adults with complete airway obstruction. *Resuscitation.* 2000;44:105–108.

155. Redding JS. The choking controversy: critique of evidence on the Heimlich maneuver. *Crit Care Med.* 1979;7:475–479.

156. Guildner CW, Williams D, Subitch T. Airway obstructed by foreign material: the Heimlich maneuver. *JACEP.* 1976;5:675–677.

157. Kabbani M, Goodwin SR. Traumatic epiglottis following blind finger sweep to remove a pharyngeal foreign body. *Clin Pediatr (Phila).* 1995;34:495–497.

158. Hartrey R, Bingham RM. Pharyngeal trauma as a result of blind finger sweeps in the choking child. *J Accid Emerg Med.* 1995;12:52–54.

159. Gjoni D, Mbamalu D, Banerjee A, James K. An unusual complication of an attempt to open the airway in a choking child. *Br J Hosp Med (Lond).* 2009;70:595.

160. Spaite DW, Conroy C, Tibbitts M, Karriker KJ, Seng M, Battaglia N, Criss EA, Valenzuela TD, Meislin HW. Use of emergency medical services by children with special health care needs. *Prehosp Emerg Care.* 2000;4:19–23.

161. Schultz-Grant LD, Young-Cureton V, Kataoka-Yahiro M. Advance directives and do not resuscitate orders: nurses' knowledge and the level of practice in school settings. *J Sch Nurs.* 1998;14:4–10, 12–13.

162. Policy statement–emergency information forms and emergency preparedness for children with special health care needs. *Pediatrics.* 2010; 125:829–837.

163. Herzenberg JE, Hensinger RN, Dedrick DK, Phillips WA. Emergency transport and positioning of young children who have an injury of the cervical spine. The standard backboard may be hazardous. *J Bone Joint Surg Am.* 1989;71:15–22.

164. Nypaver M, Treloar D. Neutral cervical spine positioning in children. *Ann Emerg Med.* 1994;23:208–211.

165. Graf WD, Cummings P, Quan L, Brutocao D. Predicting outcome in pediatric submersion victims. *Ann Emerg Med.* 1995;26:312–319.

166. Modell JH, Idris AH, Pineda JA, Silverstein JH. Survival after prolonged submersion in freshwater in Florida. *Chest.* 2004;125: 1948–1951.

167. Mehta SR, Srinivasan KV, Bindra MS, Kumar MR, Lahiri AK. Near drowning in cold water. *J Assoc Physicians India.* 2000;48:674–676.

168. Szpilman D, Soares M. In-water resuscitation–is it worthwhile? *Resuscitation.* 2004;63:25–31.

KEY WORDS: automatic external defibrillator ■ cardiopulmonary resuscitation ■ pediatrics

# Part 14: Pediatric Advanced Life Support

## 2010 American Heart Association Guidelines for Cardiopulmonary Resuscitation and Emergency Cardiovascular Care

Monica E. Kleinman, Chair; Leon Chameides; Stephen M. Schexnayder; Ricardo A. Samson;
Mary Fran Hazinski; Dianne L. Atkins; Marc D. Berg; Allan R. de Caen; Ericka L. Fink;
Eugene B. Freid; Robert W. Hickey; Bradley S. Marino; Vinay M. Nadkarni; Lester T. Proctor;
Faiqa A. Qureshi; Kennith Sartorelli; Alexis Topjian; Elise W. van der Jagt; Arno L. Zaritsky

In contrast to adults, cardiac arrest in infants and children does not usually result from a primary cardiac cause. More often it is the terminal result of progressive respiratory failure or shock, also called an asphyxial arrest. Asphyxia begins with a variable period of systemic hypoxemia, hypercapnea, and acidosis, progresses to bradycardia and hypotension, and culminates with cardiac arrest.[1]

Another mechanism of cardiac arrest, ventricular fibrillation (VF) or pulseless ventricular tachycardia (VT), is the initial cardiac rhythm in approximately 5% to 15% of pediatric in-hospital and out-of-hospital cardiac arrests;[2–9] it is reported in up to 27% of pediatric in-hospital arrests at some point during the resuscitation.[6] The incidence of VF/pulseless VT cardiac arrest rises with age.[2,4] Increasing evidence suggests that sudden unexpected death in young people can be associated with genetic abnormalities in myocyte ion channels resulting in abnormalities in ion flow (see "Sudden Unexplained Deaths," below).

Since 2010 marks the 50th anniversary of the introduction of cardiopulmonary resuscitation (CPR),[10] it seems appropriate to review the progressive improvement in outcome of pediatric resuscitation from cardiac arrest. Survival from in-hospital cardiac arrest in infants and children in the 1980s was around 9%.[11,12] Approximately 20 years later, that figure had increased to 17%,[13,14] and by 2006, to 27%.[15–17] In contrast to those favorable results from in-hospital cardiac arrest, overall survival to discharge from out-of-hospital cardiac arrest in infants and children has not changed substantially in 20 years and remains at about 6% (3% for infants and 9% for children and adolescents).[7,9]

It is unclear why the improvement in outcome from in-hospital cardiac arrest has occurred, although earlier recognition and management of at-risk patients on general inpatient units and more aggressive implementation of evidence-based resuscitation guidelines may have played a role. Implementation of a formal pediatric medical emergency team (MET) or rapid response team (RRT) as part of an emergency response system for a deteriorating inpatient has been shown to significantly decrease the incidence of cardiac and respiratory arrests, as well as hospital mortality rates in some large children's hospitals.[18–21] Such teams, often consisting of providers with expertise in assessment and initial management of acutely ill patients (critical-care nurses, respiratory therapists, and critical-care physicians), decreased the number of cardiac and respiratory arrests by as much as 72%[18] and hospital mortality by as much as 35% in institutions where the effect was studied.[19] Although it is possible that most of the impact is due to a decrease in respiratory arrests, this cannot be confirmed by the available published data. Implementation of a pediatric MET/RRT may be beneficial in facilities where children with high risk illnesses are present on general inpatient units (Class IIa, LOE B).

Despite the improved outcome of in-hospital CPR, a majority of children with in-hospital cardiac arrest and an even larger percentage of children with out-of-hospital cardiac arrest do not survive, or they are severely incapacitated if they do. Several studies, discussed later in this document, showed that the presence of family members during resuscitation has helped them deal with the inevitable trauma and grief following the death of a child. Therefore, whenever possible, provide family members with the option of being present during resuscitation of an infant or child (Class I, LOE B).

## BLS Considerations During PALS

Pediatric advanced life support (PALS) usually takes place in the setting of an organized response in an advanced healthcare environment. In these circumstances, multiple responders are rapidly mobilized and are capable of simultaneous coordinated action. Resuscitation teams may also have access to invasive patient monitoring that may provide additional information during the performance of basic life support (BLS).

The American Heart Association requests that this document be cited as follows: Kleinman ME, Chameides L, Schexnayder SM, Samson RA, Hazinski MF, Atkins DL, Berg MD, de Caen AR, Fink EL, Freid EB, Hickey RW, Marino BS, Nadkarni VM, Proctor LT, Qureshi FA, Sartorelli K, Topjian A, van der Jagt EW, Zaritsky AL. Part 14: pediatric advanced life support: 2010 American Heart Association Guidelines for Cardiopulmonary Resuscitation and Emergency Cardiovascular Care. Circulation. 2010;122(suppl 3):S876–S908.

(*Circulation.* **2010;122[suppl 3]:S876–S908.**)

*Circulation* is available at http://circ.ahajournals.org

DOI: 10.1161/CIRCULATIONAHA.110.971101

## Simultaneous Actions

BLS (whether for a child or adult) is presented as a series of sequential events with the assumption that there is only one responder, but PALS usually takes place in an environment where many rescuers are rapidly mobilized and actions are performed simultaneously. The challenge is to organize the rescuers into an efficient team. Important considerations for the greatest chance of a successful resuscitation from cardiac arrest include the following:

- Chest compressions should be immediately started by one rescuer, while a second rescuer prepares to start ventilations with a bag and mask. Ventilation is extremely important in pediatrics because of the large percentage of asphyxial arrests in which best results are obtained by a combination of chest compressions and ventilations.[8] Unfortunately ventilations are sometimes delayed because equipment (bag, mask, oxygen, airway) must be mobilized. Chest compressions require only the hands of a willing rescuer. Therefore, start CPR with chest compressions immediately, while a second rescuer prepares to provide ventilations (Class I, LOE C).
- The effectiveness of PALS is dependent on high-quality CPR, which requires an adequate compression rate (at least 100 compressions/min), an adequate compression depth (at least one third of the AP diameter of the chest or approximately 1 ½ inches [4 cm] in infants and approximately 2 inches [5 cm] in children), allowing complete recoil of the chest after each compression, minimizing interruptions in compressions, and avoiding excessive ventilation. Reasons for not performing high-quality CPR include rescuer inattention to detail, rescuer fatigue, and long or frequent interruptions to secure the airway, check the heart rhythm, and move the patient.[22] Optimal chest compressions are best delivered with the victim on a firm surface.[23,24]
- While one rescuer performs chest compressions and another performs ventilations, other rescuers should obtain a monitor/defibrillator, establish vascular access, and calculate and prepare the anticipated medications.

## Monitored Patients

Many in-hospital patients, especially if they are in an ICU, are monitored and some have an advanced airway and are receiving mechanical ventilation. If the patient has an indwelling arterial catheter, use the waveform as feedback to evaluate hand position and chest compression depth. A minor adjustment of hand position or depth of compression can significantly improve the amplitude of the arterial waveform, reflecting better chest compression-induced stroke volume. The arterial waveform may also be useful in identification of return of spontaneous circulation (ROSC). If the patient's end-tidal $CO_2$ ($PETCO_2$) is being monitored, it can be used to evaluate the quality of chest compressions; it can also provide an indication of ROSC (see below).

## Respiratory Failure

Respiratory failure is characterized by inadequate ventilation, insufficient oxygenation, or both. Anticipate respiratory failure if any of the following signs is present:

- An increased respiratory rate, particularly with signs of distress (eg, increased respiratory effort including nasal flaring, retractions, seesaw breathing, or grunting)
- An inadequate respiratory rate, effort, or chest excursion (eg, diminished breath sounds or gasping), especially if mental status is depressed
- Cyanosis with abnormal breathing despite supplementary oxygen

## Shock

Shock results from inadequate blood flow and oxygen delivery to meet tissue metabolic demands. The most common type of shock in children is hypovolemic, including shock due to hemorrhage. Distributive, cardiogenic, and obstructive shock occur less frequently. Shock progresses over a continuum of severity, from a compensated to a decompensated state. Compensatory mechanisms include tachycardia and increased systemic vascular resistance (vasoconstriction) in an effort to maintain cardiac output and perfusion pressure respectively. Decompensation occurs when compensatory mechanisms fail and results in hypotensive shock.

Typical signs of compensated shock include

- Tachycardia
- Cool and pale distal extremities
- Prolonged (>2 seconds) capillary refill (despite warm ambient temperature)
- Weak peripheral pulses compared with central pulses
- Normal systolic blood pressure

As compensatory mechanisms fail, signs of inadequate end-organ perfusion develop. In addition to the above, these signs include

- Depressed mental status
- Decreased urine output
- Metabolic acidosis
- Tachypnea
- Weak central pulses
- Deterioration in color (eg, mottling, see below)

Decompensated shock is characterized by signs and symptoms consistent with inadequate delivery of oxygen to tissues (pallor, peripheral cyanosis, tachypnea, mottling of the skin, decreased urine output, metabolic acidosis, depressed mental status), weak or absent peripheral pulses, weak central pulses, and hypotension.

Learn to integrate the signs of shock because no single sign confirms the diagnosis. For example:

- Capillary refill time alone is not a good indicator of circulatory volume, but a capillary refill time >2 seconds is a useful indicator of moderate dehydration when combined with decreased urine output, absent tears, dry mucous membranes, and a generally ill appearance. Capillary refill time is influenced by ambient temperature,[25] site, and age and its interpretation can be influenced by lighting.[26]
- Tachycardia is a common sign of shock, but it can also result from other causes, such as pain, anxiety, and fever.

- Pulses are weak in hypovolemic and cardiogenic shock, but may be bounding in anaphylactic, neurogenic, and septic shock.
- Blood pressure may be normal in a child with compensated shock but may decline rapidly when the child decompensates. Like the other signs, hypotension must be interpreted within the context of the entire clinical picture.

There are several sources of data that use large populations to identify the 5th percentile for systolic blood pressure at various ages.[27,28] For purposes of these guidelines, hypotension is defined as a *systolic* blood pressure:

- <60 mm Hg in term neonates (0 to 28 days)
- <70 mm Hg in infants (1 month to 12 months)
- <70 mm Hg + (2 × age in years) in children 1 to 10 years
- <90 mm Hg in children ≥10 years of age

### Airway

#### Oropharyngeal and Nasopharyngeal Airways

Oropharyngeal and nasopharyngeal airways help maintain an open airway by displacing the tongue or soft palate from the pharyngeal air passages. Oropharyngeal airways are used in unresponsive victims who do not have a gag reflex. Make sure to select the correct size: an oropharyngeal airway that is too small may push the base of the tongue farther into the airway; one that is too large may obstruct the airway.

Nasopharyngeal airways can be used in children who do have a gag reflex. Pay careful attention to proper diameter and length. A nasopharyngeal airway that is too short may not maintain an open airway, while one that is too long may obstruct it. A small-diameter nasopharyngeal airway may be obstructed easily by secretions. It may therefore require frequent suctioning.

#### Laryngeal Mask Airway (LMA)

Although several supraglottic devices have been used in children, clinical studies of devices other than the LMA in pediatric patients are limited. When bag-mask ventilation (see "Bag-Mask Ventilation," below) is unsuccessful and when endotracheal intubation is not possible, the LMA is acceptable when used by experienced providers to provide a patent airway and support ventilation (Class IIa, LOE C).[29–37] LMA insertion is associated with a higher incidence of complications in young children compared with older children and adults.[38–43]

### Oxygen

It is reasonable to ventilate with 100% oxygen during CPR because there is insufficient information on the optimal inspired oxygen concentration (Class IIa, LOE C). Once the circulation is restored, monitor systemic oxygen saturation. It may be reasonable, when the appropriate equipment is available, to titrate oxygen administration to maintain the oxyhemoglobin saturation ≥94%. Provided appropriate equipment is available, once ROSC is achieved, adjust the $F_{IO_2}$ to the minimum concentration needed to achieve an arterial oxyhemoglobin saturation at least 94%, with the goal of avoiding hyperoxia while ensuring adequate oxygen delivery. Since an arterial oxyhemoglobin saturation of 100%

may correspond to a $PaO_2$ anywhere between ~80 and 500 mmHg, in general it is appropriate to wean the $F_{IO_2}$ when saturation is 100%, provided the oxyhemoglobin saturation can be maintained ≥94% (Class IIb, LOE C). Remember that adequate oxygen delivery requires not only adequate arterial oxyhemoglobin saturation but also adequate hemoglobin concentration and cardiac output.

### Pulse Oximetry

If the patient has a perfusing rhythm, monitor oxyhemoglobin saturation continuously with a pulse oximeter because clinical recognition of hypoxemia is not reliable.[44] Pulse oximetry may, however, also be unreliable in patients with poor peripheral perfusion, carbon monoxide poisoning, or methemoglobinemia.

### Bag-Mask Ventilation

Bag-mask ventilation can be as effective, and may be safer, than endotracheal tube ventilation for short periods during out-of-hospital resuscitation.[45–52] In the prehospital setting it is reasonable to ventilate and oxygenate infants and children with a bag-mask device, especially if transport time is short (Class IIa, LOE B). Bag-mask ventilation requires training and periodic retraining in selecting a correct mask size, maintaining an open airway, providing a tight seal between mask and face, providing ventilation, and assessing effectiveness of ventilation (see Part 13, "Pediatric Basic Life Support").

#### Precautions

Use only the force and tidal volume needed to just make the chest rise visibly (Class I, LOE C); avoid delivering excessive ventilation during cardiac arrest (Class III, LOE C). Evidence shows that cardiac arrest victims frequently receive excessive ventilation.[22,53–55] Excessive ventilation during cardiac arrest increases intrathoracic pressure, which impedes venous return, thus reducing cardiac output and cerebral and coronary blood flow. These effects will reduce the likelihood of ROSC.[54] In addition, excessive ventilation may cause air trapping and barotrauma in patients with small airway obstruction. It also increases the risk of stomach inflation, regurgitation, and aspiration.

If the infant or child is not intubated, pause after 30 chest compressions (1 rescuer) or after 15 chest compressions (2 rescuers) to give 2 ventilations (mouth-to-mouth, mouth-to-mask, or bag-mask). Deliver each breath with an inspiratory time of approximately 1 second. If the infant or child is intubated, ventilate at a rate of about 1 breath every 6 to 8 seconds (8 to 10 times per minute) without interrupting chest compressions (Class I, LOE C). It may be reasonable to do the same if an LMA is in place (Class IIb, LOE C).

In the victim with a perfusing rhythm but absent or inadequate respiratory effort, give 1 breath every 3 to 5 seconds (12 to 20 breaths per minute), using the higher rate for the younger child (Class I, LOE C). One way to achieve that rate with a ventilating bag is to use the mnemonic "squeeze-release-release" at a normal speaking rate.[45,56]

### Two-Person Bag-Mask Ventilation

A 2-person ventilation technique may be preferable when personnel are available and may be more effective than ventilation by a single rescuer if the patient has significant airway obstruction, poor lung compliance, or the rescuer has difficulty in creating a tight mask-to-face seal.[57,58] One rescuer uses both hands to maintain an open airway with a jaw thrust and a tight mask-to-face seal while the other compresses the ventilation bag. Both rescuers should observe the victim's chest to ensure chest rise.

## Gastric Inflation

Gastric inflation may interfere with effective ventilation[59] and cause regurgitation, aspiration of stomach contents, and further ventilatory compromise. The risk of gastric inflation can be decreased by

- Avoiding excessive peak inspiratory pressures by ventilating slowly and giving only enough tidal volume to just achieve visible chest rise.[45]
- Applying cricoid pressure in an unresponsive victim to reduce air entry into the stomach (Class IIa, LOE B).[60-62] This may require a third rescuer if cricoid pressure cannot be applied by the rescuer who is securing the bag to the face. Avoid excessive cricoid pressure so as not to obstruct the trachea (Class III, LOE B).[63]
- Passing a nasogastric or orogastric tube to relieve gastric inflation, especially if oxygenation and ventilation are compromised. Pass the tube after intubation because a gastric tube interferes with gastroesophageal sphincter function, allowing regurgitation during intubation. If a gastrostomy tube is present, vent it during bag-mask ventilation to allow gastric decompression.

## Ventilation With an Endotracheal Tube

Endotracheal intubation in infants and children requires special training because the pediatric airway anatomy differs from that of the adult. The likelihood of successful endotracheal tube placement with minimal complications is related to the length of training, supervised experience in the operating room and in the field,[64,65] adequate ongoing experience,[66] and use of rapid sequence intubation (RSI).[67,68]

## Rapid Sequence Intubation (RSI)

To facilitate emergency intubation and reduce the incidence of complications, skilled, experienced providers may use sedatives, neuromuscular blocking agents, and other medications to rapidly sedate and neuromuscularly block the pediatric patient.[69]

Use RSI only if you are trained, and have experience using these medications and are proficient in the evaluation and management of the pediatric airway. If you use RSI you must have a secondary plan to manage the airway in the event that you cannot achieve intubation.

Actual body weight, rather than ideal body weight, should be used for some non-resuscitation medications (eg, succinylcholine).[70-85]

## Cricoid Pressure During Intubation

There is insufficient evidence to recommend routine cricoid pressure application to prevent aspiration during endotracheal intubation in children. Do not continue cricoid pressure if it interferes with ventilation or the speed or ease of intubation (Class III, LOE C).[86,87]

## Cuffed Versus Uncuffed Endotracheal Tubes

Both cuffed and uncuffed endotracheal tubes are acceptable for intubating infants and children (Class IIa, LOE C). In the operating room, cuffed endotracheal tubes are associated with a higher likelihood of correct selection of tube size, thus achieving a lower reintubation rate with no increased risk of perioperative complications.[88-90] In intensive care settings the risk of complications in infants and in children is no greater with cuffed tubes than with noncuffed tubes.[91-93] Cuffed endotracheal tubes may decrease the risk of aspiration.[94] If cuffed endotracheal tubes are used, cuff inflating pressure should be monitored and limited according to manufacturer's instruction (usually less than 20 to 25 cm $H_2O$).

In certain circumstances (eg, poor lung compliance, high airway resistance, or a large glottic air leak) a cuffed endotracheal tube may be preferable to an uncuffed tube, provided that attention is paid to endotracheal tube size, position, and cuff inflation pressure (Class IIa, LOE B).[88,91,92]

## Endotracheal Tube Size

Length-based resuscitation tapes are helpful and more accurate than age-based formula estimates of endotracheal tube size for children up to approximately 35 kg,[77,95,96] even for children with short stature.[97]

In preparation for intubation with either a cuffed or an uncuffed endotracheal tube, confirm that tubes with an internal diameter (ID) 0.5 mm smaller and 0.5 mm larger than the estimated size are available. During intubation, if the endotracheal tube meets resistance, place a tube 0.5 mm smaller instead. Following intubation, if there is a large glottic air leak that interferes with oxygenation or ventilation, consider replacing the tube with one that is 0.5 mm larger, or place a cuffed tube of the same size if an uncuffed tube was used originally. Note that replacement of a functional endotracheal tube is associated with risk; the procedure should be undertaken in an appropriate setting by experienced personnel.

If an uncuffed endotracheal tube is used for emergency intubation, it is reasonable to select a 3.5-mm ID tube for infants up to one year of age and a 4.0-mm ID tube for patients between 1 and 2 years of age. After age 2, uncuffed endotracheal tube size can be estimated by the following formula:

$$\text{Uncuffed endotracheal tube ID (mm)} = 4 + (\text{age}/4)$$

If a cuffed tube is used for emergency intubation of an infant less than 1 year of age, it is reasonable to select a 3.0 mm ID tube. For children between 1 and 2 years of age, it is reasonable to use a cuffed endotracheal tube with an internal diameter of 3.5 mm (Class IIa, LOE B).[89,98-100] After age 2 it is reasonable to estimate tube size with the following formula (Class IIa, LOE B:[89,98-101]):

$$\text{Cuffed endotracheal tube ID (mm)} = 3.5 + (\text{age}/4)$$

## Verification of Endotracheal Tube Placement

There is a risk of endotracheal tube misplacement (ie, in the esophagus, the pharynx above the vocal cords, or a mainstem bronchus) and an ongoing risk of displacement or obstruction,[45,102] especially during patient transport.[103] Since no single confirmation technique, including clinical signs[104] or the presence of water vapor in the tube,[105] is completely reliable, use both clinical assessment and confirmatory devices to verify proper tube placement immediately after intubation, again after securing the endotracheal tube, during transport, and each time the patient is moved (eg, from gurney to bed) (Class I, LOE B).

The following are methods for confirming correct position:

- Look for bilateral chest movement and listen for equal breath sounds over both lung fields, especially over the axillae.
- Listen for gastric insufflation sounds over the stomach. They should *not* be present if the tube is in the trachea.[104]
- Check for exhaled $CO_2$ (see "Exhaled or End-Tidal $CO_2$ Monitoring," below).
- If there is a perfusing rhythm, check oxyhemoglobin saturation with a pulse oximeter. Remember that following hyperoxygenation, the oxyhemoglobin saturation detected by pulse oximetry may not decline for as long as 3 minutes even without effective ventilation.[106,107]
- If you are still uncertain, perform direct laryngoscopy and visualize the endotracheal tube to confirm that it lies between the vocal cords.
- In hospital settings, perform a chest x-ray to verify that the tube is not in a bronchus and to identify proper position in the midtrachea.

After intubation, secure the tube; there is insufficient evidence to recommend any single method. After securing the tube, maintain the patient's head in a neutral position; neck flexion may push the tube farther into the airway, and extension may pull the tube out of the airway.[108,109]

If an intubated patient's condition deteriorates, consider the following possibilities (mnemonic DOPE):

- **D**isplacement of the tube
- **O**bstruction of the tube
- **P**neumothorax
- **E**quipment failure

## Exhaled or End-Tidal $CO_2$ Monitoring

When available, exhaled $CO_2$ detection (capnography or colorimetry) is recommended as confirmation of tracheal tube position for neonates, infants, and children with a perfusing cardiac rhythm in all settings (eg, prehospital, emergency department [ED], ICU, ward, operating room) (Class I, LOE C)[110–114] and during intrahospital or interhospital transport (Class IIb, LOE C).[115,116] Remember that a color change or the presence of a capnography waveform confirms tube position in the airway but does not rule out right mainstem bronchus intubation. During cardiac arrest, if exhaled $CO_2$ is not detected, confirm tube position with direct laryngoscopy (Class IIa, LOE C)[110,117–120] because the absence of $CO_2$ may reflect very low pulmonary blood flow rather than tube misplacement.

Confirmation of endotracheal tube position by colorimetric end-tidal $CO_2$ detector may be altered by the following:

- If the detector is contaminated with gastric contents or acidic drugs (eg, endotracheally administered epinephrine),

a consistent color rather than a breath-to-breath color change may be seen.
- An intravenous (IV) bolus of epinephrine[121] may transiently reduce pulmonary blood flow and exhaled $CO_2$ below the limits of detection.[120]
- Severe airway obstruction (eg, status asthmaticus) and pulmonary edema may impair $CO_2$ elimination below the limits of detection.[120,122–124]
- A large glottic air leak may reduce exhaled tidal volume through the tube and dilute $CO_2$ concentration.

## Esophageal Detector Device (EDD)

If capnography is not available, an esophageal detector device (EDD) may be considered to confirm endotracheal tube placement in children weighing >20 kg with a perfusing rhythm (Class IIb, LOE B),[125,126] but the data are insufficient to make a recommendation for or against its use in children during cardiac arrest.

## Transtracheal Catheter Oxygenation and Ventilation

Transtracheal catheter oxygenation and ventilation may be considered for patients with severe airway obstruction above the level of the cricoid cartilage if standard methods to manage the airway are unsuccessful. Note that transtracheal ventilation primarily supports oxygenation as tidal volumes are usually too small to effectively remove carbon dioxide. This technique is intended for temporary use while a more effective airway is obtained. Attempt this procedure only after proper training and with appropriate equipment (Class IIb, LOE C).[127]

## Suction Devices

A properly sized suction device with an adjustable suction regulator should be available. Do not insert the suction catheter beyond the end of the endotracheal tube to avoid injuring the mucosa. Use a maximum suction force of -80 to -120 mm Hg for suctioning the airway via an endotracheal tube. Higher suction pressures applied through large-bore noncollapsible suction tubing and semirigid pharyngeal tips are used to suction the mouth and pharynx.

## CPR Guidelines for Newborns With Cardiac Arrest of Cardiac Origin

Recommendations for infants differ from those for the newly born (ie, in the delivery room and during the first hours after birth) and newborns (during their initial hospitalization and in the NICU). The compression-to-ventilation ratio differs (newly born and newborns – 3:1; infant two rescuer - 15:2) and how to provide ventilations in the presence of an advanced airway differs (newly born and newborns – pause after 3 compressions; infants – no pauses for ventilations). This presents a dilemma for healthcare providers who may also care for newborns outside the NICU. Because there are no definitive scientific data to help resolve this dilemma, for ease of training we recommend that newborns (intubated or not) who require CPR in the newborn nursery or NICU receive CPR using the same technique as for the newly born in the delivery room (ie, 3:1 compression-to-ventilation ratio with a pause for ventilation). Newborns who require CPR in other settings (eg, prehospital, ED, pediatric intensive care unit [PICU], etc.), should receive CPR according to infant guidelines: 2 rescuers provide continuous chest compressions with asynchronous ventilations if an advanced airway is in place and a 15:2 ventilation-to-compression ratio if no advanced airway is in place (Class IIb, LOE C). It is reasonable to resuscitate newborns with a primary cardiac etiology of arrest, regardless of location, according to infant guidelines, with emphasis on chest compressions (Class IIa, LOE C). For further information, please refer to Part 13, "Pediatric Basic Life Support," and Part 15, "Neonatal Resuscitation."

## Extracorporeal Life Support (ECLS)

Extracorporeal life support (ECLS) is a modified form of cardiopulmonary bypass used to provide prolonged delivery of oxygen to tissues. Consider early activation of ECLS for a cardiac arrest that occurs in a highly supervised environment, such as an ICU, with the clinical protocols in place and the expertise and equipment available to initiate it rapidly. ECLS should be considered only for children in cardiac arrest refractory to standard resuscitation attempts, with a potentially reversible cause of arrest (Class IIa, LOE C).[128–154] When ECLS is employed during cardiac arrest, outcome for children with underlying cardiac disease is better than the outcome for children with noncardiac disease. With underlying cardiac disease, long-term survival when ECLS is initiated in a critical-care setting has been reported even after >50 minutes of standard CPR.[128,129,139,147]

## Monitoring

### Electrocardiography

Monitor cardiac rhythm as soon as possible so both normal and abnormal cardiac rhythms are identified and followed. Continuous monitoring is helpful in tracking responses to treatment and changes in clinical condition.

### Echocardiography

There is insufficient evidence for or against the routine use of echocardiography in pediatric cardiac arrest. When appropriately trained personnel are available, echocardiography may be considered to identify patients with potentially treatable causes of the arrest, particularly pericardial tamponade and inadequate ventricular filling (Class IIb, LOE C).[155–162] Minimize interruption of CPR while performing echocardiography.

### End-Tidal CO$_2$ (P$_{ETCO_2}$)

Continuous capnography or capnometry monitoring, if available, may be beneficial during CPR, to help guide therapy, especially the effectiveness of chest compressions (Class IIa, LOE C). Animal and adult studies show a strong correlation between P$_{ETCO_2}$ and interventions that increase cardiac output during CPR or shock.[53,163–169] If the P$_{ETCO_2}$ is consistently <10 to 15 mm Hg, focus efforts on improving chest compressions and make sure that the victim does not receive excessive ventilation. An abrupt and sustained rise in P$_{ETCO_2}$ in adults[170,171] and animals[110] is observed just prior to clinical identification of ROSC, so use of P$_{ETCO_2}$ may spare the rescuer from interrupting chest compressions for a pulse check. P$_{ETCO_2}$ must be interpreted with caution for 1 to 2 minutes after administration of epinephrine or other vasoconstrictive medications because these medications may decrease the end-tidal CO$_2$ level by reducing pulmonary blood flow.

## Vascular Access

Vascular access is essential for administering medications and drawing blood samples. Obtaining peripheral venous access can be challenging in infants and children during an emergency; intraosseous (IO) access can be quickly established with minimal complications by providers with varied levels of training.[172–179] Limit the time spent attempting to establish peripheral venous access in a critically ill or injured child.[180]

## Intraosseous (IO) Access

IO access is a rapid, safe, effective, and acceptable route for vascular access in children,[172–179,181] and it is useful as the initial vascular access in cases of cardiac arrest (Class I, LOE C). All intravenous medications can be administered intraosseously, including epinephrine, adenosine, fluids, blood products,[182,183] and catecholamines.[184] Onset of action and drug levels for most drugs are comparable to venous administration.[185] IO access can be used to obtain blood samples for analysis including for type and cross match and blood gases during CPR,[186] but acid-base analysis is inaccurate after sodium bicarbonate administration via the IO cannula.[187] Use manual pressure or an infusion pump to administer viscous drugs or rapid fluid boluses;[188,189] follow each medication with a saline flush to promote entry into the central circulation.

## Venous Access

Peripheral IV access is acceptable during resuscitation if it can be placed rapidly, but placement may be difficult in a critically ill child. Although a central venous catheter can provide more secure long-term access, its placement requires training and experience, and the procedure can be time-consuming. Therefore central venous access is not recommended as the initial route of vascular access during an emergency. If both central and peripheral accesses are available, administer medications into the central circulation since some medications (eg, adenosine) are more effective when administered closer to the heart, and others (eg, calcium, amiodarone, procainamide, sympathomimetics) may be irritating when infused into a peripheral vein. The length of a central catheter can contribute to increased resistance, making it more difficult to push boluses of fluid rapidly through a multilumen central than a peripheral catheter.

## Endotracheal Drug Administration

Vascular access (IO or IV) is the preferred method for drug delivery during CPR, but if it is not possible, lipid-soluble drugs, such as lidocaine, epinephrine, atropine, and naloxone (mnemonic "LEAN")[190,191] can be administered via an endotracheal tube.[192] However, the effects may not be uniform with tracheal as compared with intravenous administration. One study of children in cardiac arrest[193] demonstrated similar ROSC and survival rates regardless of the method of

**Table 1.  Medications for Pediatric Resuscitation**

| Medication | Dose | Remarks |
|---|---|---|
| Adenosine | 0.1 mg/kg (maximum 6 mg)<br>Second dose: 0.2 mg/kg (maximum 12 mg) | Monitor ECG<br>Rapid IV/IO bolus with flush |
| Amiodarone | 5 mg/kg IV/IO; may repeat twice up to 15 mg/kg<br>Maximum single dose 300 mg | Monitor ECG and blood pressure; adjust administration rate to urgency (IV push during cardiac arrest, more slowly–over 20–60 minutes with perfusing rhythm). Expert consultation strongly recommended prior to use when patient has a perfusing rhythm<br>Use caution when administering with other drugs that prolong QT (obtain expert consultation) |
| Atropine | 0.02 mg/kg IV/IO<br>0.04–0.06 mg/kg ET*<br>Repeat once if needed<br>Minimum dose: 0.1 mg<br>Maximum single dose:<br>0.5 mg | Higher doses may be used with organophosphate poisoning |
| Calcium Chloride (10%) | 20 mg/kg IV/IO (0.2 mL/kg)<br>Maximum single dose 2 g | Administer slowly |
| Epinephrine | 0.01 mg/kg (0.1 mL/kg 1:10,000) IV/IO<br>0.1 mg/kg (0.1 mL/kg 1:1000) ET*<br>Maximum dose 1 mg IV/IO; 2.5 mg ET | May repeat every 3–5 minutes |
| Glucose | 0.5–1 g/kg IV/IO | Newborn: 5–10 mL/kg $D_{10}$W<br>Infants and Children: 2–4 mL/kg $D_{25}$W<br>Adolescents: 1–2 mL/kg $D_{50}$W |
| Lidocaine | Bolus: 1 mg/kg IV/IO<br>Infusion: 20–50 mcg/kg/minute | |
| Magnesium Sulfate | 25–50 mg/kg IV/IO over 10–20 minutes, faster in torsades de pointes<br>Maximum dose 2 g | |
| Naloxone | Full Reversal:<br><5 y or ≤20 kg: 0.1 mg/kg IV/IO/ET*<br>≥5y or >20 kg: 2 mg IV/IO/ET* | Use lower doses to reverse respiratory depression associated with therapeutic opioid use (1–5 mcg/kg titrate to effect) |
| Procainamide | 15 mg/kg IV/IO<br>Adult Dose: 20 mg/min IV infusion to total maximum dose of 17 mg/kg | Monitor ECG and blood pressure;<br>Give slowly–over 30–60 minutes. Use caution when administering with other drugs that prolong QT (obtain expert consultation) |
| Sodium bicarbonate | 1 mEq/kg per dose IV/IO slowly | After adequate ventilation |

IV indicates intravenous; IO, intraosseous; and ET, via endotracheal tube.
*Flush with 5 mL of normal saline and follow with 5 ventilations.

drug delivery, while three studies of adults in cardiac arrest[194–196] demonstrated reduced ROSC and survival to hospital discharge with tracheal administration of epinephrine compared to vascular delivery. If CPR is in progress, stop chest compressions briefly, administer the medications, and follow with a flush of at least 5 mL of normal saline and 5 consecutive positive-pressure ventilations.[197] Optimal endotracheal doses of medications are unknown; in general expert consensus recommends doubling or tripling the dose of lidocaine, atropine or naloxone given via the ETT. For epinephrine, a dose ten times the intravenous dose (0.1 mg/kg or 0.1 mL/kg of 1:1000 concentration) is recommended (see Table 1).

The effectiveness of endotracheal epinephrine during cardiac arrest is controversial. Some studies showed it to be as effective as vascular administration[193,198,199] while other studies have not found it to be as effective.[194–196,200] Animal studies[201–206] suggested that a higher dose of epinephrine is required for endotracheal than for intravascular administration because the lower epinephrine concentrations achieved when the drug is delivered by the endotracheal route may produce predominant transient peripheral $\beta_2$-adrenergic vasodilating effects. These effects can be detrimental, and cause hypotension, lower coronary artery perfusion pressure and flow, and a reduced potential for ROSC.

Non-lipid-soluble drugs (eg, sodium bicarbonate and calcium) may injure the airway; they should not be administered via the endotracheal route.

## Emergency Fluids and Medications

### Estimating Weight

In the out-of-hospital setting, a child's weight is often unknown, and even experienced personnel may not be able to estimate it accurately.[74] Tapes with precalculated doses printed at various patient lengths have been clinically validated[74,77,95] and are more accurate than age-based or observer (parent or provider) estimate-based methods in the prediction of body weight.[70–77] Body habitus may also be an important consideration.[70,72,78,79]

## Medication Dose Calculation

To calculate the dose of resuscitation medications, use the child's weight if it is known. If the child's weight is unknown, it is reasonable to use a body length tape with precalculated doses (Class IIa, LOE C).[70–77]

It is unclear if an adjustment in the calculation of resuscitation medications is needed in obese children. Use of the actual body weight in calculation of drug doses in obese patients may result in potentially toxic doses. Length-based tapes estimate the 50th percentile weight for length (ie, ideal body weight), which may, theoretically, result in inadequate doses of some medications in obese patients. Despite these theoretical considerations, there are no data regarding the safety or efficacy of adjusting the doses of resuscitation medications in obese patients. Therefore, regardless of the patient's habitus, use the actual body weight for calculating initial resuscitation drug doses or use a body length tape with precalculated doses (Class IIb, LOE C).

For subsequent doses of resuscitation drugs in both non-obese and obese patients, expert providers may consider adjusting doses to achieve the desired therapeutic effect. In general, the dose administered to a child should not exceed the standard dose recommended for adult patients.

## Medications (See Table 1)

### Adenosine

Adenosine causes a temporary atrioventricular (AV) nodal conduction block and interrupts reentry circuits that involve the AV node. The drug has a wide safety margin because of its short half-life. Adenosine should be given only IV or IO, followed by a rapid saline flush to promote drug delivery to the central circulation. If adenosine is given IV, it should be administered as close to the heart as possible. (See also "Arrhythmia.")

### Amiodarone

Amiodarone slows AV conduction, prolongs the AV refractory period and QT interval, and slows ventricular conduction (widens the QRS). Expert consultation is strongly recommended prior to administration of amiodarone to a pediatric patient with a perfusing rhythm. (See also "Arrhythmia.")

#### Precautions

Monitor blood pressure and electrocardiograph (ECG) during intravenous administration of amiodarone. If the patient has a perfusing rhythm, administer the drug as slowly (over 20 to 60 minutes) as the patient's clinical condition allows; if the patient is in VF/pulseless VT, give the drug as a rapid bolus. Amiodarone causes hypotension through its vasodilatory property, and the severity is related to the infusion rate; hypotension is less common with the aqueous form of amiodarone.[207] Decrease the infusion rate if there is prolongation of the QT interval or heart block; stop the infusion if the QRS widens to >50% of baseline or hypotension develops. Other potential complications of amiodarone include bradycardia and torsades de pointes ventricular tachycardia. Amiodarone should not be administered together with another drug that causes QT prolongation, such as procainamide, without expert consultation.

### Atropine

Atropine sulfate is a parasympatholytic drug that accelerates sinus or atrial pacemakers and increases the speed of AV conduction.

#### Precautions

Small doses of atropine (<0.1 mg) may produce paradoxical bradycardia because of its central effect.[208] Larger than recommended doses may be required in special circumstances such as organophosphate poisoning[209] or exposure to nerve gas agents.

### Calcium

Calcium administration is not recommended for pediatric cardiopulmonary arrest in the absence of documented hypocalcemia, calcium channel blocker overdose, hypermagnesemia, or hyperkalemia (Class III, LOE B). Routine calcium administration in cardiac arrest provides no benefit[210–221] and may be harmful.[210–212]

If calcium administration is indicated during cardiac arrest, either calcium chloride or calcium gluconate may be considered. Hepatic dysfunction does not appear to alter the ability of calcium gluconate to raise serum calcium levels.[222] In critically ill children, calcium chloride may be preferred because it results in a greater increase in ionized calcium during the treatment of hypocalcemia.[222A] In the nonarrest setting, if the only venous access is peripheral, calcium gluconate is recommended because it has a lower osmolality than calcium chloride and is therefore less irritating to the vein.

### Epinephrine

The α-adrenergic-mediated vasoconstriction of epinephrine increases aortic diastolic pressure and thus coronary perfusion pressure, a critical determinant of successful resuscitation from cardiac arrest.[223,224] At low doses, the β-adrenergic effects may predominate, leading to decreased systemic vascular resistance; in the doses used during cardiac arrest, the vasoconstrictive α-effects predominate.

#### Precautions

- Do not administer catecholamines and sodium bicarbonate simultaneously through an IV catheter or tubing because alkaline solutions such as the bicarbonate inactivate the catecholamines.
- In patients with a perfusing rhythm, epinephrine causes tachycardia; it may also cause ventricular ectopy, tachyarrhythmias, vasoconstriction, and hypertension.

### Glucose

Because infants have a relatively high glucose requirement and low glycogen stores, they may develop hypoglycemia when energy requirements rise.[225] Check blood glucose concentration during the resuscitation and treat hypoglycemia promptly (Class I, LOE C).[226]

### Lidocaine

Lidocaine decreases automaticity and suppresses ventricular arrhythmias,[227] but is not as effective as amiodarone for improving ROSC or survival to hospital admission among adult patients with VF refractory to shocks and epinephrine.[228] Neither lidocaine nor amiodarone has been shown to improve survival to hospital discharge.

### Precautions

Lidocaine toxicity includes myocardial and circulatory depression, drowsiness, disorientation, muscle twitching, and seizures, especially in patients with poor cardiac output and hepatic or renal failure.[229,230]

### Magnesium

Magnesium is indicated for the treatment of documented hypomagnesemia or for torsades de pointes (polymorphic VT associated with long QT interval). There is insufficient evidence to recommend for or against the routine administration of magnesium during cardiac arrest.[231–233]

### Precautions

Magnesium produces vasodilation and may cause hypotension if administered rapidly.

### Procainamide

Procainamide prolongs the refractory period of the atria and ventricles and depresses conduction velocity.

### Precautions

There is limited clinical data on using procainamide in infants and children.[234–236] Infuse procainamide very slowly (over 30 to 60 minutes) while monitoring the ECG and blood pressure. Decrease the infusion rate if there is prolongation of the QT interval, or heart block; stop the infusion if the QRS widens to >50% of baseline or hypotension develops. Do not administer together with another drug causing QT prolongation, such as amiodarone, without expert consultation. Prior to using procainamide for a hemodynamically stable patient, expert consultation is strongly recommended.

### Sodium Bicarbonate

Routine administration of sodium bicarbonate is not recommended in cardiac arrest (Class III, LOE B).[212,237,238] Sodium bicarbonate may be administered for treatment of some toxidromes (see "Toxicological Emergencies," below) or special resuscitation situations such as hyperkalemic cardiac arrest.

### Precautions

During cardiac arrest or severe shock, arterial blood gas analysis may not accurately reflect tissue and venous acidosis.[239,240] Excessive sodium bicarbonate may impair tissue oxygen delivery;[241] cause hypokalemia, hypocalcemia, hypernatremia, and hyperosmolality;[242,243] decrease the VF threshold;[244] and impair cardiac function.

### Vasopressin

There is insufficient evidence to make a recommendation for or against the routine use of vasopressin during cardiac arrest. Pediatric[245–247] and adult[248,249] case series/reports suggested that vasopressin[245] or its long-acting analog, terlipressin,[246,247] may be effective in refractory cardiac arrest when standard therapy fails. A large pediatric NRCPR case series, however, suggested that vasopressin is associated with lower

ROSC, and a trend toward lower 24-hour and discharge survival.[250] A preponderance of controlled trials in adults do not demonstrate a benefit.[251–256]

## Pulseless Arrest

In the text below, box numbers identify the corresponding step in the algorithm (Figure 1).

- (Step 1) As soon as the child is found to be unresponsive with no breathing, call for help, send for a defibrillator (manual or AED), and start CPR (with supplementary oxygen if available). Attach ECG monitor or AED pads as soon as available. Throughout resuscitation, emphasis should be placed on provision of high-quality CPR (providing chest compressions of adequate rate and depth, allowing complete chest recoil after each compression, minimizing interruptions in compressions and avoiding excessive ventilation).

- While CPR is being given, determine the child's cardiac rhythm from the ECG or, if you are using an AED, the device will tell you whether the rhythm is "shockable" (eg, VF or rapid VT) or "not shockable" (eg, asystole or PEA). It may be necessary to temporarily interrupt chest compressions to determine the child's rhythm. Asystole and bradycardia with a wide QRS are most common in asphyxial arrest.[1] VF and PEA are less common[13] but VF is more likely to be present in older children with sudden witnessed arrest.

### "Nonshockable Rhythm": Asystole/PEA (Step 9)

PEA is an organized electric activity—most commonly slow, wide QRS complexes—without palpable pulses. Less frequently there is a sudden impairment of cardiac output with an initially normal rhythm but without pulses and with poor perfusion. This subcategory, formerly known as electromechanical dissociation (EMD), may be more reversible than asystole. For asystole and PEA:

- (Step 10) Continue CPR with as few interruptions in chest compressions as possible. A second rescuer obtains vascular access and delivers epinephrine, 0.01 mg/kg (0.1 mL/kg of 1:10 000 solution) maximum of 1 mg (10 mL), while CPR is continued. The same epinephrine dose is repeated every 3 to 5 minutes (Class I, LOE B). There is no survival benefit from high-dose epinephrine, and it may be harmful, particularly in asphyxia (Class III, LOE B).[257–261] High-dose epinephrine may be considered in exceptional circumstances, such as β-blocker overdose (Class IIb, LOE C).

- Once an advanced airway is in place, 1 rescuer should give continuous chest compressions at a rate of at least 100 per minute without pause for ventilation. The second rescuer delivers ventilations at a rate of 1 breath every 6 to 8 seconds (about 8 to 10 breaths per minute). Rotate the compressor role approximately every 2 minutes to prevent compressor fatigue and deterioration in quality and rate of chest compressions. Check rhythm every 2 minutes with minimal interruptions in chest compressions. If the rhythm is "nonshockable" continue with cycles of CPR and epinephrine administration until there is evidence of ROSC or you decide to terminate the effort. If at any time the rhythm

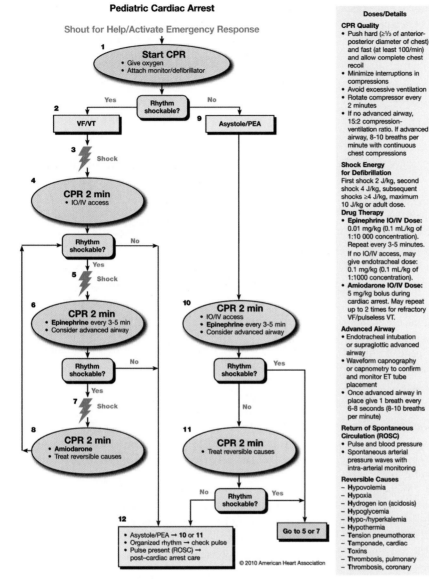

Figure 1. PALS Pulseless Arrest Algorithm.

becomes "shockable," give a shock (Step 7) and immediately resume chest compressions for 2 minutes before rechecking the rhythm. Minimize time between chest compressions and shock delivery (ie, check rhythm and deliver shocks immediately after compressions rather than after rescue breaths, if possible) and between shock delivery and resumption of chest compressions.

• Search for and treat reversible causes.

## "Shockable Rhythm": VF/Pulseless VT (Step 2)

Defibrillation is the definitive treatment for VF (Class I, LOE B) with an overall survival rate of 17% to 20%.[4,262,263] Survival is better in primary than in secondary VF.[6] In adults, the probability of survival declines by 7% to 10% for each minute of arrest without CPR and defibrillation.[264] Survival is better if early, high-quality CPR is provided with minimal interruptions. Outcome of shock delivery is best if rescuers minimize the time between last compression and shock delivery, so rescuers should be prepared to coordinate (brief) interruptions in chest compressions to deliver shocks, and

should resume compressions immediately after shock delivery.

## Defibrillators

Defibrillators are either manual or automated (AED), with monophasic or biphasic waveforms. For further information see Part 6, "Electrical Therapies: Automated External Defibrillators, Defibrillation, Cardioversion, and Pacing."

AEDs in institutions caring for children at risk for arrhythmias and cardiac arrest (eg, hospitals, EDs) must be capable of recognizing pediatric cardiac rhythms and should ideally have a method of adjusting the energy level for children.

The following should be considered when using a manual defibrillator:

## Paddle Size

In general, manual defibrillators have two sizes of hand-held paddles: adult and infant. The infant paddles may slide over or be located under the adult paddles. Manual defibrillators can also be used with hands-free pads that are self adhesive.

Use the largest paddles or self-adhering electrodes[265–267] that will fit on the child's chest without touching (when possible, leave about 3 cm between the paddles or electrodes). Paddles and self-adhering pads appear to be equally effective.[268] Self-adhering pads should be pressed firmly on the chest so that the gel on the pad completely touches the child's chest. An appropriate paddle or self-adhesive pad size is

- "Adult" size (8 to 10 cm) for children >10 kg (> approximately 1 year)
- "Infant" size for infants <10 kg

## Interface
The electrode–chest wall interface is part of the self-adhesive pad; in contrast, electrode gel must be applied liberally on manually applied paddles. Do not use saline-soaked pads, ultrasound gel, bare paddles, or alcohol pads.

## Paddle Position
Follow package directions for placement of self-adhesive AED or monitor/defibrillator pads.

Place manual paddles over the right side of the upper chest and the apex of the heart (to the left of the nipple over the left lower ribs) so the heart is between the two paddles. Apply firm pressure. There is no advantage in an anterior-posterior position of the paddles.[268]

## Energy Dose
The lowest energy dose for effective defibrillation and the upper limit for safe defibrillation in infants and children are not known; more data are needed. It has been observed that in children with VF, an initial monophasic dose of 2 J/kg is only effective in terminating ventricular fibrillation 18% to 50% of the time,[269,270] while similar doses of biphasic shocks are effective 48% of the time.[268] Children with out-of-hospital VF cardiac arrest often receive more than 2 J/kg,[271,272] and one in-hospital cardiac arrest study[268] showed that children received doses between 2.5 and 3.2 J/kg to achieve ROSC. Energy doses >4 J/kg (up to 9 J/kg) have effectively defibrillated children[272–274] and pediatric animals[275] with negligible adverse effects. Based on data from adult studies[276,277] and pediatric animal models,[278–280] biphasic shocks appear to be at least as effective as monophasic shocks and less harmful.

It is acceptable to use an initial dose of 2 to 4 J/kg (Class IIa, LOE C), but for ease of teaching an initial dose of 2 J/kg may be considered (Class IIb, LOE C). For refractory VF, it is reasonable to increase the dose to 4 J/kg (Class IIa, LOE C). Subsequent energy levels should be at least 4 J/kg, and higher energy levels may be considered, not to exceed 10 J/kg or the adult maximum dose (Class IIb, LOE C).

## AEDs
Many AEDs can accurately detect VF in children of all ages.[271,281–283] They can differentiate "shockable" from "nonshockable" rhythms with a high degree of sensitivity and specificity.[281,282] It is recommended that systems and institutions that have AED programs and that care for children should use AEDs with a high specificity to recognize pediatric shockable rhythms and a pediatric attenuating system

that can be used for infants and children up to approximately 25 kg (approximately 8 years of age).[274,284] If an AED with an attenuator is not available, use an AED with standard electrodes (Class IIa, LOE C).

In infants <1 year of age a manual defibrillator is preferred. If a manual defibrillator is not available, an AED with a dose attenuator may be used. An AED without a dose attenuator may be used if neither a manual defibrillator nor one with a dose attenuator is available (Class IIb, LOE C).

## Integration of Defibrillation With Resuscitation Sequence
The following are important considerations:

- Provide CPR until the defibrillator is ready to deliver a shock; after shock delivery, resume CPR, beginning with chest compressions. Minimize interruptions of chest compressions. In adults with prolonged arrest[285,286] and in animal models,[287] defibrillation is more likely to be successful after a period of effective chest compressions. Ideally chest compressions should be interrupted only for ventilations (until an advanced airway is in place), rhythm check, and shock delivery. If a "shockable" rhythm is still present, continue chest compressions after a rhythm check (when possible) while the defibrillator is charging (so chest compressions are delivered until shock delivery).
- (Step 3) Give 1 shock (2 J/kg) as quickly as possible and immediately resume CPR, beginning with chest compressions. If 1 shock fails to eliminate VF, the incremental benefit of another immediate shock is low, and resumption of CPR is likely to confer a greater value than another shock. CPR may provide coronary perfusion, increasing the likelihood of defibrillation with a subsequent shock. It is important to minimize the time between chest compressions and shock delivery and between shock delivery and resumption of postshock compressions.
- (Step 4) Continue CPR for about 2 minutes. In in-hospital settings with continuous invasive monitoring, this sequence may be modified at the expert provider's discretion (see, also Part 8.2: "Management of Cardiac Arrest"). If sufficient rescuers are present, obtain vascular (IO or IV) access.
- After 2 minutes of CPR, check the rhythm; recharge the defibrillator to a higher dose (4 J/kg).
- (Step 5) If a "shockable" rhythm persists, give another shock (4 J/kg). If rhythm is "nonshockable," continue with the asystole/PEA algorithm (Steps 10 and 11).
- (Step 6) Immediately resume chest compressions. Continue CPR for approximately 2 minutes. During CPR give epinephrine 0.01 mg/kg (0.1 mL/kg of 1:10 000 concentration), maximum of 1 mg (Class I, LOE B) **every 3 to 5 minutes.** It is helpful if a third rescuer prepares the drug doses *before* the rhythm is checked so epinephrine can be administered as soon as possible. Epinephrine should be administered during chest compressions, but the timing of drug administration is less important than the need to minimize interruptions in chest compressions. Just prior to the rhythm check, the rescuer operating the defibrillator should prepare to recharge the defibrillator (4 J/kg or more

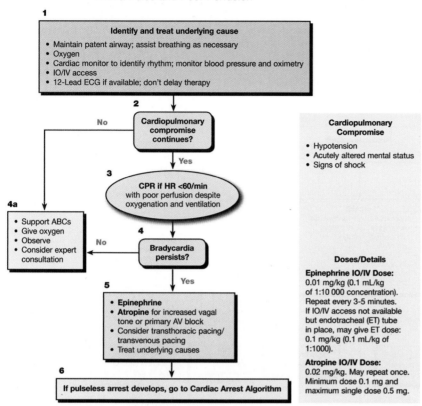

**Pediatric Bradycardia**
With a Pulse and Poor Perfusion

**1**

**Identify and treat underlying cause**
- Maintain patent airway; assist breathing as necessary
- Oxygen
- Cardiac monitor to identify rhythm; monitor blood pressure and oximetry
- IO/IV access
- 12-Lead ECG if available; don't delay therapy

**2**  No ← **Cardiopulmonary compromise continues?**

Yes ↓

**3** **CPR if HR <60/min** with poor perfusion despite oxygenation and ventilation

**4a**
- Support ABCs
- Give oxygen
- Observe
- Consider expert consultation

No ← **4** **Bradycardia persists?**

Yes ↓

**5**
- **Epinephrine**
- **Atropine** for increased vagal tone or primary AV block
- Consider transthoracic pacing/transvenous pacing
- Treat underlying causes

**6**
**If pulseless arrest develops, go to Cardiac Arrest Algorithm**

**Cardiopulmonary Compromise**
- Hypotension
- Acutely altered mental status
- Signs of shock

**Doses/Details**
**Epinephrine IO/IV Dose:**
0.01 mg/kg (0.1 mL/kg of 1:10 000 concentration). Repeat every 3-5 minutes. If IO/IV access not available but endotracheal (ET) tube in place, may give ET dose: 0.1 mg/kg (0.1 mL/kg of 1:1000).

**Atropine IO/IV Dose:**
0.02 mg/kg. May repeat once. Minimum dose 0.1 mg and maximum single dose 0.5 mg.

**Figure 2.** PALS Bradycardia Algorithm.

with a maximum dose not to exceed 10 J/kg or the adult dose, whichever is lower).

- Check the rhythm
- (Step 7) If the rhythm is "shockable," deliver another shock (4 J/kg or more with a maximum dose not to exceed 10 J/kg or the adult dose, whichever is lower) and immediately resume CPR (beginning with chest compressions).
- (Step 8) While continuing CPR, give amiodarone (Class IIb, LOE C)[228,288–290] or lidocaine if amiodarone is not available.
- If at any time the rhythm check shows a "nonshockable" rhythm, proceed to the "Pulseless Arrest" sequence (Steps 10 or 11).
- Once an advanced airway is in place, 2 rescuers no longer deliver cycles of CPR (ie, compressions interrupted by pauses for ventilation). Instead, the compressing rescuer gives continuous chest compressions at a rate of at least 100 per minute without pause for ventilation. The rescuer delivering ventilation provides about 1 breath every 6 to 8 seconds (8 to 10 breaths per minute). Two or more rescuers should rotate the compressor role approximately every 2 minutes to prevent compressor fatigue and deterioration in quality and rate of chest compressions.
- If defibrillation successfully restores an organized rhythm (or there is other evidence of ROSC, such as an abrupt rise in Petco₂ or visible pulsations on an arterial waveform), check the child's pulse to determine if a perfusing rhythm is present. If a pulse is present, continue with postresuscitation care.

- If defibrillation is successful but VF recurs, resume CPR and give another bolus of amiodarone before trying to defibrillate with the previously successful shock dose.
- Search for and treat reversible causes

## Torsades de Pointes

This polymorphic VT is associated with a long QT interval, which may be congenital or may result from toxicity with type IA antiarrhythmics (eg, procainamide, quinidine, and disopyramide) or type III antiarrhythmics (eg, sotalol and amiodarone), tricyclic antidepressants (see below), digitalis, or drug interactions.[291,292]

### Treatment

Torsades de pointes VT typically deteriorates rapidly to VF or pulseless VT, so providers should initiate CPR and proceed with defibrillation when pulseless arrest develops (see above). Regardless of the cause, treat torsades de pointes with a rapid (several minutes) IV infusion of magnesium sulfate (25 to 50 mg/kg; maximum single dose 2 g).

## Bradycardia

Box numbers in the text below refer to the corresponding boxes in the PALS Bradycardia Algorithm (see Figure 2). This algorithm applies to the care of the infant or child with bradycardia and cardiorespiratory compromise, but a palpable pulse. If at any time the patient develops pulseless arrest, see the PALS Pulseless Arrest Algorithm.

Emergency treatment of bradycardia is indicated when the rhythm results in hemodynamic compromise.

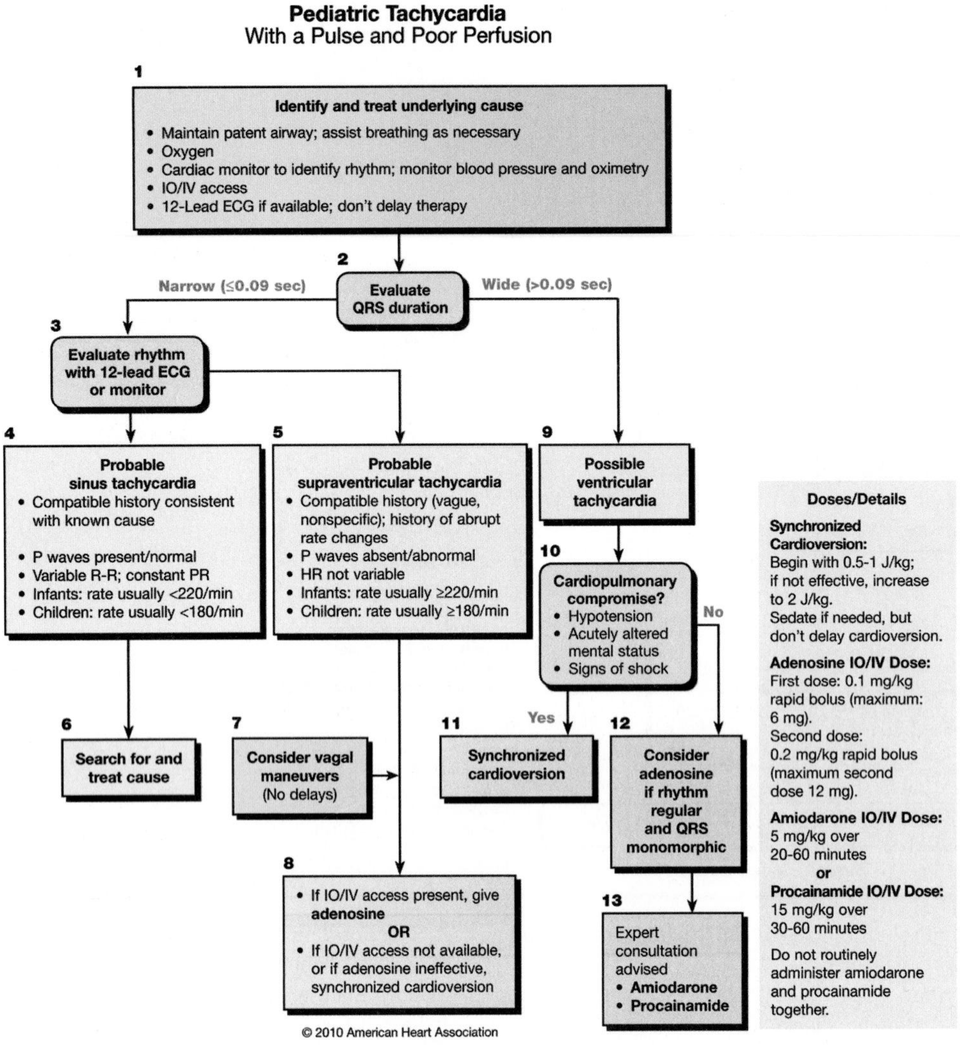

**Pediatric Tachycardia**
With a Pulse and Poor Perfusion

**1**
**Identify and treat underlying cause**
- Maintain patent airway; assist breathing as necessary
- Oxygen
- Cardiac monitor to identify rhythm; monitor blood pressure and oximetry
- IO/IV access
- 12-Lead ECG if available; don't delay therapy

**2** Narrow (≤0.09 sec) ← **Evaluate QRS duration** → Wide (>0.09 sec)

**3** **Evaluate rhythm with 12-lead ECG or monitor**

**4**
**Probable sinus tachycardia**
- Compatible history consistent with known cause
- P waves present/normal
- Variable R-R; constant PR
- Infants: rate usually <220/min
- Children: rate usually <180/min

**5**
**Probable supraventricular tachycardia**
- Compatible history (vague, nonspecific); history of abrupt rate changes
- P waves absent/abnormal
- HR not variable
- Infants: rate usually ≥220/min
- Children: rate usually ≥180/min

**9**
**Possible ventricular tachycardia**

**10**
**Cardiopulmonary compromise?**
- Hypotension
- Acutely altered mental status
- Signs of shock

→ No

**6**
**Search for and treat cause**

**7**
**Consider vagal maneuvers**
(No delays)

**11**
Yes → **Synchronized cardioversion**

**12**
**Consider adenosine if rhythm regular and QRS monomorphic**

**8**
- If IO/IV access present, give **adenosine**
OR
- If IO/IV access not available, or if adenosine ineffective, synchronized cardioversion

**13**
**Expert consultation advised**
- **Amiodarone**
- **Procainamide**

**Doses/Details**

**Synchronized Cardioversion:**
Begin with 0.5-1 J/kg; if not effective, increase to 2 J/kg. Sedate if needed, but don't delay cardioversion.

**Adenosine IO/IV Dose:**
First dose: 0.1 mg/kg rapid bolus (maximum: 6 mg).
Second dose: 0.2 mg/kg rapid bolus (maximum second dose 12 mg).

**Amiodarone IO/IV Dose:**
5 mg/kg over 20-60 minutes
**or**
**Procainamide IO/IV Dose:**
15 mg/kg over 30-60 minutes

Do not routinely administer amiodarone and procainamide together.

© 2010 American Heart Association

**Figure 3.** PALS Tachycardia Algorithm.

- (Box 1) Support a patent airway, breathing, and circulation as needed. Administer oxygen, attach an ECG monitor/defibrillator, and obtain vascular access.
- (Box 2) Reassess the patient to determine if bradycardia persists and is still causing cardiorespiratory symptoms despite adequate oxygenation and ventilation.
- (Box 4a) If pulses, perfusion, and respirations are adequate, no emergency treatment is necessary. Monitor and proceed with evaluation.
- (Box 3) If heart rate is <60 beats per minute with poor perfusion despite effective ventilation with oxygen, start CPR.
- (Box 4) After 2 minutes reevaluate the patient to determine if bradycardia and signs of hemodynamic compromise persist. Verify that the support is adequate (eg, check airway, oxygen source, and effectiveness of ventilation).
- (Box 5) Medications and pacing:
  - Continue to support airway, ventilation, oxygenation, and chest compressions (Class I, LOE B). If bradycardia persists or responds only transiently, give epinephrine IV (or IO) 0.01 mg/kg (0.1 mL/kg of 1:10,000 solution) or if IV/IO access not available, give endotracheally 0.1 mg/kg (0.1 mL/kg of 1:1,000 solution) (Class I, LOE B).

  - If bradycardia is due to increased vagal tone or primary AV conduction block (ie, not secondary to factors such as hypoxia), give IV/IO atropine 0.02 mg/kg or an endotracheal dose of 0.04 to 0.06 mg/kg (Class I, LOE C).
  - Emergency transcutaneous pacing may be lifesaving if the bradycardia is due to complete heart block or sinus node dysfunction unresponsive to ventilation, oxygenation, chest compressions, and medications, especially if it is associated with congenital or acquired heart disease (Class IIb, LOE C).[293] Pacing is not useful for asystole[293,294] or bradycardia due to postarrest hypoxic/ischemic myocardial insult or respiratory failure.

### Tachycardia

The box numbers in the text below correspond to the numbered boxes in the Tachycardia Algorithm (see Figure 3).

- If there are signs of poor perfusion and pulses are not palpable, proceed with the PALS Pulseless Arrest Algorithm (see Figure 1).
- (Box 1) If pulses are palpable and the patient has adequate perfusion

–Assess and support airway, breathing, and circulation
–Provide oxygen.
–Attach monitor/defibrillator.
–Obtain vascular access.
–Evaluate 12-lead ECG and assess QRS duration (Box 2).

## Narrow-Complex (≤0.09 Second) Tachycardia

Evaluation of a 12-lead ECG (Box 3) and the patient's clinical presentation and history (Boxes 4 and 5) should help differentiate sinus tachycardia from supraventricular tachycardia (SVT). If the rhythm is sinus tachycardia, search for and treat reversible causes.

## Supraventricular Tachycardia (Box 5)

- Monitor rhythm during therapy to evaluate the effect of interventions. The choice of therapy is determined by the patient's degree of hemodynamic instability.
- Attempt vagal stimulation (Box 7) first, unless the patient is hemodynamically unstable or the procedure will unduly delay chemical or electric cardioversion (Class IIa, LOE C). In infants and young children, apply ice to the face without occluding the airway.[295,296]
- In older children, carotid sinus massage or Valsalva maneuvers are safe.[297–299]
- One method for performing a Valsalva maneuver is to have the child blow through a narrow straw.[298] Do not apply pressure to the eye because this can damage the retina.
- Pharmacologic cardioversion with adenosine (Box 8) is very effective with minimal and transient side effects.[300–304] If IV/IO access is readily available, adenosine is the drug of choice (Class I, LOE C). Side effects are usually transient.[300–304] Administer IV/IO adenosine 0.1 mg/kg using 2 syringes connected to a T-connector or stopcock; give adenosine rapidly with 1 syringe and immediately flush with ≥5 mL of normal saline with the other. An IV/IO dose of Verapamil, 0.1 to 0.3 mg/kg is also effective in terminating SVT in older children,[305,306] but it should not be used in infants without expert consultation (Class III, LOE C) because it may cause potential myocardial depression, hypotension, and cardiac arrest.[306,307]
- If the patient is hemodynamically unstable or if adenosine is ineffective, perform electric synchronized cardioversion (Box 8). Use sedation, if possible. Start with a dose of 0.5 to 1 J/kg. If unsuccessful, increase the dose to 2 J/kg (Class IIb, LOE C). If a second shock is unsuccessful or the tachycardia recurs quickly, consider amiodarone or procainamide before a third shock.
- Consider amiodarone 5 mg/kg IO/IV[308,309] or procainamide 15 mg/kg IO/IV[236] for a patient with SVT unresponsive to vagal maneuvers and adenosine and/or electric cardioversion; for hemodynamically stable patients, expert consultation is strongly recommended prior to administration (Class IIb, LOE C). Both amiodarone and procainamide must be infused slowly (amiodarone over 20 to 60 minutes and procainamide over 30 to 60 minutes), depending on the urgency, while the ECG and blood pressure are monitored. If there is no effect and there are no signs of toxicity, give

additional doses (Table 1). Avoid the simultaneous use of amiodarone and procainamide without expert consultation.

## Wide-Complex (>0.09 Second) Tachycardia (Box 9)

Wide-complex tachycardia often originates in the ventricles (ventricular tachycardia) but may be supraventricular in origin.[310]

Because all arrhythmia therapies have a potential for serious adverse effects, consultation with an expert in pediatric arrhythmias is strongly recommended before treating children who are hemodynamically stable.

The following are important considerations in treating wide-complex tachycardia in hemodynamically stable patients:

- Adenosine may be useful in differentiating SVT from VT and converting wide-complex tachycardia of supraventricular origin (Box 12). Adenosine should be considered only if the rhythm is regular and the QRS is monomorphic. Do not use adenosine in patients with known Wolff-Parkinson-White syndrome and wide-complex tachycardia.
- Consider electric cardioversion after sedation using a starting energy dose of 0.5 to 1 J/kg. If that fails, increase the dose to 2 J/kg (Class IIb, LOE C) (Box 11).
- Consider pharmacologic conversion with either intravenous amiodarone (5 mg/kg over 20 to 60 minutes) or procainamide (15 mg/kg given over 30 to 60 minutes) while monitoring ECG and blood pressure. Stop or slow the infusion if there is a decline in blood pressure or the QRS widens (Box 13). Expert consultation is strongly recommended prior to administration.

In hemodynamically unstable patients:

- Electric cardioversion is recommended using a starting energy dose of 0.5 to 1 J/kg. If that fails, increase the dose to 2 J/kg (Class 1, LOE C).

## Special Resuscitation Situations

### Septic Shock

- There appears to be no clinically important difference in survival of children who are treated for septic shock with colloid compared with those who are treated with isotonic crystalloid solutions.[311–314] Although colloid may be beneficial as part of a protocol-driven strategy,[315] it is reasonable to use isotonic crystalloid solution as the initial fluid for the treatment of septic shock (Class IIa, LOE C).
- Monitoring the central venous (superior vena cava) oxygen saturation (ScvO2) may be useful to titrate therapy in infants and children with septic shock. Protocol-driven or "goal-directed" therapy, with a target ScvO2 ≥70% appears to improve patient survival in severe sepsis (Class IIb, LOE B).[316–318]
- Early assisted ventilation may be considered as part of a protocol-driven strategy for septic shock (Class IIb, LOE C).[315,319]
- Etomidate has been shown to facilitate endotracheal intubation in infants and children with minimal hemodynamic effect,[320–322] but do not use it routinely in pediatric patients with evidence of septic shock (Class III, LOE B). Adrenal

suppression is seen after administration of etomidate in children[323] and adults.[324] In children and adults with septic shock, etomidate administration is associated with a higher mortality rate.[323,325]

## Hypovolemic Shock

- Use an isotonic crystalloid solution (eg, lactated Ringer's solution or normal saline)[326,327] as the initial fluid for the treatment of shock (Class I, LOE A). There is no added benefit in using colloid (eg, albumin) during the early phase of resuscitation.[328,329]
- Treat signs of shock with a bolus of 20 mL/kg of isotonic crystalloid even if blood pressure is normal (Class IIb, LOE C). Crystalloids may have an associated survival benefit over colloid for children with shock secondary to general trauma, traumatic brain injury, and burns.[329–332] There is no evidence to support the use of a specific isotonic crystalloid. Give additional boluses (20 mL/kg) if systemic perfusion fails to improve. There are insufficient data to make a recommendation for or against use of hypertonic saline for shock associated with head injuries or hypovolemia.[333,334]
- There is insufficient evidence in infants and children to make a recommendation about the best timing or extent of volume resuscitation for children with hemorrhagic shock following trauma.

## Trauma

Some aspects of trauma resuscitation require emphasis because improperly performed resuscitation is a major cause of preventable pediatric deaths.[335]

Common errors in pediatric trauma resuscitation include failure to open and maintain the airway, failure to provide appropriate fluid resuscitation, and failure to recognize and treat internal bleeding. Involve a qualified surgeon early and, if possible, transport a child with multisystem trauma to a trauma center with pediatric expertise.

The following are special aspects of trauma resuscitation:

- When the mechanism of injury is compatible with cervical spinal injury, restrict motion of the cervical spine and avoid traction or movement of the head and neck. Open and maintain the airway with a jaw thrust, and do not tilt the head.
- If the airway cannot be opened with a jaw thrust, use a head tilt–chin lift because you must establish a patent airway. Because of the disproportionately large head of infants and young children, optimal positioning may require recessing the occiput[336] or elevating the torso to avoid undesirable backboard-induced cervical flexion.[336,337]
- Do not routinely hyperventilate even in case of head injury (Class III, LOE C).[338,339] Intentional brief hyperventilation may be used as a temporizing rescue therapy if there are signs of impending brain herniation (eg, sudden rise in measured intracranial pressure, dilation of one or both pupils with decreased response to light, bradycardia, and hypertension).
- Suspect thoracic injury in all thoraco-abdominal trauma, even in the absence of external injuries. Tension pneumo-thorax, hemothorax, or pulmonary contusion may impair oxygenation and ventilation.
- If the patient has maxillofacial trauma or if you suspect a basilar skull fracture, insert an orogastric rather than a nasogastric tube (Class IIa, LOE C).[340]
- In the very select circumstances of children with cardiac arrest from penetrating trauma with short transport times, consider performing resuscitative thoracotomy (Class IIb, LOE C).[341,342]
- Consider intra-abdominal hemorrhage, tension pneumothorax, pericardial tamponade, and spinal cord injury in infants and children, and intracranial hemorrhage in infants, as causes of shock.[343,344]

## Single Ventricle

Standard prearrest and arrest resuscitation procedures should be followed for infants and children with single ventricle anatomy following Stage I palliation or in the infant or neonate with a univentricular heart and a shunt to augment pulmonary blood flow. Heparin may be considered for infants with a systemic-pulmonary artery shunt or right ventricular-pulmonary artery shunt. Following resuscitation from cardiac arrest, oxygen administration should be adjusted to balance systemic and pulmonary blood flow, targeting an oxyhemoglobin saturation ($SpO_2$) of approximately 80%. End-tidal $CO_2$ ($PETCO_2$) in the single-ventricle patient during cardiac arrest may not be a reliable indicator of CPR quality because pulmonary blood flow changes rapidly and does not necessarily reflect cardiac output during CPR.[345]

Neonates in a prearrest state due to elevated pulmonary-to-systemic flow ratio prior to Stage I repair might benefit from a $PaCO_2$ of 50 to 60 mm Hg, which can be achieved during mechanical ventilation by reducing minute ventilation, increasing the inspired fraction of $CO_2$, or administering opioids with or without chemical paralysis (Class IIb, LOE B).[346,347] Neonates in a low cardiac output state following stage I repair may benefit from systemic vasodilators such as $\alpha$-adrenergic antagonists (eg, phenoxybenzamine) to treat or ameliorate increased systemic vascular resistance, improve systemic oxygen delivery, and reduce the likelihood of cardiac arrest (Class IIa, LOE B).[348–350] Other drugs that reduce systemic vascular resistance (eg, milrinone or nipride)[351] may also be considered for patients with excessive Qp:Qs (Class IIa, LOE B).[352] Following Stage I repair, evaluation of oxygen delivery and extraction (eg, using central venous oxygen saturation [$ScvO_2$] and near-infrared spectroscopy) may help identify evolving changes in hemodynamics that may herald impending cardiac arrest.[353–355] During cardiopulmonary arrest, it is reasonable to consider extracorporeal membrane oxygenation (ECMO) for patients with single ventricle anatomy who have undergone Stage I procedure (Class IIa, LOE B).[129,132,152,356,357]

Hypoventilation may improve oxygen delivery in patients in a prearrest state with Fontan or hemi-Fontan/bidirectional Glenn (BDG) physiology (Class IIa, LOE B).[358–361] Negative-pressure ventilation may improve cardiac output (Class IIa, LOE C).[362,363] During cardiopulmonary arrest, it is reasonable to consider extracorporeal membrane oxygenation (ECMO) for patients with Fontan physiology (Class IIa, LOE C).[364] It is unclear at this time whether patients with hemi-Fontan/BDG physiology in cardiac arrest might benefit from ECMO.

## Pulmonary Hypertension

Standard PALS, including oxygenation and ventilation, should be provided to patients with pulmonary hypertension and a cardiopulmonary arrest. It may be beneficial to attempt to correct hypercarbia. Administration of a bolus of isotonic fluid may be useful to maintain preload to the systemic ventricle. If intravenous or inhaled therapy to decrease pulmonary hypertension has been interrupted, reinstitute it (Class IIa, LOE C). Consider administering inhaled nitric oxide (iNO) or aerosolized prostacyclin or analogue to reduce pulmonary vascular resistance (Class IIa, LOE C). If iNO is not available, consider giving an intravenous bolus of prostacyclin (Class IIa, LOE C).[365–367] ECMO may be beneficial if instituted early in the resuscitation (Class IIa, LOE C).[368]

## Children With Special Healthcare Needs

Children with special healthcare needs[369] may require emergency care for chronic conditions (eg, obstruction of a tracheostomy), failure of support technology (eg, ventilator failure), progression of their underlying disease, or events unrelated to those special needs.[370]

For additional information about CPR see Part 13: "Pediatric Basic Life Support."

## Ventilation With a Tracheostomy or Stoma

Parents, school nurses, and home healthcare providers should know how to assess patency of the airway, clear the airway, replace the tracheostomy tube, and perform CPR using the artificial airway in a child with a tracheostomy.

Parents and providers should be able to ventilate via a tracheostomy tube and verify effectiveness by assessing chest expansion. If, after suctioning, the chest does not expand with ventilation, remove the tracheostomy tube and replace it or insert a same-sized endotracheal tube, if available, into the tracheal stoma. If a clean tube is unavailable, perform mouth-to-stoma or mask-to-stoma ventilations. If the upper airway is patent, bag-mask ventilation via the nose and mouth may be effective if the tracheal stoma is manually occluded.

## Toxicological Emergencies

Overdose with local anesthetics, cocaine, narcotics, tricyclic antidepressants, calcium channel blockers, and β-adrenergic blockers may require specific treatment modalities in addition to the usual resuscitative measures.

## Local Anesthetic

Local anesthetics are used topically, intravenously, subcutaneously, and in epidural or other catheters for delivery of regional analgesia. The toxicity of local anesthetics is well recognized in children; they may cause changes in mental status, seizures, arrhythmias, or even cardiac arrest in settings of overdose or inadvertent vascular administration. Multiple case reports, including some pediatric reports, have described successful treatment of local anesthetic toxicity with intravenous lipid emulsion.[371]

## Cocaine

Acute coronary syndrome, manifested by chest pain and cardiac rhythm disturbances (including VT and VF), is the most frequent cocaine-related reason for hospitalization in adults.[372,373] Cocaine also may prolong the action potential and QRS duration and impairs myocardial contractility.[374,375]

### Treatment

- Hyperthermia, which may result from cocaine-induced hypermetabolism, is associated with an increase in toxicity;[376] therefore treat elevated temperature aggressively.
- For coronary vasospasm consider nitroglycerin (Class IIa, LOE C),[377,378] a benzodiazepine, and phentolamine (an α-adrenergic antagonist) (Class IIb, LOE C).[379,380]
- *Do not* give β-adrenergic blockers (Class III, LOE C),[376]
- For ventricular arrhythmia, consider sodium bicarbonate (1 to 2 mEq/kg) administration (Class IIb, LOE C)[381,382] in addition to standard treatment.
- To prevent arrhythmias secondary to myocardial infarction, consider a lidocaine bolus followed by a lidocaine infusion (Class IIb, LOE C).

## Tricyclic Antidepressants and Other Sodium Channel Blockers

Toxic doses cause cardiovascular abnormalities, including intraventricular conduction delays, heart block, bradycardia, prolongation of the QT interval, ventricular arrhythmias (including torsades de pointes, VT, and VF), hypotension, seizures,[375,383] and a depressed level of consciousness.

### Treatment

- Give 1 to 2 mEq/kg intravenous boluses of sodium bicarbonate until arterial pH is >7.45; then provide an infusion of 150 mEq NaHCO3 per liter of D5W to maintain alkalosis. In cases of severe intoxication increase the pH to 7.50 to 7.55.[375,384] Do not administer Class IA (quinidine, procainamide), Class IC (flecainide, propafenone), or Class III (amiodarone and sotalol) antiarrhythmics, which may exacerbate cardiac toxicity (Class III, LOE C).[384]
- For hypotension, give boluses (10 mL/kg each) of normal saline. If hypotension persists, epinephrine and norepinephrine are more effective than dopamine in raising blood pressure.[385,386]
- Consider ECMO if high-dose vasopressors do not maintain blood pressure.[387,388]

## Calcium Channel Blockers

Manifestations of toxicity include hypotension, ECG changes (prolongation of the QT interval, widening of the QRS, and right bundle branch block), arrhythmias (bradycardia, SVT, VT, torsades de pointes, and VF),[389] seizures, and altered mental status.

### Treatment

- Treat mild hypotension with small boluses (5 to 10 mL/kg) of normal saline because myocardial depression may limit the amount of fluid the patient can tolerate.

- The effectiveness of calcium administration is variable (Class IIb, LOE C).[389–393] Infuse 20 mg/kg (0.2 mL/kg) of 10% calcium chloride intravenously over 5 to 10 minutes; if there is a beneficial effect, give an infusion of 20 to 50 mg/kg per hour. Monitor serum ionized calcium concentration to prevent hypercalcemia. It is preferable to administer calcium chloride via a central venous catheter; use caution when infusing into a peripheral IV because infiltration can cause severe tissue injury. If no central venous catheter is available, infuse calcium gluconate through a secure peripheral IV. For bradycardia and hypotension, consider vasopressors and inotropes such as norepinephrine or epinephrine (Class IIb, LOE C).[392]
- There are insufficient data to recommend for or against an infusion of insulin and glucose[394–397] or sodium bicarbonate.

### Beta-Adrenergic Blockers

Toxic doses of β-adrenergic blockers cause bradycardia, heart block, and decreased cardiac contractility, and some (eg, propranolol and sotalol) may also prolong the QRS and the QT intervals.[397–400]

#### Treatment

- High-dose epinephrine infusion may be effective (Class IIb, LOE C).[400,401]
- Consider glucagon (Class IIb, LOE C).[397,400,402,403] In adolescents infuse 5 to 10 mg of glucagon over several minutes followed by an IV infusion of 1 to 5 mg/hour.
- Consider an infusion of glucose and insulin (Class IIb, LOE C).[394]
- There are insufficient data to make a recommendation for or against using calcium (Class IIb, LOE C).[390,404,405]
- Calcium may be considered if glucagon and catecholamines are ineffective (Class IIb, LOE C).

### Opioids

Narcotics may cause hypoventilation, apnea, bradycardia, and hypotension in addition to depressed responsiveness.

#### Treatment

- Support of oxygenation and ventilation is the initial treatment for severe respiratory depression from any cause (Class I).
- Naloxone reverses the respiratory depression of narcotic overdose (Class I, LOE B),[406–410] but in persons with long-term addictions or cardiovascular disease, naloxone may markedly increase heart rate and blood pressure and cause acute pulmonary edema, cardiac arrhythmias (including asystole), and seizures. Ventilation before administration of naloxone appears to reduce these adverse effects.[411] Intramuscular administration of naloxone may lower the risk by slowing the onset of drug effect.

### Postresuscitation Stabilization (Post Cardiac Arrest Care)

The goals of postresuscitation care are to preserve neurologic function, prevent secondary organ injury, diagnose and treat the cause of illness, and enable the patient to arrive at a pediatric tertiary-care facility in an optimal physiologic state.

Frequent reassessment of the patient is necessary because cardiorespiratory status may deteriorate.

### Respiratory System

- Data suggest that hyperoxemia (ie, a high $PaO_2$) enhances the oxidative injury observed following ischemia-reperfusion. Therefore, one goal of the postresuscitation phase is to reduce the risk of oxidative injury while maintaining adequate oxygen delivery. A practical way to achieve that goal is to reduce the $FIO_2$ to reduce the $PaO_2$ while ensuring adequate arterial oxygen content. Specifically, use the lowest inspired oxygen concentration that will maintain the arterial oxyhemoglobin saturation ≥94%. Provided appropriate equipment is available, once ROSC is achieved, adjust the $FIO_2$ to the minimum concentration needed to achieve transcutaneous or arterial oxygen saturation at least 94%, with the goal of avoiding hyperoxia while ensuring adequate oxygen delivery. Since an arterial oxyhemoglobin saturation of 100% may correspond to a $PaO_2$ anywhere between ~80 and 500 mmHg, in general it is appropriate to wean the $FIO_2$ for a saturation of 100%, provided the oxyhemoglobin saturation can be maintained ≥94%.
- In addition to the usual clinical signs of adequate perfusion, laboratory parameters of adequate oxygen delivery over time include resolution of metabolic acidosis, reduced lactate concentration, and normalization of venous oxygen saturation.
- Assist ventilation if there is significant respiratory compromise (tachypnea, respiratory distress with agitation or decreased responsiveness, poor air exchange, cyanosis, hypoxemia). If the patient is already intubated, verify tube position, patency, and security. In the hospital setting, consider obtaining arterial blood gases 10 to 15 minutes after establishing the initial mechanical ventilator settings and make appropriate adjustments. Ideally, correlate blood gases with capnographic end-tidal $CO_2$ concentration ($PETCO_2$) to enable noninvasive monitoring of ventilation.
- Control pain and discomfort with analgesics (eg, fentanyl or morphine) and sedatives (eg, lorazepam or midazolam). Neuromuscular blocking agents (eg, vecuronium or pancuronium) with analgesia or sedation, or both, may improve oxygenation and ventilation in case of patient-ventilator dyssynchrony or severely compromised pulmonary function. Neuromuscular blockers, however, can mask seizures and impede neurologic examinations.
- Monitor exhaled $CO_2$ ($PETCO_2$), especially during transport and diagnostic procedures (Class IIa, LOE B).[116,412,413]
- Insert a gastric tube to relieve and help prevent gastric inflation.

### Cardiovascular System

- Monitor heart rate and blood pressure. Repeat clinical evaluations at frequent intervals until the patient is stable. Consider monitoring urine output with an indwelling catheter. A 12-lead ECG may be helpful in establishing the cause of the cardiac arrest.
- Remove the IO access after alternative (preferably 2) secure venous catheters are placed. Monitor venous or arterial blood gas analysis and serum electrolytes, glucose,

**Table 2. Medications to Maintain Cardiac Output and for Postresuscitation Stabilization**

| Medication | Dose Range | Comment |
|---|---|---|
| Inamrinone | 0.75–1 mg/kg IV/IO over 5 minutes; may repeat × 2 then: 5–10 mcg/kg per minute | Inodilator |
| Dobutamine | 2–20 mcg/kg per minute IV/IO | Inotrope; vasodilator |
| Dopamine | 2–20 mcg/kg per minute IV/IO | Inotrope; chronotrope; renal and splanchnic vasodilator in low doses; pressor in high doses |
| Epinephrine | 0.1–1 mcg/kg per minute IV/IO | Inotrope; chronotrope; vasodilator in low doses; pressor in higher doses |
| Milrinone | Loading dose: 50 mcg/kg IV/IO over 10–60 min then 0.25–0.75 mcg/kg per minute | Inodilator |
| Norepineph- rine | 0.1–2 mcg/kg per minute | Vasopressor |
| Sodium nitroprusside | Initial: 0.5–1 mcg/kg per minute; titrate to effect up to 8 mcg/kg per minute | Vasodilator Prepare only in $D_5W$ |

IV indicates intravenous; and IO, intraosseous.

Alternative formula for verifying dose during continuous infusion: Infusion rate

$$(mL/h) = \frac{[\text{weight (kg)} \times \text{dose (mcg/kg per min)} \times 60 \text{ (min/hour)}]}{\text{concentration(mcg/mL)}}.$$

and calcium concentrations. A chest x-ray should be performed to evaluate endotracheal tube position, heart size, and pulmonary status. Consider obtaining arterial lactate and central venous oxygen saturation to assess adequacy of tissue oxygen delivery.

## Drugs Used to Maintain Cardiac Output (Table 2)

Myocardial dysfunction and vascular instability are common following resuscitation from cardiac arrest.[414–419] Systemic and pulmonary vascular resistances are often increased initially, except in some cases of septic shock.[420] The postarrest effects on the cardiovascular system may evolve over time, with an initial hyperdynamic state replaced by worsening cardiac function. Therefore in infants and children with documented or suspected cardiovascular dysfunction after cardiac arrest, it is reasonable to administer vasoactive drugs titrated to improve myocardial function and organ perfusion.

There are no studies evaluating the benefit of specific vasoactive agents after ROSC in infants and children. In animal studies after resuscitation from cardiac arrest[418,419,421–424] and post–cardiac surgical experience in children[352] and adults,[425–428] hemodynamic improvement was associated with administration of selected vasoactive agents. Each drug and dose must be tailored to the patient because clinical response is variable. Infuse all vasoactive drugs into a secure IV line. The potential adverse effects of catecholamines include local ischemia and ulceration, tachycardia, atrial and ventricular tachyarrhythmias, hypertension, and metabolic changes (hyperglycemia, increased lactate concentration,[429] and hypokalemia).

### Epinephrine

Low-dose infusions (<0.3 mcg/kg per minute) generally produce β-adrenergic actions (tachycardia, potent inotropy, and decreased systemic vascular resistance). Higher-dose infusions (>0.3 mcg/kg per minute) cause α-adrenergic vasoconstriction.[430,431] Because there is great interpatient variability in response,[432,433] titrate the drug to the desired effect. Epinephrine or norepinephrine may be preferable to dopamine in patients (especially infants) with marked circulatory instability and decompensated shock.[434]

### Dopamine

Dopamine can produce direct dopaminergic effects and indirect β- and α-adrenergic effects through stimulation of norepinephrine release. Titrate dopamine to treat shock that is unresponsive to fluids and when systemic vascular resistance is low (Class IIb, LOE C).[420,435] Typically a dose of 2 to 20 mcg/kg per minute is used. Although low-dose dopamine infusion has been frequently recommended to maintain renal blood flow or improve renal function, data do not show benefit from such therapy.[436,437] At higher doses (>5 mcg/kg per minute), dopamine stimulates cardiac β-adrenergic receptors, but this effect may be reduced in infants and in patients with chronic congestive heart failure. Infusion rates >20 mcg/kg per minute may result in excessive vasoconstriction.[430,431] In one study in single ventricle postoperative cardiac patients, dopamine increased oxygen consumption while not improving blood pressure or cardiac output.[438]

### Dobutamine Hydrochloride

Dobutamine has a relatively selective effect on β1- and β2-adrenergic receptors due to effects of the two isomers; one is an α-adrenergic agonist, and the other is an α-adrenergic antagonist.[439] Dobutamine increases myocardial contractility and can decrease peripheral vascular resistance. Titrate the infusion[432,440,441] to improve cardiac output and blood pressure due to poor myocardial function.[441]

### Norepinephrine

Norepinephrine is a potent vasopressor promoting peripheral vasoconstriction. Titrate the infusion to treat shock with low systemic vascular resistance (septic, anaphylactic, spinal, or vasodilatory) unresponsive to fluid.

### Sodium Nitroprusside

Sodium nitroprusside increases cardiac output by decreasing vascular resistance (afterload). If hypotension is related to poor myocardial function, consider using a combination of sodium nitroprusside to reduce afterload and an inotrope to improve contractility. Fluid administration may be required secondary to vasodilatory effects.

### Inodilators

Inodilators (inamrinone and milrinone) augment cardiac output with little effect on myocardial oxygen demand. It is reasonable to use an inodilator in a highly monitored setting for treatment of myocardial dysfunction with increased systemic or pulmonary vascular resistance (Class IIa, LOE B[352,442–444]). Administration of fluids may be required secondary to vasodilatory effects.

Inodilators have a long half-life with a delay in reaching a steady-state hemodynamic effect after the infusion rate is changed (18 hours with inamrinone and 4.5 hours with milrinone). In cases of toxicity the cardiovascular effects may persist for several hours even after the infusion is discontinued.

## Neurologic System

A primary goal of resuscitation is to preserve brain function. Limit the risk of secondary neuronal injury by adhering to the following precautions:

- Do not routinely provide excessive ventilation or hyperventilation. Hyperventilation has no benefit and may impair neurologic outcome by adversely affecting cardiac output and cerebral perfusion.[445] Intentional brief hyperventilation may be used as temporizing rescue therapy in response to signs of impending cerebral herniation (eg, sudden rise in measured intracranial pressure, dilated pupil[s] not responsive to light, bradycardia, hypertension).

- Therapeutic hypothermia (32°C to 34°C) may be considered for children who remain comatose after resuscitation from cardiac arrest (Class IIb, LOE C).[446,447] It is reasonable for adolescents resuscitated from sudden, witnessed, out-of-hospital VF cardiac arrest (Class IIa, LOE C). Although there are no randomized studies in the pediatric population on the effect of therapeutic hypothermia, it is of benefit in adults following witnessed out-of-hospital VF arrest[448,449] and in asphyxiated newborns.[450,451]

- The ideal method and duration of cooling and rewarming are not known. Prevent shivering by providing sedation and, if needed, neuromuscular blockade, recognizing that this can mask seizure activity. Closely watch for signs of infection. Other potential complications of hypothermia include diminished cardiac output, arrhythmia, pancreatitis, coagulopathy, thrombocytopenia, hypophosphatemia, hypovolemia from cold diuresis, hypokalemia, and hypomagnesemia.

- Monitor temperature continuously, if possible, and treat fever (>38°C) aggressively with antipyretics and cooling devices because fever adversely influences recovery from ischemic brain injury (Class IIa, LOE C).[452–458]

- Treat postischemic seizures aggressively; search for a correctable metabolic cause such as hypoglycemia or electrolyte imbalance.

- Avoid rewarming from 32 to 34°C faster than 0.5°C per 2 hours unless the patient requires rapid rewarming for clinical reasons.

## Renal System

Decreased urine output (<1 mL/kg per hour in infants and children or <30 mL/hour in adolescents) may be caused by prerenal conditions (eg, dehydration, inadequate systemic perfusion), renal ischemic damage, or a combination of factors. Avoid nephrotoxic medications and adjust the dose of medications excreted by the kidneys until you have checked renal function.

## Interhospital Transport

Ideally postresuscitation care should be provided by a trained team from a pediatric tertiary care facility. Contact such a team as early as possible during the resuscitation attempt and coordinate transportation with the receiving unit.[459] Transport team members should be trained and experienced in the care of critically ill and injured children[103,460] and supervised by a pediatric emergency medicine or pediatric critical care physician. The mode of transport and composition of the team should be established for each system based on the care required by each patient.[461] Monitor exhaled CO2 (qualitative colorimetric detector or capnography) during interhospital or intrahospital transport of intubated patients (Class IIa, LOE B).[116,413]

## Family Presence During Resuscitation

Family presence during CPR is increasingly common, and most parents would like to be given the opportunity to be present during resuscitation of their child.[462–471] Studies show that family members who are present at a resuscitation would recommend it to others.[462,463,465,471,472] Parents of chronically ill children are comfortable with medical equipment and emergency procedures, but even family members with no medical background who were at the side of a loved one to say goodbye during the final moments of life believe that their presence was beneficial to the patient,[462–464,466,471–476] comforting for them,[462–465,468–471,476] and helpful in their adjustment[463–465,472,473,476,477] and grieving process.[477] Standardized psychological examinations suggest that, compared with those not present, family members present during attempted resuscitations have less anxiety and depression and more constructive grieving behavior.[477] Parents or family members often fail to ask, but healthcare providers should offer the opportunity in most situations.[474,478,479] Whenever possible, provide family members with the option of being present during resuscitation of an infant or child (Class I, LOE B).[474,478,479]

Family presence during resuscitation, in general, is not disruptive,[464,472,475,476,480,481] and does not create stress among staff or negatively affect their performance.[462,464,480,482] If the presence of family members creates undue staff stress or is considered detrimental to the resuscitation,[483] then family members should be respectfully asked to leave (Class IIa, LOE C). Members of the resuscitation team must be sensitive to the presence of family members, and one person should be assigned to remain with the family to comfort, answer questions, and support the family.[484]

## Termination of Resuscitative Efforts

There are no reliable predictors of outcome to guide when to terminate resuscitative efforts in children.

Clinical variables associated with survival include length of CPR, number of doses of epinephrine, age, witnessed versus unwitnessed cardiac arrest, and the first and subsequent rhythm.[6,7,11–13,15,16,151,485–489] None of these associations, however, predict outcome. Witnessed collapse, bystander CPR, and a short interval from collapse to arrival of professionals improve the chances of a successful resuscitation. Intact survival has been documented after unusually prolonged in-hospital resuscitation.[13,133,134,151,490,491]

## Sudden Unexplained Deaths

Increasing evidence demonstrates that some cases of sudden infant death syndrome (SIDS) and sudden death in older children and young adults may be associated with genetic mutations causing cardiac ion channelopathies. Channelopathies are dysfunctional myocyte ion channels that result in abnormal movement of electrolytes into and/or out of the cell and predispose the heart to arrhythmia.[492–501] Mutations causing cardiac ion channelopathies are found in 2% to 10% of victims[492–498] and in 14% to 20% of young adults with sudden death in whom the cause of death is not evident in a routine autopsy.[499–501] Clinical and laboratory (eg, ECG, molecular-genetic screening) investigations of first- and second-degree relatives of patients with sudden unexplained death reported inherited, arrhythmogenic disease in 22% to 53% of families.[502–505]

Therefore when sudden unexplained cardiac arrest occurs in children and young adults, obtain a complete past medical and family history (including a history of syncopal episodes, sei-

zures, unexplained accidents or drownings, or sudden unexpected death at <50 years old) and review previous ECGs.

All infants, children, and young adults with sudden unexpected death should, where resources allow, have an unrestricted, complete autopsy, preferably performed by a pathologist with training and experience in cardiovascular pathology. Consider appropriate preservation and genetic analysis of tissue to determine the presence of a channelopathy. Refer families of patients that do not have a cause of death found on autopsy to a healthcare provider or center with expertise in arrhythmias (Class I, LOE C).

# Disclosures

## Guidelines Part 14: PALS Writing Group Disclosures

| Writing Group Member | Employment | Research Grant | Other Research Support | Speakers' Bureau/ Honoraria | Ownership Interest | Consultant/ Advisory Board | Other |
|---|---|---|---|---|---|---|---|
| Monica E. Kleinman | Children's Hospital Anesthesia Foundation–Senior Associate in Critical Care Medicine | None | None | None | None | None | None |
| Leon Chameides | Emeritus Director Pediatric Cardiology, Clinical Professor, University of Connecticut | None | None | None | None | None | None |
| Stephen M. Schexnayder | University of Arkansas for Medical Sciences—Professor/ Division Chief; †AHA Compensated Consultant as Associate Senior Science Editor | *Pharmacokinetics of Proton Pumps inhibitors in Critically Ill patients | None | None | None | None | *Expert witness in several cases involving pediatric critical care & emergency medicine |
| Ricardo A. Samson | The University of Arizona: clinical care, teaching and research related to the field of Pediatric Cardiology in academic setting-Professor | None | None | None | None | None | None |
| Mary Fran Hazinski | Vanderbilt University School of Nursing—Professor; AHA ECC Product Development—Senior Science Editor- †Significant compensation as a paid AHA consultant to help develop and edit the 2010 AHA Guidelines for CPR and ECC. | None | None | None | None | None | None |
| Dianne L. Atkins | University of Iowa—Professor *Compensated worksheet editor for the 2010 AHA Guidelines. Money is divided 2/3 to my institution and 1/3 to me. | None | None | None | None | None | *Defense expert witness for episode of ventricular fibrillation in a 2 year old child. Attorney are Buckley and Thereoux of Princeton, New Jersey |
| Marc D. Berg | University of Arizona - Staff Intensivist; Asso. Prof. Clinical Pediatrics, Attending Intensivist, Pediatric Critical Care Medicine | None | None | Travel expenses defrayed with an honorarium of $4000 for speaking at 13th Asian Australasian Congress of Anesthesiologists, Fukuoka, Japan 6/2010 | None | None | None |
| Allan R. de Caen | Self employed, pediatric intensivist | None | None | None | None | None | *Medical expert for Canadian Medical ProtectiveAssoc |

(Continued)

**Guidelines Part 14: PALS Writing Group Disclosures,** *Continued*

| Writing Group Member | Employment | Research Grant | Other Research Support | Speakers' Bureau/ Honoraria | Ownership Interest | Consultant/ Advisory Board | Other |
|---|---|---|---|---|---|---|---|
| Ericka L. Fink | Children's Hospital of Pittsburgh of UPMC–Assistant Professor | †National Institutes of Health, NINDS K23, Laerdal Foundation, and Children's Hospital of Pittsburgh Clinical and Translational Science Institute grants to study duration of hypothermia after pediatric cardiac arrest. | None | None | None | None | None |
| Eugene B. Freid | Nemours Childrens Clinics–Anesthesiologist and Intensivist | None | None | *$1500.00 from University of North Carolina to Nemours Childrens Clinics for 3 lectures at annual anesthesiology conference-lectures related to anesthesia management of patients with cancer, operating room ventilators & postoperative nausea/vomiting. No direct conflicts with Pediatric Life support topics | None | None | None |
| Robert W. Hickey | University of Pittsburgh–Pediatric Emergency Medicine Physician | †NIH sponsored research on the effect of cyclopentenone prostaglandins upon post-ischemic brain. | None | None | None | None | *Occasional expert witness (1–2 times per year) |
| Bradley S. Marino | Cincinnati Children's Hospital Medical Center–Associate Professor of Pediatrics | None | None | None | None | None | None |
| Vinay M. Nadkarni | University of Pennsylvania, Children's Hospital of Philadelphia–Attending Physician, Pediatric Critical Care | †NIH RO1: Coinvestigator, Therapeutic Hypothermia After Pediatric Cardiac Arrest Center of Excellence Grant, PI, Laerdal Foundation for Acute Care Medicine AHRQ: Agency for Healthcare Research and Quality: PI, Tracheal Intubation Safety in Pediatric ICUs *NHTSA: Coinvestigator, Chest compression characteristics in children | None | None | None | None | *Volunteer (no salary or remuneration), World Federation of Pediatric Intensive and Critical Care Societies Volunteer (no salary), Data Safety and Monitoring Board, CIRC study |
| Lester T. Proctor | University of Wisconsin-Madison College of Medicine and Public Health–Professor | None | None | None | None | None | None |
| Faiqa A. Qureshi | Children's Specialty Group—Partner | None | None | None | None | None | None |
| Kennith Sartorelli | University of Vermont–Associate Professor of Surgery | None | None | None | None | None | None |
| Alexis Topjian | University of Pennsylvania–Assistant Professor | *Site principal investigator at the Children's hospital of Philadelphia for the "Therpaeutic Hypothermia after Pediatric Cardiac Arrest" funded via an NIH U01 | None | None | None | None | None |
| Elise W. van der Jagt | University of Rochester–Professor of Pediatrics and Critical Care | None | None | None | None | None | None |
| Arno L. Zaritsky | Childen's Hospital of The King's Daughters-Sr. VP for Clinical Services | None | None | None | None | *Data Safety Monitoring Board for NIH-funded pediatric hypothermia after cardiac arrest research project | None |

This table represents the relationships of writing group members that may be perceived as actual or reasonably perceived conflicts of interest as reported on the Disclosure Questionnaire, which all members of the writing group are required to complete and submit. A relationship is considered to be "significant" if (a) the person receives $10 000 or more during any 12-month period, or 5% or more of the person's gross income; or (b) the person owns 5% or more of the voting stock or share of the entity, or owns $10 000 or more of the fair market value of the entity. A relationship is considered to be "modest" if it is less than "significant" under the preceding definition.

*Modest.

†Significant.

# References

1. Young KD, Seidel JS. Pediatric cardiopulmonary resuscitation: a collective review. *Ann Emerg Med*. 1999;33:195–205.

2. Appleton GO, Cummins RO, Larson MP, Graves JR. CPR and the single rescuer: at what age should you "call first" rather than "call fast"? *Ann Emerg Med*. 1995;25:492–494.

3. Hickey RW, Cohen DM, Strausbaugh S, Dietrich AM. Pediatric patients requiring CPR in the prehospital setting. *Ann Emerg Med*. 1995;25:495–501.

4. Mogayzel C, Quan L, Graves JR, Tiedeman D, Fahrenbruch C, Herndon P. Out-of-hospital ventricular fibrillation in children and adolescents: causes and outcomes. *Ann Emerg Med*. 1995;25:484–491.

5. Donoghue AJ, Nadkarni V, Berg RA, Osmond MH, Wells G, Nesbitt L, Stiell IG. Out-of-hospital pediatric cardiac arrest: an epidemiologic review and assessment of current knowledge. *Ann Emerg Med*. 2005; 46:512–522.

6. Samson RA, Nadkarni VM, Meaney PA, Carey SM, Berg MD, Berg RA. Outcomes of in-hospital ventricular fibrillation in children. *N Engl J Med*. 2006;354:2328–2339.

7. Atkins DL, Everson-Stewart S, Sears GK, Daya M, Osmond MH, Warden CR, Berg RA. Epidemiology and outcomes from out-of-hospital cardiac arrest in children: the Resuscitation Outcomes Consortium Epistry-Cardiac Arrest. *Circulation*. 2009;119:1484–1491.

8. Kitamura T, Iwami T, Kawamura T, Nagao K, Tanaka H, Nadkarni VM, Berg RA, Hiraide A. Conventional and chest-compression-only cardiopulmonary resuscitation by bystanders for children who have out-of-hospital cardiac arrests: a prospective, nationwide, population-based cohort study. *Lancet*. 2010;375:1347–1354.

9. Park CB, Shin SD, Suh GJ, Ahn KO, Cha WC, Song KJ, Kim SJ, Lee EJ, Ong ME. Pediatric out-of-hospital cardiac arrest in Korea: A nationwide population-based study. *Resuscitation*. 2010;81:512–517.

10. Kouwenhoven WB, Jude JR, Knickerbocker GG. Closed-chest cardiac massage. *JAMA*. 1960;173:1064–1067.

11. Zaritsky A, Nadkarni V, Getson P, Kuehl K. CPR in children. *Ann Emerg Med*. 1987;16:1107–1111.

12. Gillis J, Dickson D, Rieder M, Steward D, Edmonds J. Results of inpatient pediatric resuscitation. *Crit Care Med*. 1986;14:469–471.

13. Reis AG, Nadkarni V, Perondi MB, Grisi S, Berg RA. A prospective investigation into the epidemiology of in-hospital pediatric cardiopulmonary resuscitation using the international Utstein reporting style. *Pediatrics*. 2002;109:200–209.

14. Suominen P, Olkkola KT, Voipio V, Korpela R, Palo R, Rasanen J. Utstein style reporting of in-hospital paediatric cardiopulmonary resuscitation. *Resuscitation*. 2000;45:17–25.

15. Nadkarni VM, Larkin GL, Peberdy MA, Carey SM, Kaye W, Mancini ME, Nichol G, Lane-Truitt T, Potts J, Ornato JP, Berg RA. First documented rhythm and clinical outcome from in-hospital cardiac arrest among children and adults. *JAMA*. 2006;295:50–57.

16. Meaney PA, Nadkarni VM, Cook EF, Testa M, Helfaer M, Kaye W, Larkin GL, Berg RA. Higher survival rates among younger patients after pediatric intensive care unit cardiac arrests. *Pediatrics*. 2006;118: 2424–2433.

17. Tibballs J, Kinney S. A prospective study of outcome of in-patient paediatric cardiopulmonary arrest. *Resuscitation*. 2006;71:310–318.

18. Sharek PJ, Parast LM, Leong K, Coombs J, Earnest K, Sullivan J, Frankel LR, Roth SJ. Effect of a rapid response team on hospital-wide mortality and code rates outside the ICU in a Children's Hospital. *JAMA*. 2007;298:2267–2274.

19. Tibballs J, Kinney S. Reduction of hospital mortality and of preventable cardiac arrest and death on introduction of a pediatric medical emergency team. *Pediatr Crit Care Med*. 2009;10:306–312.

20. Brilli RJ, Gibson R, Luria JW, Wheeler TA, Shaw J, Linam M, Kheir J, McLain P, Lingsch T, Hall-Haering A, McBride M. Implementation of a medical emergency team in a large pediatric teaching hospital prevents respiratory and cardiopulmonary arrests outside the intensive care unit. *Pediatr Crit Care Med*. 2007;8:236–246.

21. Hunt EA, Zimmer KP, Rinke ML, Shilkofski NA, Matlin C, Garger C, Dickson C, Miller MR. Transition from a traditional code team to a medical emergency team and categorization of cardiopulmonary arrests in a children's center. *Arch Pediatr Adolesc Med*. 2008;162:117–122.

22. Abella BS, Alvarado JP, Myklebust H, Edelson DP, Barry A, O'Hearn N, Vanden Hoek TL, Becker LB. Quality of cardiopulmonary resuscitation during in-hospital cardiac arrest. *JAMA*. 2005;293:305–310.

23. Nishisaki A, Nysaether J, Sutton R, Maltese M, Niles D, Donoghue A, Bishnoi R, Helfaer M, Perkins GD, Berg R, Arbogast K, Nadkarni V. Effect of mattress deflection on CPR quality assessment for older children and adolescents. *Resuscitation*. 2009;80:540–545.

24. Noordergraaf GJ, Paulussen IW, Venema A, van Berkom PF, Woerlee PH, Scheffer GJ, Noordergraaf A. The impact of compliant surfaces on in-hospital chest compressions: effects of common mattresses and a backboard. *Resuscitation*. 2009;80:546–552.

25. Raju NV, Maisels MJ, Kring E, Schwarz-Warner L. Capillary refill time in the hands and feet of normal newborn infants. *Clin Pediatr*. 1999; 38:139–144.

26. Brown LH, Prasad NH, Whitley TW. Adverse lighting condition effects on the assessment of capillary refill. *Am J Emerg Med*. 1994;12:46–47.

27. Haque IU, Zaritsky AL. Analysis of the evidence for the lower limit of systolic and mean arterial pressure in children. *Pediatr Crit Care Med*. 2007;8:138–144.

28. Zubrow AB, Hulman S, Kushner H, Falkner B. Determinants of blood pressure in infants admitted to neonatal intensive care units: a prospective multicenter study. Philadelphia Neonatal Blood Pressure Study Group. *J Perinatol*. 1995;15:470–479.

29. Carenzi B, Corso RM, Stellino V, Carlino GD, Tonini C, Rossini L, Gentili G. Airway management in an infant with congenital centrofacial dysgenesia. *Br J Anaesth*. 2002;88:726–728.

30. Fraser J, Hill C, McDonald D, Jones C, Petros A. The use of the laryngeal mask airway for inter-hospital transport of infants with type 3 laryngotracheo-oesophageal clefts. *Intensive Care Med*. 1999;25: 714–716.

31. Iohom G, Lyons B, Casey W. Airway management in a baby with femoral hypoplasia-unusual facies syndrome. *Paediatr Anaesth*. 2002; 12:461–464.

32. Johr M, Berger TM, Ruppen W, Schlegel C. Congenital laryngotracheo-oesophageal cleft: successful ventilation with the Laryngeal Mask Airway. *Paediatr Anaesth*. 2003;13:68–71.

33. Leal-Pavey YR. Use of the LMA classic to secure the airway of a premature neonate with Smith-Lemli-Opitz syndrome: a case report. *AANA J*. 2004;72:427–430.

34. Russell P, Chambers N, du Plessis J, Vijayasekeran S. Emergency use of a size 1 laryngeal mask airway in a ventilated neonate with an undiagnosed type IV laryngotracheo-oesophageal cleft. *Paediatr Anaesth*. 2008;18:658–662.

35. Scheller B, Schalk R, Byhahn C, Peter N, L'Allemand N, Kessler P, Meininger D. Laryngeal tube suction II for difficult airway management in neonates and small infants. *Resuscitation*. 2009;80:805–810.

36. Stocks RM, Egerman R, Thompson JW, Peery M. Airway management of the severely retrognathic child: use of the laryngeal mask airway. *Ear Nose Throat J*. 2002;81:223–226.

37. Yao CT, Wang JN, Tai YT, Tsai TY, Wu JM. Successful management of a neonate with Pierre-Robin syndrome and severe upper airway obstruction by long term placement of a laryngeal mask airway. *Resuscitation*. 2004; 61:97–99.

38. Lopez-Gil M, Brimacombe J, Alvarez M. Safety and efficacy of the laryngeal mask airway. A prospective survey of 1400 children. *Anaesthesia*. 1996;51:969–972.

39. Lopez-Gil M, Brimacombe J, Cebrian J, Arranz J. Laryngeal mask airway in pediatric practice: a prospective study of skill acquisition by anesthesia residents. *Anesthesiology*. 1996;84:807–811.

40. Park C, Bahk JH, Ahn WS, Do SH, Lee KH. The laryngeal mask airway in infants and children. *Can J Anaesth*. 2001;48:413–417.

41. Bagshaw O. The size 1.5 laryngeal mask airway (LMA) in paediatric anaesthetic practice. *Paediatr Anaesth*. 2002;12:420–423.

42. Harnett M, Kinirons B, Heffernan A, Motherway C, Casey W. Airway complications in infants: comparison of laryngeal mask airway and the facemask-oral airway. *Can J Anaesth*. 2000;47:315–318.

43. Flick RP, Wilder RT, Pieper SF, van Koeverden K, Ellison KM, Marienau ME, Hanson AC, Schroeder DR, Sprung J. Risk factors for laryngospasm in children during general anesthesia. *Paediatr Anaesth*. 2008;18:289–296.

44. Brown LH, Manring EA, Kornegay HB, Prasad NH. Can prehospital personnel detect hypoxemia without the aid of pulse oximeters? *Am J Emerg Med*. 1996;14:43–44.

45. Gausche M, Lewis RJ, Stratton SJ, Haynes BE, Gunter CS, Goodrich SM, Poore PD, McCollough MD, Henderson DP, Pratt FD, Seidel JS. Effect of out-of-hospital pediatric endotracheal intubation on survival and neurological outcome: a controlled clinical trial. *JAMA*. 2000;283: 783–790.

46. Stockinger ZT, McSwain NE, Jr. Prehospital endotracheal intubation for trauma does not improve survival over bag-valve-mask ventilation. *J Trauma.* 2004;56:531–536.

47. Pitetti R, Glustein JZ, Bhende MS. Prehospital care and outcome of pediatric out-of-hospital cardiac arrest. *Prehosp Emerg Care.* 2002;6: 283–290.

48. Gerritse BM, Draaisma JM, Schalkwijk A, van Grunsven PM, Scheffer GJ. Should EMS-paramedics perform paediatric tracheal intubation in the field? *Resuscitation.* 2008;79:225–229.

49. A prospective multicenter evaluation of prehospital airway management performance in a large metropolitan region. *Prehosp Emerg Care.* 2009; 13:304–310.

50. Garza AG, Algren DA, Gratton MC, Ma OJ. Populations at risk for intubation nonattempt and failure in the prehospital setting. *Prehosp Emerg Care.* 2005;9:163–166.

51. Hon KL, Olsen H, Totapally B, Leung TF. Hyperventilation at referring hospitals is common before transport in intubated children with neurological diseases. *Pediatr Emerg Care.* 2005;21:662–666.

52. Wang HE, Lave JR, Sirio CA, Yealy DM. Paramedic intubation errors: isolated events or symptoms of larger problems? *Health Aff (Millwood).* 2006;25:501–509.

53. Kern KB, Sanders AB, Raife J, Milander MM, Otto CW, Ewy GA. A study of chest compression rates during cardiopulmonary resuscitation in humans: the importance of rate-directed chest compressions. *Arch Intern Med.* 1992;152:145–149.

54. Aufderheide TP, Sigurdsson G, Pirrallo RG, Yannopoulos D, McKnite S, von Briesen C, Sparks CW, Conrad CJ, Provo TA, Lurie KG. Hyperventilation-induced hypotension during cardiopulmonary resuscitation. *Circulation.* 2004;109:1960–1965.

55. Wik L, Kramer-Johansen J, Myklebust H, Sorebo H, Svensson L, Fellows B, Steen PA. Quality of cardiopulmonary resuscitation during out-of-hospital cardiac arrest. *JAMA.* 2005;293:299–304.

56. Gausche-Hill M, Lewis RJ, Gunter CS, Henderson DP, Haynes BE, Stratton SJ. Design and implementation of a controlled trial of pediatric endotracheal intubation in the out-of-hospital setting. *Ann Emerg Med.* 2000;36:356–365.

57. Jesudian MC, Harrison RR, Keenan RL, Maull KI. Bag-valve-mask ventilation; two rescuers are better than one: preliminary report. *Crit Care Med.* 1985;13:122–123.

58. Davidovic L, LaCovey D, Pitetti RD. Comparison of 1- versus 2-person bag-valve-mask techniques for manikin ventilation of infants and children. *Ann Emerg Med.* 2005;46:37–42.

59. Berg MD, Idris AH, Berg RA. Severe ventilatory compromise due to gastric distention during pediatric cardiopulmonary resuscitation. *Resuscitation.* 1998;36:71–73.

60. Moynihan RJ, Brock-Utne JG, Archer JH, Feld LH, Kreitzman TR. The effect of cricoid pressure on preventing gastric insufflation in infants and children. *Anesthesiology.* 1993;78:652–656.

61. Salem MR, Wong AY, Mani M, Sellick BA. Efficacy of cricoid pressure in preventing gastric inflation during bag-mask ventilation in pediatric patients. *Anesthesiology.* 1974;40:96–98.

62. Sellick BA. Cricoid pressure to control regurgitation of stomach contents during induction of anaesthesia. *Lancet.* 1961;2:404–406.

63. Hartsilver EL, Vanner RG. Airway obstruction with cricoid pressure. *Anaesthesia.* 2000;55:208–211.

64. Sirbaugh PE, Pepe PE, Shook JE, Kimball KT, Goldman MJ, Ward MA, Mann DM. A prospective, population-based study of the demographics, epidemiology, management, and outcome of out-of-hospital pediatric cardiopulmonary arrest. *Ann Emerg Med.* 1999;33:174–184.

65. Brownstein DR, Quan L, Orr R, Wentz KR, Copass MK. Paramedic intubation training in a pediatric operating room. *Am J Emerg Med.* 1992;10:418–420.

66. Vilke GM, Steen PJ, Smith AM, Chan TC. Out-of-hospital pediatric intubation by paramedics: the San Diego experience. *J Emerg Med.* 2002;22:71–74.

67. Ma OJ, Atchley RB, Hatley T, Green M, Young J, Brady W. Intubation success rates improve for an air medical program after implementing the use of neuromuscular blocking agents. *Am J Emerg Med.* 1998;16: 125–127.

68. Sing RF, Rotondo MF, Zonies DH, Schwab CW, Kauder DR, Ross SE, Brathwaite CC. Rapid sequence induction for intubation by an aeromedical transport team: a critical analysis. *Am J Emerg Med.* 1998;16: 598–602.

69. Sagarin MJ, Chiang V, Sakles JC, Barton ED, Wolfe RE, Vissers RJ, Walls RM. Rapid sequence intubation for pediatric emergency airway management. *Pediatr Emerg Care.* 2002;18:417–423.

70. Black K, Barnett P, Wolfe R, Young S. Are methods used to estimate weight in children accurate? *Emerg Med (Fremantle).* 2002;14: 160–165.

71. Chan GM, Moyer-Mileur L, Rallison L. An easy and accurate method of estimating newborn birthweight for resuscitation. *Am J Perinatol.* 9(5–6):371–373, 1992.

72. Garland JS, Kishaba RG, Nelson DB, Losek JD, Sobocinski KA. A rapid and accurate method of estimating body weight. *Am J Emerg Med.* 1986;4:390–393.

73. Krieser D, Nguyen K, Kerr D, Jolley D, Clooney M, Kelly AM. Parental weight estimation of their child's weight is more accurate than other weight estimation methods for determining children's weight in an emergency department? *Emerg Med J.* 2007;24:756–759.

74. Lubitz DS, Seidel JS, Chameides L, Luten RC, Zaritsky AL, Campbell FW. A rapid method for estimating weight and resuscitation drug dosages from length in the pediatric age group. *Ann Emerg Med.* 1988; 17:576–581.

75. Varghese A, Vasudevan VK, Lewin S, Indumathi CK, Dinakar C, Rao SD. Do the length-based (Broselow) Tape, APLS, Argall and Nelson's formulae accurately estimate weight of Indian children? *Indian Pediatr.* 2006;43:889–894.

76. Vilke GM, Marino A, Fisher R, Chan TC. Estimation of pediatric patient weight by EMT-PS. *J Emerg Med.* 2001;21:125–128.

77. Hofer CK, Ganter M, Tucci M, Klaghofer R, Zollinger A. How reliable is length-based determination of body weight and tracheal tube size in the paediatric age group? The Broselow tape reconsidered. *Br J Anaesth.* 2002;88:283–285.

78. DuBois D, Baldwin S, King WD. Accuracy of weight estimation methods for children. *Pediatr Emerg Care.* 2007;23:227–230.

79. Yamamoto LG, Inaba AS, Young LL, Anderson KM. Improving length-based weight estimates by adding a body habitus (obesity) icon. *Am J Emerg Med.* 2009;27:810–815.

80. Johnson TN. The problems in scaling adult drug doses to children. *Arch Dis Child.* 2008;93:207–211.

81. Mahmood I. Prediction of drug clearance in children: impact of allometric exponents, body weight, and age. *Ther Drug Monit.* 2007;29: 271–278.

82. Edginton AN, Schmitt W, Willmann S. Development and evaluation of a generic physiologically based pharmacokinetic model for children. *Clin Pharmacokinet.* 2006;45:1013–1034.

83. Gill MA, Ueda CT. Novel method for the determination of pediatric dosages. *Am J Hosp Pharm.* 1976;33:389–392.

84. Rodriguez W, Selen A, Avant D, Chaurasia C, Crescenzi T, Gieser G, Di Giacinto J, Huang SM, Lee P, Mathis L, Murphy D, Murphy S, Roberts R, Sachs HC, Suarez S, Tandon V, Uppoor RS. Improving pediatric dosing through pediatric initiatives: what we have learned. *Pediatrics.* 2008;121:530–539.

85. Traub SL, Kichen L. Estimating ideal body mass in children. *Am J Hosp Pharm.* 1983;40:107–110.

86. Ellis DY, Harris T, Zideman D. Cricoid pressure in emergency department rapid sequence tracheal intubations: a risk-benefit analysis. *Ann Emerg Med.* 2007;50:653–665.

87. Walker RW, Ravi R, Haylett K. Effect of cricoid force on airway calibre in children: a bronchoscopic assessment. *Br J Anaesth.* 2010;104:71–74.

88. Khine HH, Corddry DH, Kettrick RG, Martin TM, McCloskey JJ, Rose JB, Theroux MC, Zagnoev M. Comparison of cuffed and uncuffed endotracheal tubes in young children during general anesthesia. *Anesthesiology.* 1997; 86:627–631; discussion 627A.

89. Weiss M, Dullenkopf A, Fischer JE, Keller C, Gerber AC. Prospective randomized controlled multi-centre trial of cuffed or uncuffed endotracheal tubes in small children. *Br J Anaesth.* 2009;103:867–873.

90. Bordet F, Allaouchiche B, Lansiaux S, Combet S, Pouyau A, Taylor P, Bonnard C, Chassard D. Risk factors for airway complications during general anaesthesia in paediatric patients. *Paediatr Anaesth.* 2002;12: 762–769.

91. Newth CJ, Rachman B, Patel N, Hammer J. The use of cuffed versus uncuffed endotracheal tubes in pediatric intensive care. *J Pediatr.* 2004; 144:333–337.

92. Deakers TW, Reynolds G, Stretton M, Newth CJ. Cuffed endotracheal tubes in pediatric intensive care. *J Pediatr.* 1994;125:57–62.

93. Mhanna MJ, Zamel YB, Tichy CM, Super DM. The "air leak" test around the endotracheal tube, as a predictor of postextubation stridor, is age dependent in children. *Crit Care Med*. 2002;30:2639–2643.

94. Browning DH, Graves SA. Incidence of aspiration with endotracheal tubes in children. *J Pediatr*. 1983;102:582–584.

95. Luten RC, Wears RL, Broselow J, Zaritsky A, Barnett TM, Lee T, Bailey A, Vally R, Brown R, Rosenthal B. Length-based endotracheal tube and emergency equipment in pediatrics. *Ann Emerg Med*. 1992;21: 900–904.

96. Davis D, Barbee L, Ririe D. Pediatric endotracheal tube selection: a comparison of age-based and height-based criteria. *AANA J*. 1998;66: 299–303.

97. Daugherty RJ, Nadkarni V, Brenn BR. Endotracheal tube size estimation for children with pathological short stature. *Pediatr Emerg Care*. 2006; 22:710–717.

98. Dullenkopf A, Gerber AC, Weiss M. Fit and seal characteristics of a new paediatric tracheal tube with high volume-low pressure polyurethane cuff. *Acta Anaesthesiol Scand*. 2005;49:232–237.

99. Dullenkopf A, Kretschmar O, Knirsch W, Tomaske M, Hug M, Stutz K, Berger F, Weiss M. Comparison of tracheal tube cuff diameters with internal transverse diameters of the trachea in children. *Acta Anaesthesiol Scand*. 2006;50:201–205.

100. Salgo B, Schmitz A, Henze G, Stutz K, Dullenkopf A, Neff S, Gerber AC, Weiss M. Evaluation of a new recommendation for improved cuffed tracheal tube size selection in infants and small children. *Acta Anaesthesiol Scand*. 2006;50:557–561.

101. Duracher C, Schmautz E, Martinon C, Faivre J, Carli P, Orliaguet G. Evaluation of cuffed tracheal tube size predicted using the Khine formula in children. *Paediatr Anaesth*. 2008;18:113–118.

102. Katz SH, Falk JL. Misplaced endotracheal tubes by paramedics in an urban emergency medical services system. *Ann Emerg Med*. 2001;37: 32–37.

103. Beyer AJd, Land G, Zaritsky A. Nonphysician transport of intubated pediatric patients: a system evaluation. *Crit Care Med*. 1992;20: 961–966.

104. Andersen KH, Schultz-Lebahn T. Oesophageal intubation can be undetected by auscultation of the chest. *Acta Anaesthesiol Scand*. 1994;38: 580–582.

105. Kelly JJ, Eynon CA, Kaplan JL, de Garavilla L, Dalsey WC. Use of tube condensation as an indicator of endotracheal tube placement. *Ann Emerg Med*. 1998;31:575–578.

106. Poirier MP, Gonzalez Del-Rey JA, McAneney CM, DiGiulio GA. Utility of monitoring capnography, pulse oximetry, and vital signs in the detection of airway mishaps: a hyperoxemic animal model. *Am J Emerg Med*. 1998;16:350–352.

107. Birmingham PK, Cheney FW, Ward RJ. Esophageal intubation: a review of detection techniques. *Anesth Analg*. 1986;65:886–891.

108. Donn SM, Kuhns LR. Mechanism of endotracheal tube movement with change of head position in the neonate. *Pediatr Radiol*. 1980;9:37–40.

109. Hartrey R, Kestin IG. Movement of oral and nasal tracheal tubes as a result of changes in head and neck position. *Anaesthesia*. 1995;50: 682–687.

110. Bhende MS, Karasic DG, Karasic RB. End-tidal carbon dioxide changes during cardiopulmonary resuscitation after experimental asphyxial cardiac arrest. *Am J Emerg Med*. 1996;14:349–350.

111. Kelly JS, Wilhoit RD, Brown RE, James R. Efficacy of the FEF colorimetric end-tidal carbon dioxide detector in children. *Anesth Analg*. 1992;75:45–50.

112. Hosono S, Inami I, Fujita H, Minato M, Takahashi S, Mugishima H. A role of end-tidal CO monitoring for assessment of tracheal intubations in very low birth weight infants during neonatal resuscitation at birth. *J Perinat Med*. 2009;37:79–84.

113. O'Donnell CP, Kamlin CO, Davis PG, Morley CJ. Endotracheal intubation attempts during neonatal resuscitation: success rates, duration, and adverse effects. *Pediatrics*. 2006;117:e16–21.

114. Salthe J, Kristiansen SM, Sollid S, Oglaend B, Soreide E. Capnography rapidly confirmed correct endotracheal tube placement during resuscitation of extremely low birthweight babies (<1000 g). *Acta Anaesthesiol Scand*. 2006;50:1033–1036.

115. Campbell RC, Boyd CR, Shields RO, Odom JW, Corse KM. Evaluation of an end-tidal carbon dioxide detector in the aeromedical setting. *J Air Med Transp*. 1990;9:13–15.

116. Bhende MS, Allen WD, Jr. Evaluation of a Capno-Flo resuscitator during transport of critically ill children. *Pediatr Emerg Care*. 2002;18: 414–416.

117. Bhende MS, Thompson AE, Orr RA. Utility of an end-tidal carbon dioxide detector during stabilization and transport of critically ill children. *Pediatrics*. 89(pt 1):1042–1044, 1992.

118. Bhende MS, Thompson AE. Evaluation of an end-tidal CO2 detector during pediatric cardiopulmonary resuscitation. *Pediatrics*. 1995;95: 395–399.

119. Cardoso MM, Banner MJ, Melker RJ, Bjoraker DG. Portable devices used to detect endotracheal intubation during emergency situations: a review. *Crit Care Med*. 1998;26:957–964.

120. Ornato JP, Shipley JB, Racht EM, Slovis CM, Wrenn KD, Pepe PE, Almeida SL, Ginger VF, Fotre TV. Multicenter study of a portable, hand-size, colorimetric end-tidal carbon dioxide detection device. *Ann Emerg Med*. 1992;21:518–523.

121. Cantineau JP, Merckx P, Lambert Y, Sorkine M, Bertrand C, Duvaldestin P. Effect of epinephrine on end-tidal carbon dioxide pressure during prehospital cardiopulmonary resuscitation. *Am J Emerg Med*. 1994;12:267–270.

122. Ward KR, Yealy DM. End-tidal carbon dioxide monitoring in emergency medicine. Part 2: Clinical applications. *Acad Emerg Med*. 1998;5:637–646.

123. Hand IL, Shepard EK, Krauss AN, Auld PA. Discrepancies between transcutaneous and end-tidal carbon dioxide monitoring in the critically ill neonate with respiratory distress syndrome. *Crit Care Med*. 1989;17: 556–559.

124. Tobias JD, Meyer DJ. Noninvasive monitoring of carbon dioxide during respiratory failure in toddlers and infants: end-tidal versus transcutaneous carbon dioxide. *Anesth Analg*. 1997;85:55–58.

125. Sharieff GQ, Rodarte A, Wilton N, Bleyle D. The self-inflating bulb as an airway adjunct: is it reliable in children weighing less than 20 kilograms? *Acad Emerg Med*. 2003;10:303–308.

126. Sharieff GQ, Rodarte A, Wilton N, Silva PD, Bleyle D. The self-inflating bulb as an esophageal detector device in children weighing more than twenty kilograms: A comparison of two techniques. *Ann Emerg Med*. 2003;41:623–629.

127. Klain M, Keszler H, Brader E. High frequency jet ventilation in CPR. *Crit Care Med*. 1981;9:421–422.

128. Morris MC, Wernovsky G, Nadkarni VM. Survival outcomes after extracorporeal cardiopulmonary resuscitation instituted during active chest compressions following refractory in-hospital pediatric cardiac arrest. *Pediatr Crit Care Med*. 2004;5:440–446.

129. Alsoufi B, Al-Radi OO, Nazer RI, Gruenwald C, Foreman C, Williams WG, Coles JG, Caldarone CA, Bohn DG, Van Arsdell GS. Survival outcomes after rescue extracorporeal cardiopulmonary resuscitation in pediatric patients with refractory cardiac arrest. *J Thorac Cardiovasc Surg*. 2007;134:952–959 e952.

130. Huang SC, Wu ET, Chen YS, Chang CI, Chiu IS, Wang SS, Lin FY, Ko WJ. Extracorporeal membrane oxygenation rescue for cardiopulmonary resuscitation in pediatric patients. *Crit Care Med*. 2008;36:1607–1613.

131. Allan CK, Thiagarajan RR, Armsby LR, del Nido PJ, Laussen PC. Emergent use of extracorporeal membrane oxygenation during pediatric cardiac catheterization. *Pediatr Crit Care Med*. 2006;7:212–219.

132. Chan T, Thiagarajan RR, Frank D, Bratton SL. Survival after extracorporeal cardiopulmonary resuscitation in infants and children with heart disease. *J Thorac Cardiovasc Surg*. 2008;136:984–992.

133. del Nido PJ, Dalton HJ, Thompson AE, Siewers RD. Extracorporeal membrane oxygenator rescue in children during cardiac arrest after cardiac surgery. *Circulation*. 1992;86(5 Suppl):II300–304.

134. Duncan BW, Ibrahim AE, Hraska V, del Nido PJ, Laussen PC, Wessel DL, Mayer JE, Jr., Bower LK, Jonas RA. Use of rapid-deployment extracorporeal membrane oxygenation for the resuscitation of pediatric patients with heart disease after cardiac arrest. *J Thorac Cardiovasc Surg*. 1998;116:305–311.

135. Hoskote A, Bohn D, Gruenwald C, Edgell D, Cai S, Adatia I, Van Arsdell G. Extracorporeal life support after staged palliation of a functional single ventricle: subsequent morbidity and survival. *J Thorac Cardiovasc Surg*. 2006;131:1114–1121.

136. Ibrahim AE, Duncan BW, Blume ED, Jonas RA. Long-term follow-up of pediatric cardiac patients requiring mechanical circulatory support. *Ann Thorac Surg*. 2000;69:186–192.

137. Prodhan P, Fiser RT, Dyamenahalli U, Gossett J, Imamura M, Jaquiss RD, Bhutta AT. Outcomes after extracorporeal cardiopulmonary resuscitation (ECPR) following refractory pediatric cardiac arrest in the intensive care unit. *Resuscitation*. 2009;80:1124–1129.

138. Thiagarajan RR, Laussen PC, Rycus PT, Bartlett RH, Bratton SL. Extracorporeal membrane oxygenation to aid cardiopulmonary resuscitation in infants and children. *Circulation.* 2007;116:1693–1700.

139. Lequier L, Joffe AR, Robertson CM, Dinu IA, Wongswadiwat Y, Anton NR, Ross DB, Rebeyka IM. Two-year survival, mental, and motor outcomes after cardiac extracorporeal life support at less than five years of age. *J Thorac Cardiovasc Surg.* 2008;136:976–983 e973.

140. Mahle WT, Forbess JM, Kirshbom PM, Cuadrado AR, Simsic JM, Kanter KR. Cost-utility analysis of salvage cardiac extracorporeal membrane oxygenation in children. *J Thorac Cardiovasc Surg.* 2005; 129:1084–1090.

141. Aharon AS, Drinkwater DC, Jr., Churchwell KB, Quisling SV, Reddy VS, Taylor M, Hix S, Christian KG, Pietsch JB, Deshpande JK, Kambam J, Graham TP, Chang PA. Extracorporeal membrane oxygenation in children after repair of congenital cardiac lesions. *Ann Thorac Surg.* 72:2095–2101, 2001; discussion 2101–2092.

142. Barrett CS, Bratton SL, Salvin JW, Laussen PC, Rycus PT, Thiagarajan RR. Neurological injury after extracorporeal membrane oxygenation use to aid pediatric cardiopulmonary resuscitation. *Pediatr Crit Care Med.* 2009;10:445–451.

143. Baslaim G, Bashore J, Al-Malki F, Jamjoom A. Can the outcome of pediatric extracorporeal membrane oxygenation after cardiac surgery be predicted? *Ann Thorac Cardiovasc Surg.* 2006;12:21–27.

144. Ghez O, Feier H, Ughetto F, Fraisse A, Kreitmann B, Metras D. Postoperative extracorporeal life support in pediatric cardiac surgery: recent results. *ASAIO J.* 2005;51:513–516.

145. Cochran JB, Tecklenburg FW, Lau YR, Habib DM. Emergency cardiopulmonary bypass for cardiac arrest refractory to pediatric advanced life support. *Pediatr Emerg Care.* 1999;15:30–32.

146. Dalton HJ, Siewers RD, Fuhrman BP, Del Nido P, Thompson AE, Shaver MG, Dowhy M. Extracorporeal membrane oxygenation for cardiac rescue in children with severe myocardial dysfunction. *Crit Care Med.* 1993;21:1020–1028.

147. del Nido PJ. Extracorporeal membrane oxygenation for cardiac support in children. *Ann Thorac Surg.* 61:336–339, 1996; discussion 340–341.

148. Ghez O, Fouilloux V, Charpentier A, Fesquet P, Lion F, Lebrun L, Commandeur M, Fraisse A, Metras D, Kreitmann B. Absence of rapid deployment extracorporeal membrane oxygenation (ECMO) team does not preclude resuscitation ecmo in pediatric cardiac patients with good results. *ASAIO J.* 2007;53:692–695.

149. Jaggers JJ, Forbess JM, Shah AS, Meliones JN, Kirshbom PM, Miller CE, Ungerleider RM. Extracorporeal membrane oxygenation for infant postcardiotomy support: significance of shunt management. *Ann Thorac Surg.* 2000;69:1476–1483.

150. Kelly RB, Porter PA, Meier AH, Myers JL, Thomas NJ. Duration of cardiopulmonary resuscitation before extracorporeal rescue: how long is not long enough? *ASAIO J.* 2005;51:665–667.

151. Parra DA, Totapally BR, Zahn E, Jacobs J, Aldousany A, Burke RP, Chang AC. Outcome of cardiopulmonary resuscitation in a pediatric cardiac intensive care unit. *Crit Care Med.* 2000;28:3296–3300.

152. Ravishankar C, Dominguez TE, Kreutzer J, Wernovsky G, Marino BS, Godinez R, Priestley MA, Gruber PJ, Gaynor WJ, Nicolson SC, Spray TL, Tabbutt S. Extracorporeal membrane oxygenation after stage I reconstruction for hypoplastic left heart syndrome. *Pediatr Crit Care Med.* 2006;7:319–323.

153. Shah SA, Shankar V, Churchwell KB, Taylor MB, Scott BP, Bartilson R, Byrne DW, Christian KG, Drinkwater DC. Clinical outcomes of 84 children with congenital heart disease managed with extracorporeal membrane oxygenation after cardiac surgery. *ASAIO J.* 2005;51: 504–507.

154. Thourani VH, Kirshbom PM, Kanter KR, Simsic J, Kogon BE, Wagoner S, Dykes F, Fortenberry J, Forbess JM. Venoarterial extracorporeal membrane oxygenation (VA-ECMO) in pediatric cardiac support. *Ann Thorac Surg.* 82:138–144, 2006; discussion 144–135.

155. Blaivas M, Fox JC. Outcome in cardiac arrest patients found to have cardiac standstill on the bedside emergency department echocardiogram. *Acad Emerg Med.* 2001;8:616–621.

156. Menaker J, Cushman J, Vermillion JM, Rosenthal RE, Scalea TM. Ultrasound-diagnosed cardiac tamponade after blunt abdominal trauma-treated with emergent thoracotomy. *J Emerg Med.* 2007;32:99–103.

157. Niendorff DF, Rassias AJ, Palac R, Beach ML, Costa S, Greenberg M. Rapid cardiac ultrasound of inpatients suffering PEA arrest performed by nonexpert sonographers. *Resuscitation.* 2005;67:81–87.

158. Querellou E, Meyran D, Petitjean F, Le Dreff P, Maurin O. Ventricular fibrillation diagnosed with trans-thoracic echocardiography. *Resuscitation.* 2009;80:1211–1213.

159. Salen P, Melniker L, Chooljian C, Rose JS, Alteveer J, Reed J, Heller M. Does the presence or absence of sonographically identified cardiac activity predict resuscitation outcomes of cardiac arrest patients? *Am J Emerg Med.* 2005;23:459–462.

160. Salen P, O'Connor R, Sierzenski P, Passarello B, Pancu D, Melanson S, Arcona S, Reed J, Heller M. Can cardiac sonography and capnography be used independently and in combination to predict resuscitation outcomes? *Acad Emerg Med.* 2001;8:610–615.

161. Tayal VS, Kline JA. Emergency echocardiography to detect pericardial effusion in patients in PEA and near-PEA states. *Resuscitation.* 2003; 59:315–318.

162. Varriale P, Maldonado JM. Echocardiographic observations during inhospital cardiopulmonary resuscitation. *Crit Care Med.* 1997;25: 1717–1720.

163. Li Y, Ristagno G, Bisera J, Tang W, Deng Q, Weil MH. Electrocardiogram waveforms for monitoring effectiveness of chest compression during cardiopulmonary resuscitation. *Crit Care Med.* 2008;36: 211–215.

164. Ristagno G, Tang W, Chang YT, Jorgenson DB, Russell JK, Huang L, Wang T, Sun S, Weil MH. The quality of chest compressions during cardiopulmonary resuscitation overrides importance of timing of defibrillation. *Chest.* 2007;132:70–75.

165. Berg RA, Sanders AB, Milander M, Tellez D, Liu P, Beyda D. Efficacy of audio-prompted rate guidance in improving resuscitator performance of cardiopulmonary resuscitation on children. *Acad Emerg Med.* 1994; 1:35–40.

166. Ornato JP, Gonzalez ER, Garnett AR, Levine RL, McClung BK. Effect of cardiopulmonary resuscitation compression rate on end-tidal carbon dioxide concentration and arterial pressure in man. *Crit Care Med.* 1988;16:241–245.

167. Guly UM, Robertson CE. Active decompression improves the haemodynamic state during cardiopulmonary resuscitation. *Br Heart J.* 1995; 73:372–376.

168. Rubertsson S, Karlsten R. Increased cortical cerebral blood flow with LUCAS; a new device for mechanical chest compressions compared to standard external compressions during experimental cardiopulmonary resuscitation. *Resuscitation.* 2005;65:357–363.

169. Wik L, Naess PA, Ilebekk A, Nicolaysen G, Steen PA. Effects of various degrees of compression and active decompression on haemodynamics, end-tidal CO2, and ventilation during cardiopulmonary resuscitation of pigs. *Resuscitation.* 1996;31:45–57.

170. Grmec S, Krizmaric M, Mally S, Kozelj A, Spindler M, Lesnik B. Utstein style analysis of out-of-hospital cardiac arrest–bystander CPR and end expired carbon dioxide. *Resuscitation.* 2007;72:404–414.

171. Pokorna M, Necas E, Kratochvil J, Skripsky R, Andrlik M, Franek O. A Sudden Increase in Partial Pressure End-tidal Carbon Dioxide (P(ET)CO2) at the Moment of Return of Spontaneous Circulation. *J Emerg Med.* 2009.

172. Rosetti VA, Thompson BM, Miller J, Mateer JR, Aprahamian C. Intraosseous infusion: an alternative route of pediatric intravascular access. *Ann Emerg Med.* 1985;14:885–888.

173. Brunette DD, Fischer R. Intravascular access in pediatric cardiac arrest. *Am J Emerg Med.* 1988;6:577–579.

174. Seigler RS, Tecklenburg FW, Shealy R. Prehospital intraosseous infusion by emergency medical services personnel: a prospective study. *Pediatrics.* 1989;84:173–177.

175. Glaeser PW, Hellmich TR, Szewczuga D, Losek JD, Smith DS. Five-year experience in prehospital intraosseous infusions in children and adults. *Ann Emerg Med.* 1993;22:1119–1124.

176. Ellemunter H, Simma B, Trawoger R, Maurer H. Intraosseous lines in preterm and full term neonates. *Arch Dis Child Fetal Neonatal Ed.* 1999;80:F74–F75.

177. Claudet I, Baunin C, Laporte-Turpin E, Marcoux MO, Grouteau E, Cahuzac JP. Long-term effects on tibial growth after intraosseous infusion: a prospective, radiographic analysis. *Pediatr Emerg Care.* 2003;19:397–401.

178. Fiorito BA, Mirza F, Doran TM, Oberle AN, Cruz EC, Wendtland CL, Abd-Allah SA. Intraosseous access in the setting of pediatric critical care transport. *Pediatr Crit Care Med.* 2005;6:50–53.

179. Horton MA, Beamer C. Powered intraosseous insertion provides safe and effective vascular access for pediatric emergency patients. *Pediatr Emerg Care.* 2008;24:347–350.

180. Kanter RK, Zimmerman JJ, Strauss RH, Stoeckel KA. Pediatric emergency intravenous access. Evaluation of a protocol. *Am J Dis Child*. 1986;140:132–134.

181. Banerjee S, Singhi SC, Singh S, Singh M. The intraosseous route is a suitable alternative to intravenous route for fluid resuscitation in severely dehydrated children. *Indian Pediatr*. 1994;31:1511–1520.

182. Fiser DH. Intraosseous infusion. *N Engl J Med*. 1990;322:1579–1581.

183. Guy J, Haley K, Zuspan SJ. Use of intraosseous infusion in the pediatric trauma patient. *J Pediatr Surg*. 1993;28:158–161.

184. Berg RA. Emergency infusion of catecholamines into bone marrow. *Am J Dis Child*. 1984;138:810–811.

185. Andropoulos DB, Soifer SJ, Schreiber MD. Plasma epinephrine concentrations after intraosseous and central venous injection during cardiopulmonary resuscitation in the lamb. *J Pediatr*. 1990;116:312–315.

186. Johnson L, Kissoon N, Fiallos M, Abdelmoneim T, Murphy S. Use of intraosseous blood to assess blood chemistries and hemoglobin during cardiopulmonary resuscitation with drug infusions. *Crit Care Med*. 1999;27:1147–1152.

187. Abdelmoneim T, Kissoon N, Johnson L, Fiallos M, Murphy S. Acid-base status of blood from intraosseous and mixed venous sites during prolonged cardiopulmonary resuscitation and drug infusions. *Crit Care Med*. 1999;27:1923–1928.

188. Orlowski JP, Porembka DT, Gallagher JM, Lockrem JD, VanLente F. Comparison study of intraosseous, central intravenous, and peripheral intravenous infusions of emergency drugs. *Am J Dis Child*. 1990;144:112–117.

189. Warren DW, Kissoon N, Sommerauer JF, Rieder MJ. Comparison of fluid infusion rates among peripheral intravenous and humerus, femur, malleolus, and tibial intraosseous sites in normovolemic and hypovolemic piglets. *Ann Emerg Med*. 1993;22:183–186.

190. Ward JTJ. Endotracheal drug therapy. *Am J Emerg Med*. 1983;1:71–82.

191. Johnston C. Endotracheal drug delivery. *Pediatr Emerg Care*. 1992;8:94–97.

192. Efrati O, Ben-Abraham R, Barak A, Modan-Moses D, Augarten A, Manisterski Y, Barzilay Z, Paret G. Endobronchial adrenaline: should it be reconsidered? Dose response and haemodynamic effect in dogs. *Resuscitation*. 2003;59:117–122.

193. Guay J, Lortie L. An evaluation of pediatric in-hospital advanced life support interventions using the pediatric Utstein guidelines: a review of 203 cardiorespiratory arrests. *Can J Anaesth*. 2004;51:373–378.

194. Niemann JT, Stratton SJ. Endotracheal versus intravenous epinephrine and atropine in out-of-hospital "primary" and postcountershock asystole. *Crit Care Med*. 2000;28:1815–1819.

195. Niemann JT, Stratton SJ, Cruz B, Lewis RJ. Endotracheal drug administration during out-of-hospital resuscitation: where are the survivors? *Resuscitation*. 2002;53:153–157.

196. Quinton DN, O'Byrne G, Aitkenhead AR. Comparison of endotracheal and peripheral intravenous adrenaline in cardiac arrest: is the endotracheal route reliable? *Lancet*. 1987;1:828–829.

197. Jasani MS, Nadkarni VM, Finkelstein MS, Mandell GA, Salzman SK, Norman ME. Effects of different techniques of endotracheal epinephrine administration in pediatric porcine hypoxic-hypercarbic cardiopulmonary arrest. *Crit Care Med*. 1994;22:1174–1180.

198. Battin M, Page B, Knight D. Is there still a place for endotracheal adrenaline in neonatal resuscitation? *J Paediatr Child Health*. 2007;43:504.

199. Lindemann R. Resuscitation of the newborn. Endotracheal administration of epinephrine. *Acta Paediatr Scand*. 1984;73:210–212.

200. Barber CA, Wyckoff MH. Use and efficacy of endotracheal versus intravenous epinephrine during neonatal cardiopulmonary resuscitation in the delivery room. *Pediatrics*. 2006;118:1028–1034.

201. Efrati O, Barak A, Ben-Abraham R, Modan-Moses D, Berkovitch M, Manisterski Y, Lotan D, Barzilay Z, Paret G. Should vasopressin replace adrenaline for endotracheal drug administration? *Crit Care Med*. 2003;31:572–576.

202. Elizur A, Ben-Abraham R, Manisterski Y, Barak A, Efrati O, Lotan D, Barzilay Z, Paret G. Tracheal epinephrine or norepinephrine preceded by beta blockade in a dog model. Can beta blockade bestow any benefits? *Resuscitation*. 2003;59:271–276.

203. Manisterski Y, Vaknin Z, Ben-Abraham R, Efrati O, Lotan D, Berkovitch M, Barak A, Barzilay Z, Paret G. Endotracheal epinephrine: a call for larger doses. *Anesth Analg*. 2002;95:1037–1041.

204. Orlowski JP, Gallagher JM, Porembka DT. Endotracheal epinephrine is unreliable. *Resuscitation*. 1990;19:103–113.

205. Paret G, Vaknin Z, Ezra D, Peleg E, Rosenthal T, Vardi A, Mayan H, Barzilay Z. Epinephrine pharmacokinetics and pharmacodynamics following endotracheal administration in dogs: the role of volume of diluent. *Resuscitation*. 1997;35:77–82.

206. Vaknin Z, Manisterski Y, Ben-Abraham R, Efrati O, Lotan D, Barzilay Z, Paret G. Is endotracheal adrenaline deleterious because of the beta adrenergic effect? *Anesth Analg*. 2001;92:1408–1412.

207. Somberg JC, Bailin SJ, Haffajee CI, Paladino WP, Kerin NZ, Bridges D, Timar S, Molnar J. Intravenous lidocaine versus intravenous amiodarone (in a new aqueous formulation) for incessant ventricular tachycardia. *Am J Cardiol*. 2002;90:853–859.

208. Dauchot P, Gravenstein JS. Effects of atropine on the electrocardiogram in different age groups. *Clin Pharmacol Ther*. 1971;12:274–280.

209. Zwiener RJ, Ginsburg CM. Organophosphate and carbamate poisoning in infants and children [published correction appears in *Pediatrics*. 1988;81:683]. *Pediatrics*. 1988;81:121–126.

210. Srinivasan V, Morris MC, Helfaer MA, Berg RA, Nadkarni VM. Calcium use during in-hospital pediatric cardiopulmonary resuscitation: a report from the National Registry of Cardiopulmonary Resuscitation. *Pediatrics*. 2008;121:e1144–1151.

211. de Mos N, van Litsenburg RR, McCrindle B, Bohn DJ, Parshuram CS. Pediatric in-intensive-care-unit cardiac arrest: incidence, survival, and predictive factors. *Crit Care Med*. 2006;34:1209–1215.

212. Meert KL, Donaldson A, Nadkarni V, Tieves KS, Schleien CL, Brilli RJ, Clark RS, Shaffner DH, Levy F, Statler K, Dalton HJ, van der Jagt EW, Hackbarth R, Pretzlaff R, Hernan L, Dean JM, Moler FW. Multicenter cohort study of in-hospital pediatric cardiac arrest. *Pediatr Crit Care Med*. 2009;10:544–553.

213. Blecic S, De Backer D, Huynh CH, Deleuze M, Domb M, Luypaert P, Vincent JL. Calcium chloride in experimental electromechanical dissociation: a placebo-controlled trial in dogs. *Crit Care Med*. 1987;15:324–327.

214. Harrison EE, Amey BD. The use of calcium in cardiac resuscitation. *Am J Emerg Med*. 1983;1:267–273.

215. Niemann JT, Adomian GE, Garner D, Rosborough JP. Endocardial and transcutaneous cardiac pacing, calcium chloride, and epinephrine in postcountershock asystole and bradycardias. *Crit Care Med*. 1985;13:699–704.

216. Ornato JP, Gonzales ER, Morkunas AR, Coyne MR, Beck CL. Treatment of presumed asystole during pre-hospital cardiac arrest: superiority of electrical countershock. *Am J Emerg Med*. 1985;3:395–399.

217. Redding JS, Haynes RR, Thomas JD. Drug therapy in resuscitation from electromechanical dissociation. *Crit Care Med*. 1983;11:681–684.

218. Redding JS, Pearson JW. Evaluation of drugs for cardiac resuscitation. *Anesthesiology*. 1963;24:203–207.

219. Stueven H, Thompson BM, Aprahamian C, Darin JC. Use of calcium in prehospital cardiac arrest. *Ann Emerg Med*. 1983;12:136–139.

220. Stueven HA, Thompson B, Aprahamian C, Tonsfeldt DJ, Kastenson EH. The effectiveness of calcium chloride in refractory electromechanical dissociation. *Ann Emerg Med*. 1985;14:626–629.

221. Stueven HA, Thompson B, Aprahamian C, Tonsfeldt DJ, Kastenson EH. Lack of effectiveness of calcium chloride in refractory asystole. *Ann Emerg Med*. 1985;14:630–632.

222. Martin TJ, Kang Y, Robertson KM, Virji MA, Marquez JM. Ionization and hemodynamic effects of calcium chloride and calcium gluconate in the absence of hepatic function. *Anesthesiology*. 1990;73:62–65.

222a. Broner CW, Stidham GL, Westenkirchner DF, Watson DC. A prospective, randomized. double-blind comparison of calcium chloride and calcium gluconate therapies for hypocalcemia in critically ill children. *J Pediatr*. 1990;117:986–989.

223. Niemann JT, Criley JM, Rosborough JP, Niskanen RA, Alferness C. Predictive indices of successful cardiac resuscitation after prolonged arrest and experimental cardiopulmonary resuscitation. *Ann Emerg Med*. 1985;14:521–528.

224. Sanders A, Ewy G, Taft T. Prognostic and therapeutic importance of the aortic diastolic pressure in resuscitation from cardiac arrest. *Crit Care Med*. 1984;12:871–873.

225. Losek JD. Hypoglycemia and the ABC'S (sugar) of pediatric resuscitation. *Ann Emerg Med*. 2000;35:43–46.

226. Beiser DG, Carr GE, Edelson DP, Peberdy MA, Hoek TL. Derangements in blood glucose following initial resuscitation from in-hospital cardiac arrest: a report from the national registry of cardiopulmonary resuscitation. *Resuscitation*. 2009;80:624–630.

227. Bigger JT, Jr., Mandel WJ. Effect of lidocaine on the electrophysiological properties of ventricular muscle and purkinje fibers. *J Clin Invest.* 1970;49:63–77.

228. Dorian P, Cass D, Schwartz B, Cooper R, Gelaznikas R, Barr A. Amiodarone as compared with lidocaine for shock-resistant ventricular fibrillation. *N Engl J Med.* 2002;346:884–890.

229. Wilson FC, Harpur J, Watson T, Morrow JI. Adult survivors of severe cerebral hypoxia–case series survey and comparative analysis. *Neuro Rehabilitation.* 2003;18:291–298.

230. Thomson PD, Melmon KL, Richardson JA, Cohn K, Steinbrunn W, Cudihee R, Rowland M. Lidocaine pharmacokinetics in advanced heart failure, liver disease, and renal failure in humans. *Ann Intern Med.* 1973;78:499–508.

231. Allegra J, Lavery R, Cody R, Birnbaum G, Brennan J, Hartman A, Horowitz M, Nashed A, Yablonski M. Magnesium sulfate in the treatment of refractory ventricular fibrillation in the prehospital setting. *Resuscitation.* 2001;49:245–249.

232. Hassan TB, Jagger C, Barnett DB. A randomised trial to investigate the efficacy of magnesium sulphate for refractory ventricular fibrillation. *Emerg Med J.* 2002;19:57–62.

233. Thel MC, Armstrong AL, McNulty SE, Califf RM, O'Connor CM. Randomised trial of magnesium in in-hospital cardiac arrest. Duke Internal Medicine Housestaff. *Lancet.* 1997;350:1272–1276.

234. Luedtke SA, Kuhn RJ, McCaffrey FM. Pharmacologic management of supraventricular tachycardias in children. Part 1: Wolff-Parkinson-White and atrioventricular nodal reentry. *Ann Pharmacother.* 1997;31:1227–1243.

235. Luedtke SA, Kuhn RJ, McCaffrey FM. Pharmacologic management of supraventricular tachycardias in children, part 2: atrial flutter, atrial fibrillation, and junctional and atrial ectopic tachycardia. *Ann Pharmacother.* 1997;31:1347–1359.

236. Chang PM, Silka MJ, Moromisato DY, Bar-Cohen Y. Amiodarone versus procainamide for the acute treatment of recurrent supraventricular tachycardia in pediatric patients. *Circ Arrhythm Electrophysiol.* 2010;3:134–140.

237. Vukmir RB, Katz L. Sodium bicarbonate improves outcome in prolonged prehospital cardiac arrest. *Am J Emerg Med.* 2006;24:156–161.

238. Lokesh L, Kumar P, Murki S, Narang A. A randomized controlled trial of sodium bicarbonate in neonatal resuscitation-effect on immediate outcome. *Resuscitation.* 2004;60:219–223.

239. Weil MH, Rackow EC, Trevino R, Grundler W, Falk JL, Griffel MI. Difference in acid-base state between venous and arterial blood during cardiopulmonary resuscitation. *N Engl J Med.* 1986;315:153–156.

240. Steedman DJ, Robertson CE. Acid-base changes in arterial and central venous blood during cardiopulmonary resuscitation. *Arch Emerg Med.* 1992;9:169–176.

241. Wayne MA, Delbridge TR, Ornato JP, Swor RA, Blackwell T. Concepts and application of prehospital ventilation. *Prehosp Emerg Care.* 2001;5:73–78.

242. Mattar JA, Weil MH, Shubin H, Stein L. Cardiac arrest in the critically ill. II. Hyperosmolal states following cardiac arrest. *Am J Med.* 1974;56:162–168.

243. Aufderheide TP, Martin DR, Olson DW, Aprahamian C, Woo JW, Hendley GE, Hargarten KM, Thompson B. Prehospital bicarbonate use in cardiac arrest: a 3-year experience. *Am J Emerg Med.* 1992;10:4–7.

244. Bishop RL, Weisfeldt ML. Sodium bicarbonate administration during cardiac arrest. Effect on arterial pH PCO2, and osmolality. *JAMA.* 1976;235:506–509.

245. Mann K, Berg RA, Nadkarni V. Beneficial effects of vasopressin in prolonged pediatric cardiac arrest: a case series. *Resuscitation.* 2002;52:149–156.

246. Matok I, Vardi A, Augarten A, Efrati O, Leibovitch L, Rubinshtein M, Paret G. Beneficial effects of terlipressin in prolonged pediatric cardiopulmonary resuscitation: a case series. *Crit Care Med.* 2007;35:1161–1164.

247. Gil-Anton J, Lopez-Herce J, Morteruel E, Carrillo A, Rodriguez-Nunez A. Pediatric cardiac arrest refractory to advanced life support: is there a role for terlipressin? *Pediatr Crit Care Med.* 2010;11:139–141.

248. Lindner KH, Prengel AW, Brinkmann A, Strohmenger HU, Lindner IM, Lurie KG. Vasopressin administration in refractory cardiac arrest. *Ann Intern Med.* 1996;124:1061–1064.

249. Lee CC, Kim GW, Kim SH, Crupi RS. Cases of aminophylline and vasopressin use after failed prehospital resuscitation of cardiac arrest. *Prehosp Emerg Care.* 2001;5:304–307.

250. Duncan JM, Meaney P, Simpson P, Berg RA, Nadkarni V, Schexnayder S. Vasopressin for in-hospital pediatric cardiac arrest: results from the American Heart Association National Registry of Cardiopulmonary Resuscitation. *Pediatr Crit Care Med.* 2009;10:191–195.

251. Callaway CW, Hostler D, Doshi AA, Pinchalk M, Roth RN, Lubin J, Newman DH, Kelly LJ. Usefulness of vasopressin administered with epinephrine during out-of-hospital cardiac arrest. *Am J Cardiol.* 2006;98:1316–1321.

252. Gueugniaud PY, David JS, Chanzy E, Hubert H, Dubien PY, Mauriaucourt P, Braganca C, Billeres X, Clotteau-Lambert MP, Fuster P, Thiercelin D, Debaty G, Ricard-Hibon A, Roux P, Espesson C, Querellou E, Ducros L, Ecollan P, Halbout L, Savary D, Guillaumee F, Maupoint R, Capelle P, Bracq C, Dreyfus P, Nouguier P, Gache A, Meurisse C, Boulanger B, Lae C, Metzger J, Raphael V, Beruben A, Wenzel V, Guinhouya C, Vilhelm C, Marret E. Vasopressin and epinephrine vs. epinephrine alone in cardiopulmonary resuscitation. *N Engl J Med.* 2008;359:21–30.

253. Lindner KH, Dirks B, Strohmenger HU, Prengel AW, Lindner IM, Lurie KG. Randomised comparison of epinephrine and vasopressin in patients with out-of-hospital ventricular fibrillation. *Lancet.* 1997;349:535–537.

254. Mukoyama T, Kinoshita K, Nagao K, Tanjoh K. Reduced effectiveness of vasopressin in repeated doses for patients undergoing prolonged cardiopulmonary resuscitation. *Resuscitation.* 2009;80:755–761.

255. Stiell IG, Hebert PC, Wells GA, Vandemheen KL, Tang AS, Higginson LA, Dreyer JF, Clement C, Battram E, Watpool I, Mason S, Klassen T, Weitzman BN. Vasopressin versus epinephrine for inhospital cardiac arrest: a randomised controlled trial. *Lancet.* 2001;358:105–109.

256. Wenzel V, Krismer AC, Arntz HR, Sitter H, Stadlbauer KH, Lindner KH. A comparison of vasopressin and epinephrine for out-of-hospital cardiopulmonary resuscitation. *N Engl J Med.* 2004;350:105–113.

257. Perondi MB, Reis AG, Paiva EF, Nadkarni VM, Berg RA. A comparison of high-dose and standard-dose epinephrine in children with cardiac arrest. *N Engl J Med.* 2004;350:1722–1730.

258. Rodriguez Nunez A, Garcia C, Lopez-Herce Cid J. [Is high-dose epinephrine justified in cardiorespiratory arrest in children?]. *An Pediatr (Barc).* 2005;62:113–116.

259. Patterson MD, Boenning DA, Klein BL, Fuchs S, Smith KM, Hegenbarth MA, Carlson DW, Krug SE, Harris EM. The use of high-dose epinephrine for patients with out-of-hospital cardiopulmonary arrest refractory to prehospital interventions. *Pediatr Emerg Care.* 2005;21:227–237.

260. Dieckmann RA, Vardis R. High-dose epinephrine in pediatric out-of-hospital cardiopulmonary arrest. *Pediatrics.* 1995;95:901–913.

261. Carpenter TC, Stenmark KR. High-dose epinephrine is not superior to standard-dose epinephrine in pediatric in-hospital cardiopulmonary arrest. *Pediatrics.* 1997;99:403–408.

262. Herlitz J, Engdahl J, Svensson L, Young M, Angquist KA, Holmberg S. Characteristics and outcome among children suffering from out of hospital cardiac arrest in Sweden. *Resuscitation.* 2005;64:37–40.

263. Safranek DJ, Eisenberg MS, Larsen MP. The epidemiology of cardiac arrest in young adults. *Ann Emerg Med.* 1992;21:1102–1106.

264. Larsen MP, Eisenberg MS, Cummins RO, Hallstrom AP. Predicting survival from out-of-hospital cardiac arrest: a graphic model. *Ann Emerg Med.* 1993;22:1652–1658.

265. Atkins DL, Sirna S, Kieso R, Charbonnier F, Kerber RE. Pediatric defibrillation: importance of paddle size in determining transthoracic impedance. *Pediatrics.* 1988;82:914–918.

266. Atkins DL, Kerber RE. Pediatric defibrillation: current flow is improved by using "adult" electrode paddles. *Pediatrics.* 1994;94:90–93.

267. Samson RA, Atkins DL, Kerber RE. Optimal size of self-adhesive preapplied electrode pads in pediatric defibrillation. *Am J Cardiol.* 1995;75:544–545.

268. Tibballs J, Carter B, Kiraly NJ, Ragg P, Clifford M. External and internal biphasic direct current shock doses for pediatric ventricular fibrillation and pulseless ventricular tachycardia. *Pediatr Crit Care Med.* 2010. In press.

269. Berg MD, Samson RA, Meyer RJ, Clark LL, Valenzuela TD, Berg RA. Pediatric defibrillation doses often fail to terminate prolonged out-of-hospital ventricular fibrillation in children. *Resuscitation.* 2005;67:63–67.

270. Rodriguez-Nunez A, Lopez-Herce J, Garcia C, Dominguez P, Carrillo A, Bellon JM. Pediatric defibrillation after cardiac arrest: initial response and outcome. *Crit Care.* 2006;10:R113.

271. Atkins DL, Hartley LL, York DK. Accurate recognition and effective treatment of ventricular fibrillation by automated external defibrillators in adolescents. *Pediatrics.* 1998;101(3 Pt 1):393–397.

272. Rossano JW, Quan L, Kenney MA, Rea TD, Atkins DL. Energy doses for treatment of out-of-hospital pediatric ventricular fibrillation. *Resuscitation.* 2006;70:80–89.

273. Gurnett CA, Atkins DL. Successful use of a biphasic waveform automated external defibrillator in a high-risk child. *Am J Cardiol.* 2000;86:1051–1053.

274. Atkins DL, Jorgenson DB. Attenuated pediatric electrode pads for automated external defibrillator use in children. *Resuscitation.* 2005;66:31–37.

275. Berg RA, Chapman FW, Berg MD, Hilwig RW, Banville I, Walker RG, Nova RC, Sherrill D, Kern KB. Attenuated adult biphasic shocks compared with weight-based monophasic shocks in a swine model of prolonged pediatric ventricular fibrillation. *Resuscitation.* 2004;61:189–197.

276. Schneider T, Martens PR, Paschen H, Kuisma M, Wolcke B, Gliner BE, Russell JK, Weaver WD, Bossaert L, Chamberlain D. Multicenter, randomized, controlled trial of 150-J biphasic shocks compared with 200- to 360-J monophasic shocks in the resuscitation of out-of-hospital cardiac arrest victims. Optimized Response to Cardiac Arrest (ORCA) Investigators. *Circulation.* 2000;102:1780–1787.

277. van Alem AP, Chapman FW, Lank P, Hart AA, Koster RW. A prospective, randomised and blinded comparison of first shock success of monophasic and biphasic waveforms in out-of-hospital cardiac arrest. *Resuscitation.* 2003;58:17–24.

278. Berg RA, Samson RA, Berg MD, Chapman FW, Hilwig RW, Banville I, Walker RG, Nova RC, Anavy N, Kern KB. Better outcome after pediatric defibrillation dosage than adult dosage in a swine model of pediatric ventricular fibrillation. *J Am Coll Cardiol.* 2005;45:786–789.

279. Clark CB, Zhang Y, Davies LR, Karlsson G, Kerber RE. Pediatric transthoracic defibrillation: biphasic versus monophasic waveforms in an experimental model. *Resuscitation.* 2001;51:159–163.

280. Tang W, Weil MH, Jorgenson D, Klouche K, Morgan C, Yu T, Sun S, Snyder D. Fixed-energy biphasic waveform defibrillation in a pediatric model of cardiac arrest and resuscitation. *Crit Care Med.* 2002;30:2736–2741.

281. Atkinson E, Mikysa B, Conway JA, Parker M, Christian K, Deshpande J, Knilans TK, Smith J, Walker C, Stickney RE, Hampton DR, Hazinski MF. Specificity and sensitivity of automated external defibrillator rhythm analysis in infants and children. *Ann Emerg Med.* 2003;42:185–196.

282. Cecchin F, Jorgenson DB, Berul CI, Perry JC, Zimmerman AA, Duncan BW, Lupinetti FM, Snyder D, Lyster TD, Rosenthal GL, Cross B, Atkins DL. Is arrhythmia detection by automatic external defibrillator accurate for children? Sensitivity and specificity of an automatic external defibrillator algorithm in 696 pediatric arrhythmias. *Circulation.* 2001;103:2483–2488.

283. Atkins DL, Scott WA, Blaufox AD, Law IH, Dick M, II, Geheb F, Sobh J, Brewer JE. Sensitivity and specificity of an automated external defibrillator algorithm designed for pediatric patients. *Resuscitation.* 2008;76:168–174.

284. Samson RA, Berg RA, Bingham R, Biarent D, Coovadia A, Hazinski MF, Hickey RW, Nadkarni V, Nichol G, Tibballs J, Reis AG, Tse S, Zideman D, Potts J, Uzark K, Atkins D. Use of automated external defibrillators for children: an update: an advisory statement from the pediatric advanced life support task force, International Liaison Committee on Resuscitation. *Circulation.* 2003;107:3250–3255.

285. Cobb LA, Fahrenbruch CE, Walsh TR, Copass MK, Olsufka M, Breskin M, Hallstrom AP. Influence of cardiopulmonary resuscitation prior to defibrillation in patients with out-of-hospital ventricular fibrillation. *JAMA.* 1999;281:1182–1188.

286. Wik L, Hansen TB, Fylling F, Steen T, Vaagenes P, Auestad BH, Steen PA. Delaying defibrillation to give basic cardiopulmonary resuscitation to patients with out-of-hospital ventricular fibrillation: a randomized trial. *JAMA.* 2003;289:1389–1395.

287. Yakaitis RW, Ewy GA, Otto CW, Taren DL, Moon TE. Influence of time and therapy on ventricular defibrillation in dogs. *Crit Care Med.* 1980;8:157–163.

288. Kudenchuk PJ, Cobb LA, Copass MK, Cummins RO, Doherty AM, Fahrenbruch CE, Hallstrom AP, Murray WA, Olsufka M, Walsh T. Amiodarone for resuscitation after out-of-hospital cardiac arrest due to ventricular fibrillation. *N Engl J Med.* 1999;341:871–878.

289. Perry JC, Fenrich AL, Hulse JE, Triedman JK, Friedman RA, Lamberti JJ. Pediatric use of intravenous amiodarone: efficacy and safety in critically ill patients from a multicenter protocol. *J Am Coll Cardiol.* 1996;27:1246–1250.

290. Perry JC, Knilans TK, Marlow D, Denfield SW, Fenrich AL, Friedman RA. Intravenous amiodarone for life-threatening tachyarrhythmias in children and young adults. *J Am Coll Cardiol.* 1993;22:95–98.

291. van Haarst AD, van 't Klooster GA, van Gerven JM, Schoemaker RC, van Oene JC, Burggraaf J, Coene MC, Cohen AF. The influence of cisapride and clarithromycin on QT intervals in healthy volunteers. *Clin Pharmacol Ther.* 1998;64:542–546.

292. Ray WA, Murray KT, Meredith S, Narasimhulu SS, Hall K, Stein CM. Oral erythromycin and the risk of sudden death from cardiac causes. *N Engl J Med.* 2004;351:1089–1096.

293. Beland MJ, Hesslein PS, Finlay CD, Faerron-Angel JE, Williams WG, Rowe RD. Noninvasive transcutaneous cardiac pacing in children. *Pacing Clin Electrophysiol.* 1987;10:1262–1270.

294. Quan L, Graves JR, Kinder DR, Horan S, Cummins RO. Transcutaneous cardiac pacing in the treatment of out-of-hospital pediatric cardiac arrests. *Ann Emerg Med.* 1992;21:905–909.

295. Sreeram N, Wren C. Supraventricular tachycardia in infants: response to initial treatment. *Arch Dis Child.* 1990;65:127–129.

296. Aydin M, Baysal K, Kucukoduk S, Cetinkaya F, Yaman S. Application of ice water to the face in initial treatment of supraventricular tachycardia. *Turk J Pediatr.* 1995;37:15–17.

297. Ornato JP, Hallagan LF, Reese WA, Clark RF, Tayal VS, Garnett AR, Gonzalez ER. Treatment of paroxysmal supraventricular tachycardia in the emergency department by clinical decision analysis [published correction appears in *Am J Emerg Med.* 1990;8:85]. *Am J Emerg Med.* 1988;6:555–560.

298. Lim SH, Anantharaman V, Teo WS, Goh PP, Tan AT. Comparison of treatment of supraventricular tachycardia by Valsalva maneuver and carotid sinus massage. *Ann Emerg Med.* 1998;31:30–35.

299. Waxman MB, Wald RW, Sharma AD, Huerta F, Cameron DA. Vagal techniques for termination of paroxysmal supraventricular tachycardia. *Am J Cardiol.* 1980;46:655–664.

300. Balaguer Gargallo M, Jordan Garcia I, Caritg Bosch J, Cambra Lasaosa FJ, Prada Hermogenes F, Palomaque Rico A. [Supraventricular tachycardia in infants and children]. *An Pediatr (Barc).* 2007;67:133–138.

301. Dixon J, Foster K, Wyllie J, Wren C. Guidelines and adenosine dosing in supraventricular tachycardia. *Arch Dis Child.* 2005;90:1190–1191.

302. Moghaddam M, Mohammad Dalili S, Emkanjoo Z. Efficacy of Adenosine for Acute Treatment of Supraventricular Tachycardia in Infants and Children. *J Teh Univ Heart Ctr.* 2008;3:157–162.

303. Riccardi A, Arboscello E, Ghinatti M, Minuto P, Lerza R. Adenosine in the treatment of supraventricular tachycardia: 5 years of experience (2002–2006). *Am J Emerg Med.* 2008;26:879–882.

304. Ertan C, Atar I, Gulmez O, Atar A, Ozgul A, Aydinalp A, Muderrisoglu H, Ozin B. Adenosine-induced ventricular arrhythmias in patients with supraventricular tachycardias. *Ann Noninvasive Electrocardiol.* 2008;13:386–390.

305. Lim SH, Anantharaman V, Teo WS, Chan YH. Slow infusion of calcium channel blockers compared with intravenous adenosine in the emergency treatment of supraventricular tachycardia. *Resuscitation.* 2009;80:523–528.

306. Holdgate A, Foo A. Adenosine versus intravenous calcium channel antagonists for the treatment of supraventricular tachycardia in adults. *Cochrane Database Syst Rev.* 2006;:CD005154.

307. Ng GY, Hampson Evans DC, Murdoch LJ. Cardiovascular collapse after amiodarone administration in neonatal supraventicular tachycardia. *Eur J Emerg Med.* 2003;10:323–325.

308. Saul JP, Scott WA, Brown S, Marantz P, Acevedo V, Etheridge SP, Perry JC, Triedman JK, Burriss SW, Cargo P, Graepel J, Koskelo EK, Wang R. Intravenous amiodarone for incessant tachyarrhythmias in children: a randomized, double-blind, antiarrhythmic drug trial. *Circulation.* 2005;112:3470–3477.

309. Haas NA, Camphausen CK. Acute hemodynamic effects of intravenous amiodarone treatment in pediatric patients with cardiac surgery. *Clin Res Cardiol.* 2008;97:801–810.

310. Benson D, Jr., Smith W, Dunnigan A, Sterba R, Gallagher J. Mechanisms of regular wide QRS tachycardia in infants and children. *Am J Cardiol.* 1982;49:1778–1788.

311. Dung NM, Day NPJ, Tam DTH, Loan HT, Chau HTT, Minh LN, Diet TV, Bethell DB, Kneen R, Hien TT, White NJ, Farrar JJ. Fluid

replacement in dengue shock syndrome: A randomized, double-blind comparison of four intravenous-fluid regimens. *Clin Infect Dis.* 1999; 29:787–794.

312. Ngo NT, Cao XT, Kneen R, Wills B, Nguyen VM, Nguyen TQ, Chu VT, Nguyen TT, Simpson JA, Solomon T, White NJ, Farrar J. Acute management of dengue shock syndrome: a randomized double-blind comparison of 4 intravenous fluid regimens in the first hour. *Clin Infect Dis.* 2001;32:204–213.

313. Wills BA, Nguyen MD, Ha TL, Dong TH, Tran TN, Le TT, Tran VD, Nguyen TH, Nguyen VC, Stepniewska K, White NJ, Farrar JJ. Comparison of three fluid solutions for resuscitation in dengue shock syndrome. *N Engl J Med.* 2005;353:877–889.

314. Upadhyay M, Singhi S, Murlidharan J, Kaur N, Majumdar S. Randomized evaluation of fluid resuscitation with crystalloid (saline) and colloid (polymer from degraded gelatin in saline) in pediatric septic shock. *Indian Pediatr.* 2005;42:223–231.

315. Booy R, Habibi P, Nadel S, de Munter C, Britto J, Morrison A, Levin M. Reduction in case fatality rate from meningococcal disease associated with improved healthcare delivery. *Arch Dis Child.* 2001;85:386–390.

316. de Oliveira CF, de Oliveira DS, Gottschald AF, Moura JD, Costa GA, Ventura AC, Fernandes JC, Vaz FA, Carcillo JA, Rivers EP, Troster EJ. ACCM/PALS haemodynamic support guidelines for paediatric septic shock: an outcomes comparison with and without monitoring central venous oxygen saturation. *Intensive Care Med.* 2008;34:1065–1075.

317. Rivers E, Nguyen B, Havstad S, Ressler J, Muzzin A, Knoblich B, Peterson E, Tomlanovich M. Early goal-directed therapy in the treatment of severe sepsis and septic shock. *N Engl J Med.* 2001;345: 1368–1377.

318. Nguyen HB, Corbett SW, Steele R, Banta J, Clark RT, Hayes SR, Edwards J, Cho TW, Wittlake WA. Implementation of a bundle of quality indicators for the early management of severe sepsis and septic shock is associated with decreased mortality. *Crit Care Med.* 2007;35: 1105–1112.

319. Ledingham IM, McArdle CS. Prospective study of the treatment of septic shock. *Lancet.* 1978;1:1194–1197.

320. Zuckerbraun NS, Pitetti RD, Herr SM, Roth KR, Gaines BA, King C. Use of etomidate as an induction agent for rapid sequence intubation in a pediatric emergency department. *Acad Emerg Med.* 2006;13:602–609.

321. Sokolove PE, Price DD, Okada P. The safety of etomidate for emergency rapid sequence intubation of pediatric patients. *Pediatr Emerg Care.* 2000;16:18–21.

322. Guldner G, Schultz J, Sexton P, Fortner C, Richmond M. Etomidate for rapid-sequence intubation in young children: hemodynamic effects and adverse events. *Acad Emerg Med.* 2003;10:134–139.

323. den Brinker M, Hokken-Koelega AC, Hazelzet JA, de Jong FH, Hop WC, Joosten KF. One single dose of etomidate negatively influences adrenocortical performance for at least 24h in children with meningococcal sepsis. *Intensive Care Med.* 2008;34:163–168.

324. Jabre P, Combes X, Lapostolle F, Dhaouadi M, Ricard-Hibon A, Vivien B, Bertrand L, Beltramini A, Gamand P, Albizzati S, Perdrizet D, Lebail G, Chollet-Xemard C, Maxime V, Brun-Buisson C, Lefrant JY, Bollaert PE, Megarbane B, Ricard JD, Anguel N, Vicaut E, Adnet F. Etomidate versus ketamine for rapid sequence intubation in acutely ill patients: a multicentre randomised controlled trial. *Lancet.* 2009;374:293–300.

325. Sprung CL, Annane D, Keh D, Moreno R, Singer M, Freivogel K, Weiss YG, Benbenishty J, Kalenka A, Forst H, Laterre PF, Reinhart K, Cuthbertson BH, Payen D, Briegel J. Hydrocortisone therapy for patients with septic shock. *N Engl J Med.* 2008;358:111–124.

326. Schierhout G, Roberts I. Fluid resuscitation with colloid or crystalloid solutions in critically ill patients: a systematic review of randomised trials. *BMJ.* 1998;316:961–964.

327. Human albumin administration in critically ill patients: systematic review of randomised controlled trials. Cochrane Injuries Group Albumin Reviewers. *BMJ.* 1998;317:235–240.

328. Alderson P, Schierhout G, Roberts I, Bunn F. Colloids versus crystalloids for fluid resuscitation in critically ill patients. *In: The Cochrane Library. Oxford: Update Software.* 2003(Issue 3).

329. Finfer S, Bellomo R, Boyce N, French J, Myburgh J, Norton R. A comparison of albumin and saline for fluid resuscitation in the intensive care unit. *N Engl J Med.* 2004;350:2247–2256.

330. Choi PT, Yip G, Quinonez LG, Cook DJ. Crystalloids vs. colloids in fluid resuscitation: a systematic review. *Crit Care Med.* 1999;27: 200–210.

331. Myburgh J, Cooper DJ, Finfer S, Bellomo R, Norton R, Bishop N, Kai Lo S, Vallance S. Saline or albumin for fluid resuscitation in patients with traumatic brain injury. *N Engl J Med.* 2007;357:874–884.

332. Huang PP, Stucky FS, Dimick AR, Treat RC, Bessey PQ, Rue LW. Hypertonic sodium resuscitation is associated with renal failure and death. *Ann Surg.* 221:543–554, 1995; discussion 554–547.

333. Simma B, Burger R, Falk M, Sacher P, Fanconi S. A prospective, randomized, and controlled study of fluid management in children with severe head injury: lactated Ringer's solution versus hypertonic saline. *Crit Care Med.* 1998;26:1265–1270.

334. Bunn F, Roberts I, Tasker R, Akpa E. Hypertonic versus isotonic crystalloid for fluid resuscitation in critically ill patients. *In: The Cochrane Library. Oxford: Update Software.* 2003(Issue 3).

335. Dykes EH, Spence LJ, Young JG, Bohn DJ, Filler RM, Wesson DE. Preventable pediatric trauma deaths in a metropolitan region. *J Pediatr Surg.* 1989;24:107–110.

336. Herzenberg JE, Hensinger RN, Dedrick DK, Phillips WA. Emergency transport and positioning of young children who have an injury of the cervical spine. The standard backboard may be hazardous. *J Bone Joint Surg Am.* 1989;71:15–22.

337. Nypaver M, Treloar D. Neutral cervical spine positioning in children. *Ann Emerg Med.* 1994;23:208–211.

338. Muizelaar JP, Marmarou A, Ward JD, Kontos HA, Choi SC, Becker DP, Gruemer H, Young HF. Adverse effects of prolonged hyperventilation in patients with severe head injury: a randomized clinical trial. *J Neurosurg.* 1991;75:731–739.

339. Skippen P, Seear M, Poskitt K, Kestle J, Cochrane D, Annich G, Handel J. Effect of hyperventilation on regional cerebral blood flow in head-injured children. *Crit Care Med.* 1997;25:1402–1409.

340. Baskaya MK. Inadvertent intracranial placement of a nasogastric tube in patients with head injuries. *Surg Neurol.* 1999;52:426–427.

341. Powell RW, Gill EA, Jurkovich GJ, Ramenofsky ML. Resuscitative thoracotomy in children and adolescents. *Am Surg.* 1988;54:188–191.

342. Rothenberg SS, Moore EE, Moore FA, Baxter BT, Moore JB, Cleveland HC. Emergency Department thoracotomy in children–a critical analysis. *J Trauma.* 1989;29:1322–1325.

343. Ramenofsky ML, Luterman A, Quindlen E, Riddick L, Curreri PW. Maximum survival in pediatric trauma: the ideal system. *J Trauma.* 1984;24:818–823.

344. Luterman A, Ramenofsky M, Berryman C, Talley MA, Curreri PW. Evaluation of prehospital emergency medical service (EMS): defining areas for improvement. *J Trauma.* 1983;23:702–707.

345. Matthews IL, Bjornstad PG, Kaldestad RH, Heiberg L, Thaulow E, Gronn M. The impact of shunt size on lung function in infants with univentricular heart physiology. *Pediatr Crit Care Med.* 2009;10: 60–65.

346. Ramamoorthy C, Tabbutt S, Kurth CD, Steven JM, Montenegro LM, Durning S, Wernovsky G, Gaynor JW, Spray TL, Nicolson SC. Effects of inspired hypoxic and hypercapnic gas mixtures on cerebral oxygen saturation in neonates with univentricular heart defects. *Anesthesiology.* 2002;96:283–288.

347. Tabbutt S, Ramamoorthy C, Montenegro LM, Durning SM, Kurth CD, Steven JM, Godinez RI, Spray TL, Wernovsky G, Nicolson SC. Impact of inspired gas mixtures on preoperative infants with hypoplastic left heart syndrome during controlled ventilation. *Circulation.* 2001;104(12 Suppl 1):I159–164.

348. De Oliveira NC, Van Arsdell GS. Practical use of alpha blockade strategy in the management of hypoplastic left heart syndrome following stage one palliation with a Blalock-Taussig shunt. *Semin Thorac Cardiovasc Surg Pediatr Card Surg Annu.* 2004;7:11–15.

349. Hoffman GM, Tweddell JS, Ghanayem NS, Mussatto KA, Stuth EA, Jaquis RD, Berger S. Alteration of the critical arteriovenous oxygen saturation relationship by sustained afterload reduction after the Norwood procedure. *J Thorac Cardiovasc Surg.* 2004;127:738–745.

350. Tweddell JS, Hoffman GM, Mussatto KA, Fedderly RT, Berger S, Jaquiss RD, Ghanayem NS, Frisbee SJ, Litwin SB. Improved survival of patients undergoing palliation of hypoplastic left heart syndrome: lessons learned from 115 consecutive patients. *Circulation.* 2002; 106(12 Suppl 1):I82–89.

351. Motta P, Mossad E, Toscana D, Zestos M, Mee R. Comparison of phenoxybenzamine to sodium nitroprusside in infants undergoing surgery. *J Cardiothorac Vasc Anesth.* 2005;19:54–59.

352. Hoffman TM, Wernovsky G, Atz AM, Kulik TJ, Nelson DP, Chang AC, Bailey JM, Akbary A, Kocsis JF, Kaczmarek R, Spray TL, Wessel DL. Efficacy and safety of milrinone in preventing low cardiac output

syndrome in infants and children after corrective surgery for congenital heart disease. *Circulation*. 2003;107:996–1002.

353. Charpie JR, Dekeon MK, Goldberg CS, Mosca RS, Bove EL, Kulik TJ. Postoperative hemodynamics after Norwood palliation for hypoplastic left heart syndrome. *Am J Cardiol*. 2001;87:198–202.

354. Hoffman GM, Mussatto KA, Brosig CL, Ghanayem NS, Musa N, Fedderly RT, Jaquiss RD, Tweddell JS. Systemic venous oxygen saturation after the Norwood procedure and childhood neurodevelopmental outcome. *J Thorac Cardiovasc Surg*. 2005;130:1094–1100.

355. Johnson BA, Hoffman GM, Tweddell JS, Cava JR, Basir M, Mitchell ME, Scanlon MC, Mussatto KA, Ghanayem NS. Near-infrared spectroscopy in neonates before palliation of hypoplastic left heart syndrome. *Ann Thorac Surg*. 87:571–577, 2009; discussion 577–579.

356. Raymond TT, Cunnyngham CB, Thompson MT, Thomas JA, Dalton HJ, Nadkarni VM. Outcomes among neonates, infants, and children after extracorporeal cardiopulmonary resuscitation for refractory in-hospital pediatric cardiac arrest: A report from the National Registry of CardioPulmonary Resuscitation*. *Pediatr Crit Care Med*. 2009.

357. Tajik M, Cardarelli MG. Extracorporeal membrane oxygenation after cardiac arrest in children: what do we know? *Eur J Cardiothorac Surg*. 2008;33:409–417.

358. Hoskote A, Li J, Hickey C, Erickson S, Van Arsdell G, Stephens D, Holtby H, Bohn D, Adatia I. The effects of carbon dioxide on oxygenation and systemic, cerebral, and pulmonary vascular hemodynamics after the bidirectional superior cavopulmonary anastomosis. *J Am Coll Cardiol*. 2004;44:1501–1509.

359. Li J, Hoskote A, Hickey C, Stephens D, Bohn D, Holtby H, Van Arsdell G, Redington AN, Adatia I. Effect of carbon dioxide on systemic oxygenation, oxygen consumption, and blood lactate levels after bidirectional superior cavopulmonary anastomosis. *Crit Care Med*. 2005;33:984–989.

360. Fogel MA, Durning S, Wernovsky G, Pollock AN, Gaynor JW, Nicolson S. Brain versus lung: hierarchy of feedback loops in single-ventricle patients with superior cavopulmonary connection. *Circulation*. 2004;110(11 Suppl 1):II147–152.

361. Bradley SM, Simsic JM, Mulvihill DM. Hypoventilation improves oxygenation after bidirectional superior cavopulmonary connection. *J Thorac Cardiovasc Surg*. 2003;126:1033–1039.

362. Shekerdemian LS, Shore DF, Lincoln C, Bush A, Redington AN. Negative-pressure ventilation improves cardiac output after right heart surgery. *Circulation*. 1996;94(9 Suppl):II49–55.

363. Shekerdemian LS, Bush A, Shore DF, Lincoln C, Redington AN. Cardiopulmonary interactions after Fontan operations: augmentation of cardiac output using negative pressure ventilation. *Circulation*. 1997;96:3934–3942.

364. Booth KL, Roth SJ, Thiagarajan RR, Almodovar MC, del Nido PJ, Laussen PC. Extracorporeal membrane oxygenation support of the Fontan and bidirectional Glenn circulations. *Ann Thorac Surg*. 2004;77:1341–1348.

365. Rimensberger PC, Spahr-Schopfer I, Berner M, Jaeggi E, Kalangos A, Friedli B, Beghetti M. Inhaled nitric oxide versus aerosolized iloprost in secondary pulmonary hypertension in children with congenital heart disease: vasodilator capacity and cellular mechanisms. *Circulation*. 2001;103:544–548.

366. Limsuwan A, Wanitkul S, Khosithset A, Attanavanich S, Samankatiwat P. Aerosolized iloprost for postoperative pulmonary hypertensive crisis in children with congenital heart disease. *Int J Cardiol*. 2008;129:333–338.

367. Morris K, Beghetti M, Petros A, Adatia I, Bohn D. Comparison of hyperventilation and inhaled nitric oxide for pulmonary hypertension after repair of congenital heart disease. *Crit Care Med*. 2000;28:2974–2978.

368. Dhillon R, Pearson GA, Firmin RK, Chan KC, Leanage R. Extracorporeal membrane oxygenation and the treatment of critical pulmonary hypertension in congenital heart disease. *Eur J Cardiothorac Surg*. 1995;9:553–556.

369. Policy statement–emergency information forms and emergency preparedness for children with special health care needs. *Pediatrics*. 2010;125:829–837.

370. Spaite DW, Conroy C, Tibbitts M, Karriker KJ, Seng M, Battaglia N, Criss EA, Valenzuela TD, Meislin HW. Use of emergency medical services by children with special health care needs. *Prehosp Emerg Care*. 2000;4:19–23.

371. Ludot H, Tharin JY, Belouadah M, Mazoit JX, Malinovsky JM. Successful resuscitation after ropivacaine and lidocaine-induced ventricular

arrhythmia following posterior lumbar plexus block in a child [published erratum appears in *Anesth Analg*. 2008;107:238]. *Anesth Analg*. 2008;106:1572–1574.

372. Hollander JE, Hoffman RS, Gennis P, Fairweather P, DiSano MJ, Schumb DA, Feldman JA, Fish SS, Dyer S, Wax P, et al. Prospective multicenter evaluation of cocaine-associated chest pain. Cocaine Associated Chest Pain (COCHPA) Study Group. *Acad Emerg Med*. 1994;1:330–339.

373. Brody SL, Slovis CM, Wrenn KD. Cocaine-related medical problems: consecutive series of 233 patients. *Am J Med*. 1990;88:325–331.

374. Bauman JL, Grawe JJ, Winecoff AP, Hariman RJ. Cocaine-related sudden cardiac death: a hypothesis correlating basic science and clinical observations. *J Clin Pharmacol*. 1994;34:902–911.

375. Kolecki PF, Curry SC. Poisoning by sodium channel blocking agents. *Crit Care Clin*. 1997;13:829–848.

376. Lange RA, Cigarroa RG, Flores ED, McBride W, Kim AS, Wells PJ, Bedotto JB, Danziger RS, Hillis LD. Potentiation of cocaine-induced coronary vasoconstriction by beta-adrenergic blockade. *Ann Intern Med*. 1990;112:897–903.

377. Brogan WCI, Lange RA, Kim AS, Moliterno DJ, Hillis LD. Alleviation of cocaine-induced coronary vasoconstriction by nitroglycerin. *J Am Coll Cardiol*. 1991;18:581–586.

378. Hollander JE, Hoffman RS, Gennis P, Fairweather P, DiSano MJ, Schumb DA, Feldman JA, Fish SS, Dyer S, Wax P, et al. Nitroglycerin in the treatment of cocaine associated chest pain–clinical safety and efficacy. *J Toxicol Clin Toxicol*. 1994;32:243–256.

379. Hoffman RS, Hollander JE. Evaluation of patients with chest pain after cocaine use. *Crit Care Clin*. 1997;13:809–828.

380. Lange RA, Cigarroa RG, Yancy CW, Jr., Willard JE, Popma JJ, Sills MN, McBride W, Kim AS, Hillis LD. Cocaine-induced coronary-artery vasoconstriction. *N Engl J Med*. 1989;321:1557–1562.

381. Kerns W, II, Garvey L, Owens J. Cocaine-induced wide complex dysrhythmia. *J Emerg Med*. 1997;15:321–329.

382. Beckman KJ, Parker RB, Hariman RJ, Gallastegui JL, Javaid JI, Bauman JL. Hemodynamic and electrophysiological actions of cocaine: effects of sodium bicarbonate as an antidote in dogs. *Circulation*. 1991;83:1799–1807.

383. Dziukas LJ, Vohra J. Tricyclic antidepressant poisoning. *Med J Aust*. 1991;154:344–350.

384. Liebelt EL. Targeted management strategies for cardiovascular toxicity from tricyclic antidepressant overdose: the pivotal role for alkalinization and sodium loading. *Pediatr Emerg Care*. 1998;14:293–298.

385. Teba L, Schiebel F, Dedhia HV, Lazzell VA. Beneficial effect of norepinephrine in the treatment of circulatory shock caused by tricyclic antidepressant overdose. *Am J Emerg Med*. 1988;6:566–568.

386. Tran TP, Panacek EA, Rhee KJ, Foulke GE. Response to dopamine vs norepinephrine in tricyclic antidepressant-induced hypotension. *Acad Emerg Med*. 1997;4:864–868.

387. Williams JM, Hollingshed MJ, Vasilakis A, Morales M, Prescott JE, Graeber GM. Extracorporeal circulation in the management of severe tricyclic antidepressant overdose. *Am J Emerg Med*. 1994;12:456–458.

388. Larkin GL, Graeber GM, Hollingsed MJ. Experimental amitriptyline poisoning: treatment of severe cardiovascular toxicity with cardiopulmonary bypass. *Ann Emerg Med*. 1994;23:480–486.

389. Ramoska EA, Spiller HA, Winter M, Borys D. A one-year evaluation of calcium channel blocker overdoses: toxicity and treatment. *Ann Emerg Med*. 1993;22:196–200.

390. Henry M, Kay MM, Viccellio P. Cardiogenic shock associated with calcium-channel and beta blockers: reversal with intravenous calcium chloride. *Am J Emerg Med*. 1985;3:334–336.

391. Howarth DM, Dawson AH, Smith AJ, Buckley N, Whyte IM. Calcium channel blocking drug overdose: an Australian series. *Hum Exp Toxicol*. 1994;13:161–166.

392. Horowitz BZ, Rhee KJ. Massive verapamil ingestion: a report of two cases and a review of the literature. *Am J Emerg Med*. 1989;7:624–631.

393. Watling SM, Crain JL, Edwards TD, Stiller RA. Verapamil overdose: case report and review of the literature. *Ann Pharmacother*. 1992;26:1373–1378.

394. Kerns W, II, Schroeder D, Williams C, Tomaszewski C, Raymond R. Insulin improves survival in a canine model of acute beta-blocker toxicity. *Ann Emerg Med*. 1997;29:748–757.

395. Kline JA, Tomaszewski CA, Schroeder JD, Raymond RM. Insulin is a superior antidote for cardiovascular toxicity induced by verapamil in the anesthetized canine. *J Pharmacol Exp Ther*. 1993;267:744–750.

396. Yuan TH, Kerns WPI, Tomaszewski CA, Ford MD, Kline JA. Insulin-glucose as adjunctive therapy for severe calcium channel antagonist poisoning. *J Toxicol Clin Toxicol.* 1999;37:463–474.

397. Kerns W, II, Kline J, Ford MD. Beta-blocker and calcium channel blocker toxicity. *Emerg Med Clin North Am.* 1994;12:365–390.

398. Lewis M, Kallenbach J, Germond C, Zaltzman M, Muller F, Steyn J, Zwi S. Survival following massive overdose of adrenergic blocking agents (acebutolol and labetalol). *Eur Heart J.* 1983;4:328–332.

399. Cruickshank JM, Neil-Dwyer G, Cameron MM, McAinsh J. beta-Adrenoreceptor-blocking agents and the blood-brain barrier. *Clin Sci.* 1980; 59(suppl 6):453s–455s.

400. Weinstein RS. Recognition and management of poisoning with beta-adrenergic blocking agents. *Ann Emerg Med.* 1984;13:1123–1131.

401. Avery GJd, Spotnitz HM, Rose EA, Malm JR, Hoffman BF. Pharmacologic antagonism of beta-adrenergic blockade in dogs, I: hemodynamic effects of isoproterenol, dopamine, and epinephrine in acute propranolol administration. *J Thorac Cardiovasc Surg.* 1979;77:267–276.

402. Zaritsky AL, Horowitz M, Chernow B. Glucagon antagonism of calcium channel blocker-induced myocardial dysfunction. *Crit Care Med.* 1988; 16:246–251.

403. Mofenson HC, Caraccio TR, Laudano J. Glucagon for propranolol overdose. *JAMA.* 1986;255:2025–2026.

404. Love JN, Hanfling D, Howell JM. Hemodynamic effects of calcium chloride in a canine model of acute propranolol intoxication. *Ann Emerg Med.* 1996;28:1–6.

405. Haddad LM. Resuscitation after nifedipine overdose exclusively with intravenous calcium chloride. *Am J Emerg Med.* 1996;14:602–603.

406. McGuire W, Fowlie PW. Naloxone for narcotic exposed newborn infants: systematic review. *Arch Dis Child Fetal Neonatal Ed.* 2003;88: F308–F311.

407. Chernick V, Manfreda J, De Booy V, Davi M, Rigatto H, Seshia M. Clinical trial of naloxone in birth asphyxia. *J Pediatr.* 1988;113: 519–525.

408. Fischer CG, Cook DR. The respiratory and narcotic antagonistic effects of naloxone in infants. *Anesth Analg.* 1974;53:849–852.

409. Kattwinkel J, Niermeyer S, Nadkarni V, Tibballs J, Phillips B, Zideman D, Van Reempts P, Osmond M. An advisory statement from the Pediatric Working Group of the International Liaison Committee on Resuscitation. *Middle East J Anesthesiol.* 2001;16:315–351.

410. Am Academy of Pediatrics Committee on Drugs: Naloxone dosage and route of administration for infants and children: addendum to emergency drug doses for infants and children. *Pediatrics.* 1990;86:484–485.

411. Mills CA, Flacke JW, Flacke WE, Bloor BC, Liu MD. Narcotic reversal in hypercapnic dogs: comparison of naloxone and nalbuphine. *Can J Anaesth.* 1990;37:238–244.

412. Tobias JD, Lynch A, Garrett J. Alterations of end-tidal carbon dioxide during the intrahospital transport of children. *Pediatr Emerg Care.* 1996;12:249–251.

413. Singh S, Allen WD, Jr., Venkataraman ST, Bhende MS. Utility of a novel quantitative handheld microstream capnometer during transport of critically ill children. *Am J Emerg Med.* 2006;24:302–307.

414. Hildebrand CA, Hartmann AG, Arcinue EL, Gomez RJ, Bing RJ. Cardiac performance in pediatric near-drowning. *Crit Care Med.* 1988;16:331–335.

415. Checchia PA, Sehra R, Moynihan J, Daher N, Tang W, Weil MH. Myocardial injury in children following resuscitation after cardiac arrest. *Resuscitation.* 2003;57:131–137.

416. Laurent I, Monchi M, Chiche JD, Joly LM, Spaulding C, Bourgeois B, Cariou A, Rozenberg A, Carli P, Weber S, Dhainaut JF. Reversible myocardial dysfunction in survivors of out-of-hospital cardiac arrest. *J Am Coll Cardiol.* 2002;40:2110–2116.

417. Mayr V, Luckner G, Jochberger S, Wenzel V, Ulmer H, Pajk W, Knotzer H, Friesenecker B, Lindner K, Hasibeder W, Dunser M. Arginine vasopressin in advanced cardiovascular failure during the post-resuscitation phase after cardiac arrest. *Resuscitation.* 2007;72:35–44.

418. Kern KB, Hilwig RW, Berg RA, Rhee KH, Sanders AB, Otto CW, Ewy GA. Postresuscitation left ventricular systolic and diastolic dysfunction: treatment with dobutamine. *Circulation.* 1997;95:2610–2613.

419. Meyer RJ, Kern KB, Berg RA, Hilwig RW, Ewy GA. Post-resuscitation right ventricular dysfunction: delineation and treatment with dobutamine. *Resuscitation.* 2002;55:187–191.

420. Ceneviva G, Paschall JA, Maffei F, Carcillo JA. Hemodynamic support in fluid-refractory pediatric septic shock. *Pediatrics.* 1998;102:e19.

421. Huang L, Weil MH, Sun S, Cammarata G, Cao L, Tang W. Levosimendan improves postresuscitation outcomes in a rat model of CPR. *J Lab Clin Med.* 2005;146:256–261.

422. Huang L, Weil MH, Tang W, Sun S, Wang J. Comparison between dobutamine and levosimendan for management of postresuscitation myocardial dysfunction. *Crit Care Med.* 2005;33:487–491.

423. Studer W, Wu X, Siegemund M, Marsch S, Seeberger M, Filipovic M. Influence of dobutamine on the variables of systemic haemodynamics, metabolism, and intestinal perfusion after cardiopulmonary resuscitation in the rat. *Resuscitation.* 2005;64:227–232.

424. Vasquez A, Kern KB, Hilwig RW, Heidenreich J, Berg RA, Ewy GA. Optimal dosing of dobutamine for treating post-resuscitation left ventricular dysfunction. *Resuscitation.* 2004;61:199–207.

425. Alvarez J, Bouzada M, Fernandez AL, Caruezo V, Taboada M, Rodriguez J, Ginesta V, Rubio J, Garcia-Bengoechea JB, Gonzalez-Juanatey JR. [Hemodynamic effects of levosimendan compared with dobutamine in patients with low cardiac output after cardiac surgery]. *Rev Esp Cardiol.* 2006;59:338–345.

426. Jorgensen K, Bech-Hanssen O, Houltz E, Ricksten SE. Effects of levosimendan on left ventricular relaxation and early filling at maintained preload and afterload conditions after aortic valve replacement for aortic stenosis. *Circulation.* 2008;117:1075–1081.

427. Lobato EB, Willert JL, Looke TD, Thomas J, Urdaneta F. Effects of milrinone versus epinephrine on left ventricular relaxation after cardiopulmonary bypass following myocardial revascularization: assessment by color m-mode and tissue Doppler. *J Cardiothorac Vasc Anesth.* 2005;19:334–339.

428. Nijhawan N, Nicolosi AC, Montgomery MW, Aggarwal A, Pagel PS, Warltier DC. Levosimendan enhances cardiac performance after cardiopulmonary bypass: a prospective, randomized placebo-controlled trial. *J Cardiovasc Pharmacol.* 1999;34:219–228.

429. Levy B, Bollaert PE, Charpentier C, Nace L, Audibert G, Bauer P, Nabet P, Larcan A. Comparison of norepinephrine and dobutamine to epinephrine for hemodynamics, lactate metabolism, and gastric tonometric variables in septic shock: a prospective, randomized study. *Intensive Care Med.* 1997;23:282–287.

430. Zaritsky A, Chernow B. Use of catecholamines in pediatrics. *J Pediatr.* 1984;105:341–350.

431. Steinberg C, Notterman DA. Pharmacokinetics of cardiovascular drugs in children. Inotropes and vasopressors. *Clin Pharmacokinet.* 1994;27: 345–367.

432. Berg RA, Padbury JF. Sulfoconjugation and renal excretion contribute to the interpatient variation of exogenous catecholamine clearance in critically ill children. *Crit Care Med.* 1997;25:1247–1251.

433. Fisher DG, Schwartz PH, Davis AL. Pharmacokinetics of exogenous epinephrine in critically ill children. *Crit Care Med.* 1993;21:111–117.

434. De Backer D, Biston P, Devriendt J, Madl C, Chochrad D, Aldecoa C, Brasseur A, Defrance P, Gottignies P, Vincent JL. Comparison of dopamine and norepinephrine in the treatment of shock. *N Engl J Med.* 2010;362:779–789.

435. Ushay HM, Notterman DA. Pharmacology of pediatric resuscitation. *Pediatr Clin North Am.* 1997;44:207–233.

436. Bellomo R, Chapman M, Finfer S, Hickling K, Myburgh J. Low-dose dopamine in patients with early renal dysfunction: a placebo-controlled randomised trial. Australian and New Zealand Intensive Care Society (ANZICS) Clinical Trials Group. *Lancet.* 2000;356:2139–2143.

437. Zacharias M, Conlon NP, Herbison GP, Sivalingam P, Walker RJ, Hovhannisyan K. Interventions for protecting renal function in the perioperative period. *Cochrane Database Syst Rev.* 2008;:CD003590.

438. Li J, Zhang G, Holtby H, Humpl T, Caldarone CA, Van Arsdell GS, Redington AN. Adverse effects of dopamine on systemic hemodynamic status and oxygen transport in neonates after the Norwood procedure. *J Am Coll Cardiol.* 2006;48:1859–1864.

439. Ruffolo RR, Jr., Spradlin TA, Pollock GD, Waddell JE, Murphy PJ. Alpha and beta adrenergic effects of the stereoisomers of dobutamine. *J Pharmacol Exp Ther.* 1981;219:447–452.

440. Habib DM, Padbury JF, Anas NG, Perkin RM, Minegar C. Dobutamine pharmacokinetics and pharmacodynamics in pediatric intensive care patients. *Crit Care Med.* 1992;20:601–608.

441. Martinez AM, Padbury JF, Thio S. Dobutamine pharmacokinetics and cardiovascular responses in critically ill neonates. *Pediatrics.* 1992;89: 47–51.

442. Barton P, Garcia J, Kouatli A, Kitchen L, Zorka A, Lindsay C, Lawless S, Giroir B. Hemodynamic effects of i.v. milrinone lactate in pediatric

patients with septic shock: a prospective, double-blinded, randomized, placebo-controlled, interventional study. *Chest*. 1996;109:1302–1312.

443. Bailey JM, Miller BE, Lu W, Tosone SR, Kanter KR, Tam VK. The pharmacokinetics of milrinone in pediatric patients after cardiac surgery. *Anesthesiology*. 1999;90:1012–1018.

444. Abdallah I, Shawky H. A randomised controlled trial comparing milrinone and epinephrine as inotropes in paediatric patients undergoing total correction of Tetralogy of Fallot. *Egyptian Journal of Anaesthesia*. 2003;19:323–329.

445. Buunk G, van der Hoeven JG, Meinders AE. Cerebrovascular reactivity in comatose patients resuscitated from a cardiac arrest. *Stroke*. 1997;28: 1569–1573.

446. Doherty DR, Parshuram CS, Gaboury I, Hoskote A, Lacroix J, Tucci M, Joffe A, Choong K, Farrell R, Bohn DJ, Hutchison JS. Hypothermia therapy after pediatric cardiac arrest. *Circulation*. 2009;119:1492–1500.

447. Fink EL, Clark RS, Kochanek PM, Bell MJ, Watson RS. A tertiary care center's experience with therapeutic hypothermia after pediatric cardiac arrest. *Pediatr Crit Care Med*. 2010;11:66–74.

448. Bernard SA, Gray TW, Buist MD, Jones BM, Silvester W, Gutteridge G, Smith K. Treatment of comatose survivors of out-of-hospital cardiac arrest with induced hypothermia. *N Engl J Med*. 2002;346:557–563.

449. Hypothermia After Cardiac Arrest Study Group. Mild therapeutic hypothermia to improve the neurologic outcome after cardiac arrest. *N Engl J Med*. 2002;346:549–556.

450. Gluckman PD, Wyatt JS, Azzopardi D, Ballard R, Edwards AD, Ferriero DM, Polin RA, Robertson CM, Thoresen M, Whitelaw A, Gunn AJ. Selective head cooling with mild systemic hypothermia after neonatal encephalopathy: multicentre randomised trial. *Lancet*. 2005;365: 663–670.

451. Shankaran S, Laptook AR, Ehrenkranz RA, Tyson JE, McDonald SA, Donovan EF, Fanaroff AA, Poole WK, Wright LL, Higgins RD, Finer NN, Carlo WA, Duara S, Oh W, Cotten CM, Stevenson DK, Stoll BJ, Lemons JA, Guillet R, Jobe AH. Whole-body hypothermia for neonates with hypoxic-ischemic encephalopathy. *N Engl J Med*. 2005;353: 1574–1584.

452. Zeiner A, Holzer M, Sterz F, Schorkhuber W, Eisenburger P, Havel C, Kliegel A, Laggner AN. Hyperthermia after cardiac arrest is associated with an unfavorable neurologic outcome. *Arch Intern Med*. 2001;161: 2007–2012.

453. Takasu A, Saitoh D, Kaneko N, Sakamoto T, Okada Y. Hyperthermia: is it an ominous sign after cardiac arrest? *Resuscitation*. 2001;49: 273–277.

454. Ginsberg MD, Busto R. Combating hyperthermia in acute stroke: a significant clinical concern. *Stroke*. 1998;29:529–534.

455. Hickey RW, Kochanek PM, Ferimer H, Alexander HL, Garman RH, Graham SH. Induced hyperthermia exacerbates neurologic neuronal histologic damage after asphyxial cardiac arrest in rats. *Crit Care Med*. 2003;31:531–535.

456. Laptook A, Tyson J, Shankaran S, McDonald S, Ehrenkranz R, Fanaroff A, Donovan E, Goldberg R, O'Shea TM, Higgins RD, Poole WK. Elevated temperature after hypoxic-ischemic encephalopathy: risk factor for adverse outcomes. *Pediatrics*. 2008;122:491–499.

457. Kim Y, Busto R, Dietrich WD, Kraydieh S, Ginsberg MD. Delayed postischemic hyperthermia in awake rats worsens the histopathological outcome of transient focal cerebral ischemia. *Stroke*. 27:2274–2280, 1996; discussion 2281.

458. Baena RC, Busto R, Dietrich WD, Globus MY, Ginsberg MD. Hyperthermia delayed by 24 hours aggravates neuronal damage in rat hippocampus following global ischemia. *Neurology*. 1997;48:768–773.

459. Henning R. Emergency transport of critically ill children: stabilisation before departure. *Med J Aust*. 1992;156:117–124.

460. Edge WE, Kanter RK, Weigle CG, Walsh RF. Reduction of morbidity in interhospital transport by specialized pediatric staff. *Crit Care Med*. 1994;22:1186–1191.

461. Woodward G, ed. *Guidelines for Air and Ground Transport of Neonatal and Pediatric Patients*. III ed; 2006. Am Academy of Pediatrics Section on Transport Medicine.

462. Dudley NC, Hansen KW, Furnival RA, Donaldson AE, Van Wagenen KL, Scaife ER. The effect of family presence on the efficiency of pediatric trauma resuscitations. *Ann Emerg Med*. 2009;53:777–784 e773.

463. Tinsley C, Hill JB, Shah J, Zimmerman G, Wilson M, Freier K, Abd-Allah S, Tinsley C, Hill JB, Shah J, Zimmerman G, Wilson M, Freier K, Abd-Allah S. Experience of families during cardiopulmonary

464. Mangurten J, Scott SH, Guzzetta CE, Clark AP, Vinson L, Sperry J, Hicks B, Voelmeck W, Mangurten J, Scott SH, Guzzetta CE, Clark AP, Vinson L, Sperry J, Hicks B, Voelmeck W. Effects of family presence during resuscitation and invasive procedures in a pediatric emergency department. *Journal of Emergency Nursing*. 2006;32:225–233.

465. McGahey-Oakland PR, Lieder HS, Young A, Jefferson LS, McGahey-Oakland PR, Lieder HS, Young A, Jefferson LS. Family experiences during resuscitation at a children's hospital emergency department. *Journal of Pediatric Health Care*. 2007;21:217–225.

466. Jones M, Qazi M, Young KD. Ethnic differences in parent preference to be present for painful medical procedures. *Pediatrics*. 2005;116:e191–197.

467. Boie ET, Moore GP, Brummett C, Nelson DR. Do parents want to be present during invasive procedures performed on their children in the emergency department? A survey of 400 parents. *Ann Emerg Med*. 1999;34:70–74.

468. Andrews R, Andrews R. Family presence during a failed major trauma resuscitation attempt of a 15-year-old boy: lessons learned.[see comment]. *Journal of Emergency Nursing*. 2004;30:556–558.

469. Dill K, Gance-Cleveland B, Dill K, Gance-Cleveland B. With you until the end: family presence during failed resuscitation. *Journal for Specialists in Pediatric Nursing: JSPN*. 2005;10:204–207.

470. Gold KJ, Gorenflo DW, Schwenk TL, Bratton SL, Gold KJ, Gorenflo DW, Schwenk TL, Bratton SL. Physician experience with family presence during cardiopulmonary resuscitation in children.[see comment]. *Pediatr Crit Care Med*. 2006;7:428–433.

471. Duran CR, Oman KS, Abel JJ, Koziel VM, Szymanski D. Attitudes Toward and Beliefs About Family Presence: A Survey of Healthcare Providers, Patients' Families, and Patients. *Am Journal of Critical Care*. 2007;16:270–279.

472. Doyle CJ, Post H, Burney RE, Maino J, Keefe M, Rhee KJ. Family participation during resuscitation: an option. *Ann Emerg Med*. 1987;16: 673–675.

473. Hanson C, Strawser D. Family presence during cardiopulmonary resuscitation: Foote Hospital emergency department's nine-year perspective. *J Emerg Nurs*. 1992;18:104–106.

474. Meyers TA, Eichhorn DJ, Guzzetta CE. Do families want to be present during CPR? A retrospective survey. *J Emerg Nurs*. 1998;24:400–405.

475. Meyers TA, Eichhorn DJ, Guzzetta CE, Clark AP, Klein JD, Taliaferro E, Calvin A. Family presence during invasive procedures and resuscitation. *Am J Nurs*. 100:32–42, 2000; quiz 43.

476. Holzhauser K, Finucane J, De Vries S. Family Presence During Resuscitation: A Randomised Controlled Trial Of The Impact Of Family Presence. *Australasian Emergency Nursing Journal*. 2005;8:139–147.

477. Robinson SM, Mackenzie-Ross S, Campbell Hewson GL, Egleston CV, Prevost AT. Psychological effect of witnessed resuscitation on bereaved relatives. *Lancet*. 1998;352:614–617.

478. Boyd R. Witnessed resuscitation by relatives. *Resuscitation*. 2000;43: 171–176.

479. Offord RJ. Should relatives of patients with cardiac arrest be invited to be present during cardiopulmonary resuscitation? *Intensive Crit Care Nurs*. 1998;14:288–293.

480. O'Connell KJ, Farah MM, Spandorfer P, Zorc JJ, O'Connell KJ, Farah MM, Spandorfer P, Zorc JJ. Family presence during pediatric trauma team activation: an assessment of a structured program. *Pediatrics*. 2007;120:e565–574.

481. Engel KG, Barnosky AR, Berry-Bovia M, Desmond JS, Ubel PA, Engel KG, Barnosky AR, Berry-Bovia M, Desmond JS, Ubel PA. Provider experience and attitudes toward family presence during resuscitation procedures. *Journal of Palliative Medicine*. 2007;10:1007–1009.

482. Boyd R, White S, Does witnessed cardiopulmonary resuscitation alter perceived stress in accident and emergency staff? *Eur J Emerg Med*. 2000;7:51–53.

483. Compton S, Madgy A, Goldstein M, Sandhu J, Dunne R, Swor R. Emergency medical service providers' experience with family presence during cardiopulmonary resuscitation. *Resuscitation*. 2006;70:223–228.

484. Eichhorn DJ, Meyers TA, Mitchell TG, Guzzetta CE. Opening the doors: family presence during resuscitation. *J Cardiovasc Nurs*. 1996; 10:59–70.

485. Innes PA, Summers CA, Boyd IM, Molyneux EM. Audit of paediatric cardiopulmonary resuscitation. *Arch Dis Child*. 1993;68:487–491.

486. Slonim AD, Patel KM, Ruttimann UE, Pollack MM. Cardiopulmonary resuscitation in pediatric intensive care units. *Crit Care Med*. 1997;25: 1951–1955.

487. Young KD, Gausche-Hill M, McClung CD, Lewis RJ. A prospective, population-based study of the epidemiology and outcome of out-of-hospital pediatric cardiopulmonary arrest. *Pediatrics*. 2004;114:157–164.

488. Suominen P, Baillie C, Korpela R, Rautanen S, Ranta S, Olkkola KT. Impact of age, submersion time and water temperature on outcome in near-drowning. *Resuscitation*. 2002;52:247–254.

489. Rodriguez-Nunez A, Lopez-Herce J, Garcia C, Carrillo A, Dominguez P, Calvo C, Delgado MA. Effectiveness and long-term outcome of cardiopulmonary resuscitation in paediatric intensive care units in Spain. *Resuscitation*. 2006;71:301–309.

490. Lopez-Herce J, Garcia C, Dominguez P, Carrillo A, Rodriguez-Nunez A, Calvo C, Delgado MA. Characteristics and outcome of cardiorespiratory arrest in children. *Resuscitation*. 2004;63:311–320.

491. Lopez-Herce J, Garcia C, Rodriguez-Nunez A, Dominguez P, Carrillo A, Calvo C, Delgado MA. Long-term outcome of paediatric cardiorespiratory arrest in Spain. *Resuscitation*. 2005;64:79–85.

492. Ackerman MJ, Siu BL, Sturner WQ, Tester DJ, Valdivia CR, Makielski JC, Towbin JA. Postmortem molecular analysis of SCN5A defects in sudden infant death syndrome. *JAMA*. 2001;286:2264–2269.

493. Arnestad M, Crotti L, Rognum TO, Insolia R, Pedrazzini M, Ferrandi C, Vege A, Wang DW, Rhodes TE, George AL, Jr., Schwartz PJ. Prevalence of long-QT syndrome gene variants in sudden infant death syndrome. *Circulation*. 2007;115:361–367.

494. Cronk LB, Ye B, Kaku T, Tester DJ, Vatta M, Makielski JC, Ackerman MJ. Novel mechanism for sudden infant death syndrome: persistent late sodium current secondary to mutations in caveolin-3. *Heart Rhythm*. 2007;4:161–166.

495. Millat G, Kugener B, Chevalier P, Chahine M, Huang H, Malicier D, Rodriguez-Lafrasse C, Rousson R. Contribution of long-QT syndrome genetic variants in sudden infant death syndrome. *Pediatr Cardiol*. 2009;30:502–509.

496. Otagiri T, Kijima K, Osawa M, Ishii K, Makita N, Matoba R, Umetsu K, Hayasaka K. Cardiac ion channel gene mutations in sudden infant death syndrome. *Pediatr Res*. 2008;64:482–487.

497. Plant LD, Bowers PN, Liu Q, Morgan T, Zhang T, State MW, Chen W, Kittles RA, Goldstein SA. A common cardiac sodium channel variant associated with sudden infant death in African Americans, SCN5A S1103Y. *J Clin Invest*. 2006;116:430–435.

498. Tester DJ, Dura M, Carturan E, Reiken S, Wronska A, Marks AR, Ackerman MJ. A mechanism for sudden infant death syndrome (SIDS): stress-induced leak via ryanodine receptors. *Heart Rhythm*. 2007;4:733–739.

499. Albert CM, Nam EG, Rimm EB, Jin HW, Hajjar RJ, Hunter DJ, MacRae CA, Ellinor PT. Cardiac sodium channel gene variants and sudden cardiac death in women. *Circulation*. 2008;117:16–23.

500. Chugh SS, Senashova O, Watts A, Tran PT, Zhou Z, Gong Q, Titus JL, Hayflick SJ. Postmortem molecular screening in unexplained sudden death. *J Am Coll Cardiol*. 2004;43:1625–1629.

501. Tester DJ, Spoon DB, Valdivia HH, Makielski JC, Ackerman MJ. Targeted mutational analysis of the RyR2-encoded cardiac ryanodine receptor in sudden unexplained death: a molecular autopsy of 49 medical examiner/coroner's cases. *Mayo Clin Proc*. 2004;79:1380–1384.

502. Behr E, Wood DA, Wright M, Syrris P, Sheppard MN, Casey A, Davies MJ, McKenna W. Cardiological assessment of first-degree relatives in sudden arrhythmic death syndrome. *Lancet*. 2003;362:1457–1459.

503. Behr ER, Dalageorgou C, Christiansen M, Syrris P, Hughes S, Tome Esteban MT, Rowland E, Jeffery S, McKenna WJ. Sudden arrhythmic death syndrome: familial evaluation identifies inheritable heart disease in the majority of families. *Eur Heart J*. 2008;29:1670–1680.

504. Hofman N, Tan HL, Clur SA, Alders M, van Langen IM, Wilde AA. Contribution of inherited heart disease to sudden cardiac death in childhood. *Pediatrics*. 2007;120:e967–973.

505. Tan HL, Hofman N, van Langen IM, van der Wal AC, Wilde AA. Sudden unexplained death: heritability and diagnostic yield of cardiological and genetic examination in surviving relatives. *Circulation*. 2005;112:207–213.

KEY WORDS: arrhythmia ■ cardiopulmonary resuscitation ■ pediatrics

# Part 15: Neonatal Resuscitation

## 2010 American Heart Association Guidelines for Cardiopulmonary Resuscitation and Emergency Cardiovascular Care

John Kattwinkel, Co-Chair*; Jeffrey M. Perlman, Co-Chair*; Khalid Aziz; Christopher Colby; Karen Fairchild; John Gallagher; Mary Fran Hazinski; Louis P. Halamek; Praveen Kumar; George Little; Jane E. McGowan; Barbara Nightengale; Mildred M. Ramirez; Steven Ringer; Wendy M. Simon; Gary M. Weiner; Myra Wyckoff; Jeanette Zaichkin

The following guidelines are an interpretation of the evidence presented in the *2010 International Consensus on Cardiopulmonary Resuscitation and Emergency Cardiovascular Care Science With Treatment Recommendations*[1]). They apply primarily to newly born infants undergoing transition from intrauterine to extrauterine life, but the recommendations are also applicable to neonates who have completed perinatal transition and require resuscitation during the first few weeks to months following birth. Practitioners who resuscitate infants at birth or at any time during the initial hospital admission should consider following these guidelines. For the purposes of these guidelines, the terms *newborn* and *neonate* are intended to apply to any infant during the initial hospitalization. The term *newly born* is intended to apply specifically to an infant at the time of birth.

Approximately 10% of newborns require some assistance to begin breathing at birth. Less than 1% require extensive resuscitative measures.[2,3] Although the vast majority of newly born infants do not require intervention to make the transition from intrauterine to extrauterine life, because of the large total number of births, a sizable number will require some degree of resuscitation.

Those newly born infants who do not require resuscitation can generally be identified by a rapid assessment of the following 3 characteristics:

- Term gestation?
- Crying or breathing?
- Good muscle tone?

If the answer to all 3 of these questions is "yes," the baby does not need resuscitation and should not be separated from the mother. The baby should be dried, placed skin-to-skin with the mother, and covered with dry linen to maintain temperature. Observation of breathing, activity, and color should be ongoing.

If the answer to any of these assessment questions is "no," the infant should receive one or more of the following 4 categories of action in sequence:

A. Initial steps in stabilization (provide warmth, clear airway if necessary, dry, stimulate)
B. Ventilation
C. Chest compressions
D. Administration of epinephrine and/or volume expansion

Approximately 60 seconds ("the Golden Minute") are allotted for completing the initial steps, reevaluating, and beginning ventilation if required (see Figure). The decision to progress beyond the initial steps is determined by simultaneous assessment of 2 vital characteristics: respirations (apnea, gasping, or labored or unlabored breathing) and heart rate (whether greater than or less than 100 beats per minute). Assessment of heart rate should be done by intermittently auscultating the precordial pulse. When a pulse is detectable, palpation of the umbilical pulse can also provide a rapid estimate of the pulse and is more accurate than palpation at other sites.[4,5]

A pulse oximeter can provide a continuous assessment of the pulse without interruption of other resuscitation measures, but the device takes 1 to 2 minutes to apply, and it may not function during states of very poor cardiac output or perfusion. Once positive pressure ventilation or supplementary oxygen administration is begun, assessment should consist of simultaneous evaluation of 3 vital characteristics: heart rate, respirations, and the state of oxygenation, the latter optimally determined by a pulse oximeter as discussed under "Assessment of Oxygen Need and Administration of Oxygen" below. The most sensitive indicator of a successful response to each step is an increase in heart rate.

## Anticipation of Resuscitation Need

Anticipation, adequate preparation, accurate evaluation, and prompt initiation of support are critical for successful neona-

---

The American Heart Association requests that this document be cited as follows: Kattwinkel J, Perlman JM, Aziz K, Colby C, Fairchild K, Gallagher J, Hazinski MF, Halamek LP, Kumar P, Little G, McGowan JE, Nightengale B, Ramirez MM, Ringer S, Simon WM, Weiner GM, Wyckoff M, Zaichkin J. Part 15: neonatal resuscitation: 2010 American Heart Association Guidelines for Cardiopulmonary Resuscitation and Emergency Cardiovascular Care. *Circulation*. 2010;122(suppl 3):S909–S919.

*Co-chairs and equal first co-authors.

(*Circulation*. 2010;122[suppl 3]:S909–S919.)

*Circulation* is available at http://circ.ahajournals.org        DOI: 10.1161/CIRCULATIONAHA.110.971119

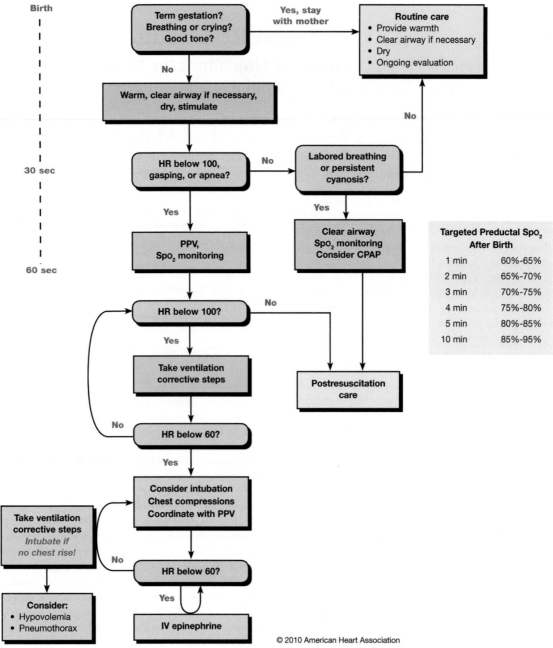

**Figure.** Newborn Resuscitation Algorithm.

tal resuscitation. At every delivery there should be at least 1 person whose primary responsibility is the newly born. This person must be capable of initiating resuscitation, including administration of positive-pressure ventilation and chest compressions. Either that person or someone else who is promptly available should have the skills required to perform a complete resuscitation, including endotracheal intubation and administration of medications.[6] Several studies have demonstrated that a cesarean section performed under regional anesthesia at 37 to 39 weeks, without antenatally identified risk factors, versus a similar vaginal delivery performed at term, does not increase the risk of the baby requiring endotracheal intubation.[7–10]

With careful consideration of risk factors, the majority of newborns who will need resuscitation can be identified before

birth. If the possible need for resuscitation is anticipated, additional skilled personnel should be recruited and the necessary equipment prepared. Identifiable risk factors and the necessary equipment for resuscitation are listed in the *Textbook of Neonatal Resuscitation, 6th Edition* (American Academy of Pediatrics, *in press*).[11] If a preterm delivery (<37 weeks of gestation) is expected, special preparations will be required. Preterm babies have immature lungs that may be more difficult to ventilate and are also more vulnerable to injury by positive-pressure ventilation. Preterm babies also have immature blood vessels in the brain that are prone to hemorrhage; thin skin and a large surface area, which contribute to rapid heat loss; increased susceptibility to infection; and increased risk of hypovolemic shock related to small blood volume.

## Initial Steps

The initial steps of resuscitation are to provide warmth by placing the baby under a radiant heat source, positioning the head in a "sniffing" position to open the airway, clearing the airway if necessary with a bulb syringe or suction catheter, drying the baby, and stimulating breathing. Recent studies have examined several aspects of these initial steps. These studies are summarized below.

### Temperature Control

Very low-birth-weight (<1500 g) preterm babies are likely to become hypothermic despite the use of traditional techniques for decreasing heat loss.[12] For this reason additional warming techniques are recommended (eg, prewarming the delivery room to 26°C,[13] covering the baby in plastic wrapping (food or medical grade, heat-resistant plastic) (Class I, LOE A[14,15]), placing the baby on an exothermic mattress (Class IIb, LOE B[16]), and placing the baby under radiant heat (Class IIb, LOE C[17]). The infant's temperature must be monitored closely because of the slight, but described risk of hyperthermia when these techniques are used in combination (Class IIb, LOE B[16]). Other techniques for maintaining temperature during stabilization of the baby in the delivery room have been used (eg, prewarming the linen, drying and swaddling, placing the baby skin-to-skin with the mother and covering both with a blanket) and are recommended, but they have not been studied specifically (Class IIb, LOE C). All resuscitation procedures, including endotracheal intubation, chest compression, and insertion of intravenous lines, can be performed with these temperature-controlling interventions in place (Class IIb, LOE C).

Infants born to febrile mothers have been reported to have a higher incidence of perinatal respiratory depression, neonatal seizures, and cerebral palsy and an increased risk of mortality.[18,19] Animal studies indicate that hyperthermia during or after ischemia is associated with progression of cerebral injury. Lowering the temperature reduces neuronal damage.[20] Hyperthermia should be avoided (Class IIb, LOE C). The goal is to achieve normothermia and avoid iatrogenic hyperthermia.

### Clearing the Airway

#### When Amniotic Fluid Is Clear

There is evidence that suctioning of the nasopharynx can create bradycardia during resuscitation[21,22] and that suctioning of the trachea in intubated babies receiving mechanical ventilation in the neonatal intensive care unit (NICU) can be associated with deterioration of pulmonary compliance and oxygenation and reduction in cerebral blood flow velocity when performed routinely (ie, in the absence of obvious nasal or oral secretions).[23,24] However, there is also evidence that suctioning in the presence of secretions can decrease respiratory resistance.[25] Therefore it is recommended that suctioning immediately following birth (including suctioning with a bulb syringe) should be reserved for babies who have obvious obstruction to spontaneous breathing or who require positive-pressure ventilation (PPV) (Class IIb, LOE C).

#### When Meconium is Present

Aspiration of meconium before delivery, during birth, or during resuscitation can cause severe meconium aspiration syndrome (MAS). Historically a variety of techniques have been recommended to reduce the incidence of MAS. Suctioning of the oropharynx before delivery of the shoulders was considered routine until a randomized controlled trial demonstrated it to be of no value.[26] Elective and routine endotracheal intubation and direct suctioning of the trachea were initially recommended for all meconium-stained newborns until a randomized controlled trial demonstrated that there was no value in performing this procedure in babies who were vigorous at birth.[27] Although depressed infants born to mothers with meconium-stained amniotic fluid (MSAF) are at increased risk to develop MAS,[28,29] tracheal suctioning has not been associated with reduction in the incidence of MAS or mortality in these infants.[30,31] The only evidence that direct tracheal suctioning of meconium may be of value was based on comparison of suctioned babies with historic controls, and there was apparent selection bias in the group of intubated babies included in those studies.[32–34]

In the absence of randomized, controlled trials, there is insufficient evidence to recommend a change in the current practice of performing endotracheal suctioning of nonvigorous babies with meconium-stained amniotic fluid (Class IIb, LOE C). However, if attempted intubation is prolonged and unsuccessful, bag-mask ventilation should be considered, particularly if there is persistent bradycardia.

### Assessment of Oxygen Need and Administration of Oxygen

There is a large body of evidence that blood oxygen levels in uncompromised babies generally do not reach extrauterine values until approximately 10 minutes following birth. Oxyhemoglobin saturation may normally remain in the 70% to 80% range for several minutes following birth, thus resulting in the appearance of cyanosis during that time. Other studies have shown that clinical assessment of skin color is a very poor indicator of oxyhemoglobin saturation during the immediate neonatal period and that lack of cyanosis appears to be a very poor indicator of the state of oxygenation of an uncompromised baby following birth.

Optimal management of oxygen during neonatal resuscitation becomes particularly important because of the evidence that either insufficient or excessive oxygenation can be harmful to the newborn infant. Hypoxia and ischemia are known to result in injury to multiple organs. Conversely there is growing experimental evidence, as well as evidence from studies of babies receiving resuscitation, that adverse outcomes may result from even brief exposure to excessive oxygen during and following resuscitation.

### Pulse Oximetry

Numerous studies have defined the percentiles of oxygen saturation as a function of time from birth in uncompromised babies born at term (see table in Figure). This includes saturations measured from both preductal and postductal sites, following both operative and vaginal deliveries, and those occurring at sea level and at altitude.[35–40]

Newer pulse oximeters, which employ probes designed specifically for neonates, have been shown to provide reliable readings within 1 to 2 minutes following birth.[41–43] These oximeters are reliable in the large majority of newborns, both term and preterm, and requiring resuscitation or not, as long as there is sufficient cardiac output and skin blood flow for the oximeter to detect a pulse. It is recommended that oximetry be used when resuscitation can be anticipated,[2] when positive pressure is administered for more than a few breaths, when cyanosis is persistent, or when supplementary oxygen is administered (Class I, LOE B).

To appropriately compare oxygen saturations to similar published data, the probe should be attached to a preductal location (ie, the right upper extremity, usually the wrist or medial surface of the palm).[43] There is some evidence that attaching the probe to the baby before connecting the probe to the instrument facilitates the most rapid acquisition of signal (Class IIb, LOE C).[42]

## Administration of Supplementary Oxygen

Two meta-analyses of several randomized controlled trials comparing neonatal resuscitation initiated with room air versus 100% oxygen showed increased survival when resuscitation was initiated with air.[44,45] There are no studies in term infants comparing outcomes when resuscitations are initiated with different concentrations of oxygen other than 100% or room air. One study in preterm infants showed that initiation of resuscitation with a blend of oxygen and air resulted in less hypoxemia or hyperoxemia, as defined by the investigators, than when resuscitation was initiated with either air or 100% oxygen followed by titration with an adjustable blend of air and oxygen.[46]

In the absence of studies comparing outcomes of neonatal resuscitation initiated with other oxygen concentrations or targeted at various oxyhemoglobin saturations, it is recommended that the goal in babies being resuscitated at birth, whether born at term or preterm, should be an oxygen saturation value in the interquartile range of preductal saturations (see table in Figure) measured in healthy term babies following vaginal birth at sea level (Class IIb, LOE B). These targets may be achieved by initiating resuscitation with air or a blended oxygen and titrating the oxygen concentration to achieve an SpO$_2$ in the target range as described above using pulse oximetry (Class IIb, LOE C). If blended oxygen is not available, resuscitation should be initiated with air (Class IIb, LOE B). If the baby is bradycardic (HR <60 per minute) after 90 seconds of resuscitation with a lower concentration of oxygen, oxygen concentration should be increased to 100% until recovery of a normal heart rate (Class IIb, LOE B).

## Positive-Pressure Ventilation (PPV)

If the infant remains apneic or gasping, or if the heart rate remains <100 per minute after administering the initial steps, start PPV.

## Initial Breaths and Assisted Ventilation

Initial inflations following birth, either spontaneous or assisted, create a functional residual capacity (FRC).[47–50] The optimal pressure, inflation time, and flow rate required to establish an effective FRC when PPV is administered during resuscitation have not been determined. Evidence from animal studies indicates that preterm lungs are easily injured by large-volume inflations immediately after birth.[51,52] Assisted ventilation rates of 40 to 60 breaths per minute are commonly used, but the relative efficacy of various rates has not been investigated.

The primary measure of adequate initial ventilation is prompt improvement in heart rate.[53] Chest wall movement should be assessed if heart rate does not improve. The initial peak inflating pressures needed are variable and unpredictable and should be individualized to achieve an increase in heart rate or movement of the chest with each breath. Inflation pressure should be monitored; an initial inflation pressure of 20 cm H$_2$O may be effective, but ≥30 to 40 cm H$_2$O may be required in some term babies without spontaneous ventilation (Class IIb, LOE C).[48,50,54] If circumstances preclude the use of pressure monitoring, the minimal inflation required to achieve an increase in heart rate should be used. There is insufficient evidence to recommend an optimum inflation time. In summary, assisted ventilation should be delivered at a rate of 40 to 60 breaths per minute to promptly achieve or maintain a heart rate >100 per minute (Class IIb, LOE C).

The use of colorimetric CO$_2$ detectors during mask ventilation of small numbers of preterm infants in the intensive care unit and in the delivery room has been reported, and such detectors may help to identify airway obstruction.[55,56] However, it is unclear whether the use of CO$_2$ detectors during mask ventilation confers additional benefit above clinical assessment alone (Class IIb, LOE C).

## End-Expiratory Pressure

Many experts recommend administration of continuous positive airway pressure (CPAP) to infants who are breathing spontaneously, but with difficulty, following birth, although its use has been studied only in infants born preterm. A multicenter randomized clinical trial of newborns at 25 to 28 weeks gestation with signs of respiratory distress showed no significant difference in the outcomes of death or oxygen requirement at 36 weeks postmenstrual age between infants started on CPAP versus those intubated and placed on mechanical ventilation in the delivery room. Starting infants on CPAP reduced the rates of intubation and mechanical ventilation, surfactant use, and duration of ventilation, but increased the rate of pneumothorax.[57] Spontaneously breathing preterm infants who have respiratory distress may be supported with CPAP or with intubation and mechanical ventilation (Class IIb, LOE B). The most appropriate choice may be guided by local expertise and preferences. There is no evidence to support or refute the use of CPAP in the delivery room in the term baby with respiratory distress.

Although positive end–expiratory pressure (PEEP) has been shown to be beneficial and its use is routine during mechanical ventilation of neonates in intensive care units, there have been no studies specifically examining PEEP versus no PEEP when PPV is used during establishment of an FRC following birth. Nevertheless, PEEP is likely to be beneficial and should be used if suitable equipment is available (Class IIb, LOE C). PEEP can easily be given with a flow-inflating bag or T-piece resuscitator, but it cannot be given with a self-inflating bag unless an optional PEEP valve is used. There is, however, some evidence that such valves often deliver inconsistent end-expiratory pressures.[58,59]

## Assisted-Ventilation Devices

Effective ventilation can be achieved with either a flow-inflating or self-inflating bag or with a T-piece mechanical device designed to regulate pressure.[60-63] The pop-off valves of self-inflating bags are dependent on the flow rate of incoming gas, and pressures generated may exceed the value specified by the manufacturer. Target inflation pressures and long inspiratory times are more consistently achieved in mechanical models when T-piece devices are used rather than bags,[60,61] although the clinical implications of these findings are not clear (Class IIb, LOE C). It is likely that inflation pressures will need to change as compliance improves following birth, but the relationship of pressures to delivered volume and the optimal volume to deliver with each breath as FRC is being established have not been studied. Resuscitators are insensitive to changes in lung compliance, regardless of the device being used (Class IIb, LOE C).[64]

### Laryngeal Mask Airways

Laryngeal mask airways that fit over the laryngeal inlet have been shown to be effective for ventilating newborns weighing more than 2000 g or delivered $\geq$34 weeks gestation (Class IIb, LOE B[65-67]). There are limited data on the use of these devices in small preterm infants, ie, < 2000 g or <34 weeks (Class IIb, LOE C[65-67]). A laryngeal mask should be considered during resuscitation if facemask ventilation is unsuccessful and tracheal intubation is unsuccessful or not feasible (Class IIa, LOE B). The laryngeal mask has not been evaluated in cases of meconium-stained fluid, during chest compressions, or for administration of emergency intratracheal medications.

### Endotracheal Tube Placement

Endotracheal intubation may be indicated at several points during neonatal resuscitation:

- Initial endotracheal suctioning of nonvigorous meconium-stained newborns
- If bag-mask ventilation is ineffective or prolonged
- When chest compressions are performed
- For special resuscitation circumstances, such as congenital diaphragmatic hernia or extremely low birth weight

The timing of endotracheal intubation may also depend on the skill and experience of the available providers.

After endotracheal intubation and administration of intermittent positive pressure, a prompt increase in heart rate is the best indicator that the tube is in the tracheobronchial tree and providing effective ventilation.[53] Exhaled $CO_2$ detection is effective for confirmation of endotracheal tube placement in infants, including very low-birth-weight infants (Class IIa, LOE B[68-71]). A positive test result (detection of exhaled $CO_2$) in patients with adequate cardiac output confirms placement of the endotracheal tube within the trachea, whereas a negative test result (ie, no $CO_2$ detected) strongly suggests esophageal intubation.[68-72] Exhaled $CO_2$ detection is the recommended method of confirmation of endotracheal tube placement (Class IIa, LOE B). However, it should be noted that poor or absent pulmonary blood flow may give false-negative results (ie, no $CO_2$ detected despite tube placement in the trachea). A false-negative result may thus lead to unnecessary extubation and reintubation of critically ill infants with poor cardiac output.

Other clinical indicators of correct endotracheal tube placement are condensation in the endotracheal tube, chest movement, and presence of equal breath sounds bilaterally, but these indicators have not been systematically evaluated in neonates (Class 11b, LOE C).

## Chest Compressions

Chest compressions are indicated for a heart rate that is <60 per minute despite adequate ventilation with supplementary oxygen for 30 seconds. Because ventilation is the most effective action in neonatal resuscitation and because chest compressions are likely to compete with effective ventilation, rescuers should ensure that assisted ventilation is being delivered optimally before starting chest compressions.

Compressions should be delivered on the lower third of the sternum to a depth of approximately one third of the anterior-posterior diameter of the chest (Class IIb, LOE C[73-75]). Two techniques have been described: compression with 2 thumbs with fingers encircling the chest and supporting the back (the 2 thumb–encircling hands technique) or compression with 2 fingers with a second hand supporting the back. Because the 2 thumb–encircling hands technique may generate higher peak systolic and coronary perfusion pressure than the 2-finger technique,[76-80] the 2 thumb–encircling hands technique is recommended for performing chest compressions in newly born infants (Class IIb, LOE C). The 2-finger technique may be preferable when access to the umbilicus is required during insertion of an umbilical catheter, although it is possible to administer the 2 thumb–encircling hands technique in intubated infants with the rescuer standing at the baby's head, thus permitting adequate access to the umbilicus (Class IIb, LOE C).

Compressions and ventilations should be coordinated to avoid simultaneous delivery.[81] The chest should be permitted to reexpand fully during relaxation, but the rescuer's thumbs should not leave the chest (Class IIb, LOE C). There should be a 3:1 ratio of compressions to ventilations with 90 compressions and 30 breaths to achieve approximately 120 events per minute to maximize ventilation at an achievable rate. Thus each event will be allotted approximately 1/2 second, with exhalation occurring during the first compression after each ventilation (Class IIb, LOE C).

There is evidence from animals and non-neonatal studies that sustained compressions or a compression ratio of 15:2 or even 30:2 may be more effective when the arrest is of primary cardiac etiology. One study in children suggests that CPR with rescue breathing is preferable to chest compressions alone when the arrest is of noncardiac etiology.[82] It is recommended that a 3:1 compression to ventilation ratio be used for neonatal resuscitation where compromise of ventilation is nearly always the primary cause, but rescuers should consider using higher ratios (eg, 15:2) if the arrest is believed to be of cardiac origin (Class IIb, LOE C).

Respirations, heart rate, and oxygenation should be reassessed periodically, and coordinated chest compressions and ventilations should continue until the spontaneous heart rate is ≥60 per minute (Class IIb, LOE C). However, frequent interruptions of compressions should be avoided, as they will compromise artificial maintenance of systemic perfusion and maintenance of coronary blood flow (Class IIb, LOE C).

## Medications

Drugs are rarely indicated in resuscitation of the newly born infant. Bradycardia in the newborn infant is usually the result of inadequate lung inflation or profound hypoxemia, and establishing adequate ventilation is the most important step toward correcting it. However, if the heart rate remains <60 per minute despite adequate ventilation (usually with endotracheal intubation) with 100% oxygen and chest compressions, administration of epinephrine or volume expansion, or both, may be indicated. Rarely, buffers, a narcotic antagonist, or vasopressors may be useful after resuscitation, but these are not recommended in the delivery room.

### Rate and Dose of Epinephrine Administration

Epinephrine is recommended to be administered intravenously (Class IIb, LOE C). Past guidelines recommended that initial doses of epinephrine be given through an endotracheal tube because the dose can be administered more quickly than when an intravenous route must be established. However, animal studies that showed a positive effect of endotracheal epinephrine used considerably higher doses than are currently recommended,[83,84] and the one animal study that used currently recommended doses via endotracheal tube showed no effect.[85] Given the lack of supportive data for endotracheal epinephrine, the IV route should be used as soon as venous access is established (Class IIb, LOE C).

The recommended IV dose is 0.01 to 0.03 mg/kg per dose. Higher IV doses are not recommended because animal[86,87] and pediatric[88,89] studies show exaggerated hypertension, decreased myocardial function, and worse neurological function after administration of IV doses in the range of 0.1 mg/kg. If the endotracheal route is used, doses of 0.01 or 0.03 mg/kg will likely be ineffective. Therefore, IV administration of 0.01 to 0.03 mg/kg per dose is the preferred route. While access is being obtained,

administration of a higher dose (0.05 to 0.1 mg/kg) through the endotracheal tube may be considered, but the safety and efficacy of this practice have not been evaluated (Class IIb, LOE C). The concentration of epinephrine for either route should be 1:10,000 (0.1 mg/mL).

## Volume Expansion

Volume expansion should be considered when blood loss is known or suspected (pale skin, poor perfusion, weak pulse) and the baby's heart rate has not responded adequately to other resuscitative measures (Class IIb, LOE C).[90] An isotonic crystalloid solution or blood is recommended for volume expansion in the delivery room (Class IIb, LOE C). The recommended dose is 10 mL/kg, which may need to be repeated. When resuscitating premature infants, care should be taken to avoid giving volume expanders rapidly, because rapid infusions of large volumes have been associated with intraventricular hemorrhage (Class IIb, LOE C).

## Postresuscitation Care

Babies who require resuscitation are at risk for deterioration after their vital signs have returned to normal. Once adequate ventilation and circulation have been established, the infant should be maintained in, or transferred to an environment where close monitoring and anticipatory care can be provided.

### Naloxone

Administration of naloxone is not recommended as part of initial resuscitative efforts in the delivery room for newborns with respiratory depression. Heart rate and oxygenation should be restored by supporting ventilation.

### Glucose

Newborns with lower blood glucose levels are at increased risk for brain injury and adverse outcomes after a hypoxic-ischemic insult, although no specific glucose level associated with worse outcome has been identified.[91,92] Increased glucose levels after hypoxia or ischemia were not associated with adverse effects in a recent pediatric series[93] or in animal studies,[94] and they may be protective.[95] However, there are no randomized controlled trials that examine this question. Due to the paucity of data, no specific target glucose concentration range can be identified at present. Intravenous glucose infusion should be considered as soon as practical after resuscitation, with the goal of avoiding hypoglycemia (Class IIb, LOE C).

### Induced Therapeutic Hypothermia

Several randomized controlled multicenter trials of induced hypothermia (33.5°C to 34.5°C) of newborns ≥36 weeks gestational age, with moderate to severe hypoxic-ischemic encephalopathy as defined by strict criteria, showed that those babies who were cooled had significantly lower mortality and less neurodevelopmental disability at 18-month follow-up than babies who were not cooled.[96–98] The randomized trials produced similar results using different methods of cooling (selective head versus systemic).[96–100] It is recommended that infants born at ≥36 weeks gestation with evolving moderate to severe hypoxic-ischemic encephalopathy should be offered therapeutic hypothermia. The treatment should be implemented according to the studied protocols, which currently include commencement within 6 hours following birth, continuation for 72 hours, and slow rewarming over at least 4 hours. Therapeutic hypothermia should be administered under clearly defined protocols similar to those used in published clinical trials and in facilities with the capabilities for multidisciplinary care and longitudinal follow-up (Class IIa, LOE A). Studies suggest that there may be some associated adverse effects, such as thrombocytopenia and increased need for inotropic support.

## Guidelines for Withholding and Discontinuing Resuscitation

For neonates at the margins of viability or those with conditions which predict a high risk of mortality or morbidity, attitudes and practice vary according to region and availability of resources. Studies indicate that parents desire a larger role in decisions to initiate resuscitation and continue life support of severely compromised newborns. Opinions among neonatal providers vary widely regarding the benefits and disadvantages of aggressive therapies in such newborns.

### Withholding Resuscitation

It is possible to identify conditions associated with high mortality and poor outcome in which withholding resuscitative efforts may be considered reasonable, particularly when there has been the opportunity for parental agreement (Class IIb, LOE C[101,102]).

A consistent and coordinated approach to individual cases by the obstetric and neonatal teams and the parents is an important goal. Noninitiation of resuscitation and discontinuation of life-sustaining treatment during or after resuscitation are ethically equivalent, and clinicians should not hesitate to withdraw support when functional survival is highly unlikely.[103] The following guidelines must be interpreted according to current regional outcomes:

- When gestation, birth weight, or congenital anomalies are associated with almost certain early death and when unacceptably high morbidity is likely among the rare survivors, resuscitation is not indicated. Examples include extreme prematurity (gestational age <23 weeks or birth weight <400 g), anencephaly, and some major chromosomal abnormalities, such as trisomy 13 (Class IIb, LOE C).

- In conditions associated with a high rate of survival and acceptable morbidity, resuscitation is nearly always indicated. This will generally include babies with gestational age ≥25 weeks and those with most congenital malformations (Class IIb, LOE C).

- In conditions associated with uncertain prognosis in which survival is borderline, the morbidity rate is relatively high, and the anticipated burden to the child is high, parental desires concerning initiation of resuscitation should be supported (Class IIb, LOE C).

Assessment of morbidity and mortality risks should take into consideration available data, and may be augmented by use of published tools based on data from specific populations. Decisions should also take into account changes in medical practice that may occur over time.

Mortality and morbidity data by gestational age compiled from data collected by perinatal centers in the US and several other countries may be found on the Neonatal Resuscitation Program (NRP) website (www.aap.org/nrp). A link to a computerized tool to estimate mortality and morbidity from a population of extremely low-birth-weight babies born in a network of regional perinatal centers may be found at that site. However, unless conception occurred via in vitro fertilization, techniques used for obstetric dating are accurate to only ±3 to 4 days if applied in the first trimester and to only ±1 to 2 weeks subsequently. Estimates of fetal weight are accurate to only ±15% to 20%. Even small discrepancies of 1 or 2 weeks between estimated and actual gestational age or a 100- to 200-g difference in birth weight may have implications for survival and long-term morbidity. Also, fetal weight can be misleading if there has been intrauterine growth restriction, and outcomes may be less predictable. These uncertainties underscore the importance of not making firm commitments about withholding or providing resuscitation until you have the opportunity to examine the baby after birth.

### Discontinuing Resuscitative Efforts

In a newly born baby with no detectable heart rate, it is appropriate to consider stopping resuscitation if the heart rate remains undetectable for 10 minutes (Class IIb, LOE C[104–106]). The decision to continue resuscitation efforts beyond 10 minutes with no heart rate should take into consideration factors such as the presumed etiology of the arrest, the gestation of the baby, the presence or absence of complications, the potential role of therapeutic hypothermia, and the parents' previously expressed feelings about acceptable risk of morbidity.

## Structure of Educational Programs to Teach Neonatal Resuscitation

Studies have demonstrated that use of simulation-based learning methodologies enhances performance in both real-life clinical situations and simulated resuscitations,[107–110] although a few studies have found no differences when compared to standard or other nonsimulated training.[111,112] Also, studies examining briefings or debriefings of resuscitation team performance have generally shown improved knowledge or skills.[113–118] Interpretation of data is complicated by the heterogeneity and limitations of the studies, including a paucity of data about clinical outcomes. Based on available evidence, it is recommended that the AAP/AHA Neonatal Resuscitation Program adopt simulation, briefing, and debriefing techniques in designing an education program for the acquisition and maintenance of the skills necessary for effective neonatal resuscitation (Class IIb, LOE C).

# Disclosures

## Guidelines Part 15: Neonatal Resuscitation Writing Group Disclosures

| Writing Group Member | Employment | Research Grant | Other Research Support | Speakers' Bureau/ Honoraria | Ownership Interest | Consultant/ Advisory Board | Other |
|---|---|---|---|---|---|---|---|
| John Kattwinkel | University of Virginia–Professor of Pediatrics | None | None | None | None | None | None |
| Jeffrey M. Perlman | Weill Cornell-Professor of Pediatrics | †NIH-NIH- Improving antimicrobial prescribing practices in the NICU | None | None | None | None | None |
| Khalid Aziz | University of Alberta– Associate Professor of Pediatrics | None | None | None | None | None | None |
| Christopher Colby | Mayo Clinic–physician | None | None | None | None | None | None |
| Karen Fairchild | University of Virginia Health System–Associate Professor of Pediatrics | None | None | None | None | None | None |
| John Gallagher | Univ. Hosp of Cleveland-Crit Care Coordinator of Ped.Resp Care | None | None | None | None | None | None |
| Mary Fran Hazinski | Vanderbilt University School of Nursing—Professor; AHA ECC Product Development-Senior Science Editor †Significant AHA compensation to write, edit and review documents such as the 2010 AHA Guidelines for CPR and ECC. | None | None | None | None | None | None |
| Louis P. Halamek | Stanford University–Associate Professor | †Laerdal Foundation: The Laerdal Foundation (not company) provided a grant to the Center for Advanced Pediatric and Perinatal Education at Packard Children's Hospital at Stanford during the academic years 2006–07, 2007–08, 2008–09; I develop simulation-based training programs and conduct research at CAPE. This support was provided directly to my institution. | None | *I have received < 10 honoraria in amounts of $500 or less from speaking at various academic meetings in the past 24 months; none of these meetings were conducted by for-profit entities. | None | *Laerdal Medical Advanced Medical Simulation Both of these companies reimburse me directly. | *I provide medical consultation to the legal profession for which I am reimbursed directly. |
| Praveen Kumar | PEDIATRIC FACULTY FOUNDATION- ATTENDING NEONATOLOGIST | None | None | None | None | None | None |
| George Little | Dartmouth College- Ped. Professor; Dartmouth Hitchcock Medfont. Center Neonatologist | None | None | None | None | None | None |
| Jane E. McGowan | St Christopher's Pediatric Associate/ Tenet Healthcare–Attending neonatologist; medical director, NICU | None | None | None | None | None | * reviewed records of cases involving neonatal resuscitation on one or two occasions over the past 5 years. *As co-editor for Textbook of Neonatal Resuscitation 6th edition, to be published by the AAP, being paid a total of $4000 over 3 years by the AAP. |
| Barbara Nightengale | Univ.Health Assoc,Nurse Practitioner | None | None | None | None | None | None |
| Mildred M. Ramirez | Univ of Texas Med School Houston-Physician | None | None | *Signed as consultant for Cytokine Pharmasciences, Inc., for a lecture in Mexico City. Product Propress for cervical rippening. $2,000 Money to Univ. | None | None | *Expert for Current expert case of triplets and preterm delivery. Money to the university &lquote;09 |
| Steven Ringer | Brigham and Women's Hospital–Chief, Newborn Medicine | None | None | *Vermont Oxford Neonatal Network, $1000, comes to me | None | *Alere $2000, consultation Dey Pharamaceutical $1000 Consultation Forrest Pharmaceuticals $1500 Grant Review Committee | †Several Attorneys, serving as expert witness in Medical malpractice cases |
| Wendy M. Simon | American Academy of Pediatrics–Director, Life Support Programs | None | None | None | None | None | None |
| Gary M. Weiner | St. Joseph Mercy Hospital-Ann Arbor Michigan–Attending Neonatologist | None | †Received equipment on-loan (3 resuscitation mannequins, 2 sets of video recording equipment) from Laerdal Medical Corporation to be used to complete a research project evaluating educational methods for teaching neonatal resuscitation. The value of the on-loan equipment is approximately $35,000. | None | None | None | None |

(Continued)

**Guidelines Part 15: Neonatal Resuscitation Writing Group Disclosures, *Continued***

| Writing Group Member | Employment | Research Grant | Other Research Support | Speakers' Bureau/ Honoraria | Ownership Interest | Consultant/ Advisory Board | Other |
|---|---|---|---|---|---|---|---|
| Myra Wyckoff | UT Southwestern Medical Center–Associate Professor of Pediatrics | †American Academy of Pediatrics Neonatal Research Grant-Ergonomics of Neonatal CPR 2008–2009 | †Received a SimNewB neonatal simulator for help in Beta testing prior to final production | *Speaker at Symposia on Neonatal Care from University of Miami-honoraria paid to me Speaker at Symposia on Neonatal Care from Columbia/Cornell-honoraria paid directly to me Speaker for Grand Rounds from University of Oklahoma-honoraria paid directly to me | None | None | None |
| Jeanette Zaichkin | Seattle Children's Hospital–Neonatal Outreach Coordinator | None | None | *I receive honoraria directly to me from the AAP as compensation for editorial activities for NRP instructor ms. | None | None | None |

This table represents the relationships of writing group members that may be perceived as actual or reasonably perceived conflicts of interest as reported on the Disclosure Questionnaire, which all members of the writing group are required to complete and submit. A relationship is considered to be "significant" if (a) the person receives $10 000 or more during any 12-month period, or 5% or more of the person's gross income; or (b) the person owns 5% or more of the voting stock or share of the entity, or owns $10 000 or more of the fair market value of the entity. A relationship is considered to be "modest" if it is less than "significant" under the preceding definition.

*Modest.

†Significant.

# References

1. 2010 International Consensus on Cardiopulmonary Resuscitation and Emergency Cardiovascular Care Science with Treatment Recommendations. *Circulation.* In Press.
2. Perlman JM, Risser R. Cardiopulmonary resuscitation in the delivery room: associated clinical events. *Arch Pediatr Adolesc Med.* 1995;149:20–25.
3. Barber CA, Wyckoff MH. Use and efficacy of endotracheal versus intravenous epinephrine during neonatal cardiopulmonary resuscitation in the delivery room. *Pediatrics.* 2006;118:1028–1034.
4. Owen CJ, Wyllie JP. Determination of heart rate in the baby at birth. *Resuscitation.* 2004;60:213–217.
5. Kamlin CO, Dawson JA, O'Donnell CP, Morley CJ, Donath SM, Sekhon J, Davis PG. Accuracy of pulse oximetry measurement of heart rate of newborn infants in the delivery room. *J Pediatr.* 2008;152:756–760.
6. Am Academy of Pediatrics, Am College of Obstetricians and Gynecologists. In: Lockwood C, Lemons J, eds. *Guidelines for Perinatal Care.* 6th ed. Elk Grove Village, IL: Am Academy of Pediatrics;2007:205.
7. Annibale DJ, Hulsey TC, Wagner CL, Southgate WM. Comparative neonatal morbidity of abdominal and vaginal deliveries after uncomplicated pregnancies. *Arch Pediatr Adolesc Med.* 1995;149:862–867.
8. Atherton N, Parsons SJ, Mansfield P. Attendance of paediatricians at elective Caesarean sections performed under regional anaesthesia: is it warranted? *J Paediatr Child Health.* 2006;42:332–336.
9. Gordon A, McKechnie EJ, Jeffery H. Pediatric presence at cesarean section: justified or not? *Am J Obstet Gynecol.* 2005;193(3 Pt 1):599–605.
10. Parsons SJ, Sonneveld S, Nolan T. Is a paediatrician needed at all Caesarean sections? *J Paediatr Child Health.* 1998;34:241–244.
11. Kattwinkel J, ed. *Textbook of Neonatal Resuscitation.* 6th ed. Elk Grove Village: Am Academy of Pediatrics; In Press.
12. Cramer K, Wiebe N, Hartling L, Crumley E, Vohra S. Heat loss prevention: a systematic review of occlusive skin wrap for premature neonates. *J Perinatol.* 2005;25:763–769.
13. Kent AL, Williams J. Increasing ambient operating theatre temperature and wrapping in polyethylene improves admission temperature in premature infants. *J Paediatr Child Health.* 2008;44:325–331.
14. Vohra S, Frent G, Campbell V, Abbott M, Whyte R. Effect of polyethylene occlusive skin wrapping on heat loss in very low birth weight infants at delivery: a randomized trial. *J Pediatr.* 1999;134:547–551.
15. Vohra S, Roberts RS, Zhang B, Janes M, Schmidt B. Heat Loss Prevention (HeLP) in the delivery room: A randomized controlled trial of polyethylene occlusive skin wrapping in very preterm infants. *J Pediatr.* 2004;145:750–753.
16. Singh A, Duckett J, Newton T, Watkinson M. Improving neonatal unit admission temperatures in preterm babies: exothermic mattresses, polythene bags or a traditional approach? *J Perinatol.* 2010;30:45–49.
17. Meyer MP, Bold GT. Admission temperatures following radiant warmer or incubator transport for preterm infants <28 weeks: a randomised study. *Arch Dis Child Fetal Neonatal Ed.* 2007;92:F295–F297.
18. Petrova A, Demissie K, Rhoads GG, Smulian JC, Marcella S, Ananth CV. Association of maternal fever during labor with neonatal and infant morbidity and mortality. *Obstet Gynecol.* 2001;98:20–27.
19. Lieberman E, Lang J, Richardson DK, Frigoletto FD, Heffner LJ, Cohen A. Intrapartum maternal fever and neonatal outcome. *Pediatrics.* 2000;105(1 Pt 1):8–13.
20. Coimbra C, Boris-Moller F, Drake M, Wieloch T. Diminished neuronal damage in the rat brain by late treatment with the antipyretic drug dipyrone or cooling following cerebral ischemia. *Acta Neuropathol.* 1996;92:447–453.
21. Gungor S, Kurt E, Teksoz E, Goktolga U, Ceyhan T, Baser I. Oronasopharyngeal suction versus no suction in normal and term infants delivered by elective cesarean section: a prospective randomized controlled trial. *Gynecol Obstet Invest.* 2006;61:9–14.
22. Waltman PA, Brewer JM, Rogers BP, May WL. Building evidence for practice: a pilot study of newborn bulb suctioning at birth. *J Midwifery Womens Health.* 2004;49:32–38.
23. Perlman JM, Volpe JJ. Suctioning in the preterm infant: effects on cerebral blood flow velocity, intracranial pressure, and arterial blood pressure. *Pediatrics.* 1983;72:329–334.
24. Simbruner G, Coradello H, Fodor M, Havelec L, Lubec G, Pollak A. Effect of tracheal suction on oxygenation, circulation, and lung mechanics in newborn infants. *Arch Dis Child.* 1981;56:326–330.
25. Prendiville A, Thomson A, Silverman M. Effect of tracheobronchial suction on respiratory resistance in intubated preterm babies. *Arch Dis Child.* 1986;61:1178–1183.
26. Vain NE, Szyld EG, Prudent LM, Wiswell TE, Aguilar AM, Vivas NI. Oropharyngeal and nasopharyngeal suctioning of meconium-stained neonates before delivery of their shoulders: multicentre, randomised controlled trial. *Lancet.* 2004;364:597–602.
27. Wiswell TE, Gannon CM, Jacob J, Goldsmith L, Szyld E, Weiss K, Schutzman D, Cleary GM, Filipov P, Kurlat I, Caballero CL, Abassi S, Sprague D, Oltorf C, Padula M. Delivery room management of the apparently vigorous meconium-stained neonate: results of the multicenter, international collaborative trial. *Pediatrics.* 2000;105(1 Pt 1):1–7.
28. Rossi EM, Philipson EH, Williams TG, Kalhan SC. Meconium aspiration syndrome: intrapartum and neonatal attributes. *Am J Obstet Gynecol.* 1989;161:1106–1110.
29. Usta IM, Mercer BM, Sibai BM. Risk factors for meconium aspiration syndrome. *Obstet Gynecol.* 1995;86:230–234.
30. Gupta V, Bhatia BD, Mishra OP. Meconium stained amniotic fluid: antenatal, intrapartum and neonatal attributes. *Indian Pediatr.* 1996;33:293–297.
31. Al Takroni AM, Parvathi CK, Mendis KB, Hassan S, Reddy I, Kudair HA. Selective tracheal suctioning to prevent meconium aspiration syndrome. *Int J Gynaecol Obstet.* 1998;63:259–263.
32. Carson BS, Losey RW, Bowes WA, Jr, Simmons MA. Combined obstetric and pediatric approach to prevent meconium aspiration syndrome. *Am J Obstet Gynecol.* 1976;126:712–715.

33. Ting P, Brady JP. Tracheal suction in meconium aspiration. *Am J Obstet Gynecol*. 1975;122:767–771.

34. Gregory GA, Gooding CA, Phibbs RH, Tooley WH. Meconium aspiration in infants–a prospective study. *J Pediatr*. 1974;85:848–852.

35. Toth B, Becker A, Seelbach-Gobel B. Oxygen saturation in healthy newborn infants immediately after birth measured by pulse oximetry. *Arch Gynecol Obstet*. 2002;266:105–107.

36. Gonzales GF, Salirrosas A. Arterial oxygen saturation in healthy newborns delivered at term in Cerro de Pasco (4340 m) and Lima (150 m). *Reprod Biol Endocrinol*. 2005;3:46.

37. Altuncu E, Ozek E, Bilgen H, Topuzoglu A, Kavuncuoglu S. Percentiles of oxygen saturations in healthy term newborns in the first minutes of life. *Eur J Pediatr*. 2008;167:687–688.

38. Kamlin CO, O'Donnell CP, Davis PG, Morley CJ. Oxygen saturation in healthy infants immediately after birth. *J Pediatr*. 2006;148:585–589.

39. Mariani G, Dik PB, Ezquer A, Aguirre A, Esteban ML, Perez C, Fernandez Jonusas S, Fustinana C. Pre-ductal and post-ductal O2 saturation in healthy term neonates after birth. *J Pediatr*. 2007;150:418–421.

40. Rabi Y, Yee W, Chen SY, Singhal N. Oxygen saturation trends immediately after birth. *J Pediatr*. 2006;148:590–594.

41. Hay WW, Jr, Rodden DJ, Collins SM, Melara DL, Hale KA, Fashaw LM. Reliability of conventional and new pulse oximetry in neonatal patients. *J Perinatol*. 2002;22:360–366.

42. O'Donnell CP, Kamlin CO, Davis PG, Morley CJ. Feasibility of and delay in obtaining pulse oximetry during neonatal resuscitation. *J Pediatr*. 2005;147:698–699.

43. Dawson JA, Kamlin CO, Wong C, te Pas AB, O'Donnell CP, Donath SM, Davis PG, Morley CJ. Oxygen saturation and heart rate during delivery room resuscitation of infants <30 weeks' gestation with air or 100% oxygen. *Arch Dis Child Fetal Neonatal Ed*. 2009;94:F87–F91.

44. Davis PG, Tan A, O'Donnell CP, Schulze A. Resuscitation of newborn infants with 100% oxygen or air: a systematic review and meta-analysis. *Lancet*. 2004;364:1329–1333.

45. Rabi Y, Rabi D, Yee W. Room air resuscitation of the depressed newborn: a systematic review and meta-analysis. *Resuscitation*. 2007; 72:353–363.

46. Escrig R, Arruza L, Izquierdo I, Villar G, Saenz P, Gimeno A, Moro M, Vento M. Achievement of targeted saturation values in extremely low gestational age neonates resuscitated with low or high oxygen concentrations: a prospective, randomized trial. *Pediatrics*. 2008;121:875–881.

47. Karlberg P, Koch G. Respiratory studies in newborn infants. III. Development of mechanics of breathing during the first week of life. A longitudinal study. *Acta Paediatr*. 1962;(Suppl 135):121–129.

48. Vyas H, Milner AD, Hopkin IE, Boon AW. Physiologic responses to prolonged and slow-rise inflation in the resuscitation of the asphyxiated newborn infant. *J Pediatr*. 1981;99:635–639.

49. Vyas H, Field D, Milner AD, Hopkin IE. Determinants of the first inspiratory volume and functional residual capacity at birth. *Pediatr Pulmonol*. 1986;2:189–193.

50. Boon AW, Milner AD, Hopkin IE. Lung expansion, tidal exchange, and formation of the functional residual capacity during resuscitation of asphyxiated neonates. *J Pediatr*. 1979;95:1031–1036.

51. Hillman NH, Moss TJ, Kallapur SG, Bachurski C, Pillow JJ, Polglase GR, Nitsos I, Kramer BW, Jobe AH. Brief, large tidal volume ventilation initiates lung injury and a systemic response in fetal sheep. *Am J Respir Crit Care Med*. 2007;176:575–581.

52. Polglase GR, Hooper SB, Gill AW, Allison BJ, McLean CJ, Nitsos I, Pillow JJ, Kluckow M. Cardiovascular and pulmonary consequences of airway recruitment in preterm lambs. *J Appl Physiol*. 2009;106:1347–1355.

53. Dawes GS. Foetal and Neonatal Physiology. A Comparative Study of the Changes at Birth. Chicago: Year Book Medical Publishers, Inc; 1968.

54. Lindner W, Vossbeck S, Hummler H, Pohlandt F. Delivery room management of extremely low birth weight infants: spontaneous breathing or intubation? *Pediatrics*. 1999;103(5 Pt 1):961–967.

55. Leone TA, Lange A, Rich W, Finer NN. Disposable colorimetric carbon dioxide detector use as an indicator of a patent airway during noninvasive mask ventilation. *Pediatrics*. 2006;118:e202–204.

56. Finer NN, Rich W, Wang C, Leone T. Airway obstruction during mask ventilation of very low birth weight infants during neonatal resuscitation. *Pediatrics*. 2009;123:865–869.

57. Morley CJ, Davis PG, Doyle LW, Brion LP, Hascoet JM, Carlin JB. Nasal CPAP or intubation at birth for very preterm infants. *N Engl J Med*. 2008;358:700–708.

58. Kelm M, Proquitte H, Schmalisch G, Roehr CC. Reliability of two common PEEP-generating devices used in neonatal resuscitation. *Klin Padiatr*. 2009;221:415–418.

59. Morley CJ, Dawson JA, Stewart MJ, Hussain F, Davis PG. The effect of a PEEP valve on a Laerdal neonatal self-inflating resuscitation bag. *J Paediatr Child Health*. 46(1–2):51–56, 2010.

60. Oddie S, Wyllie J, Scally A. Use of self-inflating bags for neonatal resuscitation. *Resuscitation*. 2005;67:109–112.

61. Hussey SG, Ryan CA, Murphy BP. Comparison of three manual ventilation devices using an intubated mannequin. *Arch Dis Child Fetal Neonatal Ed*. 2004;89:F490–493.

62. Finer NN, Rich W, Craft A, Henderson C. Comparison of methods of bag and mask ventilation for neonatal resuscitation. *Resuscitation*. 2001; 49:299–305.

63. Bennett S, Finer NN, Rich W, Vaucher Y. A comparison of three neonatal resuscitation devices. *Resuscitation*. 2005;67:113–118.

64. Kattwinkel J, Stewart C, Walsh B, Gurka M, Paget-Brown A. Responding to compliance changes in a lung model during manual ventilation: perhaps volume, rather than pressure, should be displayed. *Pediatrics*. 2009;123:e465–470.

65. Trevisanuto D, Micaglio M, Pitton M, Magarotto M, Piva D, Zanardo V. Laryngeal mask airway: is the management of neonates requiring positive pressure ventilation at birth changing? *Resuscitation*. 2004;62:151–157.

66. Gandini D, Brimacombe JR. Neonatal resuscitation with the laryngeal mask airway in normal and low birth weight infants. *Anesth Analg*. 1999;89:642–643.

67. Esmail N, Saleh M, et al. Laryngeal mask airway versus endotracheal intubation for Apgar score improvement in neonatal resuscitation. *Egyptian Journal of Anesthesiology*. 2002;18:115–121.

68. Hosono S, Inami I, Fujita H, Minato M, Takahashi S, Mugishima H. A role of end-tidal CO monitoring for assessment of tracheal intubations in very low birth weight infants during neonatal resuscitation at birth. *J Perinat Med*. 2009;37:79–84.

69. Repetto JE, Donohue P-CP, Baker SF, Kelly L, Nogee LM. Use of capnography in the delivery room for assessment of endotracheal tube placement. *J Perinatol*. 2001;21:284–287.

70. Roberts WA, Maniscalco WM, Cohen AR, Litman RS, Chhibber A. The use of capnography for recognition of esophageal intubation in the neonatal intensive care unit. *Pediatr Pulmonol*. 1995;19:262–268.

71. Aziz HF, Martin JB, Moore JJ. The pediatric disposable end-tidal carbon dioxide detector role in endotracheal intubation in newborns. *J Perinatol*. 1999;19:110–113.

72. Garey DM, Ward R, Rich W, Heldt G, Leone T, Finer NN. Tidal volume threshold for colorimetric carbon dioxide detectors available for use in neonates. *Pediatrics*. 2008;121:e1524–1527.

73. Orlowski JP. Optimum position for external cardiac compression in infants and young children. *Ann Emerg Med*. 1986;15:667–673.

74. Phillips GW, Zideman DA. Relation of infant heart to sternum: its significance in cardiopulmonary resuscitation. *Lancet*. 1986;1:1024–1025.

75. Braga MS, Dominguez TE, Pollock AN, Niles D, Meyer A, Myklebust H, Nysaether J, Nadkarni V. Estimation of optimal CPR chest compression depth in children by using computer tomography. *Pediatrics*. 2009;124:e69–e74.

76. Menegazzi JJ, Auble TE, Nicklas KA, Hosack GM, Rack L, Goode JS. Two-thumb versus two-finger chest compression during CRP in a swine infant model of cardiac arrest. *Ann Emerg Med*. 1993;22:240–243.

77. Houri PK, Frank LR, Menegazzi JJ, Taylor R. A randomized, controlled trial of two-thumb vs two-finger chest compression in a swine infant model of cardiac arrest. *Prehosp Emerg Care*. 1997;1:65–67.

78. Udassi JP, Udassi S, Theriaque DW, Shuster JJ, Zaritsky AL, Haque IU. Effect of alternative chest compression techniques in infant and child on rescuer performance. *Pediatr Crit Care Med*. 2009;10:328–333.

79. David R. Closed chest cardiac massage in the newborn infant. *Pediatrics*. 1988;81:552–554.

80. Thaler MM, Stobie GH. An improved technique of external caridac compression in infants and young children. *N Engl J Med*. 1963;269: 606–610.

81. Berkowitz ID, Chantarojanasiri T, Koehler RC, Schleien CL, Dean JM, Michael JR, Rogers MC, Traystman RJ. Blood flow during cardiopulmonary resuscitation with simultaneous compression and ventilation in infant pigs. *Pediatr Res*. 1989;26:558–564.

82. Kitamura T, Iwami T, Kawamura T, Nagao K, Tanaka H, Nadkarni VM, Berg RA, Hiraide A. Conventional and chest-compression-only cardiopulmonary resuscitation by bystanders for children who have out-of-

hospital cardiac arrests: a prospective, nationwide, population-based cohort study. *Lancet.* 2010;375:1347–1354.

83. Mielke LL, Frank C, Lanzinger MJ, Wilhelm MG, Entholzner EK, Hargasser SR, Hipp RF. Plasma catecholamine levels following tracheal and intravenous epinephrine administration in swine. *Resuscitation.* 1998;36:187–192.

84. Roberts JR, Greenberg MI, Knaub MA, Kendrick ZV, Baskin SI. Blood levels following intravenous and endotracheal epinephrine administration. *JACEP.* 1979;8:53–56.

85. Hornchen U, Schuttler J, Stoeckel H, Eichelkraut W, Hahn N. Endo-bronchial instillation of epinephrine during cardiopulmonary resuscitation. *Crit Care Med.* 1987;15:1037–1039.

86. Berg RA, Otto CW, Kern KB, Hilwig RW, Sanders AB, Henry CP, Ewy GA. A randomized, blinded trial of high-dose epinephrine versus standard-dose epinephrine in a swine model of pediatric asphyxial cardiac arrest. *Crit Care Med.* 1996;24:1695–1700.

87. Burchfield DJ, Preziosi MP, Lucas VW, Fan J. Effects of graded doses of epinephrine during asphyxia-induced bradycardia in newborn lambs. *Resuscitation.* 1993;25:235–244.

88. Perondi MB, Reis AG, Paiva EF, Nadkarni VM, Berg RA. A comparison of high-dose and standard-dose epinephrine in children with cardiac arrest. *N Engl J Med.* 2004;350:1722–1730.

89. Patterson MD, Boenning DA, Klein BL, Fuchs S, Smith KM, Hegenbarth MA, Carlson DW, Krug SE, Harris EM. The use of high-dose epinephrine for patients with out-of-hospital cardiopulmonary arrest refractory to pre-hospital interventions. *Pediatr Emerg Care.* 2005;21:227–237.

90. Wyckoff MH, Perlman JM, Laptook AR. Use of volume expansion during delivery room resuscitation in near-term and term infants. *Pediatrics.* 2005;115:950–955.

91. Salhab WA, Wyckoff MH, Laptook AR, Perlman JM. Initial hypoglycemia and neonatal brain injury in term infants with severe fetal acidemia. *Pediatrics.* 2004;114:361–366.

92. Ondoa-Onama C, Tumwine JK. Immediate outcome of babies with low Apgar score in Mulago Hospital, Uganda. *East Afr Med J.* 2003;80:22–29.

93. Klein GW, Hojsak JM, Schmeidler J, Rapaport R. Hyperglycemia and outcome in the pediatric intensive care unit. *J Pediatr.* 2008;153:379–384.

94. LeBlanc MH, Huang M, Patel D, Smith EE, Devidas M. Glucose given after hypoxic ischemia does not affect brain injury in piglets. *Stroke.* 25:1443–1447, 1994; discussion 1448.

95. Hattori H, Wasterlain CG. Posthypoxic glucose supplement reduces hypoxic-ischemic brain damage in the neonatal rat. *Ann Neurol.* 1990; 28:122–128.

96. Gluckman PD, Wyatt JS, Azzopardi D, Ballard R, Edwards AD, Ferriero DM, Polin RA, Robertson CM, Thoresen M, Whitelaw A, Gunn AJ. Selective head cooling with mild systemic hypothermia after neonatal encephalopathy: multicentre randomised trial. *Lancet.* 2005;365:663–670.

97. Shankaran S, Laptook AR, Ehrenkranz RA, Tyson JE, McDonald SA, Donovan EF, Fanaroff AA, Poole WK, Wright LL, Higgins RD, Finer NN, Carlo WA, Duara S, Oh W, Cotten CM, Stevenson DK, Stoll BJ, Lemons JA, Guillet R, Jobe AH. Whole-body hypothermia for neonates with hypoxic-ischemic encephalopathy. *N Engl J Med.* 2005;353:1574–1584.

98. Azzopardi DV, Strohm B, Edwards AD, Dyet L, Halliday HL, Juszczak E, Kapellou O, Levene M, Marlow N, Porter E, Thoresen M, Whitelaw A, Brocklehurst P. Moderate hypothermia to treat perinatal asphyxial encephalopathy. *N Engl J Med.* 2009;361:1349–1358.

99. Eicher DJ, Wagner CL, Katikaneni LP, Hulsey TC, Bass WT, Kaufman DA, Horgan MJ, Languani S, Bhatia JJ, Givelichian LM, Sankaran K, Yager JY. Moderate hypothermia in neonatal encephalopathy: safety outcomes. *Pediatr Neurol.* 2005;32:18–24.

100. Lin ZL, Yu HM, Lin J, Chen SQ, Liang ZQ, Zhang ZY. Mild hypothermia via selective head cooling as neuroprotective therapy in term neonates with perinatal asphyxia: an experience from a single neonatal intensive care unit. *J Perinatol.* 2006;26:180–184.

101. Field DJ, Dorling JS, Manktelow BN, Draper ES. Survival of extremely premature babies in a geographically defined population: prospective cohort study of 1994–9 compared with 2000–5. *BMJ.* 2008;336: 1221–1223.

102. Tyson JE, Parikh NA, Langer J, Green C, Higgins RD. Intensive care for extreme prematurity–moving beyond gestational age. *N Engl J Med.* 2008;358:1672–1681.

103. Paris JJ. What standards apply to resuscitation at the borderline of gestational age? *J Perinatol.* 2005;25:683–684.

104. Jain L, Ferre C, Vidyasagar D, Nath S, Sheftel D. Cardiopulmonary resuscitation of apparently stillborn infants: survival and long-term outcome. *J Pediatr.* 1991;118:778–782.

105. Casalaz DM, Marlow N, Speidel BD. Outcome of resuscitation following unexpected apparent stillbirth. *Arch Dis Child Fetal Neonatal Ed.* 1998;78:F112–F115.

106. Laptook AR, Shankaran S, Ambalavanan N, Carlo WA, McDonald SA, Higgins RD, Das A. Outcome of term infants using apgar scores at 10 minutes following hypoxic-ischemic encephalopathy. *Pediatrics.* 2009; 124:1619–1626.

107. Knudson MM, Khaw L, Bullard MK, Dicker R, Cohen MJ, Staudenmayer K, Sadjadi J, Howard S, Gaba D, Krummel T. Trauma training in simulation: translating skills from SIM time to real time. *J Trauma.* 64:255–263, 2008; discussion 263–254.

108. Wayne DB, Didwania A, Feinglass J, Fudala MJ, Barsuk JH, McGaghie WC. Simulation-based education improves quality of care during cardiac arrest team responses at an academic teaching hospital: a case-control study. *Chest.* 2008;133:56–61.

109. Kory PD, Eisen LA, Adachi M, Ribaudo VA, Rosenthal ME, Mayo PH. Initial airway management skills of senior residents: simulation training compared with traditional training. *Chest.* 2007;132:1927–1931.

110. Schwid HA, Rooke GA, Michalowski P, Ross BK. Screen-based anesthesia simulation with debriefing improves performance in a mannequin-based anesthesia simulator. *Teach Learn Med.* 2001;13:92–96.

111. Shapiro MJ, Morey JC, Small SD, Langford V, Kaylor CJ, Jagminas L, Suner S, Salisbury ML, Simon R, Jay GD. Simulation based teamwork training for emergency department staff: does it improve clinical team performance when added to an existing didactic teamwork curriculum? *Qual Saf Health Care.* 2004;13:417–421.

112. Cherry RA, Williams J, George J, Ali J. The effectiveness of a human patient simulator in the ATLS shock skills station. *J Surg Res.* 2007; 139:229–235.

113. Savoldelli GL, Naik VN, Park J, Joo HS, Chow R, Hamstra SJ. Value of debriefing during simulated crisis management: oral versus video-assisted oral feedback. *Anesthesiology.* 2006;105:279–285.

114. Edelson DP, Litzinger B, Arora V, Walsh D, Kim S, Lauderdale DS, Vanden Hoek TL, Becker LB, Abella BS. Improving in-hospital cardiac arrest process and outcomes with performance debriefing. *Arch Intern Med.* 2008;168:1063–1069.

115. DeVita MA, Schaefer J, Lutz J, Wang H, Dongilli T. Improving medical emergency team (MET) performance using a novel curriculum and a computerized human patient simulator. *Qual Saf Health Care.* 2005;14: 326–331.

116. Wayne DB, Butter J, Siddall VJ, Fudala MJ, Linquist LA, Feinglass J, Wade LD, McGaghie WC. Simulation-based training of internal medicine residents in advanced cardiac life support protocols: a randomized trial. *Teach Learn Med.* 2005;17:210–216.

117. Clay AS, Que L, Petrusa ER, Sebastian M, Govert J. Debriefing in the intensive care unit: a feedback tool to facilitate bedside teaching. *Crit Care Med.* 2007;35:738–754.

118. Blum RH, Raemer DB, Carroll JS, Dufresne RL, Cooper JB. A method for measuring the effectiveness of simulation-based team training for improving communication skills. *Anesth Analg.* 2005;100:1375–1380,.

KEY WORDS: cardiopulmonary resuscitation

# Part 16: Education, Implementation, and Teams
## 2010 American Heart Association Guidelines for Cardiopulmonary Resuscitation and Emergency Cardiovascular Care

Farhan Bhanji, Chair; Mary E. Mancini; Elizabeth Sinz; David L. Rodgers; Mary Ann McNeil; Theresa A. Hoadley; Reylon A. Meeks; Melinda Fiedor Hamilton; Peter A. Meaney; Elizabeth A. Hunt; Vinay M. Nadkarni; Mary Fran Hazinski

Cardiac arrest occurs in a wide variety of settings, from the unanticipated event in the out-of-hospital setting to anticipated arrests in the intensive care unit. Outcome from cardiac arrest is a function of many factors including the willingness of bystanders to perform cardiopulmonary resuscitation (CPR), the ability of rescuers to integrate knowledge and psychomotor skills, the quality of performance delivered by individual rescuers and teams, and the efficiency and effectiveness of post–cardiac arrest care.

The Chain of Survival is a metaphor used to organize and describe the integrated set of time-sensitive, coordinated actions necessary to maximize survival from cardiac arrest. The use of evidence-based education and implementation strategies can optimize the links of that chain.

Strengthening the Chain of Survival in the prehospital setting requires focus on prevention and immediate recognition of cardiac arrest, increasing the likelihood of high-quality bystander CPR and early defibrillation, and improving regional systems of care. In the hospital setting, organized efforts targeting early identification and prevention of deterioration in patients at risk can decrease the incidence of cardiac arrest. The challenge for resuscitation programs is twofold: to ensure that providers acquire and maintain the necessary knowledge, skills, and team behavior to maximize resuscitation outcome; and to assist response systems in developing, implementing, and sustaining an evidence-based Chain of Survival.

Maximizing survival from cardiac arrest requires improvement in resuscitation education and the implementation of systems that support the delivery of high-quality resuscitation and postarrest care, including mechanisms to systematically evaluate resuscitation performance. Well-designed resuscitation education can encourage the delivery of high-quality CPR. In addition continuous quality improvement processes should close the feedback loop and narrow the gap between ideal and actual performance. Community- and hospital-based resuscitation programs should systematically monitor cardiac arrests, the level of resuscitation care provided, and outcomes. The cycle of measurement, benchmarking, feedback, and change provides fundamental information necessary to optimize resuscitation care and maximize survival.

This chapter reviews key educational issues that affect the quality of resuscitation performance and describes major implementation and team-related issues shown to improve outcomes. The information is organized into four major categories: willingness to perform CPR, educational design, improving resuscitation quality, and issues related to implementation and outcomes.

While important concepts identified in the 2010 International Liaison Committee on Resuscitation (ILCOR) and American Heart Association (AHA) evidence evaluation process are applied below,[1,2] this document does not include all education, implementation, and team-related topics contained within the *2010 International Consensus on Cardiopulmonary Resuscitation and Emergency Cardiac Care Science With Treatment Recommendations.*[1,2]

## Willingness to Perform

Without immediate initiation of CPR, most victims of cardiac arrest will die. Bystander CPR can significantly improve survival rates from cardiac arrest,[3] but recent evidence indicates that only 15% to 30% of victims of out-of-hospital arrest receive CPR before EMS arrival.[4] Strategies to increase the incidence of bystander-initiated CPR and the use of automated external defibrillators (AEDs) are addressed in this section.

### Barriers to Bystander CPR

Commonly cited reasons for reluctance to perform lifesaving maneuvers include concern for injuring the victim,[5–7] fear of performing CPR incorrectly,[6,8–11] physical limitations,[12] fear of liability,[12] fear of infection,[10] or victim characteristics.[13–16] Opportunities exist to overcome many of these barriers through education and encouragement to perform when the bystander is faced with a victim in cardiac arrest.

In a study of actual bystanders interviewed following a 911 call in which the EMS dispatcher encouraged performance of CPR, nonresponders most frequently cited panic (37.5%) and

The American Heart Association requests that this document be cited as follows: Bhanji F, Mancini ME, Sinz E, Rodgers DL, McNeil MA, Hoadley TA, Meeks RA, Hamilton MF, Meaney PA, Hunt EA, Nadkarni VM, Hazinski MF. Part 16: education, implementation, and teams: 2010 American Heart Association Guidelines for Cardiopulmonary Resuscitation and Emergency Cardiovascular Care. *Circulation.* 2010;122(suppl 3):S920–S933.

(*Circulation.* 2010;122[suppl 3]:S920–S933.)

*Circulation* is available at http://circ.ahajournals.org

DOI: 10.1161/CIRCULATIONAHA.110.971135

fear of hurting the patient (9.1%) as the reasons they were unable to perform.[6] In 2 studies reviewing actual emergencies, bystanders encountered practical and understandable barriers to performance (eg, physical limitations, inability to listen to instructions and perform skills at the same time, and system delays) more often than panic or stress, although both were important factors.[17,18] Because panic can significantly impair a bystander's ability to perform in an emergency, it may be reasonable for CPR training to address the possibility of panic and encourage learners to consider how they will overcome it (Class IIb LOE C).

Actual bystanders[6] and surveys of the general public report that people more recently trained in CPR techniques expressed greater willingness to attempt resuscitation than those without recent training.[16,19–21] Short, self-directed video instruction is an effective and cost-efficient strategy for training rescuers.[22–33]

Fear of harming the victim or fear of personal injury may reduce willingness to undertake basic life support training or to perform CPR. However infection resulting from CPR performance is extremely rare and limited to a few case reports.[34–44] Educating the public about the low risks to the rescuer and victim may increase willingness to perform CPR.

Some rescuers, including healthcare providers, may be more likely to initiate CPR if they have access to barrier devices. Despite the low risk of infections, it is reasonable to teach rescuers about the use of barrier devices emphasizing that CPR should not be delayed for their use (Class IIa, LOE C).

Rescuers who are not willing to perform mouth-to-mouth ventilations may be willing to perform Hands-Only (chest compression-only) CPR.[5,9,10,13,19,21,45–47] CPR training programs should teach compression-only CPR as an alternative to conventional CPR for rescuers when they are unwilling or unable to provide conventional CPR (Class I, LOE B).

## Barriers to Recognition of Cardiac Arrest
Victims of out-of-hospital cardiac arrest who are gasping have a higher survival rate compared to victims who are not gasping.[48] Gasping is commonly misinterpreted as a sign of life that may prevent rescuers from initiating resuscitation. Potential rescuers can be taught to recognize gasping and initiate CPR.[49] Rescuers should be taught to initiate CPR if the adult victim is unresponsive and is not breathing or not breathing normally (eg, only gasping) (Class I, LOE B).

Dispatcher telephone instructions and support has been shown to increase willingness to perform CPR.[16,50,51] In order to increase bystander willingness to perform CPR, dispatchers should provide telephone CPR instructions to callers reporting an adult who is unresponsive and not breathing or not breathing normally (ie, only gasping) (Class I, LOE B).

## Physical and Psychological Concerns for Rescuers
Correct performance of chest compressions is physically demanding.[52–54] In the few reports of injuries to CPR providers, most of the injuries are musculoskeletal in nature.[55–59] Case reports have described occasional complaints of shortness of breath[60–62]; other isolated events[63,64]; hand puncture wound from a sternal wire[65]; nerve injury[66]; pneumothorax[67]; and one death due to a myocardial infarction.[68] It is reason-able that participants undertaking CPR training be advised of the vigorous physical activity required during the skills portion of the training program (Class IIa, LOE B).

CPR training and performance are positive experiences for most providers.[69] However, firsthand observation of an actual cardiac arrest and attempting resuscitation can be stressful.[17,55,56,70] Rescuers who suffer postevent adverse psychological effects may benefit from support or psychological counseling.

## Barriers to AED Use
Some rescuers may be intimidated by the idea of delivering a shock, but AEDs are safe,[71,72] and adverse events are rare.[55,73–77] Although AEDs can be used effectively with no prior training, even brief training increases the willingness of a bystander to use an AED and improves his or her performance.[78–80] To maximize willingness to use an AED, public-access defibrillation training should continue to be encouraged for the lay public (Class I, LOE B).

In summary, although the factors influencing willingness to perform CPR are myriad, many obstacles can be overcome with education. Although the precise number of trained volunteers needed to optimize the chance that a specific victim will receive CPR is not known, it is reasonable to assume that maximizing the number of people trained in a community and providing instructions and encouragement at the time an event occurs will improve the odds that a bystander will engage in resuscitation efforts.

# Education Design
Evidence-based guidelines for instruction, as well as the development of cost-effective courses, are required to improve training of providers and ultimately improve resuscitation performance and patient outcomes.

## Course Design
The appropriate application of learning theories combined with research into program effectiveness has resulted in substantial changes to the AHA Emergency Cardiovascular Care (ECC) courses over the past quarter century. Since the development of the first ECC Guidelines in 1966,[81] the AHA has established itself as a leader in resuscitation science. However, the AHA's involvement in resuscitation education and training programs predates the development of formal ECC guidelines. In 1973, the AHA first endorsed training of the lay public in CPR.[82] Subsequently, Advanced Cardiac Life Support (ACLS) was introduced in 1974,[83,84] followed by Pediatric Advanced Life Support (PALS) in 1988.[85]

In 2004 the AHA established the ECC Education Subcommittee with members including experts in curriculum and instructional design. Over time, the Education Subcommittee endorsed several educational principles as core concepts (see Table 1). Consistent with established methodologies for program evaluation,[86] the effectiveness of resuscitation courses should be evaluated (Class I, LOE C). Although participant satisfaction is important, program evaluation should extend beyond this end point and assess learners' acquisition and retention of knowledge and skills. Evidence that learners integrate what they learn into actual practice and

**Table 1.   Core AHA ECC Educational Concepts**

- Simplification - Course content should be simplified in both the presentation of the content and the breadth of content in a single course in order to facilitate accomplishment of course objectives.[22,24,25]

- Consistency - Course content and skill demonstrations should be presented in a consistent manner. Video-mediated, practice-while-watching instruction is the preferred method for basic psychomotor skill training because it reduces instructor variability and potential distractions that deviate from the intended course agenda.[22–24,27–29,33]

- Objectives-Based - Cognitive,[87] psychomotor,[88] and affective objectives[89] should be included in all courses.

- Hands-on Practice - Substantial hands-on practice is needed to meet psychomotor skill performance objectives.[22,24,26,28,33,90,91]

- Contextual - Adult learning principles[92] should be applied to all ECC courses with emphasis on creating relevant training scenarios that can be applied practically to the learners' real-world setting, such as having hospital-based learners practice CPR on a bed instead of the floor.

- Competency-based - Successful course completion should be based on the ability of the learner to demonstrate achievement of course objectives rather than attendance in a course/program for a specific time period.[27]

- Practice to Mastery - Key skills and course content should be repeated with deliberate practice[93] to build toward mastery.[94,95]

- Assessment - Evaluative strategies should assess competence and promote learning. Learning objectives[96] must be clear and measurable and serve as the basis of evaluation.

whether that ultimately improves patient outcomes would constitute more robust forms of program evaluation.

## Strategies for Basic Life Support (BLS) Courses

Studies have demonstrated that lay rescuer CPR skills can be acquired and retained at least as well (sometimes better) through interactive computer- and video-based synchronous practice instruction when compared with instructor-led courses.[22–33] Short video instruction combined with synchronous hands-on practice is an effective alternative to instructor-led basic life support courses (Class I, LOE A).

## AED Training Requirement

Manikin-based studies have demonstrated that AEDs can be correctly operated without prior training.[79,97] Allowing the use of AEDs by untrained bystanders can be beneficial and may be lifesaving (Class IIa, LOE B). Because even minimal training has been shown to improve performance in simulated cardiac arrests,[26,78–80,98] training opportunities should be made available and promoted for the lay rescuer (Class I, LOE B).

## Strategies for Advanced Life Support (ALS) Courses

Resuscitation and education literature have demonstrated that precourse preparatory strategies including computer-assisted learning tutorials,[99–104] written self-instructional materials,[105,106] video reviews,[105] preparatory courses,[107,108] textbook reading,[109] and pretests[110,111] enhance knowledge acquisition or reduce classroom time. It is reasonable to include precourse preparatory strategies in advanced life support courses (Class IIa, LOE B).

Teamwork has been reported to impact patient outcomes in a variety of clinical situations.[112–117] Teamwork and leader-ship training have been shown to improve subsequent resuscitation performance in simulation studies[118–123] and actual clinical performance.[124] As a result teamwork and leadership skills training should be included in advanced life support courses (Class I, LOE B).

## Realistic Manikins

Some manikins utilized in resuscitation training have realistic features such as the ability to replicate chest expansion and breath sounds, to provide exhaled carbon dioxide, to generate a pulse and blood pressure, and to speak or make sounds. Two studies reported that training with such manikins improved clinical performance.[125,126] Thirteen studies showed an improvement in end-of-course skills when realistic manikins were used,[49,125,127–137] while six studies showed equal performance with lower technology manikins.[138–143] Use of more realistic manikins in training may incur substantially higher financial costs.[144]

Eight studies showed equal knowledge acquisition with realistic manikins when compared with lower-technology manikins.[128,130,138,142–146] Three studies indicated that learner satisfaction was greater with realistic manikins.[130,138,142]

There is insufficient evidence to recommend for or against the routine use of more realistic manikins to improve skills performance in actual resuscitations. Realistic manikins may be useful for integrating the knowledge, skills, and behaviors in ALS training (Class IIa, LOE B). Further research is needed to confirm if such technology improves resuscitation performance in the clinical setting and to determine if it can improve survival from cardiac arrest.

## Course Delivery Formats

Course delivery formats other than the standard 2-day ACLS or PALS provider course may achieve equivalent or better knowledge or skills acquisition. These formats include interactive multimedia courses[99,147,148]; case-based presentations[149]; integration of ACLS or PALS content into a larger curriculum such as medical student or resident training[137,150,151]; noncomputer-based, self-directed learning[152]; problem-based learning[153,154]; or combination of resuscitation courses with other programs such as Advanced Trauma Life Support (ATLS).[155] It is reasonable to consider alternative course scheduling formats for advanced life support courses (eg, ACLS or PALS), provided acceptable programmatic evaluation is conducted and learners meet course objectives (Class IIa, LOE B).

## Post-Course Assessment

Studies have shown poor correlation between written tests used in resuscitation courses and clinical skills evaluations.[156–159] A written test should not be used exclusively to assess learner competence following an advanced life support course (Class I, LOE B).

Assessment used as an instructional tool at the end of resuscitation training has been shown to improve retention of skills at 2 weeks[160] and showed a trend toward improvement at six months.[161] End-of-course assessment may be useful in helping learners retain skills (Class IIb, LOE C).

## Training Intervals

Training intervals for AHA basic and advanced life support programs have traditionally been time-specific, with a maximum 2-year interval recommended. The *AHA ECC Program Administration Manual*[162] notes that the course completion card "certifies that the individual has successfully completed the objectives and skills evaluations in accordance with the curriculum of the AHA for (*course title*)."

Reflecting the emerging trends supporting continuous maintenance of competence and continuing professional development in the healthcare professions,[163,164] there is support to move away from a time-related certification standard and toward a more competency-based approach to resuscitation education.

There is substantial evidence that basic and advanced life support skills decay rapidly after initial training. Basic skills have been shown to deteriorate when assessed at 1 to 6 months[24,27,165–167] or 7 to 12 months[168,169] following training. Advanced life support providers demonstrated similar decays in knowledge or skills when assessed at 3 to 6 months,[165,170–178] 7 to 12 months,[179,180] and more than 12 months.[181] These studies were heterogeneous with respect to participant composition, course length, course format, instructor type, and frequency of participant involvement in actual resuscitations. The majority reflected teaching methodologies in use prior to the most recent AHA course design updates in 2005.

In one study a 2-hour class was sufficient for participants to acquire and retain BLS skills for an extended time period, provided a brief re-evaluation was performed after 6 months.[182] Four studies showed minimal or no deterioration of skills or knowledge at 6,[79] 12,[183,184] or 17 months[185] after course completion.

While the optimal mechanism for maintenance of competence is not known, the need to move toward more frequent assessment and reinforcement of skills is clear. Skill performance should be assessed during the 2-year certification with reinforcement provided as needed (Class I, LOE B). The optimal timing and method for this assessment and reinforcement are not known.

Further research is needed to determine if modifications to initial training will alter the decay curve of CPR skills. Additional research is also needed to determine what time interval, mechanism of assessment, and method for refresher training will minimize decay in CPR skills. Innovative concepts to reduce the decay of skills and knowledge may include continuous maintenance of competency programs that employ frequent short-duration interactions with content and skills after an initial course, or they may include guided debriefings after real-life events that focus on response improvement.

Instructors and participants should be aware that successful completion of any AHA ECC course is only the first step toward attaining and maintaining competence. AHA ECC courses should be part of a larger continuing education and continuous quality improvement process that reflects the needs and practices of individuals or systems.

## Improving Resuscitation Skills

### Checklists/Cognitive Aids

The quality of resuscitation is a major determinant of patient outcome. Simulation studies of basic life support,[186–190] advanced life support,[191,192] and anesthetic emergencies[193,194] demonstrated improved performance when checklists or cognitive aids were used. However, 1 simulation study demonstrated delayed completion of 2 cycles of CPR[195] when individuals not adept at cell phone operation used a cell phone-based cognitive aid. In clinical practice, physicians perceived checklists to be useful.[196,197] The impact of cognitive aids or checklists on patient outcomes is unknown.

Checklists or cognitive aids, such as the AHA algorithms, may be considered for use during actual resuscitation (Class IIb, LOE C). Specific checklists and cognitive aids should be evaluated to determine if they achieve the desired effect and do not result in negative consequences such as delayed response. Further research on the optimal design is warranted.

### CPR Prompt or Feedback Devices

Training in CPR skills using a feedback device improves learning and/or retention.[167,183,198–203] The use of a CPR feedback device can be effective for training (Class IIa, LOE A).

The use of feedback devices or prompts, such as metronomes, has consistently improved performance of CPR in manikin-based studies.[204–215] In clinical practice, the use of feedback devices has resulted in improved CPR performance compared to historic or concurrent nonrandomized controls.[216–220] However, two manikin-based studies demonstrated variable reliability of feedback devices depending on the support surface (eg, floor or mattress) on which CPR is performed.[221,222] CPR prompt and feedback devices can be useful as part of an overall strategy to improve the quality of CPR during actual resuscitations (Class IIa, LOE B); effect on patient survival has not been demonstrated.

### Debriefing

Debriefing is a learner-focused, nonthreatening technique to assist individual rescuers or teams to reflect on, and improve, performance.[223] In manikin-based studies, debriefing as part of the learning strategy resulted in improved performance in post-debriefing simulated scenarios,[121,203,224–226] and it improved adherence to resuscitation guidelines in clinical settings.[126] Debriefing as a technique to facilitate learning should be included in all advanced life support courses (Class I, LOE B).

Debriefing of cardiac arrest events, either in isolation[124] or as part of an organized response system,[227] improves subsequent CPR performance in-hospital and results in higher rate of return of spontaneous circulation (ROSC). Debriefing of actual resuscitation events can be a useful strategy to improve future performance (Class IIa, LOE C). Additional research on how best to teach and implement postevent debriefing is warranted.

## Implementation and Outcomes

### Systems Approach and Feedback Loop

Organized, cohesive resuscitation programs can improve survival from cardiac arrest by strengthening the links in the

**Table 2.    System Components to Prevent or Improve Survival from In-Hospital Cardiac Arrest**

System-level components to reduce the incidence of, and improving survival from, in-hospital cardiac arrest may include[231,260]:

- Systematic education on patient deterioration and its detection.
- Frequent monitoring of vital signs and assessment of at-risk hospitalized patients.
- Consistent use of predefined calling criteria or early warning scores.
- A notification system of calling for assistance.
- Rapid and effective clinical response to calls.
- Administrative support for program initiation and continuous quality improvement.

chain of survival.[228–230] In this section some of the key systems-based initiatives that may improve patient outcomes are presented.

## Rapid Response Teams (RRTs) and Medical Emergency Teams (METs)

RRTs and METs respond to patients who are deteriorating in noncritical-care settings; such teams may represent one piece of a rapid response *system* (RRS). A RRS has several components,[231] including an "afferent arm" (ie, event detection and response triggering arm); an "efferent arm" (ie, a planned response arm, such as the RRT); a quality-monitoring arm; and an administrative support arm.

Some studies have demonstrated a reduction in cardiac arrest rates for adult patients after implementation of various components of a RRS,[232–247] while others have failed to show such a difference.[248–253]

In pediatric settings the implementation of RRSs has resulted in the prevention of respiratory arrest,[254] a decreased total number of arrests,[255,256] better survival from cardiac arrest,[256–258] and reduction in hospital-wide mortality.[256,257,259] Implementation of a pediatric MET/RRT may be beneficial in facilities where children with high-risk illnesses are present on general inpatient units (Class IIa, LOE B).

Although conflicting evidence exists, expert consensus recommends the systematic identification of patients at risk of cardiac arrest, an organized response to such patients, and evaluation of outcomes to foster continuous quality improvement (Class I, LOE C). System components that are potentially important in reducing the incidence of, and improving survival from, in-hospital cardiac arrest are summarized in Table 2.

## Regional Systems of (Emergency) Cardiovascular Care

There is wide variability in survival to hospital discharge, one-month survival, and length of critical-care stay among hospitals caring for patients after resuscitation from cardiac arrest.[261–267] Hospitals with larger patient volumes (>50 ICU cardiac arrest admissions/year) had a better survival to hospital discharge than low-volume centers (<20 ICU–cardiac arrest admissions/yr) for patients treated for either in- or out-of-hospital cardiac arrest.[265]

Implementation of comprehensive packages of post–cardiac arrest care that included therapeutic hypothermia and percutaneous coronary intervention[268–270] has been shown to improve survival from cardiac arrest. Two small studies demonstrated trends toward improved survival that were not statistically significant when comprehensive packages of post–cardiac arrest care were introduced.[271,272]

Although there is no direct evidence that regional systems of care for cardiac resuscitation improve outcome, extrapolation from research in other time-sensitive conditions, such as acute coronary syndromes,[273] stroke,[274,275] and trauma,[276] suggests there may be a benefit to such a system. In 2010 the AHA published a policy statement calling for the development of regional systems of care as a strategy to reduce the variability in survival for out-of-hospital cardiac arrest.[277] It is reasonable that regional systems of care be considered as part of an overall approach to improve survival from cardiac arrest (Class IIa, LOE C).

## Resuscitation Training in Limited-Resource Communities

Many AHA instructors are involved in training in limited-resource environments in the United States and throughout the world. The vast majority of participants enjoy training and feel more comfortable after educational programs regardless of the type of training provided.[278–290]

Improvements in provider performance and patient outcomes following training in resource-limited environments are inconsistent, and important characteristics of students and training environment, as well as outcomes (cognitive, psychomotor skills, operational performance, patient outcome, and cost-effectiveness), are inconsistently measured. Resuscitation training, when appropriately adapted to the local providers' clinical environment and resources, has significantly reduced mortality in developing countries.[284,291–294] The evidence from the trauma education is most compelling, and less clear with neonatal[295,296] and adult cardiac resuscitation training programs.[297] Patient outcome studies were often limited by study design, but 1 large, multicenter trial failed to show improvement in neonatal survival after newborn resuscitation training.[298]

There is no strong evidence to support any specific instruction method as preferable for all clinical environments and training subject experience. There is anecdotal evidence that successful resuscitation training in developing countries requires local adaptation to clinical environments,[280,299–301] utilizing existing and sustainable resources for both care and training,[282,300–302] and a dedicated local infrastructure.[289,299]

## Summary

Optimizing the links in the Chain of Survival improves outcomes and saves lives. The use of evidence-based education and implementation strategies will allow organizations and communities to strengthen these links in the most effective and efficient manner.

## Acknowledgments

The writing group would like to thank the members of the Education Subcommittee of American Heart Association Emergency Cardiovascular Care for their valuable contributions in the development of this manuscript.

# Disclosures

## Guidelines Part 16: Education Implementation and Teams Writing Group Disclosures

| Writing Group Member | Employment | Research Grant | Other Research Support | Speakers' Bureau/Honoraria | Ownership Interest | Consultant/Advisory Board | Other |
|---|---|---|---|---|---|---|---|
| Farhan Bhanji | Montreal Children's Hospital, McGill University–Assistant Professor of Pediatrics | None | None | None | None | None | None |
| Mary E. Mancini | University of Texas at Arlington—Professor | None | None | *In the past two years have received honoraria from Datascope for presentations at two national teaching institutes for the American Association of Critical Care Nurses and Emergency Nursing Association–Topic = Improving The Chain of Survival. | *I am listed on a patent held by my University for a sensing device that could be used for CPR. Device has not been produced. I receive no royalties. | None | None |
| Elizabeth Sinz | Penn State Hershey Medical Center–Professor of Anesthesiology and Neurosurgery; *American Heart Association; Associate Science Editor | None | None | None | None | None | None |
| David L. Rodgers | | Clinical Educator, the Center for Simulation, Advanced Education and Innovation, Children's Hospital of Philadelphia | None | None | None | None | †Spouse (Robin Roberts) is an employee of the American Heart Association. |
| Mary Ann McNeil | University of Minnesota Medical school- Director, Department of Emergency Medicine | None | None | None | None | None | None |
| Theresa A. Hoadley | OSF St Francis College of Nursing; Assist. Professor; Proctor Hosp-TC coordinator | None | None | None | None | None | None |
| Reylon A. Meeks | Blank Children's Hosp./Pleasant Hill FD/Southwest CC, DMACC | None | None | None | None | None | None |
| Melinda Fiedor Hamilton | Children's Hospital of Pittsburgh of UPMC–Assistant Professor of CCM and Pediatrics | None | None | None | None | None | None |
| Peter A. Meaney | University of Pennsylvania, Children's Hospital of Philadelphia– Assistant Professor | *Laerdal Foundation, Research grant"Development and Validation of a Quantitative Measurement Device to Assess Technical Basic Life Support Skills in Resource Limited Settings." No direct support to investigator Operation Smile, Educational development grant, "Pilot Training Proposal: Acute Care Training for the Peri-Operative Pediatrician". No direct support to investigator | *Laerdal Corporation, Research equipment (study mankins) for "Development and Validation of a Quantitative Measurement Device to Assess Technical Basic Life Support Skills in Resource Limited Settings." No direct support to investigator | None | None | None | None |
| Elizabeth A. Hunt | Johns Hopkins University School of Medicine– Director, Johns Hopkins Medicine Simulation Center | None | None | None | None | None | None |
| Vinay M. Nadkarni | University of Pennsylvania School of Medicine, Children's Hospital of Philadelphia– Attending Physician, Anesthesia, Critical Care and Pediatrics | †AHRQ: Agency for Healthcare, Research and Quality: PI, Grant for Evaluation of Safety of Pediatric Tracheal Intubation and Just in Time Simulation Education Intervention | None | None | None | None | None |

*(Continued)*

**Guidelines Part 16: Education Implementation and Teams Writing Group Disclosures, *Continued***

| Writing Group Member | Employment | Research Grant | Other Research Support | Speakers' Bureau/Honoraria | Ownership Interest | Consultant/Advisory Board | Other |
|---|---|---|---|---|---|---|---|
| Mary Fran Hazinski | Vanderbilt Univ. School of Nursing—Professor; AHA ECC Product Development—Senior Science Editor †I receive significant compensation as a consultant and senior science editor for the AHA ECC Product Development | None | None | None | None | None | None |

This table represents the relationships of writing group members that may be perceived as actual or reasonably perceived conflicts of interest as reported on the Disclosure Questionnaire, which all members of the writing group are required to complete and submit. A relationship is considered to be "significant" if (a) the person receives $10 000 or more during any 12-month period, or 5% or more of the person's gross income; or (b) the person owns 5% or more of the voting stock or share of the entity, or owns $10 000 or more of the fair market value of the entity. A relationship is considered to be "modest" if it is less than "significant" under the preceding definition.

*Modest.

†Significant.

# References

1. Morley PT, Atkins DL, Billi JE, Bossaert L, Callaway CW, de Caen AR, Deakin CD, Eigel B, Hazinski MF, Hickey RW, Jacobs I, Kleinman ME, Koster RW, Mancini ME, Montgomery WH, Morrison LJ, Nadkarni VM, Nolan JP, O'Connor RE, Perlman JM, Sayre MR, Semenko TI, Shuster M, Soar J, Wyllie J, Zideman D. Part 3: evidence evaluation process: 2010 International Consensus on Cardiopulmonary Resuscitation and Emergency Cardiovascular Care Science With Treatment Recommendations. *Circulation.* 2010;122(suppl 2):S283–S290.

2. Hazinski MF, Nolan JP, Billi JE, Böttiger BW, Bossaert L, De Caen AR, Deakin CD, Drajer S, Eigel B, Hickey RW, Jacobs I, Kleinman ME, Kloeck W, Koster RW, Lim SH, Mancini ME, Montgomery WH, Morley PT, Morrison LJ, Nadkarni VM, O'Connor RE, Okada K, Perlman JM, Sayre MR, Shuster M, Soar J, Sunde K, Travers AH, Wyllie J, Zideman D. Part 1: executive summary: 2010 International Consensus on Cardiopulmonary Resuscitation and Emergency Cardiovascular Care Science With Treatment Recommendations. *Circulation.* 2010;122(suppl 2):S250–S275.

3. Sasson C, Rogers MA, Dahl J, Kellermann AL. Predictors of survival from out-of-hospital cardiac arrest: a systematic review and meta-analysis. *Circ Cardiovasc Qual Outcomes.* 2010;3:63–81.

4. Abella BS, Aufderheide TP, Eigel B, Hickey RW, Longstreth WT Jr, Nadkarni V, Nichol G, Sayre MR, Sommargren CE, Hazinski MF. Reducing barriers for implementation of bystander-initiated cardiopulmonary resuscitation: a scientific statement from the American Heart Association for healthcare providers, policymakers, and community leaders regarding the effectiveness of cardiopulmonary resuscitation. *Circulation.* 2008;117:704–709.

5. Hubble MW, Bachman M, Price R, Martin N, Huie D. Willingness of high school students to perform cardiopulmonary resuscitation and automated external defibrillation. *Prehosp Emerg Care.* 2003;7:219–224.

6. Swor R, Khan I, Domeier R, Honeycutt L, Chu K, Compton S. CPR training and CPR performance: do CPR-trained bystanders perform CPR? *Acad Emerg Med.* 2006;13:596–601.

7. Moser DK, Dracup K, Doering LV. Effect of cardiopulmonary resuscitation training for parents of high-risk neonates on perceived anxiety, control, and burden. *Heart Lung.* 1999;28:326–333.

8. Omi W, Taniguchi T, Kaburaki T, Okajima M, Takamura M, Noda T, Ohta K, Itoh H, Goto Y, Kaneko S, Inaba H. The attitudes of Japanese high school students toward cardiopulmonary resuscitation. *Resuscitation.* 2008;78:340–345.

9. Shibata K, Taniguchi T, Yoshida M, Yamamoto K. Obstacles to bystander cardiopulmonary resuscitation in Japan. *Resuscitation.* 2000;44:187–193.

10. Taniguchi T, Omi W, Inaba H. Attitudes toward the performance of bystander cardiopulmonary resuscitation in Japan. *Resuscitation.* 2007;75:82–87.

11. Dwyer T. Psychological factors inhibit family members' confidence to initiate CPR. *Prehosp Emerg Care.* 2008;12:157–161.

12. Coons SJ, Guy MC. Performing bystander CPR for sudden cardiac arrest: behavioral intentions among the general adult population in Arizona. *Resuscitation.* 2009;80:334–340.

13. Caves ND, Irwin MG. Attitudes to basic life support among medical students following the 2003 SARS outbreak in Hong Kong. *Resuscitation.* 2006;68:93–100.

14. Johnston TC, Clark MJ, Dingle GA, FitzGerald G. Factors influencing Queenslanders' willingness to perform bystander cardiopulmonary resuscitation. *Resuscitation.* 2003;56:67–75.

15. Boucek CD, Phrampus P, Lutz J, Dongilli T, Bircher NG. Willingness to perform mouth-to-mouth ventilation by health care providers: a survey. *Resuscitation.* 2009;80:849–853.

16. Axelsson A, Thoren A, Holmberg S, Herlitz J. Attitudes of trained Swedish lay rescuers toward CPR performance in an emergency: a survey of 1012 recently trained CPR rescuers. *Resuscitation.* 2000;44:27–36.

17. Riegel B, Mosesso VN, Birnbaum A, Bosken L, Evans LM, Feeny D, Holohan J, Jones CD, Peberdy MA, Powell J. Stress reactions and perceived difficulties of lay responders to a medical emergency. *Resuscitation.* 2006;70:98–106.

18. Lerner EB, Sayre MR, Brice JH, White LJ, Santin AJ, Billittier AJ IV, Cloud SD. Cardiac arrest patients rarely receive chest compressions before ambulance arrival despite the availability of pre-arrival CPR instructions. *Resuscitation.* 2008;77:51–56.

19. Donohoe RT, Haefeli K, Moore F. Public perceptions and experiences of myocardial infarction, cardiac arrest and CPR in London. *Resuscitation.* 2006;71:70–79.

20. Kuramoto N, Morimoto T, Kubota Y, Maeda Y, Seki S, Takada K, Hiraide A. Public perception of and willingness to perform bystander CPR in Japan. *Resuscitation.* 2008;79:475–481.

21. Jelinek GA, Gennat H, Celenza T, O'Brien D, Jacobs I, Lynch D. Community attitudes towards performing cardiopulmonary resuscitation in Western Australia. *Resuscitation.* 2001;51:239–246.

22. Lynch B, Einspruch EL, Nichol G, Becker LB, Aufderheide TP, Idris A. Effectiveness of a 30-min CPR self-instruction program for lay responders: a controlled randomized study. *Resuscitation.* 2005;67:31–43.

23. Todd KH, Braslow A, Brennan RT, Lowery DW, Cox RJ, Lipscomb LE, Kellermann AL. Randomized, controlled trial of video self-instruction versus traditional CPR training. *Ann Emerg Med.* 1998;31:364–369.

24. Einspruch EL, Lynch B, Aufderheide TP, Nichol G, Becker L. Retention of CPR skills learned in a traditional AHA Heartsaver course versus 30-min video self-training: a controlled randomized study. *Resuscitation.* 2007;74:476–486.

25. Todd KH, Heron SL, Thompson M, Dennis R, O'Connor J, Kellermann AL. Simple CPR: a randomized, controlled trial of video self-instructional cardiopulmonary resuscitation training in an African American church congregation. *Ann Emerg Med.* 1999;34:730–737.

26. Reder S, Cummings P, Quan L. Comparison of three instructional methods for teaching cardiopulmonary resuscitation and use of an automatic external defibrillator to high school students. *Resuscitation.* 2006;69:443–453.

27. Roppolo LP, Pepe PE, Campbell L, Ohman K, Kulkarni H, Miller R, Idris A, Bean L, Bettes TN, Idris AH. Prospective, randomized trial of the effectiveness and retention of 30-min layperson training for cardio-pulmonary resuscitation and automated external defibrillators: the American Airlines Study. *Resuscitation*. 2007;74:276–285.

28. Batcheller AM, Brennan RT, Braslow A, Urrutia A, Kaye W. Cardiopul-monary resuscitation performance of subjects over forty is better fol-lowing half-hour video self-instruction compared to traditional four-hour classroom training. *Resuscitation*. 2000;43:101–110.

29. Isbye DL, Rasmussen LS, Lippert FK, Rudolph SF, Ringsted CV. Laypersons may learn basic life support in 24 min using a personal resuscitation manikin. *Resuscitation*. 2006;69:435–442.

30. Moule P, Albarran JW, Bessant E, Brownfield C, Pollock J. A non-randomized comparison of e-learning and classroom delivery of basic life support with automated external defibrillator use: a pilot study. *Int J Nurs Pract*. 2008;14:427–434.

31. Liberman M, Golberg N, Mulder D, Sampalis J. Teaching cardiopul-monary resuscitation to CEGEP students in Quebec: a pilot project. *Resuscitation*. 2000;47:249–257.

32. Jones I, Handley AJ, Whitfield R, Newcombe R, Chamberlain D. A preliminary feasibility study of a short DVD-based distance-learning package for basic life support. *Resuscitation*. 2007;75:350–356.

33. Braslow A, Brennan RT, Newman MM, Bircher NG, Batcheller AM, Kaye W. CPR training without an instructor: development and eval-uation of a video self-instructional system for effective performance of cardiopulmonary resuscitation. *Resuscitation*. 1997;34:207–220.

34. Ahmad F, Senadhira DCA, Charters J, Acquilla S. Transmission of salmonella via mouth-to-mouth resuscitation. *Lancet*. 1990;335: 787–788.

35. Chalumeau M, Bidet P, Lina G, Mokhtari M, Andre MC, Gendrel D, Bingen E, Raymond J. Transmission of Panton-Valentine leukocidin-producing Staphylococcus aureus to a physician during resuscitation of a child. *Clin Infect Dis*. 2005;41:e29–e30.

36. Christian MD, Loutfy M, McDonald LC, Martinez KF, Ofner M, Wong T, Wallington T, Gold WL, Mederski B, Green K, Low DE. Possible SARS coronavirus transmission during cardiopulmonary resuscitation. *Emerg Infect Dis*. 2004;10:287–293.

37. Feldman HA. Some recollections of the meningococcal diseases: the first Harry F. Dowling lecture. *JAMA*. 1972;220:1107–1112.

38. Finkelhor RS, Lampman JH. Herpes simplex infection following car-diopulmonary resuscitation. *JAMA*. 1980;243:650.

39. Heilman KM, Muschenheim C. Primary cutaneous tuberculosis resulting from mouth-to-mouth respiration. *N Engl J Med*. 1965;273: 1035–1036.

40. Hendricks AA, Shapiro EP. Primary herpes simplex infection following mouth-to-mouth resuscitation. *JAMA*. 1980;243:257–258.

41. Todd MA, Bell JS. Shigellosis from cardiopulmonary resuscitation. *JAMA*. 1980;243:331.

42. Valenzuela TD, Hooton TM, Kaplan EL, Schlievert P. Transmission of "toxic strep" syndrome from an infected child to a firefighter during CPR. *Ann Emerg Med*. 1991;20:90–92.

43. Neiman R. Post manikin resuscitation stomatitis. *J Ky Med Assoc*. 1982;80:813–814.

44. Nicklin G. Manikin tracheitis. *JAMA*. 1980;244:2046–2047.

45. Lam KK, Lau FL, Chan WK, Wong WN. Effect of severe acute respi-ratory syndrome on bystander willingness to perform cardiopulmonary resuscitation (CPR): is compression-only preferred to standard CPR? *Prehosp Disaster Med*. 2007;22:325–329.

46. Locke CJ, Berg RA, Sanders AB, Davis MF, Milander MM, Kern KB, Ewy GA. Bystander cardiopulmonary resuscitation: concerns about mouth-to-mouth contact. *Arch Intern Med*. 1995;155:938–943.

47. Hamasu S, Morimoto T, Kuramoto N, Horiguchi M, Iwami T, Nishiyama C, Takada K, Kubota Y, Seki S, Maeda Y, Sakai Y, Hiraide A. Effects of BLS training on factors associated with attitude toward CPR in college students. *Resuscitation*. 2009;80:359–364.

48. Bobrow BJ, Zuercher M, Ewy GA, Clark L, Chikani V, Donahue D, Sanders AB, Hilwig RW, Berg RA, Kern KB. Gasping during cardiac arrest in humans is frequent and associated with improved survival. *Circulation*. 2008;118:2550–2554.

49. Perkins GD, Walker G, Christensen K, Hulme J, Monsieurs KG. Teaching recognition of agonal breathing improves accuracy of diag-nosing cardiac arrest. *Resuscitation*. 2006;70:432–437.

50. Culley LL, Clark JJ, Eisenberg MS, Larsen MP. Dispatcher-assisted telephone CPR: common delays and time standards for delivery. *Ann Emerg Med*. 1991;20:362–366.

51. Vaillancourt C, Stiell IG, Wells GA. Understanding and improving low bystander CPR rates: a systematic review of the literature. *CJEM*. 2008;10:51–65.

52. Van Hoeyweghen RJ, Verbruggen G, Rademakers F, Bossaert LL. The physiologic response of CPR training. *Ann Emerg Med*. 1991;20: 279–282.

53. Lonergan JH, Youngberg JZ, Kaplan JA. Cardiopulmonary resusci-tation: physical stress on the rescuer. *Crit Care Med*. 1981;9:793–795.

54. Tsou JY, Chi CH, Hsu RM, Wu HF, Su FC. Mechanical loading of the low back during cardiopulmonary resuscitation. *Resuscitation*. 2009;80: 1181–1186.

55. Peberdy MA, Ottingham LV, Groh WJ, Hedges J, Terndrup TE, Pirrallo RG, Mann NC, Sehra R. Adverse events associated with lay emergency response programs: the Public Access Defibrillation Trial experience. *Resuscitation*. 2006;70:59–65.

56. Hallstrom AP, Ornato JP, Weisfeldt M, Travers A, Christenson J, McBurnie MA, Zalenski R, Becker LB, Schron EB, Proschan M. Public-access defibrillation and survival after out-of-hospital cardiac arrest. *N Engl J Med*. 2004;351:637–646.

57. Cheung W, Gullick J, Thanakrishnan G, Jacobs R, Au W, Uy J, Fick M, Narayan P, Ralston S, Tan J. Injuries occurring in hospital staff attending medical emergency team (MET) calls: a prospective, obser-vational study. *Resuscitation*. 2009;80:1351–1356.

58. Jones AY. Can cardiopulmonary resuscitation injure the back? *Resuscitation*. 2004;61:63–67.

59. Jones AY, Lee RY. Cardiopulmonary resuscitation and back injury in ambulance officers. *Int Arch Occup Environ Health*. 2005;78:332–336.

60. Thierbach AR, Piepho T, Kunde M, Wolcke BB, Golecki N, Kleine-Weischede B, Werner C. Two-rescuer CPR results in hyperventilation in the ventilating rescuer. *Resuscitation*. 2005;65:185–190.

61. Thierbach AR, Wolcke BB, Krummenauer F, Kunde M, Janig C, Dick WF. Artificial ventilation for basic life support leads to hyperventilation in first aid providers. *Resuscitation*. 2003;57:269–277.

62. Walker GM, Liddle R. Prolonged two-man basic life support may result in hypocarbia in the ventilating rescuer. *Resuscitation*. 2001;50: 179–183.

63. Greenberg M. CPR: a report of observed medical complications during training. *Ann Emerg Med*. 1983;12:194–195.

64. Macauley CA, Todd CT. Physical disability among cardiopulmonary resuscitation students. *Occup Health Nurs*. 1978;26:17–19.

65. Steinhoff JP, Pattavina C, Renzi R. Puncture wound during CPR from sternotomy wires: case report and discussion of periresuscitation infection risks. *Heart Lung*. 2001;30:159–160.

66. Shimokawa A, Tateyama S, Shimizu Y, Muramatsu I, Takasaki M. Anterior interosseous nerve palsy after cardiopulmonary resuscitation in a resuscitator with undiagnosed muscle anomaly. *Anesth Analg*. 2001; 93:290–291.

67. Sullivan F, Avstreih D. Pneumothorax during CPR training: case report and review of the CPR literature. *Prehosp Disaster Med*. 2000;15: 64–69.

68. Memon AM, Salzer JE, Hillman EC Jr, Marshall CL. Fatal myocardial infarct following CPR training: the question of risk. *Ann Emerg Med*. 1982;11:322–323.

69. Axelsson A, Herlitz J, Ekstrom L, Holmberg S. Bystander-initiated cardiopulmonary resuscitation out-of-hospital: a first description of the bystanders and their experiences. *Resuscitation*. 1996;33:3–11.

70. Gamble M. A debriefing approach to dealing with the stress of CPR attempts. *Prof Nurse*. 2001;17:157–160.

71. Lyster T, Jorgenson D, Morgan C. The safe use of automated external defibrillators in a wet environment. *Prehosp Emerg Care*. 2003;7: 307–311.

72. Lloyd MS, Heeke B, Walter PF, Langberg JJ. Hands-on defibrillation: an analysis of electrical current flow through rescuers in direct contact with patients during biphasic external defibrillation. *Circulation*. 2008; 117:2510–2514.

73. Capucci A, Aschieri D, Piepoli MF. Improving survival with early defibrillation. *Cardiol Rev*. 2003;20:12–14.

74. Page RL, Joglar JA, Kowal RC, Zagrodzky JD, Nelson LL, Ramaswamy K, Barbera SJ, Hamdan MH, McKenas DK. Use of automated external defibrillators by a U.S. airline. *N Engl J Med*. 2000;343:1210–1216.

75. Jorgenson DB, Skarr T, Russell JK, Snyder DE, Uhrbrock K. AED use in businesses, public facilities and homes by minimally trained first responders. *Resuscitation*. 2003;59:225–233.

76. Hoke RS, Heinroth K, Trappe HJ, Werdan K. Is external defibrillation an electric threat for bystanders? *Resuscitation*. 2009;80:395–401.

77. Schratter A, Weihs W, Holzer M, Janata A, Behringer W, Losert UM, Ohley WJ, Schock RB, Sterz F. External cardiac defibrillation during wet-surface cooling in pigs. *Am J Emerg Med.* 2007;25:420–424.

78. Beckers S, Fries M, Bickenbach J, Derwall M, Kuhlen R, Rossaint R. Minimal instructions improve the performance of laypersons in the use of semiautomatic and automatic external defibrillators. *Crit Care.* 2005; 9:R110–R116.

79. Beckers SK, Fries M, Bickenbach J, Skorning MH, Derwall M, Kuhlen R, Rossaint R. Retention of skills in medical students following minimal theoretical instructions on semi and fully automated external defibrillators. *Resuscitation.* 2007;72:444–450.

80. Mitchell KB, Gugerty L, Muth E. Effects of brief training on use of automated external defibrillators by people without medical expertise. *Hum Factors.* 2008;50:301–310.

81. Cardiopulmonary resuscitation. *JAMA.* 1966;198:372–379.

82. Paraskos JA. History of CPR and the role of the national conference. *Ann Emerg Med.* 1993;22(part 2):275–280.

83. Carveth S. Standards for cardiopulmonary resuscitation and emergency cardiac care. *JAMA.* 1974;227:796–797. Editorial.

84. Carveth SW, Burnap TK, Bechtel J, McIntyre K, Donegan J, Buchman RJ, Reese HE. Training in advanced cardiac life support. *JAMA.* 1976; 235:2311–2315.

85. Chameides L, ed. *Textbook of Pediatric Advanced Life Support.* Dallas, Tex: American Heart Association; 1988.

86. Kirkpatrick D, Kirkpatrick J. *Implementing the Four Levels: A Practical Guide for the Evaluation of Training Programs.* San Francisco, Calif: Berrett-Koehler; 2007.

87. Bloom B, Englehart M, et al. *Taxonomy of Educational Objectives: The Classification of Educational Goals. Handbook I: Cognitive Domain.* New York, NY: Longmans; 1956.

88. Dave RH. *Developing and Writing Behavioral Objectives.* Tucson, Ariz: Educational Innovators Press; 1970.

89. Krathwohl DR, Bloom B, et al. *Taxonomy of Educational Objectives, the Classification of Educational Goals: Handbook II: Affective Domain.* New York, NY: David McKay Co; 1964.

90. Nishiyama C, Iwami T, Kawamura T, Ando M, Kajino K, Yonemoto N, Fukuda R, Yuasa H, Yokoyama H, Nonogi H. Effectiveness of simplified chest compression-only CPR training program with or without preparatory self-learning video: a randomized controlled trial. *Resuscitation.* 2009;80: 1164–1168.

91. Monsieurs KG, Vogels C, Bossaert LL, Meert P, Manganas A, Tsiknakis M, Leisch E, Calle PA, Giorgini F. Learning effect of a novel interactive basic life support CD: the JUST system. *Resuscitation.* 2004;62: 159–165.

92. Knowles MS, Holton EF III, et al. *The Adult Learner.* Woburn, Mass: Butterworth-Heinemann; 1998.

93. Ericsson KA. Deliberate practice and the acquisition and maintenance of expert performance in medicine and related domains. *Acad Med.* 2004; 79(suppl):S70–S81.

94. Bloom BS. *Mastery Learning.* New York, NY: Holt Rinehart & Winston; 1971.

95. Ericsson K, Krampe RT, Tesch-Römer C. The role of deliberate practice in the acquisition of expert performance. *Psychol Rev.* 1993;100: 363–406.

96. Mager RF. *Preparing Instructional Objectives: A Critical Tool in the Development of Effective Instruction.* 3rd ed. Atlanta, Ga: Center for Effective Performance; 1997.

97. Gundry JW, Comess KA, DeRook FA, Jorgenson D, Bardy GH. Comparison of naive sixth-grade children with trained professionals in the use of an automated external defibrillator. *Circulation.* 1999;100: 1703–1707.

98. Mattei LC, McKay U, Lepper MW, Soar J. Do nurses and physiotherapists require training to use an automated external defibrillator? *Resuscitation.* 2002;53:277–280.

99. Clark LJ, Watson J, Cobbe SM, Reeve W, Swann IJ, Macfarlane PW. CPR '98: a practical multimedia computer-based guide to cardiopulmonary resuscitation for medical students. *Resuscitation.* 2000;44: 109–117.

100. Hudson JN. Computer-aided learning in the real world of medical education: does the quality of interaction with the computer affect student learning? *Med Educ.* 2004;38:887–895.

101. Jang KS, Hwang SY, Park SJ, Kim YM, Kim MJ. Effects of a Web-based teaching method on undergraduate nursing students' learning of electrocardiography. *J Nurs Educ.* 2005;44:35–39.

102. Leong SL, Baldwin CD, Adelman AM. Integrating Web-based computer cases into a required clerkship: development and evaluation. *Acad Med.* 2003;78:295–301.

103. Rosser JC, Herman B, Risucci DA, Murayama M, Rosser LE, Merrell RC. Effectiveness of a CD-ROM multimedia tutorial in transferring cognitive knowledge essential for laparoscopic skill training. *Am J Surg.* 2000;179:320–324.

104. Schwid HA, Rooke GA, Ross BK, Sivarajan M. Use of a computerized advanced cardiac life support simulator improves retention of advanced cardiac life support guidelines better than a textbook review. *Crit Care Med.* 1999;27:821–824.

105. Flynn ER, Wolf ZR, McGoldrick TB, Jablonski RA, Dean LM, McKee EP. Effect of three teaching methods on a nursing staff's knowledge of medication error risk reduction strategies. *J Nurs Staff Dev.* 1996;12: 19–26.

106. Goldrick B, Appling-Stevens S, Larson E. Infection control programmed instruction: an alternative to classroom instruction in baccalaureate nursing education. *J Nurs Educ.* 1990;29:20–25.

107. Eliot CR, Williams KA, Woolf BP. An intelligent learning environment for advanced cardiac life support. *Proc AMIA Annu Fall Symp.* 1996;7–11.

108. Patterson NG. Preparation techniques for ACLS exam. Dimens Crit Care Nurs. 1989;8:244–249.

109. Kim JH, Kim WO, Min KT, Yang JY, Nam YT. Learning by computer simulation does not lead to better test performance than textbook study in the diagnosis and treatment of dysrhythmias. *J Clin Anesth.* 2002;14: 395–400.

110. Denton GD, Durning SJ, Wimmer AP, Pangaro LN, Hemmer PA. Is a faculty developed pretest equivalent to pre-third year GPA or USMLE step 1 as a predictor of third-year internal medicine clerkship outcomes? *Teach Learn Med.* 2004;16:329–332.

111. Woodworth KW, Markwell LG. Bored, yawning residents falling asleep during orientation? Wake 'em up with a test! *Med Ref Serv Q.* 2005; 24:77–91.

112. Weaver SJ, Rosen MA, DiazGranados D, Lazzara EH, Lyons R, Salas E, Knych SA, McKeever M, Adler L, Barker M, King HB. Does teamwork improve performance in the operating room? A multilevel evaluation. *Jt Comm J Qual Patient Saf.* 2010;36:133–142.

113. Shetty P, Cohen T, Patel B, Patel VL. The cognitive basis of effective team performance: features of failure and success in simulated cardiac resuscitation. *AMIA Annu Symp Proc.* 2009;2009:599–603.

114. Shea-Lewis A. Teamwork: crew resource management in a community hospital. *J Healthc Qual.* 2009;31:14–18.

115. Stead K, Kumar S, Schultz TJ, Tiver S, Pirone CJ, Adams RJ, Wareham CA. Teams communicating through STEPPS. *Med J Aust.* 2009; 190(suppl):S128–S132.

116. Salas E, DiazGranados D, Klein C, Burke CS, Stagl KC, Goodwin GF, Halpin SM. Does team training improve team performance? A meta-analysis. *Hum Factors.* 2008;50:903–933.

117. Mazzocco K, Petitti DB, Fong KT, Bonacum D, Brookey J, Graham S, Lasky RE, Sexton JB, Thomas EJ. Surgical team behaviors and patient outcomes. *Am J Surg.* 2009;197:678–685.

118. Hunziker S, Buhlmann C, Tschan F, Balestra G, Legeret C, Schumacher C, Semmer NK, Hunziker P, Marsch S. Brief leadership instructions improve cardiopulmonary resuscitation in a high-fidelity simulation: a randomized controlled trial. *Crit Care Med.* 2010;38:1086–1091.

119. Thomas EJ, Taggart B, Crandell S, Lasky RE, Williams AL, Love LJ, Sexton JB, Tyson JE, Helmreich RL. Teaching teamwork during the Neonatal Resuscitation Program: a randomized trial. *J Perinatol.* 2007; 27:409–414.

120. Gilfoyle E, Gottesman R, Razack S. Development of a leadership skills workshop in paediatric advanced resuscitation. *Med Teach.* 2007;29: e276–e283.

121. DeVita MA, Schaefer J, Lutz J, Wang H, Dongilli T. Improving medical emergency team (MET) performance using a novel curriculum and a computerized human patient simulator. *Qual Saf Health Care.* 2005;14: 326–331.

122. Makinen M, Aune S, Niemi-Murola L, Herlitz J, Varpula T, Nurmi J, Axelsson AB, Thoren AB, Castren M. Assessment of CPR-D skills of nurses in Goteborg, Sweden and Espoo, Finland: teaching leadership makes a difference. *Resuscitation.* 2007;72:264–269.

123. Morey JC, Simon R, Jay GD, Wears RL, Salisbury M, Dukes KA, Berns SD. Error reduction and performance improvement in the emergency department through formal teamwork training: evaluation results of the MedTeams project. *Health Serv Res.* 2002;37:1553–1581.

124. Edelson DP, Litzinger B, Arora V, Walsh D, Kim S, Lauderdale DS, Vanden Hoek TL, Becker LB, Abella BS. Improving in-hospital cardiac arrest process and outcomes with performance debriefing. *Arch Intern Med*. 2008;168:1063–1069.

125. Mayo PH, Hackney JE, Mueck JT, Ribaudo V, Schneider RF. Achieving house staff competence in emergency airway management: results of a teaching program using a computerized patient simulator. *Crit Care Med*. 2004;32:2422–2427.

126. Wayne DB, Didwania A, Feinglass J, Fudala MJ, Barsuk JH, McGaghie WC. Simulation-based education improves quality of care during cardiac arrest team responses at an academic teaching hospital: a case-control study. *Chest*. 2008;133:56–61.

127. Donoghue AJ, Durbin DR, Nadel FM, Stryjewski GR, Kost SI, Nadkarni VM. Effect of high-fidelity simulation on Pediatric Advanced Life Support training in pediatric house staff: a randomized trial. *Pediatr Emerg Care*. 2009;25:139–144.

128. Owen H, Mugford B, Follows V, Plummer JL. Comparison of three simulation-based training methods for management of medical emergencies. *Resuscitation*. 2006;71:204–211.

129. Wayne DB, Butter J, Siddall VJ, Fudala MJ, Linquist LA, Feinglass J, Wade LD, McGaghie WC. Simulation-based training of internal medicine residents in advanced cardiac life support protocols: a randomized trial. *Teach Learn Med*. 2005;17:210–216.

130. Campbell DM, Barozzino T, Farrugia M, Sgro M. High-fidelity simulation in neonatal resuscitation. *Paediatr Child Health*. 2009;14:19–23.

131. Hunt EA, Vera K, Diener-West M, Haggerty JA, Nelson KL, Shaffner DH, Pronovost PJ. Delays and errors in cardiopulmonary resuscitation and defibrillation by pediatric residents during simulated cardiopulmonary arrests. *Resuscitation*. 2009;80:819–825.

132. Rodgers D, Securro SJ, Pauley R. The effect of high-fidelity simulation on educational outcomes in an Advanced Cardiovascular Life Support course. *Simul Healthc*. 2009;4:200–206.

133. Barsuk D, Ziv A, Lin G, Blumenfeld A, Rubin O, Keidan I, Munz Y, Berkenstadt H. Using advanced simulation for recognition and correction of gaps in airway and breathing management skills in prehospital trauma care. *Anesth Analg*. 2005;100:803–809.

134. Kory PD, Eisen LA, Adachi M, Ribaudo VA, Rosenthal ME, Mayo PH. Initial airway management skills of senior residents: simulation training compared with traditional training. *Chest*. 2007;132:1927–1931.

135. Marshall RL, Smith JS, Gorman PJ, Krummel TM, Haluck RS, Cooney RN. Use of a human patient simulator in the development of resident trauma management skills. *J Trauma*. 2001;51:17–21.

136. Wayne DB, Siddall VJ, Butter J, Fudala MJ, Wade LD, Feinglass J, McGaghie WC. A longitudinal study of internal medicine residents' retention of advanced cardiac life support skills. *Acad Med*. 2006;81(suppl):S9–S12.

137. Wayne DB, Butter J, Siddall VJ, Fudala MJ, Wade LD, Feinglass J, McGaghie WC. Mastery learning of advanced cardiac life support skills by internal medicine residents using simulation technology and deliberate practice. *J Gen Intern Med*. 2006;21:251–256.

138. Cherry RA, Williams J, George J, Ali J. The effectiveness of a human patient simulator in the ATLS shock skills station. *J Surg Res*. 2007;139:229–235.

139. Schwartz LR, Fernandez R, Kouyoumjian SR, Jones KA, Compton S. A randomized comparison trial of case-based learning versus human patient simulation in medical student education. *Acad Emerg Med*. 2007;14:130–137.

140. Wang XP, Martin SM, Li YL, Chen J, Zhang YM. Effect of emergency care simulator combined with problem-based learning in teaching of cardiopulmonary resuscitation [in Chinese]. *Zhonghua Yi Xue Za Zhi*. 2008;88:1651–1653.

141. Friedman Z, You-Ten KE, Bould MD, Naik V. Teaching lifesaving procedures: the impact of model fidelity on acquisition and transfer of cricothyrotomy skills to performance on cadavers. *Anesth Analg*. 2008;107:1663–1669.

142. Curran VR, Aziz K, O'Young S, Bessell C. Evaluation of the effect of a computerized training simulator (ANAKIN) on the retention of neonatal resuscitation skills. *Teach Learn Med*. 2004;16:157–164.

143. Hoadley TA. Learning advanced cardiac life support: a comparison study of the effects of low- and high-fidelity simulation. *Nurs Educ Perspect*. 2009;30:91–95.

144. Iglesias-Vazquez JA, Rodriguez-Nunez A, Penas-Penas M, Sanchez-Santos L, Cegarra-Garcia M, Barreiro-Diaz MV. Cost-efficiency assessment of Advanced Life Support (ALS) courses based on the comparison of advanced simulators with conventional manikins. *BMC Emerg Med*. 2007;7:18.

145. Cavaleiro AP, Guimaraes H, Calheiros F. Training neonatal skills with simulators? *Acta Paediatr*. 2009;98:636–639.

146. Knudson MM, Khaw L, Bullard MK, Dicker R, Cohen MJ, Staudenmayer K, Sadjadi J, Howard S, Gaba D, Krummel T. Trauma training in simulation: translating skills from SIM time to real time. *J Trauma*. 2008;64:255–263.

147. Christenson J, Parrish K, Barabe S, Noseworthy R, Williams T, Geddes R, Chalmers A. A comparison of multimedia and standard advanced cardiac life support learning. *Acad Emerg Med*. 1998;5:702–708.

148. Gerard JM, Scalzo AJ, Laffey SP, Sinks G, Fendya D, Seratti P. Evaluation of a novel Web-based pediatric advanced life support course. *Arch Pediatr Adolesc Med*. 2006;160:649–655.

149. Crocco TJ, Moreno R, Jauch EC, Racine AN, Pio BJ, Liu T, Kothari RU. Teaching ACLS stroke objectives to prehospital providers: a case-based approach. *Prehosp Emerg Care*. 2003;7:229–234.

150. Dagnone JD, McGraw RC, Pulling CA, Patteson AK. Interprofessional resuscitation rounds: a teamwork approach to ACLS education. *Med Teach*. 2008;30:e49–e54.

151. Dyche WJ, Walsh JH, Nelson JA. An ACLS laboratory rotation for undergraduate medical students. *Ann Emerg Med*. 1983;12:208–211.

152. Herrin TJ, Norman PF, Hill C, Crosby R. Modular approach to CPR training. *South Med J*. 1980;73:742–744.

153. Kim HS, Hwang SY, Oh EG, Lee JE. Development and evaluation of a PBL-based continuing education for clinical nurses: a pilot study. *Taehan Kanho Hakhoe Chi*. 2006;36:1308–1314.

154. Polglase RF, Parish DC, Buckley RL, Smith RW, Joiner TA. Problem-based ACLS instruction: a model approach for undergraduate emergency medical education. *Ann Emerg Med*. 1989;18:997–1000.

155. Mehne PR, Allison EJ Jr, Williamson JE, Landis SS, Brinson HM. A required, combined ACLS/ATLS provider course for senior medical students at East Carolina University. *Ann Emerg Med*. 1987;16:666–668.

156. Nadel FM, Lavelle JM, Fein JA, Giardino AP, Decker JM, Durbin DR. Assessing pediatric senior residents' training in resuscitation: fund of knowledge, technical skills, and perception of confidence. *Pediatr Emerg Care*. 2000;16:73–76.

157. Napier F, Davies RP, Baldock C, Stevens H, Lockey AS, Bullock I, Perkins GD. Validation for a scoring system of the ALS cardiac arrest simulation test (CASTest). *Resuscitation*. 2009;80:1034–1038.

158. Rodgers DL, Bhanji F, McKee BR. Written evaluation is not a predictor for skills performance in an Advanced Cardiovascular Life Support course. *Resuscitation*. 2010;81:453–456.

159. White JR, Shugerman R, Brownlee C, Quan L. Performance of advanced resuscitation skills by pediatric housestaff. *Arch Pediatr Adolesc Med*. 1998;152:1232–1235.

160. Kromann CB, Jensen ML, Ringsted C. The effect of testing on skills learning. *Med Educ*. 2009;43:21–27.

161. Kromann CB, Bohnstedt C, Jensen ML, Ringsted C. The testing effect on skills learning might last 6 months. *Adv Health Sci Educ Theory Pract*. Published online before print October 17, 2009. doi:10.1007/s10459-009-9207-x. Available at: http://www.springerlink.com/content/168g5v75v55r0207/.

162. *Program Administration Manual*. 4th ed. Dallas, Tex: American Heart Association; 2008.

163. Weiss KB. Future of board certification in a new era of public accountability. *J Am Board Fam Med*. 2010;23(suppl 1):S32–S39.

164. Miles PV. Maintenance of certification: the role of the American Board of Pediatrics in improving children's health care. *Pediatr Clin North Am*. 2009;56:987–994.

165. Smith KK, Gilcreast D, Pierce K. Evaluation of staff's retention of ACLS and BLS skills. *Resuscitation*. 2008;78:59–65.

166. Woollard M, Whitfeild R, Smith A, Colquhoun M, Newcombe RG, Vetteer N, Chamberlain D. Skill acquisition and retention in automated external defibrillator (AED) use and CPR by lay responders: a prospective study. *Resuscitation*. 2004;60:17–28.

167. Spooner BB, Fallaha JF, Kocierz L, Smith CM, Smith SC, Perkins GD. An evaluation of objective feedback in basic life support (BLS) training. *Resuscitation*. 2007;73:417–424.

168. Berden HJ, Willems FF, Hendrick JM, Pijls NH, Knape JT. How frequently should basic cardiopulmonary resuscitation training be repeated to maintain adequate skills? *BMJ*. 1993;306:1576–1577.

169. Woollard M, Whitfield R, Newcombe RG, Colquhoun M, Vetter N, Chamberlain D. Optimal refresher training intervals for AED and CPR skills: a randomised controlled trial. *Resuscitation.* 2006;71:237–247.

170. Duran R, Aladag N, Vatansever U, Kucukugurluoglu Y, Sut N, Acunas B. Proficiency and knowledge gained and retained by pediatric residents after neonatal resuscitation course. *Pediatr Int.* 2008;50:644–647.

171. Anthonypillai F. Retention of advanced cardiopulmonary resuscitation knowledge by intensive care trained nurses. *Intensive Crit Care Nurs.* 1992;8:180–184.

172. Boonmak P, Boonmak S, Srichaipanha S, Poomsawat S. Knowledge and skill after brief ACLS training. *J Med Assoc Thai.* 2004;87:1311–1314.

173. Kaye W, Wynne G, Marteau T, Dubin HG, Rallis SF, Simons RS, Evans TR. An advanced resuscitation training course for preregistration house officers. *J R Coll Physicians Lond.* 1990;24:51–54.

174. Skidmore MB, Urquhart H. Retention of skills in neonatal resuscitation. *Paediatr Child Health.* 2001;6:31–35.

175. Semeraro F, Signore L, Cerchiari EL. Retention of CPR performance in anaesthetists. *Resuscitation.* 2006;68:101–108.

176. Trevisanuto D, Ferrarese P, Cavicchioli P, Fasson A, Zanardo V, Zacchello F. Knowledge gained by pediatric residents after neonatal resuscitation program courses. *Paediatr Anaesth.* 2005;15:944–947.

177. Young R, King L. An evaluation of knowledge and skill retention following an in-house advanced life support course. *Nurs Crit Care.* 2000;5:7–14.

178. Duran R, Sen F, N A, Vatansever U, Acunaçs B. Knowledge gained and retained by neonatal nurses following neonatal resuscitation program course. *Turk Pediatr Ars.* 2007;42:153–155.

179. Grant EC, Marczinski CA, Menon K. Using pediatric advanced life support in pediatric residency training: does the curriculum need resuscitation? *Pediatr Crit Care Med.* 2007;8:433–439.

180. O'Steen DS, Kee CC, Minick MP. The retention of advanced cardiac life support knowledge among registered nurses. *J Nurs Staff Dev.* 1996;12:66–72.

181. Hammond F, Saba M, Simes T, Cross R. Advanced life support: retention of registered nurses' knowledge 18 months after initial training. *Aust Crit Care.* 2000;13:99–104.

182. Andresen D, Arntz HR, Grafling W, Hoffmann S, Hofmann D, Kraemer R, Krause-Dietering B, Osche S, Wegscheider K. Public access resuscitation program including defibrillator training for laypersons: a randomized trial to evaluate the impact of training course duration. *Resuscitation.* 2008;76:419–424.

183. Wik L, Myklebust H, Auestad BH, Steen PA. Twelve-month retention of CPR skills with automatic correcting verbal feedback. *Resuscitation.* 2005;66:27–30.

184. Christenson J, Nafziger S, Compton S, Vijayaraghavan K, Slater B, Ledingham R, Powell J, McBurnie MA. The effect of time on CPR and automated external defibrillator skills in the Public Access Defibrillation Trial. *Resuscitation.* 2007;74:52–62.

185. Riegel B, Nafziger SD, McBurnie MA, Powell J, Ledingham R, Sehra R, Mango L, Henry MC. How well are cardiopulmonary resuscitation and automated external defibrillator skills retained over time? Results from the Public Access Defibrillation (PAD) Trial. *Acad Emerg Med.* 2006;13:254–263.

186. Choa M, Park I, Chung HS, Yoo SK, Shim H, Kim S. The effectiveness of cardiopulmonary resuscitation instruction: animation versus dispatcher through a cellular phone. *Resuscitation.* 2008;77:87–94.

187. Choa M, Cho J, Choi YH, Kim S, Sung JM, Chung HS. Animation-assisted CPRII program as a reminder tool in achieving effective one-person-CPR performance. *Resuscitation.* 2009;80:680–684.

188. Ertl L, Christ F. Significant improvement of the quality of bystander first aid using an expert system with a mobile multimedia device. *Resuscitation.* 2007;74:286–295.

189. Ward P, Johnson LA, Mulligan NW, Ward MC, Jones DL. Improving cardiopulmonary resuscitation skills retention: effect of two checklists designed to prompt correct performance. *Resuscitation.* 1997;34:221–225.

190. Merchant RM, Abella BS, Abotsi EJ, Smith TM, Long JA, Trudeau ME, Leary M, Groeneveld PW, Becker LB, Asch DA. Cell telephone cardiopulmonary resuscitation: audio instructions when needed by lay rescuers: a randomized, controlled trial. *Ann Emerg Med.* 2010;55:538–543.e1.

191. Lerner C, Gaca AM, Frush DP, Hohenhaus S, Ancarana A, Seelinger TA, Frush K. Enhancing pediatric safety: assessing and improving resident competency in life-threatening events with a computer-based interactive resuscitation tool. *Pediatr Radiol.* 2009;39:703–709.

192. Schneider AJ, Murray WB, Mentzer SC, Miranda F, Vaduva S. "Helper": a critical events prompter for unexpected emergencies. *J Clin Monit.* 1995;11:358–364.

193. Berkenstadt H, Yusim Y, Ziv A, Ezri T, Perel A. An assessment of a point-of-care information system for the anesthesia provider in simulated malignant hyperthermia crisis. *Anesth Analg.* 2006;102:530–532.

194. Harrison TK, Manser T, Howard SK, Gaba DM. Use of cognitive aids in a simulated anesthetic crisis. *Anesth Analg.* 2006;103:551–556.

195. Zanner R, Wilhelm D, Feussner H, Schneider G. Evaluation of M-AID, a first aid application for mobile phones. *Resuscitation.* 2007;74:487–494.

196. Mills PD, DeRosier JM, Neily J, McKnight SD, Weeks WB, Bagian JP. A cognitive aid for cardiac arrest: you can't use it if you don't know about it. *Jt Comm J Qual Saf.* 2004;30:488–496.

197. Neily J, DeRosier JM, Mills PD, Bishop MJ, Weeks WB, Bagian JP. Awareness and use of a cognitive aid for anesthesiology. *Jt Comm J Qual Patient Saf.* 2007;33:502–511.

198. Beckers SK, Skorning MH, Fries M, Bickenbach J, Beuerlein S, Derwall M, Kuhlen R, Rossaint R. CPREzy improves performance of external chest compressions in simulated cardiac arrest. *Resuscitation.* 2007;72:100–107.

199. Monsieurs KG, De Regge M, Vogels C, Calle PA. Improved basic life support performance by ward nurses using the CAREvent Public Access Resuscitator (PAR) in a simulated setting. *Resuscitation.* 2005;67:45–50.

200. Sutton RM, Donoghue A, Myklebust H, Srikantan S, Byrne A, Priest M, Zoltani Z, Helfaer MA, Nadkarni V. The voice advisory manikin (VAM): an innovative approach to pediatric lay provider basic life support skill education. *Resuscitation.* 2007;75:161–168.

201. Wik L, Thowsen J, Steen PA. An automated voice advisory manikin system for training in basic life support without an instructor: a novel approach to CPR training. *Resuscitation.* 2001;50:167–172.

202. Wik L, Myklebust H, Auestad BH, Steen PA. Retention of basic life support skills 6 months after training with an automated voice advisory manikin system without instructor involvement. *Resuscitation.* 2002;52:273–279.

203. Dine CJ, Gersh RE, Leary M, Riegel BJ, Bellini LM, Abella BS. Improving cardiopulmonary resuscitation quality and resuscitation training by combining audiovisual feedback and debriefing. *Crit Care Med.* 2008;36:2817–2822.

204. Boyle AJ, Wilson AM, Connelly K, McGuigan L, Wilson J, Whitbourn R. Improvement in timing and effectiveness of external cardiac compressions with a new non-invasive device: the CPR-Ezy. *Resuscitation.* 2002;54:63–67.

205. Elding C, Baskett P, Hughes A. The study of the effectiveness of chest compressions using the CPR-plus. *Resuscitation.* 1998;36:169–173.

206. Handley AJ, Handley SA. Improving CPR performance using an audible feedback system suitable for incorporation into an automated external defibrillator. *Resuscitation.* 2003;57:57–62.

207. Jantti H, Silfvast T, Turpeinen A, Kiviniemi V, Uusaro A. Influence of chest compression rate guidance on the quality of cardiopulmonary resuscitation performed on manikins. *Resuscitation.* 2009;80:453–457.

208. Noordergraaf GJ, Drinkwaard BW, van Berkom PF, van Hemert HP, Venema A, Scheffer GJ, Noordergraaf A. The quality of chest compressions by trained personnel: the effect of feedback, via the CPREzy, in a randomized controlled trial using a manikin model. *Resuscitation.* 2006;69:241–252.

209. Oh JH, Lee SJ, Kim SE, Lee KJ, Choe JW, Kim CW. Effects of audio tone guidance on performance of CPR in simulated cardiac arrest with an advanced airway. *Resuscitation.* 2008;79:273–277.

210. Perkins GD, Augre C, Rogers H, Allan M, Thickett DR. CPREzy: an evaluation during simulated cardiac arrest on a hospital bed. *Resuscitation.* 2005;64:103–108.

211. Thomas SH, Stone CK, Austin PE, March JA, Brinkley S. Utilization of a pressure-sensing monitor to improve in-flight chest compressions. *Am J Emerg Med.* 1995;13:155–157.

212. Williamson LJ, Larsen PD, Tzeng YC, Galletly DC. Effect of automatic external defibrillator audio prompts on cardiopulmonary resuscitation performance. *Emerg Med J.* 2005;22:140–143.

213. Kern KB, Stickney RE, Gallison L, Smith RE. Metronome improves compression and ventilation rates during CPR on a manikin in a randomized trial. *Resuscitation.* 2010;81:206–210.

214. Peberdy MA, Silver A, Ornato JP. Effect of caregiver gender, age, and feedback prompts on chest compression rate and depth. *Resuscitation.* 2009;80:1169–1174.

215. Rawlins L, Woollard M, Williams J, Hallam P. Effect of listening to Nellie the Elephant during CPR training on performance of chest compressions by lay people: randomised crossover trial. *BMJ*. 2009;339: b4707.

216. Abella BS, Edelson DP, Kim S, Retzer E, Myklebust H, Barry AM, O'Hearn N, Hoek TL, Becker LB. CPR quality improvement during in-hospital cardiac arrest using a real-time audiovisual feedback system. *Resuscitation*. 2007;73:54–61.

217. Chiang WC, Chen WJ, Chen SY, Ko PC, Lin CH, Tsai MS, Chang WT, Chen SC, Tsan CY, Ma MH. Better adherence to the guidelines during cardiopulmonary resuscitation through the provision of audio-prompts. *Resuscitation*. 2005;64:297–301.

218. Fletcher D, Galloway R, Chamberlain D, Pateman J, Bryant G, Newcombe RG. Basics in advanced life support: a role for download audit and metronomes. *Resuscitation*. 2008;78:127–134.

219. Kramer-Johansen J, Myklebust H, Wik L, Fellows B, Svensson L, Sorebo H, Steen PA. Quality of out-of-hospital cardiopulmonary resuscitation with real time automated feedback: a prospective interventional study. *Resuscitation*. 2006;71:283–292.

220. Niles D, Nysaether J, Sutton R, Nishisaki A, Abella BS, Arbogast K, Maltese MR, Berg RA, Helfaer M, Nadkarni V. Leaning is common during in-hospital pediatric CPR, and decreased with automated corrective feedback. *Resuscitation*. 2009;80:553–557.

221. Nishisaki A, Nysaether J, Sutton R, Maltese M, Niles D, Donoghue A, Bishnoi R, Helfaer M, Perkins GD, Berg R, Arbogast K, Nadkarni V. Effect of mattress deflection on CPR quality assessment for older children and adolescents. *Resuscitation*. 2009;80:540–545.

222. Perkins GD, Boyle W, Bridgestock H, Davies S, Oliver Z, Bradburn S, Green C, Davies RP, Cooke MW. Quality of CPR during advanced resuscitation training. *Resuscitation*. 2008;77:69–74.

223. O'Donnell J, Rodgers D, Lee W, Edelson D, Haag J, Hamilton M, Hoadley T, McCullough A, Meeks R. *Structured and Supported Debriefing*. Dallas, Tex: American Heart Association; 2009.

224. Savoldelli GL, Naik VN, Park J, Joo HS, Chow R, Hamstra SJ. Value of debriefing during simulated crisis management: oral versus video-assisted oral feedback. *Anesthesiology*. 2006;105:279–285.

225. Morgan PJ, Tarshis J, LeBlanc V, Cleave-Hogg D, DeSousa S, Haley MF, Herold-McIlroy J, Law JA. Efficacy of high-fidelity simulation debriefing on the performance of practicing anaesthetists in simulated scenarios. *Br J Anaesth*. 2009;103:531–537.

226. Falcone RA Jr, Daugherty M, Schweer L, Patterson M, Brown RL, Garcia VF. Multidisciplinary pediatric trauma team training using high-fidelity trauma simulation. *J Pediatr Surg*. 2008;43:1065–1071.

227. Weng TI, Huang CH, Ma MH, Chang WT, Liu SC, Wang TD, Chen WJ. Improving the rate of return of spontaneous circulation for out-of-hospital cardiac arrests with a formal, structured emergency resuscitation team. *Resuscitation*. 2004;60:137–142.

228. Nichol G, Thomas E, Callaway CW, Hedges J, Powell JL, Aufderheide TP, Rea T, Lowe R, Brown T, Dreyer J, Davis D, Idris A, Stiell I. Regional variation in out-of-hospital cardiac arrest incidence and outcome. *JAMA*. 2008;300:1423–1431.

229. White RD, Bunch TJ, Hankins DG. Evolution of a community-wide early defibrillation programme experience over 13 years using police/fire personnel and paramedics as responders. *Resuscitation*. 2005; 65:279–283.

230. Neumar RW, Nolan JP, Adrie C, Aibiki M, Berg RA, Bottiger BW, Callaway C, Clark RS, Geocadin RG, Jauch EC, Kern KB, Laurent I, Longstreth WT Jr, Merchant RM, Morley P, Morrison LJ, Nadkarni V, Peberdy MA, Rivers EP, Rodriguez-Nunez A, Sellke FW, Spaulding C, Sunde K, Vanden Hoek T. Post-cardiac arrest syndrome: epidemiology, pathophysiology, treatment, and prognostication: a consensus statement from the International Liaison Committee on Resuscitation (American Heart Association, Australian and New Zealand Council on Resuscitation, European Resuscitation Council, Heart and Stroke Foundation of Canada, InterAmerican Heart Foundation, Resuscitation Council of Asia, and the Resuscitation Council of Southern Africa); the American Heart Association Emergency Cardiovascular Care Committee; the Council on Cardiovascular Surgery and Anesthesia; the Council on Cardiopulmonary, Perioperative, and Critical Care; the Council on Clinical Cardiology; and the Stroke Council. *Circulation*. 2008;118: 2452–2483.

231. Devita MA, Bellomo R, Hillman K, Kellum J, Rotondi A, Teres D, Auerbach A, Chen WJ, Duncan K, Kenward G, Bell M, Buist M, Chen J, Bion J, Kirby A, Lighthall G, Ovreveit J, Braithwaite RS, Gosbee J, Milbrandt E, Peberdy M, Savitz L, Young L, Harvey M, Galhotra S.

Findings of the first consensus conference on medical emergency teams. *Crit Care Med*. 2006;34:2463–2478.

232. Baxter AD, Cardinal P, Hooper J, Patel R. Medical emergency teams at The Ottawa Hospital: the first two years. *Can J Anaesth*. 2008;55: 223–231.

233. Bellomo R, Goldsmith D, Uchino S, Buckmaster J, Hart GK, Opdam H, Silvester W, Doolan L, Gutteridge G. A prospective before-and-after trial of a medical emergency team. *Med J Aust*. 2003;179:283–287.

234. Benson L, Mitchell C, Link M, Carlson G, Fisher J. Using an advanced practice nursing model for a rapid response team. *Jt Comm J Qual Patient Saf*. 2008;34:743–747.

235. Bertaut Y, Campbell A, Goodlett D. Implementing a rapid-response team using a nurse-to-nurse consult approach. *J Vasc Nurs*. 2008;26: 37–42.

236. Buist MD, Moore GE, Bernard SA, Waxman BP, Anderson JN, Nguyen TV. Effects of a medical emergency team on reduction of incidence of and mortality from unexpected cardiac arrests in hospital: preliminary study. *BMJ*. 2002;324:387–390.

237. Buist M, Harrison J, Abaloz E, Van Dyke S. Six year audit of cardiac arrests and medical emergency team calls in an Australian outer metropolitan teaching hospital. *BMJ*. 2007;335:1210–1212.

238. Chamberlain B, Donley K, Maddison J. Patient outcomes using a rapid response team. *Clin Nurse Spec*. 2009;23:11–12.

239. Dacey MJ, Mirza ER, Wilcox V, Doherty M, Mello J, Boyer A, Gates J, Brothers T, Baute R. The effect of a rapid response team on major clinical outcome measures in a community hospital. *Crit Care Med*. 2007;35:2076–2082.

240. DeVita MA, Braithwaite RS, Mahidhara R, Stuart S, Foraida M, Simmons RL. Use of medical emergency team responses to reduce hospital cardiopulmonary arrests. *Qual Saf Health Care*. 2004;13: 251–254.

241. Gould D. Promoting patient safety: the rapid medical response team. *Perm J*. 2007;11:26–34.

242. Hatler C, Mast D, Bedker D, Johnson R, Corderella J, Torres J, King D, Plueger M. Implementing a rapid response team to decrease emergencies outside the ICU: one hospital's experience. *Medsurg Nurs*. 2009;18: 84–90, 126.

243. Jolley J, Bendyk H, Holaday B, Lombardozzi KA, Harmon C. Rapid response teams: do they make a difference? *Dimens Crit Care Nurs*. 2007;26:253–260.

244. Jones D, Bellomo R, Bates S, Warrillow S, Goldsmith D, Hart G, Opdam H, Gutteridge G. Long term effect of a medical emergency team on cardiac arrests in a teaching hospital. *Crit Care*. 2005;9:R808–R815.

245. Jones D, Bellomo R, Bates S, Warrillow S, Goldsmith D, Hart G, Opdam H. Patient monitoring and the timing of cardiac arrests and medical emergency team calls in a teaching hospital. *Intensive Care Med*. 2006;32:1352–1356.

246. Moldenhauer K, Sabel A, Chu ES, Mehler PS. Clinical triggers: an alternative to a rapid response team. *Jt Comm J Qual Patient Saf*. 2009;35:164–174.

247. Offner PJ, Heit J, Roberts R. Implementation of a rapid response team decreases cardiac arrest outside of the intensive care unit. *J Trauma*. 2007;62:1223–1227.

248. Chan PS, Khalid A, Longmore LS, Berg RA, Kosiborod M, Spertus JA. Hospital-wide code rates and mortality before and after implementation of a rapid response team. *JAMA*. 2008;300:2506–2513.

249. Hillman K, Chen J, Cretikos M, Bellomo R, Brown D, Doig G, Finfer S, Flabouris A. Introduction of the medical emergency team (MET) system: a cluster-randomised controlled trial. *Lancet*. 2005;365: 2091–2097.

250. Kenward G, Castle N, Hodgetts T, Shaikh L. Evaluation of a medical emergency team one year after implementation. *Resuscitation*. 2004;61: 257–263.

251. King E, Horvath R, Shulkin DJ. Establishing a rapid response team (RRT) in an academic hospital: one year's experience. *J Hosp Med*. 2006;1:296–305.

252. McFarlan SJ, Hensley S. Implementation and outcomes of a rapid response team. *J Nurs Care Qual*. 2007;22:307–313.

253. Rothschild JM, Woolf S, Finn KM, Friedberg MW, Lemay C, Furbush KA, Williams DH, Bates DW. A controlled trial of a rapid response system in an academic medical center. *Jt Comm J Qual Patient Saf*. 2008;34:417–425, 365.

254. Hunt EA, Zimmer KP, Rinke ML, Shilkofski NA, Matlin C, Garger C, Dickson C, Miller MR. Transition from a traditional code team to a

medical emergency team and categorization of cardiopulmonary arrests in a children's center. *Arch Pediatr Adolesc Med.* 2008;162:117–122.

255. Brilli RJ, Gibson R, Luria JW, Wheeler TA, Shaw J, Linam M, Kheir J, McLain P, Lingsch T, Hall-Haering A, McBride M. Implementation of a medical emergency team in a large pediatric teaching hospital prevents respiratory and cardiopulmonary arrests outside the intensive care unit. *Pediatr Crit Care Med.* 2007;8:236–246.

256. Sharek PJ, Parast LM, Leong K, Coombs J, Earnest K, Sullivan J, Frankel LR, Roth SJ. Effect of a rapid response team on hospital-wide mortality and code rates outside the ICU in a children's hospital. *JAMA.* 2007;298:2267–2274.

257. Tibballs J, Kinney S. Reduction of hospital mortality and of preventable cardiac arrest and death on introduction of a pediatric medical emergency team. *Pediatr Crit Care Med.* 2009;10:306–312.

258. Tibballs J, Kinney S, Duke T, Oakley E, Hennessy M. Reduction of paediatric in-patient cardiac arrest and death with a medical emergency team: preliminary results. *Arch Dis Child.* 2005;90:1148–1152.

259. Chan PS, Jain R, Nallmothu BK, Berg RA, Sasson C. Rapid response teams: a systematic review and meta-analysis. *Arch Intern Med.* 2010; 170:18–26.

260. DeVita MA, Smith GB, Adam SK, Adams-Pizarro I, Buist M, Bellomo R, Bonello R, Cerchiari E, Farlow B, Goldsmith D, Haskell H, Hillman K, Howell M, Hravnak M, Hunt EA, Hvarfner A, Kellett J, Lighthall GK, Lippert A, Lippert FK, Mahroof R, Myers JS, Rosen M, Reynolds S, Rotondi A, Rubulotta F, Winters B. "Identifying the hospitalised patient in crisis": a consensus conference on the afferent limb of rapid response systems. *Resuscitation.* 2010;81:375–382.

261. Engdahl J, Abrahamsson P, Bang A, Lindqvist J, Karlsson T, Herlitz J. Is hospital care of major importance for outcome after out-of-hospital cardiac arrest? Experience acquired from patients with out-of-hospital cardiac arrest resuscitated by the same Emergency Medical Service and admitted to one of two hospitals over a 16-year period in the municipality of Goteborg. *Resuscitation.* 2000;43:201–211.

262. Langhelle A, Tyvold SS, Lexow K, Hapnes SA, Sunde K, Steen PA. In-hospital factors associated with improved outcome after out-of-hospital cardiac arrest: a comparison between four regions in Norway. *Resuscitation.* 2003;56:247–263.

263. Carr BG, Goyal M, Band RA, Gaieski DF, Abella BS, Merchant RM, Branas CC, Becker LB, Neumar RW. A national analysis of the relationship between hospital factors and post-cardiac arrest mortality. *Intensive Care Med.* 2009;35:505–511.

264. Liu JM, Yang Q, Pirrallo RG, Klein JP, Aufderheide TP. Hospital variability of out-of-hospital cardiac arrest survival. *Prehosp Emerg Care.* 2008;12:339–346.

265. Carr BG, Kahn JM, Merchant RM, Kramer AA, Neumar RW. Interhospital variability in post-cardiac arrest mortality. *Resuscitation.* 2009; 80:30–34.

266. Herlitz J, Engdahl J, Svensson L, Angquist KA, Silfverstolpe J, Holmberg S. Major differences in 1-month survival between hospitals in Sweden among initial survivors of out-of-hospital cardiac arrest. *Resuscitation.* 2006;70:404–409.

267. Keenan SP, Dodek P, Martin C, Priestap F, Norena M, Wong H. Variation in length of intensive care unit stay after cardiac arrest: where you are is as important as who you are. *Crit Care Med.* 2007;35: 836–841.

268. Oddo M, Schaller MD, Feihl F, Ribordy V, Liaudet L. From evidence to clinical practice: effective implementation of therapeutic hypothermia to improve patient outcome after cardiac arrest. *Crit Care Med.* 2006;34: 1865–1873.

269. Sunde K, Pytte M, Jacobsen D, Mangschau A, Jensen LP, Smedsrud C, Draegni T, Steen PA. Implementation of a standardised treatment protocol for post resuscitation care after out-of-hospital cardiac arrest. *Resuscitation.* 2007;73:29–39.

270. Knafelj R, Radsel P, Ploj T, Noc M. Primary percutaneous coronary intervention and mild induced hypothermia in comatose survivors of ventricular fibrillation with ST-elevation acute myocardial infarction. *Resuscitation.* 2007;74:227–234.

271. Wolfrum S, Pierau C, Radke PW, Schunkert H, Kurowski V. Mild therapeutic hypothermia in patients after out-of-hospital cardiac arrest due to acute ST-segment elevation myocardial infarction undergoing immediate percutaneous coronary intervention. *Crit Care Med.* 2008; 36:1780–1786.

272. Gaieski DF, Band RA, Abella BS, Neumar RW, Fuchs BD, Kolansky DM, Merchant RM, Carr BG, Becker LB, Maguire C, Klair A, Hylton J, Goyal M. Early goal-directed hemodynamic optimization combined

with therapeutic hypothermia in comatose survivors of out-of-hospital cardiac arrest. *Resuscitation.* 2009;80:418–424.

273. Bradley EH, Herrin J, Wang Y, Barton BA, Webster TR, Mattera JA, Roumanis SA, Curtis JP, Nallamothu BK, Magid DJ, McNamara RL, Parkosewich J, Loeb JM, Krumholz HM. Strategies for reducing the door-to-balloon time in acute myocardial infarction. *N Engl J Med.* 2006;355:2308–2320.

274. LaMonte MP, Bahouth MN, Magder LS, Alcorta RL, Bass RR, Browne BJ, Floccare DJ, Gaasch WR. A regional system of stroke care provides thrombolytic outcomes comparable with the NINDS stroke trial. *Ann Emerg Med.* 2009;54:319–327.

275. Organised inpatient (stroke unit) care for stroke. *Cochrane Database Syst Rev.* 2007 Oct 17;CD000197.

276. MacKenzie EJ, Rivara FP, Jurkovich GJ, Nathens AB, Frey KP, Egleston BL, Salkever DS, Scharfstein DO. A national evaluation of the effect of trauma-center care on mortality. *N Engl J Med.* 2006;354: 366–378.

277. Nichol G, Aufderheide TP, Eigel B, Neumar RW, Lurie KG, Bufalino VJ, Callaway CW, Menon V, Bass RR, Abella BS, Sayre M, Dougherty CM, Racht EM, Kleinman ME, O'Connor RE, Reilly JP, Ossmann EW, Peterson E. Regional systems of care for out-of-hospital cardiac arrest: a policy statement from the American Heart Association. *Circulation.* 2010;121:709–729.

278. Ali J, Adam R, Stedman M, Howard M, Williams J. Cognitive and attitudinal impact of the Advanced Trauma Life Support program in a developing country. *J Trauma.* 1994;36:695–702.

279. Bergman S, Deckelbaum D, Lett R, Haas B, Demyttenaere S, Munthali V, Mbembati N, Museru L, Razek T. Assessing the impact of the trauma team training program in Tanzania. *J Trauma.* 2008;65:879–883.

280. Bhat BV, Biswal N, Bhatia BD, Nalini P. Undergraduate training in neonatal resuscitation: a modified approach. *Indian J Matern Child Health.* 1993;4:87–88.

281. Carlo WA, Wright LL, Chomba E, McClure EM, Carlo ME, Bann CM, Collins M, Harris H. Educational impact of the neonatal resuscitation program in low-risk delivery centers in a developing country. *J Pediatr.* 2009;154:504–508.e5.

282. Couper ID, Thurley JD, Hugo JF. The neonatal resuscitation training project in rural South Africa. *Rural Remote Health.* 2005;5:459.

283. Ergenekon E, Koc E, Atalay Y, Soysal S. Neonatal resuscitation course experience in Turkey. *Resuscitation.* 2000;45:225–227.

284. Husum H, Gilbert M, Wisborg T. Training pre-hospital trauma care in low-income countries: the "Village University" experience. *Med Teach.* 2003;25:142–148.

285. Jabir MM, Doglioni N, Fadhil T, Zanardo V, Trevisanuto D. Knowledge and practical performance gained by Iraqi residents after participation to a neonatal resuscitation program course. *Acta Paediatr.* 2009;98: 1265–1268.

286. Kimura A, Okada K, Kobayashi K, Inaka A, Hagiwara Y, Sakamoto T, Sugimoto N, Nakamura M, Nakamura K, Horiuchi K, Hujii Y, Murota C, Emoto M. Introductory adult cardiac life support course for Vietnamese healthcare workers. *Resuscitation.* 2008;79:511–512.

287. McClure EM, Carlo WA, Wright LL, Chomba E, Uxa F, Lincetto O, Bann C. Evaluation of the educational impact of the WHO Essential Newborn Care course in Zambia. *Acta Paediatr.* 2007;96:1135–1138.

288. Trevisanuto D, Ibrahim SA, Doglioni N, Salvadori S, Ferrarese P, Zanardo V. Neonatal resuscitation courses for pediatric residents: comparison between Khartoum (Sudan) and Padova (Italy). *Paediatr Anaesth.* 2007;17:28–31.

289. Urbano J, Matamoros MM, Lopez-Herce J, Carrillo AP, Ordonez F, Moral R, Mencia S. A paediatric cardiopulmonary resuscitation training project in Honduras. *Resuscitation.* 2010;81:472–476.

290. Zaeem ul H, Qureshi F, Hafeez A, Zafar S, Mohamud BK, Southal DP. Evidence for improvement in the quality of care given during emergencies in pregnancy, infancy and childhood following training in life-saving skills: a postal survey. *J Pak Med Assoc.* 2009;59:22–26.

291. Ali J, Adam R, Butler AK, Chang H, Howard M, Gonsalves D, Pitt-Miller P, Stedman M, Winn J, Williams JI. Trauma outcome improves following the advanced trauma life support program in a developing country. *J Trauma.* 1993;34:890–898.

292. Ali J, Adam RU, Gana TJ, Williams JI. Trauma patient outcome after the Prehospital Trauma Life Support program. *J Trauma.* 1997;42: 1018–1021.

293. Arreola-Risa C, Mock C, Herrera-Escamilla AJ, Contreras I, Vargas J. Cost-effectiveness and benefit of alternatives to improve training for

prehospital trauma care in Mexico. *Prehosp Disaster Med.* 2004;19: 318–325.

294. Husum H, Gilbert M, Wisborg T, Van Heng Y, Murad M. Rural prehospital trauma systems improve trauma outcome in low-income countries: a prospective study from North Iraq and Cambodia. *J Trauma.* 2003;54:1188–1196.

295. Chomba E, McClure EM, Wright LL, Carlo WA, Chakraborty H, Harris H. Effect of WHO newborn care training on neonatal mortality by education. *Ambul Pediatr.* 2008;8:300–304.

296. Zhu XY, Fang HQ, Zeng SP, Li YM, Lin HL, Shi SZ. The impact of the Neonatal Resuscitation Program Guidelines (NRPG) on the neonatal mortality in a hospital in Zhuhai, China. *Singapore Med J.* 1997;38: 485–487.

297. Moretti MA, Cesar LA, Nusbacher A, Kern KB, Timerman S, Ramires JA. Advanced cardiac life support training improves long-term survival from in-hospital cardiac arrest. *Resuscitation.* 2007;72:458–465.

298. Carlo WA, Goudar SS, Jehan I, Chomba E, Tshefu A, Garces A, Parida S, Althabe F, McClure EM, Derman RJ, Goldenberg RL, Bose C, Krebs NF, Panigrahi P, Buekens P, Chakraborty H, Hartwell TD, Wright LL. Newborn-care training and perinatal mortality in developing countries. *N Engl J Med.* 2010;362:614–623.

299. Smith MK, Ross C. Teaching cardiopulmonary resuscitation in a developing country: using Nicaragua as a model. *Crit Care Nurs Q.* 1997;20:15–21.

300. Tennant C. Resuscitation training in Uganda. *Emerg Nurse.* 2000;8: 10–14.

301. Young S, Hutchinson A, Nguyen VT, Le TH, Nguyen DV, Vo TK. Teaching paediatric resuscitation skills in a developing country: introduction of the Advanced Paediatric Life Support course into Vietnam. *Emerg Med Australas.* 2008;20:271–275.

302. Zafar S, Hafeez A, Qureshi F, Arshad N, Southall D. Structured training in the management of emergencies in mothers, babies and children in a poorly resourced health system: logbooks to document skill use. *Resuscitation.* 2009;80:449–452.

KEY WORDS: cardiopulmonary resuscitation

# Part 17: First Aid
## 2010 American Heart Association and American Red Cross Guidelines for First Aid

David Markenson, Co-Chair*; Jeffrey D. Ferguson, Co-Chair*; Leon Chameides; Pascal Cassan; Kin-Lai Chung; Jonathan Epstein; Louis Gonzales; Rita Ann Herrington; Jeffrey L. Pellegrino; Norda Ratcliff; Adam Singer

The American Heart Association (AHA) and the American Red Cross (Red Cross) cofounded the National First Aid Science Advisory Board to review and evaluate the scientific literature on first aid in preparation for the *2005 American Heart Association (AHA) and American Red Cross Guidelines for First Aid.*[1] In preparation for the 2010 evidence evaluation process, the National First Aid Advisory Board was expanded to become the International First Aid Science Advisory Board with the addition of representatives from a number of international first aid organizations (see Table). The goal of the board is to reduce morbidity and mortality due to emergency events by making treatment recommendations based on an analysis of the scientific evidence that answers the following questions:

- In which emergency conditions can morbidity or mortality be reduced by the intervention of a first aid provider?
- How strong is the scientific evidence that interventions performed by a first aid provider are safe, effective, and feasible?

A critical review of the scientific literature by members of the International First Aid Science Advisory Board is summarized in the 2010 *International Consensus on First Aid Science With Treatment Recommendations (ILCOR 2010 CPR Consensus)*, from which these guidelines are derived.[2] That critical review evaluates the literature and identifies knowledge gaps that might be filled through future scientific research.

## Background

The history of first aid can be traced to the dawn of organized human societies. For example, Native American Sioux medicine men of the Bear Society were noted for treating battle injuries, fixing fractures, controlling bleeding, removing arrows, and using a sharp flint to cut around wounds and inflammation.[3]

Modern, organized first aid evolved from military experiences when surgeons taught soldiers how to splint and bandage battlefield wounds. Two British officers, Peter Shepherd and Francis Duncan, are said to have been the first to expand the concept to civilians and to develop the first curriculum in first aid.[4] Organized training in civilian first aid began in the United States in 1903 when Clara Barton, president of the Red Cross, formed a committee to establish instruction in first aid among the nation's industrial workers, where, under dangerous conditions, accidents and deaths were all too frequent.

### The Evidence Evaluation Process

The International First Aid Science Advisory Board first identified 38 questions in first aid practice that either were not raised in previous evidence evaluations or were in need of updating. Two or more board members volunteered to review the scientific literature independently and develop an evidence-based review worksheet summarizing the literature relevant to each question (see Part 2: "Evidence Evaluation and Management of Potential or Perceived Conflicts of Interest"). After each worksheet was presented to, and reviewed by, the full board, a summary draft of the scientific evidence and a treatment recommendation were crafted. The evidence-based review for each question was presented and discussed a second time at a subsequent board meeting. All first aid worksheets, co-copyrighted by the American Heart Association and the American Red Cross, can be viewed through hyperlinks in the 2010 American Heart Association and American Red Cross International Consensus on First Aid Science with Treatment Recommendations.[2] Each question, evidence-based review, draft summary of science, and draft treatment recommendation was presented, discussed, and debated on 2 separate occasions until a consensus was reached. These guidelines are based on the scientific consensus findings reported in the *2010 International Consensus on First Aid Science with Treatment Recommendations.*[2]

The American Heart Association and the American Red Cross request that this document be cited as follows: Markenson D, Ferguson JD, Chameides L, Cassan P, Chung K-L, Epstein J, Gonzales L, Herrington RA, Pellegrino JL, Ratcliff N, Singer A. Part 17: first aid: 2010 American Heart Association and American Red Cross Guidelines for First Aid. *Circulation.* 2010;122(suppl 3):S934–S946.

*Co-chairs and equal first co-authors.

(*Circulation.* 2010;122[suppl 3]:S934–S946.)

*Circulation* is available at http://circ.ahajournals.org

DOI: 10.1161/CIRCULATIONAHA.110.971150

**Table.    International First Aid Science Advisory Board Member Organizations**

American Academy of Pediatrics

American Burn Association

American College of Emergency Physicians

American College of Occupational and Environmental Medicine

American College of Surgeons

American Heart Association

American Pediatric Surgical Association

American Red Cross

American Red Cross Advisory Council on First Aid, Aquatics, Safety and Preparedness (ACFASP)

American Safety & Health Institute (ASHI) (Observer)

Austrian Red Cross

Canadian Red Cross

Divers Alert Network

European Reference Center on First Aid Education

Egyptian Red Crescent

French Red Cross

Grenada Red Cross

Hong Kong Red Cross

Hungarian Red Cross

International Federation of Red Cross and Red Crescent Societies

Medic First Aid International (Observer)

National Association of EMS Educators

National Association of EMS Physicians

National Athletic Trainers' Association

National Safety Council

Norwegian Red Cross

Occupational Safety and Health Administration

Red Cross Society of China

Resuscitation Council of Asia

St. John Ambulance, UK

Previous reports[5–8] have noted the paucity of scientific evidence supporting many interventions in prehospital emergency care. In reviewing the medical literature, members of the International First Aid Science Advisory Board once again found a paucity of evidence to guide first aid interventions. Very little research is being conducted in first aid, and many of the following recommendations are extrapolated from the experience of healthcare professionals. It is important to recognize the limitations of the evidence that supports many of these guidelines so that research can be undertaken and future guidelines can be based on a larger body of scientific evidence.

## Definition of First Aid

We define first aid as the assessments and interventions that can be performed by a bystander (or by the victim) with minimal or no medical equipment. A first aid provider is defined as someone with formal training in first aid, emergency care, or medicine who provides first aid. First aid assessments and interventions should be medically sound and based on scientific evidence or, in the absence of such evidence, on expert consensus. Administration of first aid must not delay activation of the emergency medical services (EMS) system or other medical assistance when required. We strongly believe that education in first aid should be universal: everyone can learn first aid and everyone should.

The scope of first aid is not purely scientific; it is influenced by both training and regulatory issues. The definition of scope is therefore variable, and should be defined according to circumstances, need, and regulatory requirements.

## Calling for Help

A first aid provider must be able to recognize when help is needed and how to get it. First aid providers should learn how and when to access the EMS system, how to activate the on-site emergency response plan (ERP), and how to contact the Poison Control Center (see "Poison Emergencies" below).

## Positioning the Victim

As a general rule a victim should not be moved, especially if you suspect, from the victim's position or the nature of the injury, that the victim may have a spinal injury (see "Spine Stabilization" below). There are times, however, when the victim should be moved:

- If the area is unsafe for the rescuer or the victim, move the victim to a safe location if it is safe to do so.
- If the victim is face down and is unresponsive, turn the victim face up.
- If the victim has difficulty breathing because of copious secretions or vomiting, or if you are alone and have to leave an unresponsive victim to get help, place the victim in a modified **H**igh **A**rm **IN** **E**ndangered **S**pine (HAINES) recovery position:[9,10] Extend one of the victim's arms above the head and roll the body to the side so the victim's head rests on the extended arm. Bend both legs to stabilize the victim (Class IIb, LOE C).
- If a victim shows evidence of shock, have the victim lie supine. If there is no evidence of trauma or injury, raise the feet about 6 to 12 inches (about 30° to 45°) (Class IIb, LOE C). Do not raise the feet if the movement or the position causes the victim any pain.

The evidence for a benefit to raising the feet is extrapolated from leg raising studies on volume expansion; there are no studies on the effect of leg raising as a first aid maneuver for shock. The results of the volume expansion studies are contradictory with some showing an increase in cardiac output,[11–13] while others show no change in cardiac output or mean arterial pressure[14–18] with leg raising.

## Oxygen

There is insufficient evidence to recommend routine use of supplementary oxygen by a first aid provider for victims complaining of chest discomfort[19,20] or shortness of breath[21]

(Class IIb, LOE C). Supplementary oxygen administration may be beneficial as part of first aid for divers with a decompression injury (Class IIb, LOE C[22]).

# Medical Emergencies

## Breathing Difficulties

The incidence of acute asthma is increasing, especially in urban populations.[23] Many victims with asthma take a prescribed bronchodilator medication and can self-administer it.[24–26] First aid providers are not expected to make a diagnosis of asthma, but they may assist the victim in using the victim's prescribed bronchodilator medication (Class IIa, LOE B) under the following conditions:

- The victim states that he or she is having an asthma attack or symptoms associated with a previously diagnosed breathing disorder, and the victim has the prescribed medications or inhaler in his or her possession.
- The victim identifies the medication and is unable to administer it without assistance.[24]

First aid providers should become familiar with inhalers so that they can assist a victim with an acute asthma attack in using the inhaler.

## Anaphylaxis

Allergies are relatively common, but only a small proportion of people with allergies develop anaphylactic reactions. An anaphylactic reaction is a progressive series of signs and symptoms characterized by swelling, breathing difficulty, an itching rash, and eventually shock, which, if left untreated, may lead to death. Some of these signs and symptoms can also be present in other conditions, and first aid rescuers should not be expected to make a diagnosis of anaphylaxis.[27–30]

Older patients who suffer from anaphylactic reactions know their signs and symptoms and many carry a lifesaving epinephrine auto-injector. With proper training, parents can be taught to correctly use an auto-injector to administer epinephrine to their allergic children.[31] All too often, however, neither the victim nor family members know how to correctly use an auto-injector.[32–34] First aid providers should be familiar with the epinephrine auto-injector so that they can help a victim with an anaphylactic reaction to self-administer it. First aid providers should also know how to administer the auto-injector if the victim is unable to do so, provided that the medication has been prescribed by a physician and state law permits it (Class IIb, LOE B).

In retrospective studies[35–37] 18% to 35% of patients having signs of anaphylaxis required a second dose of epinephrine if symptoms persisted or progressed after the first dose. Because of the difficulty in making a diagnosis of anaphylaxis[27–30,38,39] and the potential harm from epinephrine if the diagnosis is incorrect,[40–43] first aid providers are advised to seek medical assistance if symptoms persist, rather than routinely administering a second dose of epinephrine. In unusual circumstances, when advanced medical assistance is not available, a second dose of epinephrine may be given if symptoms of anaphylaxis persist (Class IIb, LOE C).

## Seizures

The general principles of first aid management of seizures are to

- Ensure an open airway.
- Prevent injury.

Do not restrain the victim during a seizure. Do not try to open the victim's mouth or try to place any object between the victim's teeth or in the mouth. Restraining the victim may cause musculoskeletal or soft-tissue injury. Placing an object in the victim's mouth may cause dental damage or aspiration (Class IIa, LOE C). It is not unusual for the victim to be unresponsive or confused for a short time after a seizure.

## Chest Discomfort

Because it is very difficult, even for the healthcare professional, to differentiate chest discomfort of cardiac origin from other chest discomfort, the first aid provider should assume that chest discomfort is cardiac until proven otherwise. Cardiac chest discomfort is often described as "crushing" or "pressing" and is often accompanied by shortness of breath or perspiration. But cardiac chest discomfort may not have these classical characteristics, especially in women. Call EMS immediately for anyone with chest discomfort. Do not delay and do not try to transport the patient to a healthcare facility yourself.

While waiting for EMS to arrive, the first aid provider may encourage the victim to chew 1 adult (not enteric coated) or 2 low-dose "baby" aspirin if the patient has no allergy to aspirin or other contraindication to aspirin, such as evidence of a stroke or recent bleeding (Class IIa, LOE A).[44–46]

# Injury Emergencies

## Bleeding

Control of bleeding is a basic skill of first aid and one of the few actions with which a first aid provider can critically influence outcome.

### Direct Pressure

Bleeding is best controlled by applying pressure until bleeding stops[47–53] or EMS rescuers arrive (Class I, LOE A). The amount of pressure applied and the time the pressure is held are the most important factors affecting successful control of bleeding. The pressure must be firm, and it must be maintained for a long time. Methods of applying pressure include

- Manual pressure on gauze or other cloth placed over the bleeding source. If bleeding continues, do not remove the gauze; add more gauze on top and apply more pressure.
- If it is not possible to provide continuous manual pressure, wrap an elastic bandage firmly over gauze to hold it in place with pressure.[54–57]

## Tourniquets

Although tourniquets have been shown to control bleeding effectively on the battlefield[58–60] and during surgery and have been used by paramedics in a civilian setting without complications,[61] there are no studies on controlling bleeding with first aid provider use of a tourniquet. Potential dangers of prolonged tourniquet application include temporary[62] or permanent[63] injury to the underlying nerves and muscles,[64] and systemic complications resulting from limb ischemia,[65] including acidemia, hyperkalemia, arrhythmias, shock, and death. Complications are related to tourniquet pressure[66] and duration of occlusion,[67] but there is insufficient evidence to determine a minimal critical time beyond which irreversible complications may occur. Because of the potential adverse effects of tourniquets and difficulty in their proper application, use of a tourniquet to control bleeding of the extremities is indicated only if direct pressure is not effective or possible (Class IIb, LOE B). Specifically designed tourniquets appear to be better than ones that are improvised,[60,68–71] but tourniquets should only be used with proper training (Class IIa, LOE B). If a tourniquet is used, make sure that you note the time it was applied and communicate that time to EMS personnel.

### Pressure Points and Elevation

Elevation and use of pressure points are not recommended to control bleeding (Class III, LOE C). This new recommendation is made because there is evidence that other ways of controlling bleeding are more effective. The hemostatic effect of elevation has not been studied. No effect on distal pulses was found in volunteers when pressure points were used.[72] Most important, these unproven procedures may compromise the proven intervention of direct pressure, so they could be harmful.

### Hemostatic Agents

Among the large number of commercially available hemostatic agents, some have been shown to be effective.[73–76] However, their routine use in first aid cannot be recommended at this time because of significant variation in effectiveness by different agents and their potential for adverse effects, including tissue destruction with induction of a proembolic state and potential thermal injury (Class IIb, LOE B).

## Wounds and Abrasions

Superficial wounds and abrasions should be thoroughly irrigated with a large volume of warm or room temperature potable water with or without soap[77–82] until there is no foreign matter in the wound (Class I, LOE A). Cold water appears to be as effective as warm water, but it is not as comfortable. If running water is unavailable, use any source of clean water. Wounds heal better with less infection if they are covered with an antibiotic ointment or cream and a clean occlusive dressing (Class IIa, LOE A).[83–85] Apply antibiotic ointment or cream only if the wound is an abrasion or a superficial injury and only if the victim has no known allergies to the antibiotic.

## Burns

### Thermal Burns

Cool thermal burns with cold (15° to 25°C) tap water as soon as possible and continue cooling at least until pain is relieved (Class I, LOE B).[86–93] Cooling reduces pain, edema, and depth of injury. It speeds healing and may reduce the need for excision and grafting of deep burns. Don't apply ice directly to a burn; it can produce tissue ischemia (Class III, LOE B). Prolonged cold exposure to small burns, and even brief exposure if the burn is large, can cause further local tissue injury[93–95] and hypothermia.

### Burn Blisters

Loosely cover burn blisters with a sterile dressing but leave blisters intact because this improves healing and reduces pain (Class IIa, LOE B).[96–99]

## Electric Injuries

The severity of electric injuries can vary widely, from an unpleasant tingling sensation caused by low-intensity current to thermal burns, cardiopulmonary arrest, and death. Thermal burns may result from burning clothing that is in contact with the skin or from electric current traversing a portion of the body. When current traverses the body, thermal burns may be present at the entry and exit points and along its internal pathway. Cardiopulmonary arrest is the primary cause of immediate death from electrocution.[100] Cardiac arrhythmias, including ventricular fibrillation, ventricular asystole, and ventricular tachycardia that progresses to ventricular fibrillation, may result from exposure to low- or high-voltage current.[101] Respiratory arrest may result from electric injury to the respiratory center in the brain or from tetanic contractions or paralysis of respiratory muscles.

Do not place yourself in danger by touching an electrocuted victim while the power is on (Class III, LOE C). Turn off the power at its source; at home the switch is usually near the fuse box. In case of high-voltage electrocutions caused by fallen power lines, immediately notify the appropriate authorities (eg, 911 or fire department). All materials conduct electricity if the voltage is high enough, so do not enter the area around the victim or try to remove wires or other materials with any object, including a wooden one, until the power has been turned off by knowledgeable personnel.

Once the power is off, assess the victim, who may need CPR, defibrillation, and treatment for shock and thermal burns. All victims of electric shock require medical assessment because the extent of injury may not be apparent.

## Spine Stabilization

There is approximately a 2% risk of injury to the cervical spine after blunt trauma that is serious enough to require spinal imaging in an emergency department,[102,103] and this risk is tripled in patients with craniofacial injury.[104] Most victims with spinal injuries are males between the ages of 10 and 30 years. Motor vehicles cause approximately half of all spinal injuries; many of the remainder are caused by falls (especially from a height or diving), sports, and assaults.[105]

If the cervical spine is injured, the spinal cord may be unprotected, and further injury (secondary spinal cord injury) could result from stresses to the cord that occur when the victim is manipulated or moved. This could result in permanent neurological damage including quadriplegia.[106,107] Only one controlled but underpowered study with some methodological problems[108] has examined this question. In the study, the group of injured victims with spinal immobilization by emergency medical technicians using equipment failed to show any neurological benefit compared with a group of injured victims without spinal immobilization.

Because of the dire consequences if secondary injury does occur, maintain spinal motion restriction by manually stabilizing the head so that the motion of head, neck, and spine is minimized (Class IIb, LOE C). First aid providers should not use immobilization devices because their benefit in first aid has not been proven and they may be harmful (Class III, LOE C). Immobilization devices may be needed in special circumstances when immediate extrication (eg, rescue of drowning victim) is required, but first aid providers should not use these devices unless they have been properly trained in their use.

First aid rescuers cannot conclusively identify a victim with a spinal injury, but they should suspect spinal injury if an injured victim has any of the following risk factors (these have been modified slightly from the *2005 American Heart Association and American Red Cross First Aid Guidelines*[103,109–114]):

- Age ≥65 years
- Driver, passenger, or pedestrian, in a motor vehicle, motorized cycle, or bicycle crash
- Fall from a greater than standing height
- Tingling in the extremities
- Pain or tenderness in the neck or back
- Sensory deficit or muscle weakness involving the torso or upper extremities
- Not fully alert or is intoxicated
- Other painful injuries, especially of the head and neck
- Children 2 years of age or older with evidence of head or neck trauma

## Musculoskeletal Trauma

### Sprains and Strains

Soft-tissue injuries include joint sprains and muscle contusions. Cold application decreases hemorrhage, edema, pain, and disability,[115–120] and it is reasonable to apply cold to a soft-tissue injury. Cooling is best accomplished with a plastic bag or damp cloth filled with a mixture of ice and water; the mixture is better than ice alone.[121–123] Refreezable gel packs do not cool as effectively as an ice-water mixture.[124,125] To prevent cold injury, limit each application of cold to periods ≤20 minutes.[126–128] If that length of time is uncomfortable, limit application to 10 minutes.[129] Place a barrier, such as a thin towel, between the cold container and the skin (Class IIb, LOE C[126,128]).

It is not clear whether a compression bandage is helpful for a joint injury. Heat application to a contusion or injured joint is not as good a first aid measure as cold application.[115]

### Fractures

Assume that any injury to an extremity includes a bone fracture. Cover open wounds with a dressing. Do not move or try to straighten an injured extremity (Class III, LOE C). There is no evidence that straightening an angulated suspected long bone fracture shortens healing time or reduces pain prior to permanent fixation. Expert opinion suggests that splinting may reduce pain[130] and prevent further injury. So, if you are far from definitive health care, stabilize the extremity with a splint in the position found (Class IIa, LOE C). If a splint is used, it should be padded to cushion the injury. If an injured extremity is blue or extremely pale, activate EMS immediately because this could be a medical emergency. A victim with an injured lower extremity should not bear weight until advised to do so by a medical professional.

## Human and Animal Bites

Irrigate human and animal bites with copious amounts of water (Class I, LOE B). This irrigation has been shown to prevent rabies from animal bites[131,132] and bacterial infection.[133]

### Snakebites

Do not apply suction as first aid for snakebites (Class III, LOE C). Suction does remove some venom, but the amount is very small.[134] Suction has no clinical benefit[135] and it may aggravate the injury.[136–138]

Applying a pressure immobilization bandage with a pressure between 40 and 70 mm Hg in the upper extremity and between 55 and 70 mm Hg in the lower extremity around the entire length of the bitten extremity is an effective and safe way to slow the dissemination of venom by slowing lymph flow (Class IIa, LOE C[139,140]). For practical purposes pressure is sufficient if the bandage is comfortably tight and snug but allows a finger to be slipped under it. Initially it was theorized that slowing lymphatic flow by external pressure would only benefit victims bitten by snakes producing neurotoxic venom, but the effectiveness of pressure immobilization has also been demonstrated for bites by non-neurotoxic American snakes.[140,141] The challenge is to find a way to teach the application of the correct snugness of the bandage because inadequate pressure is ineffective and too much pressure may cause local tissue damage. It has also been demonstrated that, once learned, retention of the skill of proper pressure and immobilization application is poor.[142,143]

### Jellyfish Stings

This section is new to the First Aid Guidelines. First aid for jellyfish stings consists of two important actions: preventing further nematocyst discharge and pain relief. To inactivate venom load and prevent further envenomation, jellyfish stings should be liberally washed with vinegar (4% to 6% acetic acid solution) as soon as possible for at least 30 seconds (Class IIa, LOE B). The inactivation of venom has been demonstrated for *Olindias sambaquiensis*[144] and for Physalia physalis (Portuguese man-of-war).[145] If vinegar is not available, a baking soda slurry may be used instead.[145]

For the treatment of pain, after the nematocysts are removed or deactivated, jellyfish stings should be treated with hot-water immersion when possible (Class IIa, LOE B). The victim should be instructed to take a hot shower or immerse the affected part in hot water (temperature as hot as tolerated, or 45°C if there is the capability to regulate temperature), as soon as possible, for at least 20 minutes or for as long as pain persists.[146–149] If hot water is not available, dry hot packs or, as a second choice, dry cold packs may be helpful in decreasing pain but these are not as effective as hot water (Class IIb, LOE B[146,150,151]). Topical application of aluminum sulfate or meat tenderizer, commercially available aerosol products, fresh water wash, and papain, an enzyme derived from papaya used as a local medicine, are even less effective in relieving pain (Class IIb, LOE B[147,152]).

Pressure immobilization bandages are not recommended for the treatment of jellyfish stings because animal studies[153,154] show that pressure with an immobilization bandage causes further release of venom, even from already fired nematocysts (Class III, LOE C).

## Dental Injuries

Traumatic dental injuries are common. The first aid for an avulsed tooth is as follows:

- Clean bleeding wound(s) with saline solution or tap water.
- Stop bleeding by applying pressure with gauze or cotton.
- Handle the tooth by the crown, not the root (ie, do not handle the part that was beneath the gum).
- Place the tooth in milk, or clean water if milk is not available.
- Contact the patient's dentist or take the tooth and victim to an emergency care center as quickly as possible (Class IIa, LOE C).[155–158]

# Environmental Emergencies

## Cold Emergencies

### Hypothermia

Hypothermia is caused by exposure to cold. The urgency of treatment depends on the length of exposure and the victim's body temperature. Begin rewarming a victim of hypothermia immediately by moving the victim to a warm environment, removing wet clothing, and wrapping all exposed body surfaces with anything at hand, such as blankets, clothing, and newspapers. If the hypothermia victim is far from definitive health care, begin active rewarming (Class IIa, LOE B[159,160]) although the effectiveness of active rewarming has not been evaluated. Active rewarming should not delay definitive care. Potential methods of active rewarming include placing the victim near a heat source and placing

containers of warm, but not hot, water in contact with the skin.

### Frostbite

Frostbite usually affects an exposed part of the body such as the extremities and nose. In case of frostbite, remove wet clothing and dry and cover the victim to prevent hypothermia. Transport the victim to an advanced medical facility as rapidly as possible. Do not try to rewarm the frostbite if there is any chance that it might refreeze[161,162] or if you are close to a medical facility (Class III, LOE C).

Minor or superficial frostbite (frostnip) can be treated with simple, rapid rewarming using skin-to-skin contact such as a warm hand.

Severe or deep frostbite should be rewarmed within 24 hours of injury and this is best accomplished by immersing the frostbitten part in warm (37° to 40°C or approximately body temperature) water for 20 to 30 minutes (Class IIb, LOE C[161–170]). Chemical warmers should not be placed directly on frostbitten tissue because they can reach temperatures that can cause burns (Class III, LOE C[171]). Following rewarming, efforts should be made to protect frostbitten parts from refreezing and to quickly evacuate the patient for further care. The effectiveness of ibuprofen or other nonsteroidal antiinflammatory drugs (NSAIDs) in frostbite has not been well established in human studies.[170,172–175]

## Heat Emergencies

Heat-induced symptoms, often precipitated by vigorous exercise, may include heat cramps, heat exhaustion, and heat stroke.

Heat cramps are painful involuntary muscle spasms that most often affect the calves, arms, abdominal muscles, and back. First aid includes rest, cooling off, and drinking an electrolyte-carbohydrate mixture, such as juice, milk, or a commercial electrolyte-carbohydrate drink.[176–185] Stretching, icing, and massaging the painful muscles may be helpful. Exercise should not be resumed until all symptoms have resolved.

Heat exhaustion is caused by a combination of exercise-induced heat and fluid and electrolyte loss as sweat. Signs and symptoms may start suddenly and include: nausea, dizziness, muscle cramps, feeling faint, headache, fatigue, and heavy sweating. Heat exhaustion is a serious condition because it can rapidly advance to the next stage, heat stroke, which can be fatal. Heat exhaustion must be vigorously treated by having the victim lie down in a cool place, taking off as many clothes as possible, cooling the victim with a cool water spray, and encouraging the victim to drink cool fluids, preferably containing carbohydrates and electrolytes.

Heat stroke includes all the symptoms of heat exhaustion plus signs of central nervous system involvement, including dizziness, syncope, confusion, or seizures. The most important action by a first aid provider for a victim of heat stroke is to begin immediate cooling, preferably by immersing the victim up to the chin in cold water.[186–189] It is also important to activate the EMS system. Heat stroke requires emergency treatment with intravenous fluids. Do not try to force the victim to drink liquids.

## Drowning

Drowning is a major cause of unintentional death. Methods of preventing drowning include isolation fencing around swimming pools (gates should be self-closing and self-latching),[190] wearing personal flotation devices (life jackets) while in, around, or on water, never swimming alone, and avoiding swimming or operating motorized watercraft while intoxicated. Outcome following drowning depends on the duration of the submersion, the water temperature, and how promptly CPR is started.[191,192] Occasional case reports have documented intact neurological survival in children following prolonged submersion in icy waters.[193,194]

Remove the victim rapidly and safely from the water, but do not place yourself in danger. If you have special training, you can start rescue breathing while the victim is still in the water[195] providing that it does not delay removing the victim from the water. There is no evidence that water acts as an obstructive foreign body, so do not waste time trying to remove it with abdominal or chest thrusts. Start CPR and, if you are alone, continue with about 5 cycles (about 2 minutes) of chest compressions and ventilations before activating EMS. If 2 rescuers are present, send 1 rescuer to activate EMS immediately.

## Poison Emergencies

If the patient exhibits any signs or symptoms of a life-threatening condition, (eg, sleepiness, seizures, difficulty breathing, vomiting) after exposure to a poison, activate the EMS immediately.

## Poison Control Centers

There are many poisonous substances in the home and worksite. It is important to understand the toxic nature of the chemical substances in the environment and the proper protective equipment and emergency procedures in case of toxic exposure. The Poison Help hotline of the American Association of Poison Control Centers (800-222-1222) is an excellent resource in the United States for information about treating ingestion of, or exposure to, a potential poison. Further information is available at www.aapcc.org. Similar resources may be available internationally, and their contact information (eg, 112 in Europe) should be standard in international first aid training. When phoning a poison control center or other emergency medical services, know the nature and time of exposure and the name of the product or toxic substance.

## Chemical Burns

Brush powdered chemicals off the skin with a gloved hand or piece of cloth. Remove all contaminated clothing from the victim, making sure you do not contaminate yourself in the process. In case of exposure to an acid or alkali on the skin[196–202] or eye,[203–208] immediately irrigate the affected area with copious amounts of water (Class I, LOE B).

## Toxic Eye Injury

Rinse eyes exposed to toxic substances immediately with a copious amount of water (Class I, LOE C[203,209,210]), unless a specific antidote is available.[203,210,211]

## Ingested Poisons

### Treatment With Milk or Water

Do not administer anything by mouth for any poison ingestion unless advised to do so by a poison control center or emergency medical personnel because it may be harmful (Class III, LOE C). There is insufficient evidence that dilution of the ingested poison with water or milk is of any benefit as a first aid measure. Animal studies[212–216] have shown that dilution or neutralization of a caustic agent with water or milk reduces tissue injury, but no human studies have shown a clinical benefit. Possible adverse effects of water or milk administration include emesis and aspiration.

### Activated Charcoal

Do not administer activated charcoal to a victim who has ingested a poisonous substance unless you are advised to do so by poison control center or emergency medical personnel (Class IIb, LOE C). There is no evidence that activated charcoal is effective as a component of first aid. It may be safe to administer,[217,218] but it has not been shown to be beneficial, and there are reports of it causing harm.[219–221] In addition the majority of children will not take the recommended dose.[222]

### Ipecac

Do not administer syrup of ipecac for ingestions of toxins (Class III, LOE B). Several studies[223–225] found that there is no clinically relevant advantage to administering syrup of ipecac; its administration is not associated with decreased healthcare utilization.[226] Untoward effects of ipecac administration include intractable emesis and delayed care in an advanced medical facility.[227,228]

# Disclosures

## Guidelines Part 17: First Aid: Writing Group Disclosures

| Writing Group Member | Employment | Research Grant | Other Research Support | Speakers' Bureau/ Honoraria | Ownership Interest | Consultant/Advisory Board | Other |
|---|---|---|---|---|---|---|---|
| David Markenson | NYMC–Interim Chair; EMA–Chief Pediatric ED | None | None | None | None | None | None |
| Jeffrey D. Ferguson | Brody School of Medicine, East Carolina University–Assistant Professor | None | None | None | None | None | *Serving as an expert witness in two ongoing lawsuits involving EMS related cases. Billing for this service has not yet occurred and will likely represent less than $10,000 per 12 months. This payment is expected to come directly to me |
| Leon Chameides | Emeritus Director Pediatric Cardiology, Connecticut Children's Medical Center, Clinical Professor, University of Connecticut | None | None | None | None | None | None |
| Pascal Cassan | French Red Cross, National Medical Advisor and Coordinator of the European Reference Centre for first aid education Coordinator of the Scientific Commission of First Aid for the French Interior Ministry (unpaid) | None | None | None | None | | None |
| Kin-Lai Chung | Hong Kong Hospital Authority Hospital Chief Executive | None | None | None | None | None | None |
| Jonathan Epstein | NorthEast Emergency Medical Services, Inc.– Regional EMS Council: Provide EMS System Oversight. Also provide education (First aid and CPR/AED) as an AHA Training Center. Executive Director; Isis Maternity: Pre-Natal and Post Partum edu.- Provide CPR and First Aid Training via AHA Curriculum. For-Profit Company—Instructor | None | None | None | None | *Volunteer: American Red Cross Advisory Council on First Aid, Aquatics, Safety and Preparedness (ACFASP) Vice-Chair | None |
| Louis Gonzales | City of Austin - Office of the Medical Director: EMS System Medical Director Staff–Performance Management & Research Coordinator *Beginning July 1, 2009, I will serve as a paid consultant to the AHA ECC Product Development Group as a Senior Science Editor. This assignment will include providing Science review of AHA First Aid Products | None | None | None | None | None | None |
| Rita Ann Herrington | Minute Clinic–Family Nurse Practitioner | None | None | None | None | None | None |
| Jeffrey Pellegrino | Kent State University–Assistant Dir Faculty Professional Dev. Center | None | None | None | None | †Wilderness First Aid consultant for StayWell publishing | None |
| Norda Ratcliff | Bloomington Hospital Prompt Care–Nurse Practitioner | None | None | None | None | None | None |
| Adam Singer | Stony Brook University–Physician | None | None | None | None | None | None |

This table represents the relationships of writing group members that may be perceived as actual or reasonably perceived conflicts of interest as reported on the Disclosure Questionnaire, which all members of the writing group are required to complete and submit. A relationship is considered to be "significant" if (a) the person receives $10 000 or more during any 12-month period, or 5% or more of the person's gross income; or (b) the person owns 5% or more of the voting stock or share of the entity, or owns $10 000 or more of the fair market value of the entity. A relationship is considered to be "modest" if it is less than "significant" under the preceding definition.

*Modest.

†Significant.

# References

1. 2005 American Heart Association guidelines for cardiopulmonary resuscitation and emergency cardiovascular care part 14: first aid. *Circulation.* 2005;112(suppl):IV-196–IV-203.

2. Markenson D, Ferguson JD, Chameides L, Cassan P, Chung KL, Epstein JL, Gonzales L, Hazinski MF, Herrington RA, Pelligrino JL, Ratcliff N, Singer AJ; on behalf of the First Aid Chapter Collaborators. Part 13: first aid: 2010 American Heart Association and American Red Cross International Consensus on First Aid Science With Treatment Recommendations. *Circulation.* 2010;(suppl 2):S582–S605.

3. Lewis TH. *The Medicine Men: Oglala Sioux Ceremony and Healing.* Lincoln, Neb: University of Nebraska Press; 1992.

4. Pearn J. The earliest days of first aid. *BMJ.* 1994;309:1718–1720.

5. The American Heart Association in collaboration with the International Liaison Committee on Resuscitation. Guidelines 2000 for cardiopulmonary resuscitation and emergency cardiovascular care, part 5: new guidelines for first aid. *Circulation.* 2000;102(suppl):I-77–I-85.

6. Neely KW, Drake ME, Moorhead JC, Schmidt TA, Skeen DT, Wilson EA. Multiple options and unique pathways: a new direction for EMS? *Ann Emerg Med.* 1997;30:797–799.

7. Callaham M. Quantifying the scanty science of prehospital emergency care. *Ann Emerg Med.* 1997;30:785–790.

8. Spaite DW, Criss EA, Valenzuela TD, Meislin HW. Developing a foundation for the evaluation of expanded-scope EMS: a window of opportunity that cannot be ignored. *Ann Emerg Med.* 1997;30:791–796.

9. Blake WE, Stillman BC, Eizenberg N, Briggs C, McMeeken JM. The position of the spine in the recovery position: an experimental comparison between the lateral recovery position and the modified HAINES position. *Resuscitation.* 2002;53:289–297.

10. Gunn BD, Eizenberg N, Silberstein M, McMeeken JM, Tully EA, Stillman BC, Brown DJ, Gutteridge GA. How should an unconscious person with a suspected neck injury be positioned? *Prehosp Disaster Med.* 1995;10:239–244.

11. Wong DH, O'Connor D, Tremper KK, Zaccari J, Thompson P, Hill D. Changes in cardiac output after acute blood loss and position change in man. *Crit Care Med.* 1989;17:979–983.

12. Boulain T, Achard JM, Teboul JL, Richard C, Perrotin D, Ginies G. Changes in BP induced by passive leg raising predict response to fluid loading in critically ill patients. *Chest.* 2002;121:1245–1252.

13. Teboul JL, Monnet X. Prediction of volume responsiveness in critically ill patients with spontaneous breathing activity. *Curr Opin Crit Care.* 2008;14:334–339.

14. Gaffney FA, Bastian BC, Thal ER, Atkins JM, Blomqvist CG. Passive leg raising does not produce a significant or sustained autotransfusion effect. *J Trauma.* 1982;22:190–193.

15. Ostrow CL. Use of the Trendelenburg position by critical care nurses: Trendelenburg survey. *Am J Crit Care.* 1997;6:172–176.

16. Shammas A, Clark AP. Trendelenburg positioning to treat acute hypotension: helpful or harmful? *Clin Nurse Spec.* 2007;21:181–187.

17. Reich DL, Konstadt SN, Raissi S, Hubbard M, Thys DM. Trendelenburg position and passive leg raising do not significantly improve cardiopulmonary performance in the anesthetized patient with coronary artery disease. *Crit Care Med.* 1989;17:313–317.

18. Johnson BA. Stark II, phase II: positive changes and lingering uncertainties. *MGMA Connex.* 2004;4:48–51, 1.

19. Rawles JM, Kenmure AC. Controlled trial of oxygen in uncomplicated myocardial infarction. *BMJ.* 1976;1:1121–1123.

20. Nicholson C. A systematic review of the effectiveness of oxygen in reducing acute myocardial ischaemia. *J Clin Nurs.* 2004;13:996–1007.

21. Austin M, Wood-Baker R. Oxygen therapy in the pre-hospital setting for acute exacerbations of chronic obstructive pulmonary disease. *Cochrane Database Syst Rev.* 2006;3:CD005534.

22. Longphre JM, Denoble PJ, Moon RE, Vann RD, Freiberger JJ. First aid normobaric oxygen for the treatment of recreational diving injuries. *Undersea Hyperb Med.* 2007;34:43–49.

23. Mannino DM, Homa DM, Pertowski CA, Ashizawa A, Nixon LL, Johnson CA, Ball LB, Jack E, Kang DS. Surveillance for asthma: United States, 1960–1995. *MMWR CDC Surveill Summ.* 1998;47:1–27.

24. Hamid S, Kumaradevan J, Cochrane GM. Single centre open study to compare patient recording of PRN salbutamol use on a daily diary card with actual use as recorded by the MDI compliance monitor. *Respir Med.* 1998;92:1188–1190.

25. O'Driscoll BR, Kay EA, Taylor RJ, Weatherby H, Chetty MC, Bernstein A. A long-term prospective assessment of home nebulizer treatment. *Respir Med.* 1992;86:317–325.

26. Simon HK. Caregiver knowledge and delivery of a commonly prescribed medication (albuterol) for children. *Arch Pediatr Adolesc Med.* 1999;153:615–618.

27. Kim JS, Sinacore JM, Pongracic JA. Parental use of EpiPen for children with food allergies. *J Allergy Clin Immunol.* 2005;116:164–168.

28. Sicherer SH, Simons FE. Quandaries in prescribing an emergency action plan and self-injectable epinephrine for first-aid management of anaphylaxis in the community. *J Allergy Clin Immunol.* 2005;115:575–583.

29. Pouessel G, Deschildre A, Castelain C, Sardet A, Sagot-Bevenot S, de Sauve-Boeuf A, Thumerelle C, Santos C. Parental knowledge and use of epinephrine auto-injector for children with food allergy. *Pediatr Allergy Immunol.* 2006;17:221–226.

30. Rainbow J, Browne GJ. Fatal asthma or anaphylaxis? *Emerg Med J.* 2002;19:415–417.

31. Dobbie A, Robertson CM. Provision of self-injectable adrenaline for children at risk of anaphylaxis: its source, frequency and appropriateness of use, and effect. *Ambul Child Health.* 1998;4:283–288.

32. Clegg SK, Ritchie JM. "Epipen" training: a survey of the provision for parents and teachers in West Lothian. *Ambul Child Health.* 2001;7:169–175.

33. Gold MS, Sainsbury R. First aid anaphylaxis management in children who were prescribed an epinephrine autoinjector device (EpiPen). *J Allergy Clin Immunol.* 2000;106(part 1):171–176.

34. Sicherer SH, Forman JA, Noone SA. Use assessment of self-administered epinephrine among food-allergic children and pediatricians. *Pediatrics.* 2000;105:359–362.

35. Korenblat P, Lundie MJ, Dankner RE, Day JH. A retrospective study of epinephrine administration for anaphylaxis: how many doses are needed? *Allergy Asthma Proc.* 1999;20:383–386.

36. Uguz A, Lack G, Pumphrey R, Ewan P, Warner J, Dick J, Briggs D, Clarke S, Reading D, Hourihane J. Allergic reactions in the community: a questionnaire survey of members of the anaphylaxis campaign. *Clin Exp Allergy.* 2005;35:746–750.

37. Rudders SA, Banerji A, Corel B, Clark S, Camargo CA Jr. Multicenter study of repeat epinephrine treatments for food-related anaphylaxis. *Pediatrics.* 2010;125:e711–e718.

38. Sicherer SH, Simons FE. Self-injectable epinephrine for first-aid management of anaphylaxis. *Pediatrics.* 2007;119:638–646.

39. Gaca AM, Frush DP, Hohenhaus SM, Luo X, Ancarana A, Pickles A, Frush KS. Enhancing pediatric safety: using simulation to assess radiology resident preparedness for anaphylaxis from intravenous contrast media. *Radiology.* 2007;245:236–244.

40. Pumphrey RS. Lessons for management of anaphylaxis from a study of fatal reactions. *Clin Exp Allergy.* 2000;30:1144–1150.

41. Horowitz BZ, Jadallah S, Derlet RW. Fatal intracranial bleeding associated with prehospital use of epinephrine. *Ann Emerg Med.* 1996;28:725–727.

42. Davis CO, Wax PM. Prehospital epinephrine overdose in a child resulting in ventricular dysrhythmias and myocardial ischemia. *Pediatr Emerg Care.* 1999;15:116–118.

43. Anchor J, Settipane RA. Appropriate use of epinephrine in anaphylaxis. *Am J Emerg Med.* 2004;22:488–490.

44. Zijlstra F, Ernst N, De Boer M-J, Nibbering E, Suryapranata H, Hoorntje JCA, Dambrink J-HE, Van't Hof AWJ, Verheugt FWA. Influence of prehospital administration of aspirin and heparin on initial patency of the infarct-related artery in patients with acute ST elevation myocardial infarction. *J Am Coll Cardiol.* 2002;39:1733–1737.

45. ISIS-2 (Second International Study of Infarct Survival) Collaborative Group. Randomised trial of intravenous streptokinase, oral aspirin, both, or neither among 17,187 cases of suspected acute myocardial infarction: ISIS-2. *Lancet.* 1988;2:349–360.

46. Barbash IM, Freimark D, Gottlieb S, Hod H, Hasin Y, Battler A, Crystal E, Matetzky S, Boyko V, Mandelzweig L, Behar S, Leor J. Outcome of myocardial infarction in patients treated with aspirin is enhanced by pre-hospital administration. *Cardiology.* 2002;98:141–147.

47. Lehmann KG, Heath-Lange SJ, Ferris ST. Randomized comparison of hemostasis techniques after invasive cardiovascular procedures. *Am Heart J.* 1999;138(part 1):1118–1125.

48. Koreny M, Riedmuller E, Nikfardjam M, Siostrzonek P, Mullner M. Arterial puncture closing devices compared with standard manual compression after cardiac catheterization: systematic review and meta-analysis. *JAMA.* 2004;291:350–357.

49. Mlekusch W, Dick P, Haumer M, Sabeti S, Minar E, Schillinger M. Arterial puncture site management after percutaneous transluminal procedures using a hemostatic wound dressing (Clo-Sur P.A.D.) versus

conventional manual compression: a randomized controlled trial. *J Endovasc Ther.* 2006;13:23–31.

50. Upponi SS, Ganeshan AG, Warakaulle DR, Phillips-Hughes J, Boardman P, Uberoi R. Angioseal versus manual compression for haemostasis following peripheral vascular diagnostic and interventional procedures: a randomized controlled trial. *Eur J Radiol.* 2007;61: 332–334.

51. Simon A, Bumgarner B, Clark K, Israel S. Manual versus mechanical compression for femoral artery hemostasis after cardiac catheterization. *Am J Crit Care.* 1998;7:308–313.

52. Walker SB, Cleary S, Higgins M. Comparison of the FemoStop device and manual pressure in reducing groin puncture site complications following coronary angioplasty and coronary stent placement. *Int J Nurs Pract.* 2001;7:366–375.

53. Yadav JS, Ziada KM, Almany S, Davis TP, Castaneda F. Comparison of the QuickSeal Femoral Arterial Closure System with manual compression following diagnostic and interventional catheterization procedures. *Am J Cardiol.* 2003;91:1463–1466, A1466.

54. Naimer SA, Chemla F. Elastic adhesive dressing treatment of bleeding wounds in trauma victims. *Am J Emerg Med.* 2000;18:816–819.

55. Pillgram-Larsen J, Mellesmo S. Not a tourniquet, but compressive dressing: experience from 68 traumatic amputations after injuries from mines [in Norwegian]. *Tidsskr Nor Laegeforen.* 1992;112:2188–2190.

56. Naimer SA, Nash M, Niv A, Lapid O. Control of massive bleeding from facial gunshot wound with a compact elastic adhesive compression dressing. *Am J Emerg Med.* 2004;22:586–588.

57. Naimer SA, Anat N, Katif G. Evaluation of techniques for treating the bleeding wound. *Injury.* 2004;35:974–979.

58. Lakstein D, Blumenfeld A, Sokolov T, Lin G, Bssorai R, Lynn M, Ben-Abraham R. Tourniquets for hemorrhage control on the battlefield: a 4-year accumulated experience. *J Trauma.* 2003;54(suppl): S221–S225.

59. Beekley AC, Sebesta JA, Blackbourne LH, Herbert GS, Kauvar DS, Baer DG, Walters TJ, Mullenix PS, Holcomb JB. Prehospital tourniquet use in Operation Iraqi Freedom: effect on hemorrhage control and outcomes. *J Trauma.* 2008;64(suppl):S28–S37.

60. Kragh JF Jr, Walters TJ, Baer DG, Fox CJ, Wade CE, Salinas J, Holcomb JB. Practical use of emergency tourniquets to stop bleeding in major limb trauma. *J Trauma.* 2008;64(suppl):S38–S49.

61. Kalish J, Burke P, Feldman J, Agarwal S, Glantz A, Moyer P, Serino R, Hirsch E. The return of tourniquets: original research evaluates the effectiveness of prehospital tourniquets for civilian penetrating extremity injuries. *JEMS.* 2008;33:44–46, 49–50, 52, 54.

62. Savvidis E, Parsch K. Prolonged transitory paralysis after pneumatic tourniquet use on the upper arm [in German]. *Unfallchirurg.* 1999;102: 141–144.

63. Kornbluth ID, Freedman MK, Sher L, Frederick RW. Femoral, saphenous nerve palsy after tourniquet use: a case report. *Arch Phys Med Rehabil.* 2003;84:909–911.

64. Landi A, Saracino A, Pinelli M, Caserta G, Facchini MC. Tourniquet paralysis in microsurgery. *Ann Acad Med Singapore.* 1995;24(suppl): 89–93.

65. Wakai A, Wang JH, Winter DC, Street JT, O'Sullivan RG, Redmond HP. Tourniquet-induced systemic inflammatory response in extremity surgery. *J Trauma.* 2001;51:922–926.

66. Mohler LR, Pedowitz RA, Lopez MA, Gershuni DH. Effects of tourniquet compression on neuromuscular function. *Clin Orthop Relat Res.* Feb 1999:213–220.

67. Kokki H, Vaatainen U, Penttila I. Metabolic effects of a low-pressure tourniquet system compared with a high-pressure tourniquet system in arthroscopic anterior crucial ligament reconstruction. *Acta Anaesthesiol Scand.* 1998;42:418–424.

68. King RB, Filips D, Blitz S, Logsetty S. Evaluation of possible tourniquet systems for use in the Canadian Forces. *J Trauma.* 2006;60:1061–1071.

69. Wenke JC, Walters TJ, Greydanus DJ, Pusateri AE, Convertino VA. Physiological evaluation of the U.S. Army one-handed tourniquet. *Mil Med.* 2005;170:776–781.

70. Calkins D, Snow C, Costello M, Bentley TB. Evaluation of possible battlefield tourniquet systems for the far-forward setting. *Mil Med.* 2000;165:379–384.

71. Walters TJ, Wenke JC, Kauvar DS, McManus JG, Holcomb JB, Baer DG. Effectiveness of self-applied tourniquets in human volunteers. *Prehosp Emerg Care.* 2005;9:416–422.

72. Swan KG Jr, Wright DS, Barbagiovanni SS, Swan BC, Swan KG. Tourniquets revisited. *J Trauma.* 2009;66:672–675.

73. Ersoy G, Kaynak MF, Yilmaz O, Rodoplu U, Maltepe F, Gokmen N. Hemostatic effects of microporous polysaccharide hemosphere in a rat model with severe femoral artery bleeding. *Adv Ther.* 2007;24:485–492.

74. McManus J, Hurtado T, Pusateri A, Knoop KJ. A case series describing thermal injury resulting from zeolite use for hemorrhage control in combat operations. *Prehosp Emerg Care.* 2007;11:67–71.

75. Rhee P, Brown C, Martin M, Salim A, Plurad D, Green D, Chambers L, Demetriades D, Velmahos G, Alam H. QuikClot use in trauma for hemorrhage control: case series of 103 documented uses. *J Trauma.* 2008;64:1093–1099.

76. Wedmore I, McManus JG, Pusateri AE, Holcomb JB. A special report on the chitosan-based hemostatic dressing: experience in current combat operations. *J Trauma.* 2006;60:655–658.

77. Dire DJ, Welsh AP. A comparison of wound irrigation solutions used in the emergency department. *Ann Emerg Med.* 1990;19:704–708.

78. Moscati R, Mayrose J, Fincher L, Jehle D. Comparison of normal saline with tap water for wound irrigation. *Am J Emerg Med.* 1998;16: 379–381.

79. Bansal BC, Wiebe RA, Perkins SD, Abramo TJ. Tap water for irrigation of lacerations. *Am J Emerg Med.* 2002;20:469–472.

80. Valente JH, Forti RJ, Freundlich LF, Zandieh SO, Crain EF. Wound irrigation in children: saline solution or tap water? *Ann Emerg Med.* 2003;41:609–616.

81. Moscati RM, Mayrose J, Reardon RF, Janicke DM, Jehle DV. A multicenter comparison of tap water versus sterile saline for wound irrigation. *Acad Emerg Med.* 2007;14:404–409.

82. Longmire AW, Broom LA, Burch J. Wound infection following high-pressure syringe and needle irrigation. *Am J Emerg Med.* 1987;5: 179–181.

83. Claus EE, Fusco CF, Ingram T, Ingersoll CD, Edwards JE, Melham TJ. Comparison of the effects of selected dressings on the healing of standardized abrasions. *J Athl Train.* 1998;33:145–149.

84. Beam JW. Occlusive dressings and the healing of standardized abrasions. *J Athl Train.* 2008;43:600–607.

85. Hinman CD, Maibach H. Effect of air exposure and occlusion on experimental human skin wounds. *Nature.* 1963;200:377–378.

86. Huang HM, Wang JH, Yang L, Yi ZH. Effect of local treatment with cooling and spray film on early edema of superficial II degree scald burns in rats [in Chinese]. *Nan Fang Yi Ke Da Xue Xue Bao.* 2009;29: 804–806.

87. Cuttle L, Kempf M, Kravchuk O, Phillips GE, Mill J, Wang XQ, Kimble RM. The optimal temperature of first aid treatment for partial thickness burn injuries. *Wound Repair Regen.* 2008;16:626–634.

88. Yuan J, Wu C, Holland AJ, Harvey JG, Martin HC, La Hei ER, Arbuckle S, Godfrey TC. Assessment of cooling on an acute scald burn injury in a porcine model. *J Burn Care Res.* 2007;28:514–520.

89. Ofeigsson OJ, Mitchell R, Patrick RS. Observations on the cold water treatment of cutaneous burns. *J Pathol.* 1972;108:145–150.

90. Nguyen NL, Gun RT, Sparnon AL, Ryan P. The importance of immediate cooling: a case series of childhood burns in Vietnam. *Burns.* 2002;28:173–176.

91. Tung KY, Chen ML, Wang HJ, Chen GS, Peck M, Yang J, Liu CC. A seven-year epidemiology study of 12,381 admitted burn patients in Taiwan: using the Internet registration system of the Childhood Burn Foundation. *Burns.* 2005;31(suppl 1):S12–S17.

92. Li C, Yu D, Li MS. Clinical and experiment study of cooling therapy on burned wound [in Chinese]. *Zhonghua Yi Xue Za Zhi.* 1997;77:586–588.

93. Matthews RN, Radakrishnan T. First-aid for burns. *Lancet.* 1987; 1:1371.

94. Purdue GF, Layton TR, Copeland CE. Cold injury complicating burn therapy. *J Trauma.* 1985;25:167–168.

95. Sawada Y, Urushidate S, Yotsuyanagi T, Ishita K. Is prolonged and excessive cooling of a scalded wound effective? *Burns.* 1997;23:55–58.

96. Swain AH, Azadian BS, Wakeley CJ, Shakespeare PG. Management of blisters in minor burns. *BMJ (Clin Res Ed).* 1987;295:181.

97. Cope O. The treatment of the surface burns. *Ann Surg.* 1943;117: 885–893.

98. Forage AV. The effects of removing the epidermis from burnt skin. *Lancet.* 1962;2:690–693.

99. Gimbel NS, Kapetansky DI, Weissman F, Pinkus HK. A study of epithelization in blistered burns. *AMA Arch Surg.* 1957;74:800–803.

100. Homma S, Gillam LD, Weyman AE. Echocardiographic observations in survivors of acute electrical injury. *Chest.* 1990;97:103–105.

101. Jensen PJ, Thomsen PE, Bagger JP, Norgaard A, Baandrup U. Electrical injury causing ventricular arrhythmias. *Br Heart J.* 1987;57:279–283.

102. Lowery DW, Wald MM, Browne BJ, Tigges S, Hoffman JR, Mower WR. Epidemiology of cervical spine injury victims. *Ann Emerg Med.* 2001;38:12–16.

103. Stiell IG, Wells GA, Vandemheen KL, Clement CM, Lesiuk H, De Maio VJ, Laupacis A, Schull M, McKnight RD, Verbeek R, Brison R, Cass D, Dreyer J, Eisenhauer MA, Greenberg GH, MacPhail I, Morrison L, Reardon M, Worthington J. The Canadian C-spine rule for radiography in alert and stable trauma patients. *JAMA.* 2001;286:1841–1848.

104. Hackl W, Hausberger K, Sailer R, Ulmer H, Gassner R. Prevalence of cervical spine injuries in patients with facial trauma. *Oral Surg Oral Med Oral Pathol Oral Radiol Endod.* 2001;92:370–376.

105. Kennedy E. *Spinal Cord Injury: The Facts and Figures.* Birmingham, Ala: University of Alabama Press; 1986.

106. Reid DC, Henderson R, Saboe L, Miller JD. Etiology and clinical course of missed spine fractures. *J Trauma.* 1987;27:980–986.

107. Davis JW, Phreaner DL, Hoyt DB, Mackersie RC. The etiology of missed cervical spine injuries. *J Trauma.* 1993;34:342–346.

108. Hauswald M, Ong G, Tandberg D, Omar Z. Out-of-hospital spinal immobilization: its effect on neurologic injury. *Acad Emerg Med.* 1998; 5:214–219.

109. Hoffman JR, Mower WR, Wolfson AB, Todd KH, Zucker MI; National Emergency X-Radiography Utilization Study Group. Validity of a set of clinical criteria to rule out injury to the cervical spine in patients with blunt trauma. *N Engl J Med.* 2000;343:94–99.

110. Viccellio P, Simon H, Pressman BD, Shah MN, Mower WR, Hoffman JR. A prospective multicenter study of cervical spine injury in children. *Pediatrics.* 2001;108:E20.

111. Touger M, Gennis P, Nathanson N, Lowery DW, Pollack CV Jr, Hoffman JR, Mower WR. Validity of a decision rule to reduce cervical spine radiography in elderly patients with blunt trauma. *Ann Emerg Med.* 2002;40:287–293.

112. Panacek EA, Mower WR, Holmes JF, Hoffman JR. Test performance of the individual NEXUS low-risk clinical screening criteria for cervical spine injury. *Ann Emerg Med.* 2001;38:22–25.

113. Pieretti-Vanmarcke R, Velmahos GC, Nance ML, Islam S, Falcone RA Jr, Wales PW, Brown RL, Gaines BA, McKenna C, Moore FO, Goslar PW, Inaba K, Barmparas G, Scaife ER, Metzger RR, Brockmeyer DL, Upperman JS, Estrada J, Lanning DA, Rasmussen SK, Danielson PD, Hirsh MP, Consani HF, Stylianos S, Pineda C, Norwood SH, Bruch SW, Drongowski R, Barraco RD, Pasquale MD, Hussain F, Hirsch EF, McNeely PD, Fallat ME, Foley DS, Iocono JA, Bennett HM, Waxman K, Kam K, Bakhos L, Petrovick L, Chang Y, Masiakos PT. Clinical clearance of the cervical spine in blunt trauma patients younger than 3 years: a multi-center study of the American Association for the Surgery of Trauma. *J Trauma.* 2009;67:543–549.

114. Domeier RM, Evans RW, Swor RA, Hancock JB, Fales W, Krohmer J, Frederiksen SM, Shork MA. The reliability of prehospital clinical evaluation for potential spinal injury is not affected by the mechanism of injury. *Prehosp Emerg Care.* 1999;3:332–337.

115. Cote DJ, Prentice WE Jr, Hooker DN, Shields EW. Comparison of three treatment procedures for minimizing ankle sprain swelling. *Phys Ther.* 1988;68:1072–1076.

116. Meeusen R, Lievens P. The use of cryotherapy in sports injuries. *Sports Med.* 1986;3:398–414.

117. Hocutt JE Jr, Jaffe R, Rylander CR, Beebe JK. Cryotherapy in ankle sprains. *Am J Sports Med.* 1982;10:316–319.

118. Airaksinen OV, Kyrklund N, Latvala K, Kouri JP, Gronblad M, Kolari P. Efficacy of cold gel for soft tissue injuries: a prospective randomized double-blinded trial. *Am J Sports Med.* 2003;31:680–684.

119. Basur RL, Shephard E, Mouzas GL. A cooling method in the treatment of ankle sprains. *Practitioner.* 1976;216:708–711.

120. Ayata R, Shiraki H, Fukuda T, Takemura M, Mukai N, Miyakawa S. The effects of icing after exercise on jumper's knee. *Jpn J Phys Fitness Sports Med.* 2007;56:125–130.

121. Merrick MA, Jutte LS, Smith ME. Cold modalities with different thermodynamic properties produce different surface and intramuscular temperatures. *J Athl Train.* 2003;38:28–33.

122. Dykstra JH, Hill HM, Miller MG, Cheatham CC, Michael TJ, Baker RJ. Comparisons of cubed ice, crushed ice, and wetted ice on intramuscular and surface temperature changes. *J Athl Train.* 2009;44: 136–141.

123. Kanlayanaphotporn R, Janwantanakul P. Comparison of skin surface temperature during the application of various cryotherapy modalities. *Arch Phys Med Rehabil.* 2005;86:1411–1415.

124. McMaster WC, Liddle S, Waugh TR. Laboratory evaluation of various cold therapy modalities. *Am J Sports Med.* 1978;6:291–294.

125. Chesterton LS, Foster NE, Ross L. Skin temperature response to cryotherapy. *Arch Phys Med Rehabil.* 2002;83:543–549.

126. Graham CA, Stevenson J. Frozen chips: an unusual cause of severe frostbite injury. *Br J Sports Med.* 2000;34:382–383.

127. Moeller JL, Monroe J, McKeag DB. Cryotherapy-induced common peroneal nerve palsy. *Clin J Sport Med.* 1997;7:212–216.

128. Bassett FH III, Kirkpatrick JS, Engelhardt DL, Malone TR. Cryotherapy-induced nerve injury. *Am J Sports Med.* 1992;20:516–518.

129. Bleakley CM, McDonough SM, MacAuley DC, Bjordal J. Cryotherapy for acute ankle sprains: a randomised controlled study of two different icing protocols. *Br J Sports Med.* 2006;40:700–705.

130. Auerbach PS, Geehr EC, Ryu RK. The Reel Splint: experience with a new traction splint apparatus in the prehospital setting. *Ann Emerg Med.* 1984;13:419–422.

131. Kaplan MM, Cohen D, Koprowski H, Dean D, Ferrigan L. Studies on the local treatment of wounds for the prevention of rabies. *Bull World Health Organ.* 1962;26:765–775.

132. Dean DJ, Baer GM, Thompson WR. Studies on the local treatment of rabies-infected wounds. *Bull World Health Organ.* 1963;28:477–486.

133. Callaham ML. Treatment of common dog bites: infection risk factors. *JACEP.* 1978;7:83–87.

134. Alberts MB, Shalit M, LoGalbo F. Suction for venomous snakebite: a study of "mock venom" extraction in a human model. *Ann Emerg Med.* 2004;43:181–186.

135. Lawrence WT, Giannopoulos A, Hansen A. Pit viper bites: rational management in locales in which copperheads and cottonmouths predominate. *Ann Plast Surg.* 1996;36:276–285.

136. Leopold RS, Huber GS. Ineffectiveness of suction in removing snake venom from open wounds. *U S Armed Forces Med J.* 1960;11:682–685.

137. Bush SP, Hegewald KG, Green SM, Cardwell MD, Hayes WK. Effects of a negative pressure venom extraction device (Extractor) on local tissue injury after artificial rattlesnake envenomation in a porcine model. *Wilderness Environ Med.* 2000;11:180–188.

138. Holstege CP, Singletary EM. Images in emergency medicine: skin damage following application of suction device for snakebite. *Ann Emerg Med.* 2006;48:105, 113.

139. Howarth DM, Southee AE, Whyte IM. Lymphatic flow rates and first-aid in simulated peripheral snake or spider envenomation. *Med J Aust.* 1994;161:695–700.

140. German BT, Hack JB, Brewer K, Meggs WJ. Pressure-immobilization bandages delay toxicity in a porcine model of eastern coral snake (Micrurus fulvius fulvius) envenomation. *Ann Emerg Med.* 2005;45: 603–608.

141. Bush SP, Green SM, Laack TA, Hayes WK, Cardwell MD, Tanen DA. Pressure immobilization delays mortality and increases intracompartmental pressure after artificial intramuscular rattlesnake envenomation in a porcine model. *Ann Emerg Med.* 2004;44:599–604.

142. Norris RL, Ngo J, Nolan K, Hooker G. Physicians and lay people are unable to apply pressure immobilization properly in a simulated snakebite scenario. *Wilderness Environ Med.* 2005;16:16–21.

143. Simpson ID, Tanwar PD, Andrade C, Kochar DK, Norris RL. The Ebbinghaus retention curve: training does not increase the ability to apply pressure immobilisation in simulated snake bite: implications for snake bite first aid in the developing world. *Trans R Soc Trop Med Hyg.* 2008;102:451–459.

144. Mianzan HW, Fenner PJ, Cornelius PF, Ramirez FC. Vinegar as a disarming agent to prevent further discharge of the nematocysts of the stinging hydromedusa Olindias sambaquiensis. *Cutis.* 2001;68:45–48.

145. Burnett JW, Rubinstein H, Calton GJ. First aid for jellyfish envenomation. *South Med J.* 1983;76:870–872.

146. Loten C, Stokes B, Worsley D, Seymour JE, Jiang S, Isbister GK. A randomised controlled trial of hot water (45 degrees C) immersion versus ice packs for pain relief in bluebottle stings. *Med J Aust.* 2006; 184:329–333.

147. Nomura JT, Sato RL, Ahern RM, Snow JL, Kuwaye TT, Yamamoto LG. A randomized paired comparison trial of cutaneous treatments for acute jellyfish (Carybdea alata) stings. *Am J Emerg Med.* 2002;20:624–626.

148. Yoshimoto CM, Yanagihara AA. Cnidarian (coelenterate) envenomations in Hawai'i improve following heat application. *Trans R Soc Trop Med Hyg.* 2002;96:300–303.

149. Atkinson PR, Boyle A, Hartin D, McAuley D. Is hot water immersion an effective treatment for marine envenomation? *Emerg Med J.* 2006;23: 503–508.

150. Thomas J. Dermatology in the new millennium. *Indian J Dermatol Venereol Leprol.* 2001;67:100–103.

151. Exton DR, Fenner PJ, Williamson JA. Cold packs: effective topical analgesia in the treatment of painful stings by Physalia and other jellyfish. *Med J Aust.* 1989;151:625–626.

152. Thomas CS, Scott SA, Galanis DJ, Goto RS. Box jellyfish (Carybdea alata) in Waikiki: the analgesic effect of sting-aid, Adolph's meat tenderizer and fresh water on their stings: a double-blinded, randomized, placebo-controlled clinical trial. *Hawaii Med J.* 2001;60:205–207, 210.

153. Pereira PL, Carrette T, Cullen P, Mulcahy RF, Little M, Seymour J. Pressure immobilisation bandages in first-aid treatment of jellyfish envenomation: current recommendations reconsidered. *Med J Aust.* 2000;173:650–652.

154. Seymour J, Carrette T, Cullen P, Little M, Mulcahy RF, Pereira PL. The use of pressure immobilization bandages in the first aid management of cubozoan envenomings. *Toxicon.* 2002;40:1503–1505.

155. Flores MT. Traumatic injuries in the primary dentition. *Dent Traumatol.* 2002;18:287–298.

156. Hiltz J, Trope M. Vitality of human lip fibroblasts in milk, Hanks balanced salt solution and Viaspan storage media. *Endod Dent Traumatol.* 1991;7:69–72.

157. Chan AW, Wong TK, Cheung GS. Lay knowledge of physical education teachers about the emergency management of dental trauma in Hong Kong. *Dent Traumatol.* 2001;17:77–85.

158. Sae-Lim V, Lim LP. Dental trauma management awareness of Singapore pre-school teachers. *Dent Traumatol.* 2001;17:71–76.

159. Greif R, Rajek A, Laciny S, Bastanmehr H, Sessler DI. Resistive heating is more effective than metallic-foil insulation in an experimental model of accidental hypothermia: a randomized controlled trial. *Ann Emerg Med.* 2000;35:337–345.

160. Steele MT, Nelson MJ, Sessler DI, Fraker L, Bunney B, Watson WA, Robinson WA. Forced air speeds rewarming in accidental hypothermia. *Ann Emerg Med.* 1996;27:479–484.

161. Mills WJ Jr, Whaley R, Fish W. Frostbite: experience with rapid rewarming and ultrasonic therapy: part II: 1960. *Alaska Med.* 1993;35:10–18.

162. Mills WJ Jr, Whaley R, Fish W. Frostbite: experience with rapid rewarming and ultrasonic therapy: part III: 1961. *Alaska Med.* 1993;35:19–27.

163. Fuhrman FA, Crismon JM. Studies on gangrene following cold injury: treatment of cold injury by means of immediate rapid warming. *J Clin Invest.* 1947;26:476–485.

164. Entin MA, Baxter H. Influence of rapid warming on frostbite in experimental animals. *Plast Reconstr Surg (1946).* 1952;9:511–524.

165. Fuhrman FA, Fuhrman GJ. The treatment of experimental frostbite by rapid thawing: a review and new experimental data. *Medicine (Baltimore).* 1957;36:465–487.

166. Malhotra MS, Mathew L. Effect of rewarming at various water bath temperatures in experimental frostbite. *Aviat Space Environ Med.* 1978;49:874–876.

167. Purkayastha SS, Chhabra PC, Verma SS, Selvamurthy W. Experimental studies on the treatment of frostbite in rats. *Indian J Med Res.* 1993;98:178–184.

168. Martinez Villen G, Garcia Bescos G, Rodriguez Sosa V, Morandeira Garcia JR. Effects of haemodilution and rewarming with regard to digital amputation in frostbite injury: an experimental study in the rabbit. *J Hand Surg Br.* 2002;27:224–228.

169. Purkayastha SS, Bhaumik G, Chauhan SK, Banerjee PK, Selvamurthy W. Immediate treatment of frostbite using rapid rewarming in tea decoction followed by combined therapy of pentoxifylline, aspirin & vitamin C. *Indian J Med Res.* 2002;116:29–34.

170. Bilgic S, Ozkan H, Ozenc S, Safaz I, Yildiz C. Treating frostbite. *Can Fam Physician.* 2008;54:361–363.

171. Sands WA, Kimmel WL, Wurtz BR, Stone MH, McNeal JR. Comparison of commercially available disposable chemical hand and foot warmers. *Wilderness Environ Med.* 2009;20:33–38.

172. Heggers JP, Robson MC, Manavalen K, Weingarten MD, Carethers JM, Boertman JA, Smith DJ Jr, Sachs RJ. Experimental and clinical observations on frostbite. *Ann Emerg Med.* 1987;16:1056–1062.

173. McCauley RL, Hing DN, Robson MC, Heggers JP. Frostbite injuries: a rational approach based on the pathophysiology. *J Trauma.* 1983;23:143–147.

174. Twomey JA, Peltier GL, Zera RT. An open-label study to evaluate the safety and efficacy of tissue plasminogen activator in treatment of severe frostbite. *J Trauma.* 2005;59:1350–1354.

175. Foray J. Mountain frostbite: current trends in prognosis and treatment (from results concerning 1261 cases). *Int J Sports Med.* 1992;13(suppl 1):S193–S196.

176. Kenefick RW, O'Moore KM, Mahood NV, Castellani JW. Rapid IV versus oral rehydration: responses to subsequent exercise heat stress. *Med Sci Sports Exerc.* 2006;38:2125–2131.

177. Michell MW, Oliveira HM, Kinsky MP, Vaid SU, Herndon DN, Kramer GC. Enteral resuscitation of burn shock using World Health Organization oral rehydration solution: a potential solution for mass casualty care. *J Burn Care Res.* 2006;27:819–825.

178. Barclay RL, Depew WT, Vanner SJ. Carbohydrate-electrolyte rehydration protects against intravascular volume contraction during colonic cleansing with orally administered sodium phosphate. *Gastrointest Endosc.* 2002;56:633–638.

179. Currell K, Urch J, Cerri E, Jentjens RL, Blannin AK, Jeukendrup AE. Plasma deuterium oxide accumulation following ingestion of different carbohydrate beverages. *Appl Physiol Nutr Metab.* 2008;33:1067–1072.

180. Jeukendrup AE, Currell K, Clarke J, Cole J, Blannin AK. Effect of beverage glucose and sodium content on fluid delivery. *Nutr Metab (Lond).* 2009;6:9.

181. Evans GH, Shirreffs SM, Maughan RJ. Postexercise rehydration in man: the effects of osmolality and carbohydrate content of ingested drinks. *Nutrition.* 2009;25:905–913.

182. Greenleaf JE, Jackson CG, Geelen G, Keil LC, Hinghofer-Szalkay H, Whittam JH. Plasma volume expansion with oral fluids in hypohydrated men at rest and during exercise. *Aviat Space Environ Med.* 1998;69:837–844.

183. Maughan RJ, Leiper JB. Sodium intake and post-exercise rehydration in man. *Eur J Appl Physiol Occup Physiol.* 1995;71:311–319.

184. Merson SJ, Maughan RJ, Shirreffs SM. Rehydration with drinks differing in sodium concentration and recovery from moderate exercise-induced hypohydration in man. *Eur J Appl Physiol.* 2008;103:585–594.

185. Shirreffs SM, Taylor AJ, Leiper JB, Maughan RJ. Post-exercise rehydration in man: effects of volume consumed and drink sodium content. *Med Sci Sports Exerc.* 1996;28:1260–1271.

186. Clapp AJ, Bishop PA, Muir I, Walker JL. Rapid cooling techniques in joggers experiencing heat strain. *J Sci Med Sport.* 2001;4:160–167.

187. Clements JM, Casa DJ, Knight J, McClung JM, Blake AS, Meenen PM, Gilmer AM, Caldwell KA. Ice-water immersion and cold-water immersion provide similar cooling rates in runners with exercise-induced hyperthermia. *J Athl Train.* 2002;37:146–150.

188. Proulx CI, Ducharme MB, Kenny GP. Effect of water temperature on cooling efficiency during hyperthermia in humans. *J Appl Physiol.* 2003;94:1317–1323.

189. Armstrong LE, Crago AE, Adams R, Roberts WO, Maresh CM. Whole-body cooling of hyperthermic runners: comparison of two field therapies. *Am J Emerg Med.* 1996;14:355–358.

190. American Academy of Pediatrics Committee on Injury, Violence, and Poison Prevention. Prevention of drowning in infants, children, and adolescents. *Pediatrics.* 2003;112:437–439.

191. Suominen P, Baillie C, Korpela R, Rautanen S, Ranta S, Olkkola KT. Impact of age, submersion time and water temperature on outcome in near-drowning. *Resuscitation.* 2002;52:247–254.

192. Graf WD, Cummings P, Quan L, Brutocao D. Predicting outcome in pediatric submersion victims. *Ann Emerg Med.* 1995;26:312–319.

193. Modell JH, Idris AH, Pineda JA, Silverstein JH. Survival after prolonged submersion in freshwater in Florida. *Chest.* 2004;125:1948–1951.

194. Mehta SR, Srinivasan KV, Bindra MS, Kumar MR, Lahiri AK. Near drowning in cold water. *J Assoc Physicians India.* 2000;48:674–676.

195. Szpilman D, Soares M. In-water resuscitation: is it worthwhile? *Resuscitation.* 2004;63:25–31.

196. Latenser BA, Lucktong TA. Anhydrous ammonia burns: case presentation and literature review. *J Burn Care Rehabil.* 2000;21(part 1):40–42.

197. Wibbenmeyer LA, Morgan LJ, Robinson BK, Smith SK, Lewis RW II, Kealey GP. Our chemical burn experience: exposing the dangers of anhydrous ammonia. *J Burn Care Rehabil.* 1999;20:226–231.

198. Yano K, Hosokawa K, Kakibuchi M, Hikasa H, Hata Y. Effects of washing acid injuries to the skin with water: an experimental study using rats. *Burns.* 1995;21:500–502.

199. Kono K, Yoshida Y, Watanabe M, Tanioka Y, Dote T, Orita Y, Bessho Y, Yoshida J, Sumi Y, Umebayashi K. An experimental study on the treatment of hydrofluoric acid burns. *Arch Environ Contam Toxicol.* 1992;22:414–418.

200. Murao M. Studies on the treatment of hydrofluoric acid burn. *Bull Osaka Med Coll.* 1989;35:39–48.

201. Lorette JJ Jr, Wilkinson JA. Alkaline chemical burn to the face requiring full-thickness skin grafting. *Ann Emerg Med.* 1988;17:739–741.

202. Leonard LG, Scheulen JJ, Munster AM. Chemical burns: effect of prompt first aid. *J Trauma.* 1982;22:420–423.

203. Kompa S, Schareck B, Tympner J, Wustemeyer H, Schrage NF. Comparison of emergency eye-wash products in burned porcine eyes. *Graefes Arch Clin Exp Ophthalmol.* 2002;240:308–313.

204. McCulley JP. Ocular hydrofluoric acid burns: animal model, mechanism of injury and therapy. *Trans Am Ophthalmol Soc.* 1990;88:649–684.

205. Hojer J, Personne M, Hulten P, Ludwigs U. Topical treatments for hydrofluoric acid burns: a blind controlled experimental study. *J Toxicol Clin Toxicol.* 2002;40:861–866.

206. Herr RD, White GL Jr, Bernhisel K, Mamalis N, Swanson E. Clinical comparison of ocular irrigation fluids following chemical injury. *Am J Emerg Med.* 1991;9:228–231.

207. Ingram TA III. Response of the human eye to accidental exposure to sodium hypochlorite. *J Endod.* 1990;16:235–238.

208. Burns FR, Paterson CA. Prompt irrigation of chemical eye injuries may avert severe damage. *Occup Health Saf.* 1989;58:33–36.

209. Kompa S, Redbrake C, Hilgers C, Wustemeyer H, Schrage N, Remky A. Effect of different irrigating solutions on aqueous humour pH changes, intraocular pressure and histological findings after induced alkali burns. *Acta Ophthalmol Scand.* 2005;83:467–470.

210. Spoler F, Frentz M, Forst M, Kurz H, Schrage NF. Analysis of hydrofluoric acid penetration and decontamination of the eye by means of time-resolved optical coherence tomography. *Burns.* 2008;34:549–555.

211. Rihawi S, Frentz M, Schrage NF. Emergency treatment of eye burns: which rinsing solution should we choose? *Graefes Arch Clin Exp Ophthalmol.* 2006;244:845–854.

212. Homan CS, Maitra SR, Lane BP, Geller ER. Effective treatment of acute alkali injury of the rat esophagus with early saline dilution therapy. *Ann Emerg Med.* 1993;22:178–182.

213. Homan CS, Maitra SR, Lane BP, Thode HC, Sable M. Therapeutic effects of water and milk for acute alkali injury of the esophagus. *Ann Emerg Med.* 1994;24:14–20.

214. Homan CS, Maitra SR, Lane BP, Thode HC Jr, Davidson L. Histopathologic evaluation of the therapeutic efficacy of water and milk dilution for esophageal acid injury. *Acad Emerg Med.* 1995;2:587–591.

215. Homan CS, Singer AJ, Henry MC, Thode HC Jr. Thermal effects of neutralization therapy and water dilution for acute alkali exposure in canines. *Acad Emerg Med.* 1997;4:27–32.

216. Homan CS, Singer AJ, Thomajan C, Henry MC, Thode HC Jr. Thermal characteristics of neutralization therapy and water dilution for strong acid ingestion: an in-vivo canine model. *Acad Emerg Med.* 1998;5:286–292.

217. Spiller HA, Rodgers GC Jr. Evaluation of administration of activated charcoal in the home. *Pediatrics.* 2001;108:E100.

218. Lamminpaa A, Vilska J, Hoppu K. Medical charcoal for a child's poisoning at home: availability and success of administration in Finland. *Hum Exp Toxicol.* 1993;12:29–32.

219. Donoso A, Linares M, Leon J, Rojas G, Valverde C, Ramirez M, Oberpaur B. Activated charcoal laryngitis in an intubated patient. *Pediatr Emerg Care.* 2003;19:420–421.

220. Dorrington CL, Johnson DW, Brant R. The frequency of complications associated with the use of multiple-dose activated charcoal. *Ann Emerg Med.* 2003;41:370–377.

221. Givens T, Holloway M, Wason S. Pulmonary aspiration of activated charcoal: a complication of its misuse in overdose management. *Pediatr Emerg Care.* 1992;8:137–140.

222. Scharman EJ, Cloonan HA, Durback-Morris LF. Home administration of charcoal: can mothers administer a therapeutic dose? *J Emerg Med.* 2001;21:357–361.

223. Kulig K, Bar-Or D, Cantrill SV, Rosen P, Rumack BH. Management of acutely poisoned patients without gastric emptying. *Ann Emerg Med.* 1985;14:562–567.

224. Pond SM, Lewis-Driver DJ, Williams GM, Green AC, Stevenson NW. Gastric emptying in acute overdose: a prospective randomised controlled trial. *Med J Aust.* 1995;163:345–349.

225. Caravati EM. Unintentional acetaminophen ingestion in children and the potential for hepatotoxicity. *J Toxicol Clin Toxicol.* 2000;38:291–296.

226. Bond G. Home syrup of ipecac use does not reduce emergency department use or improve outcome. *Pediatrics.* 2003;112:1061–1064.

227. Kornberg AE, Dolgin J. Pediatric ingestions: charcoal alone versus ipecac and charcoal. *Ann Emerg Med.* 1991;20:648–651.

228. Czajka PA, Russell SL. Nonemetic effects of ipecac syrup. *Pediatrics.* 1985;75:1101–1104.

KEY WORDS: emergency ■ injury